Comprehensive Healthcare Simulation

Series Editors
Adam I. Levine
Samuel DeMaria Jr.

More information about this series at http://www.springer.com/series/13029

Vincent J. Grant · Adam Cheng

Editors

Comprehensive Healthcare Simulation: Pediatrics

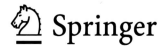

Editors
Assoc. Prof. Vincent J. Grant, MD, FRCPC
Department of Pediatrics, University of Calgary
Medical Director, KidSIM(TM)
Pediatric Simulation Program,
Alberta Children's Hospital
Co-director, Advanced Technical Skills and
Simulation Laboratory
University of Calgary
Calgary, Alberta
Canada

Assoc. Prof. Adam Cheng, MD, FRCPC
Department of Pediatrics, University of Calgary
Director of Research and Development
KidSIM-ASPIRE Simulation Research Program
Alberta Children's Hospital
Calgary, Alberta
Canada

ISSN 2366-4479   ISSN 2366-4487 (electronic)
Comprehensive Healthcare Simulation
ISBN 978-3-319-24185-2   ISBN 978-3-319-24187-6 (eBook)
DOI 10.1007/978-3-319-24187-6

Library of Congress Control Number: 2016932004

Printed on acid-free paper

Springer imprint is published by SpringerNature
The registered company is Springer International Publishing

To my wife Estée, thanks for your endless love and support. To my children Everett, Maëlle and Callum, thank you for inspiring me to help build a better and safer future for you and your children.

Vincent J. Grant

To my wife, Natalie, and my two kids, Kaeden and Chloe, for their unwavering support and love.

Adam Cheng

Foreword

The adjective "pediatric" applies to patients ranging from those born at a gestational age of 22–23 weeks with a birth weight of approximately 500 g to young adults aged 21 years standing 2 m in height and weighing more than 100 kg. Addressing many anatomic, physiologic, developmental, and psychological differences in pediatric patients creates tremendous challenges for the healthcare professionals charged with their care, and training those professionals to provide competent, compassionate, and developmentally appropriate care is similarly difficult. These and other challenges serve as a major driving force behind pediatric simulation.

Comprehensive Healthcare Simulation: Pediatrics is written by leaders in the field and encompasses many wide-ranging aspects of pediatric simulation. The first few chapters of the book focus on the importance of scenario design and debriefing as key elements of simulation-based learning methodologies. The significance of covering these core topics early while simulation technologies are discussed later should not be overlooked—indeed, unless one understands how to optimally employ simulation-based methodologies, one cannot make proper use of associated technologies. Issues unique to different pediatric subspecialties are covered in detail, providing helpful hints for the effective use of simulation in these domains. Attention is also paid to important subjects such as simulation instructor development and simulation-based research. Key themes, such as patient safety and human performance, are woven throughout the text.

Driven by the desire to improve the care of children, many of the authors who contributed to this text are also members (in some cases, founding members) of the International Pediatric Simulation Society (IPSS) and/or the International Network for Simulation-based Pediatric Innovation, Research, and Education (INSPIRE). IPSS sponsors the International Pediatric Simulation Symposia and Workshops (IPSSW)—an annual forum for the clinicians, investigators, and educators in the field of pediatric simulation—and hosts monthly webinars and publishes a quarterly newsletter. Through the INSPIRE network, investigators conduct simulation-based research, typically on a multicenter level, to advance the quality of clinical care provided to pediatric patients around the world. Taken in sum, efforts such as this text, IPSS, and INSPIRE are indicative of the passion and dedication that pediatric healthcare professionals bring to this domain.

As you can see from this body of work, the field of pediatric simulation has made tremendous progress in a relatively brief period of time. Yet many challenges remain, and we should not be content with the current state of our knowledge and expertise. Other high-risk industries are well ahead of health care in achieving a level of safety and effectiveness of which we should be envious. On the human side, we need to become more knowledgeable about the many ergonomic/human factors and issues that affect our ability to deliver care. From a technical standpoint, our physical patient simulators require better physiologic models so that their responses to interventions are more realistic. In general, more emphasis needs to be placed upon developing virtual reality-based tools and hybrid devices (physical + virtual components) to allow more flexible learning opportunities that can be tailored to meet the needs of individual healthcare professionals. In addition, the simulation research agenda should be carefully aligned with the most relevant and important clinical questions to ensure that the research that is funded and conducted actually improves clinical care. While the authors cited in this text may lead some of these initiatives, we all need to collaborate in order to push the field forward.

I look forward to seeing this progress become manifest in the coming years and reading the next edition of this comprehensive, well-organized, and practical text.

Louis Patrick Halamek, M.D., F.A.A.P.
Division of Neonatal and Developmental Medicine
Department of Pediatrics
School of Medicine
Stanford University
The Center for Advanced Pediatric and Perinatal Education
Packard Children's Hospital at Stanford

Preface

There has been tremendous growth in the field of pediatric simulation over the last couple of decades. Emerging from small pockets of simulation in neonatal care, emergency medicine, anesthesia, critical care, and transport medicine in various places around the world, pediatric simulation has evolved with the establishment of large hospital- and university-based pediatric simulation programs and the development of national and international pediatric simulation networks. Pediatric simulation programs have also evolved from delivering scenario-based simulations into sophisticated education, patient safety, and research programs, including the development of formal faculty development curricula and pediatric simulation fellowship programs. There are currently more than 125 pediatric simulation programs in over 25 countries around the world. National networks such as the Canadian Pediatric Simulation Network (CPSN) were developed to share experience and resources, promote standardization of curricula on a national scale, and collaborate on pediatric education and research projects [1]. On a global level, the development of the International Pediatric Simulation Society (IPSS) has been a remarkable step forward in consolidating the efforts of simulation educators around the world, including advocacy for regions where resources are limited. IPSS was established to promote and support interprofessional and multidisciplinary education and research for all clinical specialties and professions that care for infants, children, and adolescents. IPSS organizes an annual meeting bringing together leaders in the field of pediatric simulation. 2015 marks the seventh anniversary of the International Pediatric Simulation Symposia and Workshops (IPSSW), a conference that has been marching around the globe in various international venues, providing opportunities to collaborate and cross-fertilize across borders and to promote excellence in simulation education delivery and research [2].

The *science* of pediatric simulation has also grown dramatically in the past decade, as evidenced by both the volume of research being performed and the impact of the outcomes observed [3, 4]. Initial studies that focused primarily on whether learners felt engaged in simulation-based learning and whether it improved their confidence have been replaced by studies looking at short- and long-term clinical and behavioral performance, patient outcomes as well as the objective evaluation of various instructional design features for simulation-based education (SBE). A recent meta-analysis identified 57 studies involving over 3500 learners where SBE was used to teach pediatrics. When studies compared simulation to no intervention, effect sizes were found to be large for the outcomes of knowledge, performance in a simulated setting, behavior with patients, and time to task completion [5]. The authors suggested that future research should include comparative studies that identify optimal instructional methods (i.e., comparing SBE to other methods of education) and include pediatric-specific issues in SBE interventions.

Other areas where novel work is being done include human factors, patient safety, interprofessional education, family and patient teaching, innovative devices, and systems-based interventions [6–19]. Pediatric simulation-based research has also been buoyed by collaboration between pediatric simulation programs [20, 21]. The evolution of the International Network for Simulation-based Pediatric Innovation, Research and Education (INSPIRE) represents a major step forward in the ability to perform adequately powered research to answer many fundamental questions in the delivery and outcomes of SBE (www.inspiresim.com). As of

March 2014, INSPIRE has an active membership of more than 500 simulation educators and researchers spanning 26 countries [22].

The *art* of pediatric simulation has also advanced past the level of turning on a mannequin and running a scenario or having learners practice on a task trainer. Simulation is now being used in novel ways: to teach trainees and professionals how to conduct difficult conversations (e.g., breaking bad news to families, disclosing medical errors, disclosing non-accidental trauma (child abuse), discussions around end-of-life care and organ donation); to educate parents and other caregivers (including school faculty and staff) of patients with known medical needs (e.g., seizure disorder, tracheostomy care, anaphylaxis, among others), potentially also impacting discharge planning and hospital bed utilization; and to facilitate learning and debriefing around hospital-wide systems issues (e.g., patient safety, adequacy of clinical space, adequacy of response teams, building and outfitting of new space, testing of hospital response to large-scale disasters or child abduction/missing patients). You will read about these and many other new uses of simulation in pediatrics in the chapters of this book [23]. It appears that there is no element of health care and delivery that cannot be impacted by the use of simulation, either in training or assessment.

It is this tremendous growth and development that has provided impetus for *Comprehensive Healthcare Simulation: Pediatrics* to be written. As one of the first volumes in the new series, *Comprehensive Healthcare Simulation* (Levine and DeMaria, Series Editors), conceived to complement *The Comprehensive Textbook of Healthcare Simulation* (2013) [24], this book marks the incredible achievements of the international pediatric simulation community in working together collaboratively to remain on the "cutting edge" of simulation-based healthcare training. The authors who have contributed to this textbook are established experts in pediatric simulation, and we are proud to have their collective contribution to this volume. We hope this book will be a valuable resource to all simulation-based educators and researchers, not just for those from pediatric backgrounds. Whether you are setting up a simulation program, recruiting teachers and learners for simulation training, designing scenarios, approaching administration and donors for funding, or trying to understand and measure the impact of your work, we hope this *comprehensive* resource meets all your needs related to simulation. Although some of the content is not specifically "pediatric" in nature, all of the information is applicable to developing, growing, delivering, and measuring safe and effective simulation-based training. Part 1 covers the topics that we perceive as the *fundamentals of simulation for pediatrics,* and includes everything related to developing, organizing, and using simulation for training and assessment. Part 2 covers *simulation modalities, technologies, and environments for pediatrics,* and reviews all of the various types of simulation available to the healthcare educator. Part 3 covers *simulation for professional development in pediatrics* and includes simulation along the healthcare continuum, competency-based education, and interprofessional education. Part 4 is a complete review of simulation as it pertains to the various areas and *subspecialties of pediatrics,* including novel uses of simulation in rural environments, resource-limited settings, and for family-centered care. Part 5 is devoted to *simulation program development in pediatrics,* covering operations, administration, and education and research program development. Part 6 reviews the entire spectrum of *pediatric simulation research,* and Part 7 outlines *the future of pediatric simulation.*

We would like to thank all of the contributors for their dedication and hard work in preparing the high-quality work that forms the content of this textbook. We are honored and privileged to work with you all. We would like to thank everyone in our home simulation program (KidSIM Pediatric Simulation Program at Alberta Children's Hospital), local hospital and health authority administration (Alberta Children's Hospital and eSIM Provincial Simulation Programs of Alberta Health Services), and university department (Department of Pediatrics at the Cumming School of Medicine at the University of Calgary) for their ongoing support of all of the academic work that we do. We are privileged to represent such a dedicated group of clinical care providers, educators, researchers, and leaders. Finally, and most importantly, we would like to thank our families, who sacrifice a great deal so that we can help contribute to the growth and development of pediatric simulation on a global scale. We really believe the collective work of the pediatric simulation community is creating a safer world for our kids to grow up in.

We wish you all good fortune on your journey in simulation. Enjoy the book!

Vincent J. Grant, MD, FRCPC
Adam Cheng, MD, FRCPC

References

1. Grant VJ, Cheng A. The Canadian Pediatric Simulation Network: a report from the second national meeting in September 2009. Simul Healthc 2010;5(6):355–8.
2. International Pediatric Simulation Society [Internet]. 2014 [cited 2015 Jan 16]. Available from: http://www.ipssglobal.org.
3. Andreatta P, Saxton E, Thompson M, Annich G. Simulation-based mock codes significantly correlate with improved pediatric patient cardiopulmonary arrest survival rates. Pediatr Crit Care Med. 2011;12(1):33–8.
4. Draycott T, Sibanda T, Owen L, Akande V, Winter C, Reading S, et al. Does training in obstetric emergencies improve neonatal outcome? BJOG 2006;113(2):177–82.
5. Cheng A, Lang TR, Starr SR, Pusic M, Cook DA. Technology-enhanced simulation and pediatric education: a meta-analysis. Pediatrics 2014;133(5):e1313–23.
6. Cheng A, Grant V, Auerbach M. Using simulation to improve patient safety: dawn of a new era. 2015: JAMA Pediatrics, In Press.
7. Geis GL, Pio B, Pendergrass TL, Moyer MR, Patterson MD. Simulation to assess the safety of new healthcare teams and new facilities. Simul Healthc 2011;6(3):125–33.
8. Patterson MD, Geis GL, Falcone RA, LeMaster T, Wears RL. In situ simulation: detection of safety threats and teamwork training in a high risk emergency department. BMJ Qual Saf 2013;22(6):468–77.
9. Patterson MD, Geis GL, LeMaster T, Wears RL. Impact of multidisciplinary simulation-based training on patient safety in a paediatric emergency department. BMJ Qual Saf 2013;22(5):383–93.
10. Huang L, Norman D, Chen R. Addressing hospital-wide patient safety initiatives with high-fidelity simulation. Physician Executive Journal 2010;36(4):34–39.
11. Guise JM, Lowe NK, Deering S, Lewis PO, O'Haire C, Irwin LK et al. Mobile in situ obstetric emergency simulation and teamwork training to improve maternal-fetal safety in hospitals. Jt Comm J Qual Patient Saf 2010;36(10):443–53.
12. Wetzel EA, Lang TR, Pendergrass TL, Taylor RG, Geis GL. Identification of latent safety threats using high-fidelity simulation-based training with multidisciplinary neonatology teams. Jt Comm J Qual Patient Saf 2013;39(6):268–73.
13. Sigalet E, Donnon T, Cheng A, Cooke S, Robinson T, Bissett W, Grant V. Development of a team performance scale to assess undergraduate health professionals. Acad Med 2013;88(7):989–96.
14. Sigalet E, Donnon T, Grant V. Undergraduate students' perceptions of and attitudes toward a simulation-based interprofessional curriculum; the KidSIM ATTITUDES questionnaire. Simul Healthc 2012;7(6):353–8.
15. Sigalet EL, Donnon TL, Grant V. Insight into team competence in medical, nursing and respiratory therapy students. J Interprof Care 2014 Jul 22:1–6. [Epub ahead of print].
16. Sigalet E, Cheng A, Donnon T, Catena H, Robinson T, Chatfield J, Grant V. A simulation-based intervention teaching seizure management to caregivers: a randomized controlled study. Pediatr Child Health 2014;19(7):373–378.
17. Cheng A, Brown L, Duff J, Davidson J, Overly F, Tofil N, Peterson D, White M, Bhanji F, Bank I, Gottesman R, Adler M, Zhong J, Grant V, Grant D, Sudikoff S, Marohn K, Charnovich A, Hnt E, Kessler D, Wong H, Robertson N, Lin Y, Doan Q, Duval-Arnould J, Nadkarni V for the INSPIRE CPR Investigators. Improving cardiopulmonary resuscitation with a CPR feedback device and refresher simulations (CPR CARES Study): a multicenter, randomized trial. JAMA Pediatrics 2015;169(2):1–9. Doi:10.1001/jamapediatrics.2014.2616
18. Hunt EA, Hohenhaus SM, Luo X, Frush KS. Simulation of pediatric trauma stabilization in 35 North Carolina emergency departments: identification of targets for performance improvement. Pediatrics 2006;117(3):641–8.
19. Burton KS, Pendergrass Tl, Byczkowski TL, Taylor RG, Moyer MR, Falcone RA, et al. Impact of simulation-based extracorporeal membrane oxygenation training in the simulation laboratory and clinical environment. Simul Healthc 2011;6(5):284–91.
20. Cheng A, Auerbach M, Chang T, Hunt EA, Pusic M, Nadkarni V, Kessler D. Designing and conducting simulation-based research. Pediatrics. Published online May 12, 2014. Doi: 10.1542/peds.2013-3267.

21. Cheng A, Hunt E, Donoghue A, Nelson K, LeFlore J, Anderson J, Eppich W, Simon R, Rudolph J, Nad-karni V for the EXPRESS Pediatric Simulation Collaborative. EXPRESS—examining pediatric resusci-tation education using simulation and scripting: the birth of an international pediatric simulation research collaborative—from concept to reality. Simulation in Healthcare, 2011, 6(1):34–41.
22. International Network for Simulation-based Pediatric Innovation, Research and Education [Internet]. 2014 [cited 2015 Jan 16]. Avaiable from: http//www.inspiresim.com.
23. Grant V, Duff J, Bhanji F, Cheng A. Simulation in Pediatrics. In: Levine AI, DeMaria Jr S, Bryson EO, Schwartz AD, editors. The comprehensive textbook of healthcare simulation. New York: Springer; 2013.
24. Levine AI, DeMaria Jr S, Bryson EO, Schwartz AD, editors. The comprehensive textbook of healthcare simulation. New York: Springer; 2013.

Contents

Part III   Pediatric Simulation for Professional Development

Part IV   Pediatric Simulation Specialties

Part V   Pediatric Simulation Program Development

Contributors

Anne Ades, MD   Department of Pediatrics, Perelman School of Medicine, University of Pennsylvania, Philadelphia, PA, USA

Department of Pediatrics, Neonatology Division, The Children's Hospital of Philadelphia, Philadelphia, PA, USA

Mark Adler, MD   Department of Pediatrics and Medical Education, Northwestern University Feinberg School of Medicine, Chicago, IL, USA

Department of Pediatrics, Ann & Robert H. Lurie Children's Hospital of Chicago, Chicago, IL, USA

Dominic Allain, MD, FRCPC   Department of Emergency Medicine, Dalhousie University, Halifax, NS, Canada

Jennifer L. Arnold, MSc, MD   Simulation Center at Texas Children's Hospital, Houston, TX, USA

Division of Neonatology, Baylor College of Medicine, Houston, TX, USA

Marc Auerbach, MD, MSci   Department of Pediatrics, Section of Emergency Medicine, Yale University School of Medicine, New Haven, CT, USA

Farhan Bhanji, MD, MSc (Ed), FRCPC, FAHA   Department of Pediatrics, Centre for Medical Education, McGill University, Royal College of Physicians and Surgeons of Canada, Montreal, QC, Canada

Zia Bismilla, MD, Med, FRCPC, FAAP   Department of Paediatrics, University of Toronto, Toronto, ON, Canada

Choon Looi Bong, MBChB, FRCA   Department of Paediatric Anaesthesia, KK Women's and Children's Hospital, Duke-NUS Graduate Medical School, Yong Loo Lin School of Medicine, Singapore, Singapore

Matthew S. Braga, MD   Geisel School of Medicine at Dartmouth, Department of Pediatric Critical Care Medicine, Children's Hospital at Dartmouth, Lebanon, NH, USA

Guy F. Brisseau, MD, MEd, FAAP, FACS, FRCS(C)   Department of Pediatric Surgery, Sidra Medical & Research Center, Doha, Qatar

Linda L. Brown, MD, MSCE   Department of Pediatrics and Emergency Medicine, Alpert Medical School of Brown University, Hasbro Children's Hospital, Providence, RI, USA

Rebekah Burns, MD   Department of Pediatrics, Division of Emergency Medicine, University of Washington School of Medicine, Seattle, WA, USA

Aaron William Calhoun, MD   Department of Pediatrics, Division of Critical Care, University of Louisville School of Medicine, Kosair Children's Hospital, Louisville, KY, USA

Douglas Campbell, MSc, MD, FRCPC   Department of Pediatrics, University of Toronto, Toronto, ON, Canada

Todd P. Chang, MD, MAcM   Department of Pediatrics, Division of Emergency Medicine & Transport, University of Southern California Keck School of Medicine, Children's Hospital Los Angeles, Los Angeles, CA, USA

Adam Cheng, MD, FRCPC   Department of Pediatrics, Cumming School of Medicine, University of Calgary, Calgary, AB, Canada

KidSIM Pediatric Simulation Program, Alberta Children's Hospital, Calgary, AB, Canada

Kevin Ching, MD   Department of Pediatrics, Weill Cornell Medical College, New York Presbyterian Hospital – Weill Cornell Medical Center, New York, NY, USA

Asst. Prof. Mark X. Cicero, MD   Department of Pediatrics, Yale University School of Medicine, Yale-New Haven's Children's Hospital, New Haven, CT, USA

Suzette Cooke, MSc, MD, PhD(c)   Department of Pediatrics, University of Calgary, Calgary, AB, Canada

Ellen S. Deutsch, MD, MS   Department of Anesthesiology, Department of Critical Care Medicine, The Children's Hospital of Philadelphia, Philadelphia, PA, USA

Pennsylvania Patient Safety Authority, Plymouth Meeting, PA, USA

Maria Carmen G. Diaz, MD, FAAP, FACEP   Department of Pediatrics and Emergency Medicine, Sidney Kimmel Medical College at Thomas Jefferson University, Phliadelphia, PA, USA

Division of Emergency Medicine, Nemours Institute for Clinical Excellence, Nemours/Afred I. duPont Hospital for Children, Wilmington, DE, USA

Aaron Donoghue, MD, MSCE   Department of Pediatrics and Critical Care Medicine, Department of Emergency Medicine and Critical Care Medicine, Perelman School of Medicine of the University of Pennsylvania, Children's Hospital of Philadelphia, Philadelphia, PA, USA

Adam Dubrowski, PhD   Emergency Medicine and Pediatrics, Memorial University, Newfoundland and Labrador, Canada

Jonathan P. Duff, MD, MEd   Department of Pediatrics, Department of Pediatric Critical Care, University of Alberta, Stollery Children's Hospital, Edmonton, AB, Canada

Jordan M. Duval-Arnould, MPH, DrPHc   Department of Anesthesiology & Critical Care Medicine, Division of Health Sciences Informatics, Johns Hopkins University School of Medicine, Baltimore, MD, USA

M. Dylan Bould, MB, ChB, MRCP, FRCA, MEd Department of Anesthesiology, University of Ottawa, Children's Hospital of Eastern Ontario, Ottawa, Canada

Walter J. Eppich, MD, MEd Departments of Pediatrics and Medical Education, Department of Pediatric Emergency Medicine, Northwestern University Feinberg School of Medicine, Ann & Robert H. Lurie Children's Hospital of Chicago, Chicago, IL, USA

Tobias Everett, MBChB, FRCA Department of Anesthesia, Department of Anesthesia and Pain Medicine, The Hospital for Sick Children, University of Toronto, Toronto, ON, Canada

Marino Festa, MBBS, MRCP (UK), FCICM, MD (Res) Kids Simulation Australia & Paediatric Intensive Care, Sydney Children's Hospitals Network, Sydney, NSW, Australia

Marisa Brett Fleegler, MD Department of Pediatrics, Division of Emergency Medicine, Harvard Medical School, Boston Children's Hospital, Boston, MA, USA

Kristin Fraser, MD Department of Medicine, Division of Respirology, Cummings School of Medicine, Alberta Health Services, Calgary, AB, Canada

James Gerard, MD Department of Pediatrics, Division of Emergency Medicine, Saint Louis University School of Medicine, SSM Cardinal Glennon Children's Medical Center, St. Louis, MO, USA

Elaine Gilfoyle, MSc (Hons), MD, MMEd, FRCPC Department of Pediatrics, Department of Critical Care, University of Calgary, Alberta Children's Hospital, Calgary, AB, Canada

Ronald D. Gottesman, MD Department of Pediatrics, Department of Pediatric Critical Care, McGill University, Montreal Children's Hospital/McGill University Health Center, Montreal, QC, Canada

David J. Grant, MBChB, MRCPCH Bristol Royal Hospital for Children, University Hospitals Bristol NHS Foundation Trust, Bristol, UK

Bristol Paediatric Simulation Programme, Bristol Medical Simulation Centre, Bristol, UK

Vincent J. Grant, MD, FRCPC Department of Pediatrics, Cumming School of Medicine, University of Calgary, Calgary, AB, Canada

KidSIM Pediatric Simulation Program, Alberta Children's Hospital, Calgary, AB, Canada

Melinda Fiedor Hamilton, MD, MSc Department of Critical Care Medicine, Children's Hospital of Pittsburgh of UPMC, Pittsburgh, PA, USA

Ellen Heimberg, MD Department of Pediatric Cardiology, Pulmology, Intensive Care Medicine, University Children's Hospital, Tuebingen, Germany

Lennox Huang, MD Department of Pediatrics, McMaster University, McMaster Children's Hospital, Hamilton, ON, Canada

James L. Huffman, BSc, MD, FRCPC Department of Emergency Medicine, University of Calgary, Calgary, AB, Canada

Elizabeth A. Hunt, MD, MPH, PhD   Department of Anesthesiology & Critical Care Medicine, Pediatrics & Health Informatics, Pediatric Intensive Care Unit, Johns Hopkins University School of Medicine, Johns Hopkins Hospital, Baltimore, MD, USA

Lindsay Callahan Johnston, MD   Department of Pediatrics, Yale School of Medicine, New Haven, CT, USA

Liana Kappus, MEd   SYN:APSE Center for Learning, Transformation and Innovation, Yale New Haven Health System, New Haven, CT, USA

David O. Kessler, MD, MSc   Department of Pediatrics, Columbia University College of Physicians and Surgeons, New York Presbyterian Hospital, Columbia University Medical Center, New York, NY, USA

Susanne Kost, MD, FAAP, FACEP   Department of Pediatrics, Sidney Kimmel Medical College, Thomas Jefferson University, Philadelphia, PA, USA

Department of Anesthesia, Nemours/A.I.duPont Hospital for Children, Wilmington, DE, USA

Afrothite Kotsakis, MD, MEd, FRCPC   Department of Pediatrics, Department of Critical Care Medicine, University of Toronto, The Hospital for Sick Children, Toronto, ON, Canada

Anita Lai, MD   Department of Emergency Medicine, University of Calgary, Calgary, AB, Canada

Arielle Levy, MD, MEd, FRCPC   Department of Pediatrics Emergency, Department of Pediatrics, University of Montreal, Sainte-Justine Hospital University Centre, Montreal, QC, Canada

Yiqun Lin, MD, MHSc   Department of Community Health Science, Faculty of Medicine, KidSIM Simulation Education and Research Program, University of Calgary, Alberta's Children's Hospital, Calgary, AB, Canada

Lindsay Long, MD, FRCPC   Department of Pediatrics, University of Calgary, Calgary, AB, Canada

Joseph O. Lopreiato, MD, MPH   Val G. Hemming Simulation Center, Department of Pediatrics, Uniformed Services University of the Health Sciences, Bethesda, MD, USA

Steven R. Lopushinsky, MD, MSc, FRCSC   Section of Pediatric Surgery, Cumming School of Medicine, University of Calgary, Alberta Children's Hospital, Calgary, AB, Canada

Tensing Maa, MD   Department of Pediatrics, Department of Critical Care Medicine, Ohio State University College of Medicine, Nationwide Children's Hospital, Columbus, OH, USA

Ralph James MacKinnon, BSc (Hons), MBChB, FRCA   Faculty of Health, Psychology & Social Change, Department of Paediatric Anaesthesia & Paediatric Intensive Care, Manchester Metropolitan University, Royal Manchester Children's Hospital, North West & North Wales Paediatric Transport Service, Manchester, UK

Mary E. Mancini, RN, PhD   College of Nursing and Health Innovation, The University of Texas at Arlington, Arlington, TX, USA

Deepak Manhas, MD, FAAP, FRCP(C)   Department of Pediatrics, Department of Neonatal Intensive Care, University of British Columbia, British Columbia Children's & Women's Hospital, Vancouver, BC, Canada

Gord McNeil, MD, FRCP(C)   Department of Emergency Medicine, University of Calgary, Foothills Medical Centre and Alberta Children's Hospital, Calgary, AB, Canada

Peter A. Meaney, MD, MPH   Department of Anesthesia and Critical Care, University of Pennsylvania School of Medicine Children's Hospital of Philadelphia, Philadelphia, PA, USA

Garth D. Meckler, MD, MSHS   Department of Pediatrics and Emergency Medicine, University of British Columbia, BC Children's Hospital, Vancouver, BC, Canada

Elaine C. Meyer, PhD, RN   Department of Psychiatry, Institute for Professionalism and Ethical Practice, Harvard Medical School, Boston Children's Hospital, Boston, MA, USA

Michael Moyer, EMT-P, MS, PhD   Center for Simulation & Education, TriHealth, Cincinnati, OH, USA

Elaine Ng, MD, FRCPC, MHPE   Department of Anesthesia, Department of Anesthesia and Pain Medicine, University of Toronto, Hospital for Sick Children, Toronto, ON, Canada

Akira Nishisaki, MD, MSCE   Department of Anesthesiology and Critical Care Medicine, The Children's Hospital of Philadelphia, Philadelphia, PA, USA

Denis Oriot, MD, PhD   Simulation Laboratory, Department of Emergency Medicine, University of Poitiers, University Hospital, Poitiers, France

Frank L. Overly, MD   Department of Emergency Medicine and Pediatrics, Alpert Medical School of Brown University, Hasbro Children's Hospital, Providence, RI, USA

Janice C. Palaganas, PhD, RN, NP   Department of Anesthesia, Critical Care & Pain Medicine, Harvard University, Massachusetts General Hospital, Boston, MA, USA

Mary D. Patterson, MD, MEd   Department of Pediatrics, Northeast Ohio Medical University, Rootstown, OH, USA

Simulation Center for Safety and Reliability, Akron children's Hospital, Akron, OH, USA

Dawn Taylor Peterson, PhD   Office of Interprofessional Simulation, Department of Medical Education, University of Alabama at Birmingham, Birmingham, AL, USA

Jonathan Pirie, MD, MEd   Department of Medicine, Department of Paediatrics, University of Toronto, The Hospital for Sick Children, Toronto, ON, Canada

Martin V. Pusic, MD, PhD   Department of Emergency Medicine, New York University School of Medicine, New York, NY, USA

Jennifer R. Reid, MD   Department of Pediatrics, Division of Emergency Medicine, University of Washington School of Medicine, Seattle Children's Hospital, Seattle, WA, USA

Nicola Peiris, BSc   KidSIM Pediatric Simulation Program, University of Calgary, Alberta Children's Hospital, Calgary, AB, Canada

Traci Robinson KidSIM Pediatric Simulation Program, Alberta Children's Hospital, Calgary, AB, Canada

Taylor Sawyer, DO, MEd Department of Pediatrics, University of Washington School of Medicine, Seattle Children's Hospital, Seattle, WA, USA

Ella Scott, RN, RSCN, MA Department of Simulation, Sidra Medical & Research Center, Doha, Qatar

Allan Evan Shefrin, MD, FRCPC (pediatrics, PEM) Department of Pediatrics, Division of Pediatric Emergency Medicine, University of Ottawa, Children's Hospital of Eastern Ontario, Ottawa, ON, Canada

Yuko Shiima, MD Center for Simulation, Advanced Education and Innovation, The Children's Hospital of Philadelphia, Philadelphia, PA, USA

Nicole Ann Shilkofski, MD, MEd Departments of Pediatrics and Anesthesiology/Critical Care Medicine, Johns Hopkins University School of Medicine, Baltimore, Maryland, USA

Elaine Sigalet, RN, BSN, MN, PhD Department of Education, Sidra Research and Medical Center, Doha, Qatar

Kimberly P. Stone, MD, MS, MA Department of Pediatrics, Division of Emergency Medicine, University of Washington School of Medicine, Seattle Children's Hospital, Seattle, WA, USA

Glenn Stryjewski, MD, MPH Department of Pediatrics, Jefferson Medical College, Philadelphia, PA, USA

Division of Pediatric Critical Care, Nemours/Alfred I. duPont Hospital for Children, Wilmington, DE, USA

Stephanie N. Sudikoff, MD SYN:APSE Center for Learning, Transformation and Innovation, Yale New Haven Health System, New Haven, CT, USA

Pediatric Critical Care, Yale School of Medicine, New Haven, CT, USA

Nancy M. Tofil, MD, MEd Department of Pediatrics, University of Alabama at Birmingham, Children's of Alabama, Birmingham, AL, USA

Terry Varshney, MD, FRCPC Department of Pediatric Emergency, Children Hospital of Eastern Ontario, University of Ottawa, Ottawa, ON, Canada

Debra L. Weiner, MD, PhD Department of Pediatrics, Department of Emergency Medicine, Harvard Medical School, Boston Children's Hospital, Boston, MA, USA

Marjorie Lee White, MD, MPPM, MA Department of Pediatrics, Office of Interprofessional Simulation, Pediatric Simulation Center, University of Alabama at Birmingham, Children's of Alabama, Birmingham, AL, USA

John Zhong, MD Department of Anesthesiology and Pain Management, UTSW Medical Center, Children's Medical Center of Dallas, Dallas, TX, USA

Part I

Fundamentals of Simulation for Pediatrics

Cognitive Load and Stress in Simulation

Choon Looi Bong, Kristin Fraser and Denis Oriot

Simulation Pearls

- Simulation training induces profound biological and psychological stress responses in the learners, which can be measured using objective and subjective markers.
- The effects of stress on learning and performance in simulation varies according to task difficulty, learner's proficiency, team dynamics, individual personality traits, and coping styles, as well as socio-evaluative factors such as perceived appraisal from peers, observers, and preceptors.
- Stress that is clinically relevant and integral to the objectives of a scenario has a role in simulation design. However, stress contributes to extraneous cognitive load, an excess of which impairs the function of working memory, increasing the risk of cognitive overload and poorer learning outcomes.
- The optimal amount of stress for learning and performance is learner specific, task specific, and situation specific. One should consider the limitations of working memory when adding stress to enhance realism or learner engagement. Modification of nonessential stressors should be considered during all stages of simulation instruction.

C. L. Bong (✉)
Department of Paediatric Anaesthesia, KK Women's and Children's Hospital, Duke-NUS Graduate Medical School, Yong Loo Lin School of Medicine, 100 Bukit Timah Road, 229899 Singapore, Singapore
e-mail: bong.choon.looi@singhealth.com.sg

K. Fraser
Department of Medicine, Division of Respirology, Cumming School of Medicine, Alberta Health Services, 7007 14St SW, Calgary, AB T2V 1P9, Canada
e-mail: kristin.fraser@albertahealthservices.ca

D. Oriot
Simulation Laboratory, Department of Emergency Medicine, University of Poitiers, University Hospital, 6 rue de la Miletrie, 86000 Poitiers, France
e-mail: denis.oriot@univ-poitiers.fr

Without stress, there would be no life. (Hans Selye)

The Stress Response

Stress is a common word used in our daily conversations but is a concept that is difficult to define in scientific terms. In physics, stress refers to the pressure or tension exerted on a material object. In a medical or biological context, it refers to a physical, mental, or emotional factor that causes bodily or mental tension. In psychological terms, stress refers to the biological and emotional responses when encountering a threat that one feels that he or she may not have the resources to deal with. Stress is a highly individualistic experience that depends on specific psychological determinants that trigger a stress response [1].

Biological Stress Response

Han Selye first described the biological stress response in 1936. He defined stress as "the non-specific response of the body to any demand for change" [2] and showed that a variety of physical stressors such as fasting, extreme cold, and operative injuries all cause similar physical changes in the body, such as enlargement of the adrenal gland, atrophy of the thymus, and gastric ulceration. We now know the biological basis to this stress response. When a situation is interpreted as being stressful, it triggers the activation of the sympathetic nervous system (SNS), which produces epinephrine and norepinephrine, as well as the hypothalamic–pituitary–adrenal (HPA) axis, whereby neurons in the hypothalamus release corticotrophin-releasing hormone which triggers the release of adenocorticotrophin hormone (ACTH) from the pituitary, which in turn triggers the release of the hormone cortisol from the adrenal glands. These hormones act on the body to give rise to the fight-or-flight response, manifested

Fig. 1.1 Biological stress response. *ACTH* adenocorticotrophin hormone, *CRH* corticotropin-releasing hormone

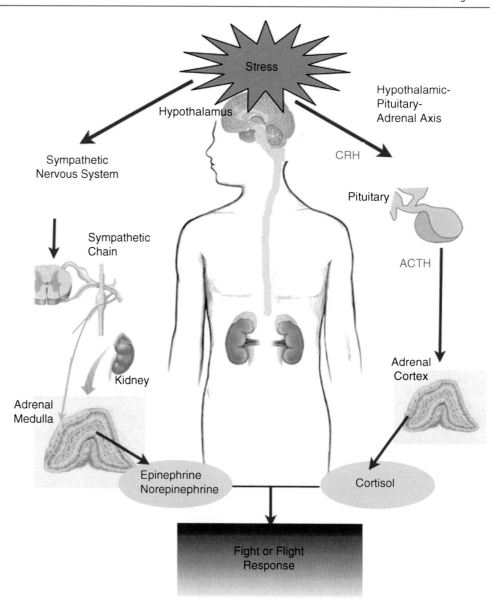

as an increase in heart rate (HR), blood pressure (BP), respiratory rate, etc. (Fig. 1.1).

Psychological Stress Response

In addition to physical stressors, the biological stress response can be triggered by a variety of psychological conditions, induced by one's interpretation of events. Stress has been described as the result of interaction between three elements: the perceived demand on an individual, the individual's perceived ability to cope, and the perception of the importance of being able to cope with the demand [3]. When one perceives that one's resources are sufficient to meet the demands, the situation is assessed as a challenge, leading to a

positive psychological state of *eustress*. When one perceives that the demands are outweighing the resources, the situation is assessed as a threat, leading to a negative psychological response of *distress* [4], causing a variety of affective states, the most common being anxiety.

Work in the 1960s [5] measured stress hormone levels in individuals subjected to various potentially stressful conditions and described three main psychological determinants that would induce a stress response. In order for a situation to induce a stress response, it has to be interpreted as being novel, unpredictable, and uncontrollable. Subsequently, a fourth element was added, namely, a threat to the ego. Simulation training contains all four of the above elements and has indeed been shown to induce a measurable physiological stress response [6, 7].

Measures of Stress Response in Simulation

No single method exists for measuring stress directly. Stress levels can only be approximated by measuring its effects, either on the subject's perceptions of themselves (subjective measures) or on their physiologic state (objective measures) [8].

Subjective Measurements

A wide variety of questionnaires have been developed to assess the psychological factors that are associated with stress. Many of these have been used for subjects' self-reporting of stress in simulation studies. The State Trait Anxiety Inventory (STAI) is a validated measure of stress and is widely used in simulation studies [9]. Other examples include the Depression, Anxiety, Stress Scale (DASS) and its short version (DASS-21) [10, 11], the Visual Analogue Scale (VAS) [12], and various Likert scales [13].

Objective Measurements

Physiological States
- *Heart rate (HR):* An increase in HR results from endogenous catecholamine release and is used in many studies as a proxy measure for stress [6, 7, 14].
- *Heart rate variability (HRV):* Changes in the interval between consecutive heartbeats and is an indicator of sympatho–vagal balance during stress. HRV changes with stress or autonomic activity and typically increases in times of stress [15].
- *Blood pressure (BP):* An increase in BP is another indirect measure of SNS activation but may be difficult to measure during simulation training.
- *Skin conductance level (SCL):* This measures the electrical conductance of the skin. An increase in stress level increases SNS activity, which increases sweat gland activity and skin moisture thus increasing skin conductance [16].
- *Electroculogram:* This utilizes an ergonomic workstation to count the number of eye blinks during surgical skills training. Increase in stress levels increases the number of eye blinks [17].

Hormone Levels
- *Salivary cortisol (SC):* Cortisol is secreted following the activation of the HPA axis and SC measurement allows the noninvasive measurement of plasma cortisol levels. SC is a well-established biomarker of stress and has been used in numerous clinical and behavioral studies over the past few decades. SC has been shown to be synchronous with serum cortisol concentration across the 24-h time frame [18] and easily measured with a simple enzyme immunoassay [19]. Cortisol levels peak at 30–40 min after the onset of stressors [20]. The concentration of SC closely approximates the plasma concentration, with a lag time of approximately 15 min. SC concentrations show a diurnal variation, with highest values in the morning, declining throughout the day towards afternoon and evening [21]. Cortisol reactivity to stressful situations can differ according to time of the day [21, 22], so studies measuring SC should ideally be conducted at similar times during the day to avoid potential confounding effects from inter- and intraindividual differences in the diurnal pattern of cortisol secretion.
- *Salivary alpha-amylase (sAA):* sAA is a digestive enzyme synthesized by the salivary glands and released in response to SNS activation [23]. sAA is increasingly used as a surrogate marker for SNS activity in current biobehavioral research. Following a psychological stressor, the increase in sAA is more rapid than SC and is significantly correlated with increases in plasma norepinephrine [24, 25]. Like SC, sAA activity also exhibits a diurnal rhythm but within a smaller range, with a pronounced decrease within 60 min after awakening and a steady increase during the course of the day [26].

Combined Measurements

- Studies on the effects of stress in simulation-based education (SBE) lack uniformity in the measurement of stress [8]. A variety of different physiological markers such as HR, SCL, eye blinks, and SC have been used to quantify stress. The use of different markers of stress in different studies renders it difficult to compare and generalize results. Most studies utilize only one objective measurement of stress, making it difficult to assess the reliability and validity. Besides, there are discrepancies between learner's perceived stress levels and their physiological stress levels. For example, there is significant correlation between STAI scores and sAA levels [25] but not SC levels [27]. There are also significant differences between perceived stress (subjects' self-report) and concurrent physiological stress responses (HR, respiratory sinus arrhythmia, and SC), as well as inverse associations between HR responsiveness and the subsequent appraisal of stress [28]. Thus, using a combination of perceived and physiological markers of stress may be more reliable than using a single measure to assess individual differences in stress responsiveness.

The Imperial Stress Assessment Tool (ISAT), comprising a combination of HR, SC, and the short version of the STAI is a nonintrusive and reliable approach combining subjective and objective methods for measuring stress in the operating room [29]. Use of such composite tools, combining subjective and objective stress measurements, may increase our understanding of the effects of stress on clinical performance and outcomes.

Studies on Stress Response in Simulation

Simulation Training Is Associated with a Measurable Stress Response over a Predictable Time Course

Several studies have demonstrated that high-fidelity SBE training is associated with a measurable stress response over a predictable time course [7, 8, 30]. Physicians participating in SBE experienced a measurable stress response, as evidenced by an increase in HR and SC over a predictable time frame from baseline to just prior to the simulation session, peaking at the end of the simulation session and decreasing, but remaining above baseline at the end of the debriefing. In contrast, physicians participating in tutorial-based training did not experience a stress response. Another study of physicians found that the stress response in 32 intensivists undergoing two different types of SBE found a significant increase in both SC and sAA levels immediately after the test scenarios [8]. Fifteen minutes after the scenario, the sAA decreased to baseline levels, but SC levels remained elevated.

All Active Participants in a Simulation Scenario Exhibit a Stress Response, Irrespective of Role

Physicians, nurses, and technicians all exhibit a stress response during SBE [7]. Measurement of stress and learning in residents and medical students undergoing difficult airway scenarios in the roles of team leader, procedure chief, or team member showed that both stress and learning appeared similar irrespective of the participant's roles in a simulation scenario [31]. There was no correlation between the stress response and learning outcomes.

Simulation Training Can Be More Stressful Than Real-Life Conditions

Simulation can be a profoundly stressful experience. The stress response of 31 medical students subjected to SBE (simulated medical crisis), laboratory stress (public speaking), and rest conditions was studied [32]. SC and psychological responses (VAS) were assessed every 15 min from

15 min prior to until 60 min after intervention. SBE was found to be a profound stressor. SC responses were similar between SBE and public speaking, but psychological stress was greater during SBE compared to public speaking. Similarly, HR and BP measured during the practical examination in an Advanced Trauma Life Support (ATLS) course and compared with the values taken during real-life clinical care in the emergency room, revealed that the stress values during the simulated scenario were higher than those measured in real cases [33]. In nurse anesthesia students, SBE raised SC levels threefold above baseline levels, while actual clinical experience in the operating room did not [34].

Stress and Learning

Cognitive Load Theory

Similar to the word *stress, cognitive load* is a term that has been used by different disciplines to describe related but slightly different concepts [35, 36]. Cognitive load theory (CLT) is a specific theory of instructional design. Its origin dates back to the sentinel work of Miller in the 1950s when he established that the human working memory is only capable of processing a limited number of novel information elements at a given time [37]. It is well established that if the capacity of working memory is exceeded then learning will be impaired. In the late 1980s, John Sweller developed CLT based on this model of human cognitive architecture to explain why some types of learning instruction are not effective in spite of excellent content [38]. Cognitive load researchers applying this concept have since derived a dozen effects that should be considered when developing instructional materials [39]. An example is the *split attention effect,* stating that when essential information is given to learners in a divided fashion, such that one piece of information must be held in working memory while awaiting the second piece, the cognitive load is increased and learning is impaired. By instructing in a non-split format (e.g., integrating text into a diagram rather than leaving it in a legend outside of a diagram), learning outcomes improve and reported cognitive load drops [40]. While the many effects described by the theory have been worked out in traditional classrooms, it is logical to apply the findings to a more complex environment such as SBE since our working memory resources remain finite, regardless of expertise. A brief description of CLT is given below, and interested readers are directed to a more extensive review of the theory applied to medical education [41]. It is important to emphasize that CLT relates only to learning and not to performance. The effects of working memory limitations on performance are presented in the next section.

Types of Cognitive Load

CLT describes two types of cognitive load: that which is *intrinsic* to the task (its difficulty depends on the expertise of the learner) and that which is *extraneous* to the task (due to ineffective instructional methods). These loads are summative and must not exceed limitations of the working memory.

Intrinsic Load

When to-be-learned materials are relatively simple with few interacting elements, intrinsic cognitive load is low and cognitive load issues are unlikely to arise. However, multiple interacting elements cause high cognitive load since they must be considered simultaneously in working memory [42]. The intrinsic load of medical simulation is necessarily high due to the complexity of medical practice where multiple sources of information are presented simultaneously for processing. Nonetheless, complex problems can be addressed by bringing previously processed, organized, and stored information from long-term memory into working memory in the form of single schemata or chunks [43]. These elements do not take up precious working memory resources as they have already been learned and can be automatically applied.

Reducing Intrinsic Load in Simulation CLT describes several strategies for reducing intrinsic load, generally methods to reduce tasks into manageable chunks and allow practice of each chunk until it is effectively stored in long-term memory. Thereafter, large amounts of information can eventually be manipulated in working memory in the form of these chunks without overloading working memory resources. An example in simulation would be learning technical skills such as intubation or defibrillation separately, prior to an immersive SBE event incorporating an advanced cardiac life support (ACLS) algorithm. Stress that is considered essential to training, such as the time pressure of securing an airway, is an intrinsic cognitive load that needs to be scaffolded into the training to prevent overloading of working memory.

Extraneous Load

Most work within a CLT framework has investigated the negative consequences of extraneous cognitive load caused by inappropriate instructional methods, such as the split-attention effect discussed above. In applying this CLT principle to the simulation setting, one could consider designing the information flow for learners in a scenario so that important patient information is consolidated on a patient chart, rather than having learners search out data from multiple sources such as patient history, chart review, or family interview. Such a format would clearly lessen the load on working memory and would be an excellent strategy for novice learners who will have a very high intrinsic load due to medical content itself. Similarly, if other features of the simulation, such as a communication challenge, were going to require significant mental resources, then reducing the extraneous load of having to search for information would be desirable. However, presenting information in such a *low extraneous load* format may not be (1) realistic, which could impair learning by reducing participant engagement; (2) possible, given the unpredictability of what learners will actually do (vs. what we expect them to do) during simulation; or (3) desirable, if demonstrating knowledge about available resources is a specific objective of the simulation session. Where possible, instructors need to predict these potential loads and if they are extraneous to the leaning objectives, try to minimize them. Extraneous load in simulation is often inadvertently generated by factors such as poor quality mannequin findings, overly emotional actors, or uncertainty about the *rules* of the simulation environment, and many of these situations can be prevented through diligent scenario planning and pre-briefing of learners. Table 1.1 lists some strategies for reducing stress and cognitive load in SBE. These strategies are particularly relevant when instructing novice learners and may be adapted as needed when instructing expert learners.

Reducing Extraneous Load in Simulation: Improving Instructional Design

Worked Example Effect There is evidence that when novice learners are presented with a problem or goal, they will typically engage in problem-solving strategies that require a high degree of mental effort, leaving inadequate cognitive resources available for actual learning [44]. Providing the solution to students in the form of worked examples has been shown to be a superior teaching strategy to problem-solving alone [45]. These worked examples are a form of scaffolding, also described as teaching within the zone of proximal development [46]. An example of providing a *worked example* during SBT is with the *call for help,* often incorporated as an opportunity for students to practice effective resource management. When the instructor enters the scenario and demonstrates the appropriate problem-solving strategy, the high cognitive load imposed on learners trying to solve the problem is reduced, and working memory resources can be reallocated to learning.

Expertise Reversal Effect This addresses a cognitive load effect caused by differing knowledge levels and states that an instructional design that is beneficial to a novice learner may be detrimental, rather than just neutral, to a more experienced learner and vice versa [47]. For example, an instructor might decide to assist junior students struggling with a case of anaphylaxis by providing a source for the dosing of IM epinephrine, aiming to reduce mental workload and free up cognitive resources for actual learning. Paradoxically,

Table 1.1 Strategies for managing stress and cognitive load in simulation

Strategy/description	Considerations	Example
Reduce intrinsic load		
Titrate the level of task difficulty to the proficiency of the learner	The learners' perception of their lack of resources/ability to deal with the challenge will lead to stress	For novices learning endotracheal intubation, choose a typical easy intubation scenario in an elective setting with minimal distraction so learners can focus on the task at hand
	Increase the level of task difficulty for proficient learners to facilitate engagement	For proficient learners, increase the level of task difficulty by worsening the laryngoscopic view, adding on time pressure (need for emergent intubation) and/or the need to deal with an anxious parent (confederate)
Reduce tasks into manageable chunks	Allow practice of each chunk until it is effectively stored in long-term memory, thus allowing subsequent manipulation of all information without overloading working memory	Teach technical skills such as intubation or defibrillation separately prior to an immersive SBE event incorporating the ACLS algorithm with a multidisciplinary team
Reduce extraneous load		
Provide worked examples	Providing part of all of the solution to a problem for learners can reduce cognitive load and enhance learning	Incorporate the opportunity to *call for help* during scenario: Instructor enters scenario and demonstrates appropriate problem-solving strategy, reducing the high cognitive load imposed on learners trying to solve the problem so working memory resources can be reallocated to learning
Respect the expertise reversal effect of CLT	Instructional strategies that are helpful for novice learners might be unhelpful or even detrimental to learning for more experienced learners (and vice versa)	For junior learners in an anaphylaxis scenario, providing an algorithm that includes the dose of epinephrine can reduce mental workload and allow them to focus on other goals such as effective resuscitation. However, if an experienced intensivist is handed the same information during a scenario he will have to exert some mental work to assess the information and likely reject it as redundant. Thus the same resource has a very different cognitive effect on learners of different levels
Expect learners to act as they would in reality	Asking learners to *pretend* to be of a different level or profession has not been proven to be beneficial and could potentially add stress for both the individual learner and the group	Asking a senior physician to participate as a learner in the role of nurse will lead to numerous difficulties with realism, learner engagement, and team dynamics. These will distract from the true objectives of the simulation scenario. Additionally, there is potential for learners to experience stress related to peer assessment and team dynamics beyond those that already exist in interprofessional teams
Reduce environmental stressors	Consider the relative importance of distractions (such as alarms, other noises) to realism vs. stress	Minimize noise, ensure appropriate temperature and lighting in physical environment
Avoid technical/equipment problems		Do a *trial run* of the scenario, ensure that the mannequin is fully functional, pertinent *clinical signs* are present, necessary equipment are available
Minimize the presence of nonessential observers	Balance the need for observers against potential increase of stress related to performance anxiety and peer assessment	The presence of observers who are not active participants of the SBE may have unpredictable effects on the psychology of the learners. Observers must also agree to confidentiality in order to maintain psychological safety
Reduce emotional stress	Pre-brief to set clear expectations	1. Ensure psychological safety of the learners. Address the issue of facilitator or peer evaluation and provide reassurance regarding confidentiality 2. Provide clarity about learning objectives, roles of the learner, facilitator, preceptors, and confederates 3. Orientate learners to the simulation environment including: mannequin capabilities and *clinical signs*, how to administer drugs or intravenous (iv) fluids, how to perform procedures, and ask for investigations or help
	Avoid unnecessary activation of the learner's emotions	1. Provide detailed scripting to actors/confederates to avoid overly emotional scenes or excessive distraction; rehearse with actors 2. Avoid *death* of the mannequin unless discussion of death is part of the SBE objectives (i.e., an intrinsic load) and adequate time and resources is set aside for debriefing
	Consider stress due to anxiety/personality traits	Provide stress-management strategies after SBE Stress inoculation training can be designed to develop coping skills for immediate problems and future stressful situations. This involves repeated exposure to SBE and providing learners with a toolkit of coping strategies, allowing them to construct a personalized coping package

SBE simulation-based education, *ACLS* advanced cardiac life support, *CLT* cognitive load theory providing the same information to a senior medical resident in this scenario could actually worsen learning if he/she already has a preexisting schema for this information. In this case, provision of this redundant information actually forces additional mental processing to decide how and whether to use such data (i.e., an extraneous load effect). Simulation instructors should understand that it is not just the way in which information is presented to learners that affects their mental resources available for completing the required exercise, but that the expected effects would vary significantly depending on the learners' prior experience.

Reducing Extraneous Load in Simulation: Managing Nonessential Stressors

If one considers the information related to the simulation environment (and not the case content) as a potential source of high cognitive load for medical learners, then adhering to a practice of routine and detailed pre-briefing of the simulation environment as part of each session will enable the creation of schemata, thereby freeing working memory resources for learning during the scenario. The pre-briefing should include a review of the mannequin capabilities and *normal* findings (with hands-on assessment) to reduce the mental workload of students trying to recall such details from prior sessions or guessing what the findings might signify (e.g., This sounds like a 'pleural rub', does this simulated patient have pleural disease, or did this sound from mechanical rubbing of the mannequin?). The plan for the simulation training session should be outlined for learners, including the time allocated to the scenario (vs. debriefing), how the case will end, and potential patient outcomes (e.g., letting junior learners know ahead of time that the mannequin will not arrest). A specific discussion regarding the roles of the students, actors, and preceptors should include identification of a source of *truth* if findings are unclear. Emotion and stress related to the peer assessment and potential for academic evaluation must be addressed with confidentiality agreements and discussions of the value of mistakes in this learning setting. An excellent pre-scenario briefing can go a long way to minimizing extraneous load for simulation participants (Table 1.1).

Measuring Cognitive Load

Most experiments involving cognitive load effects have used the validated 9-point Likert scale of Paas [48, 49] in which the learner introspects the level of mental effort required for task completion. Many other measures have been proposed including dual-task methodologies [50], HRV [51], electroencephalogram (EEG) responses [52], pupil dilation [53], functional magnetic resonance imaging, and eye tracking

[54]. To date, none of these have been found to be more reliable and discriminating than the subjective scale [55], but this research field is still in its early stages of development. The ideal measurement tool in the simulation setting would need to provide objective data that correlates with the validated subjective scale, not interfere in the simulation exercise itself, and provide continuous monitoring for detailed assessment of cognitive load across different phases of simulation training.

Effects of Stress on Memory and Learning

The effects of stress on learning are generally classified according to the phase of memory involved in the learning process when the stress is experienced [56]. Stress responses and increases in cortisol level differentially influence four distinct memory processes: sensory memory, working memory, memory consolidation, and retrieval of information from long-term memory. *Sensory memory* is the shortest-term element of memory, in which the multitude of inputs to our five senses reside for only milliseconds unless we consciously attend to the information and move it into the working memory for processing. Stress can certainly focus attention on a specific input of importance, potentially leading to enhanced learning. However, stress-induced attention can equally result in channeling or tunnelling of mental resources, whereby important peripheral information might be overlooked [57].

Working memory consists of the capacity to store and manipulate information for brief periods of time, for example, the team leader simultaneously keeps track of information gathered from multiple sources (clinical monitors, other team members) to keep previously learned information in mind (patient drug allergies) and to manipulate this information to reach clinical decisions. Elevated stress and SC levels have been shown to impair working memory capacity [58]. The focus of CLT is to respect the limitations of working memory when designing instruction. The major implication is that in the stressful environment of medical simulation, one must be especially vigilant to limit the number of novel, interacting elements in order to minimize extraneous load. However, if the task is appropriate for learner level and without extraneous load then the *stress* effects on working memory might not lead to an overloaded state. In such a situation, stress may actually be beneficial to learning through the effect of stress on memory consolidation.

Memory consolidation is the process by which new and fragile memories are rendered into more stable and permanent memories. Elevated stress responses, especially if they lead to increased cortisol levels, have been associated with the enhancement of memory consolidation through the

(+) indicates a potential benefit to learning; (-) indicates a potential impairment to learning

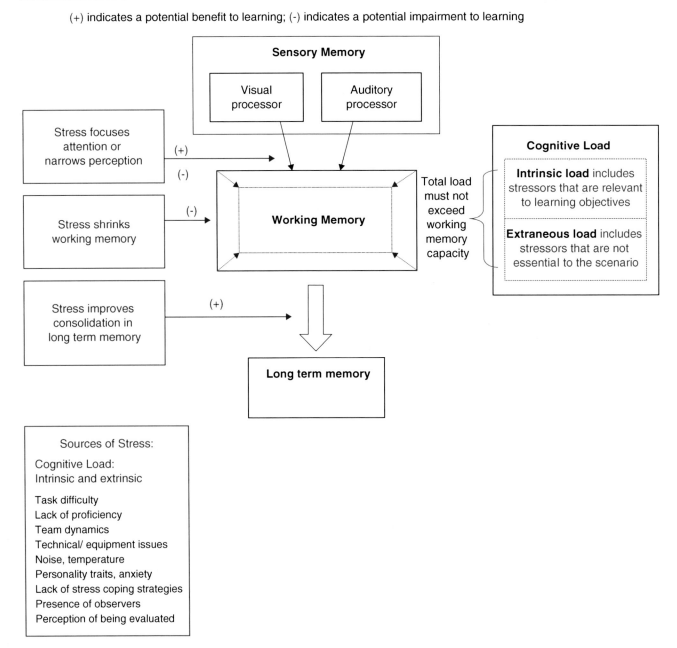

Fig. 1.2 Effects of stress on memory and learning

effects of cortical and noradrenergic activation in basolateral regions of the amygdala [58]. This is felt to be the mechanism by which clinicians often recall a very specific patient or critical event that was particularly stressful or emotional. Consolidation of information is only possible once the data has been processed and organized in working memory so the learning benefit of induced stress on memory might not be seen if working memory is overloaded.

Memory retrieval is the final phase of memory to consider. This process is also impaired by high levels of stress-related cortisol [59], likely contributing to stress-related performance decrements (Fig. 1.2).

Stress and Performance

The Yerkes–Dodson Law

The relationship between stress and performance is described theoretically in terms of an inverted U-shaped curve [60]. The *Yerkes–Dodson law* [61], rooted on the arousal theory [62, 63], states that at very low level of stress (i.e., boredom or drowsiness), performance is very low; increasing levels of stress leads to increasing arousal and performance improves until a point, after which performance decreases; at extreme levels of stress, performance is severely impaired (Fig. 1.3).

Fig. 1.3 Yerkes–Dodson curve human performance and stress curve

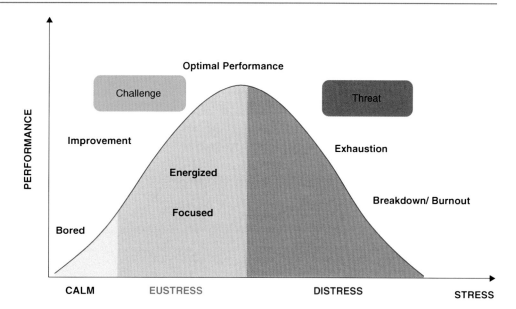

Yerke's and Dodson's static interpretation of stress—although still widely accepted in the field of psychology—might be seen as simplistic and even controversial in some situations, when emotions, environment, or different stressors modify the relationship between arousal, stress, and performance [64]. In the complex simulation environment, the learners' prior knowledge, skills, and perceived competence can determine their stress response in the simulation, yet their perception of their own performance during simulation may also modify their stress response. For example, novices may be unaware of their knowledge or performance gaps, and thus may not experience stress in the same way as proficient learners during SBT. Proficient learners may be more stressed at the beginning of SBT because of their perception of gaps in their knowledge or skills, but their stress response may be modified during the SBT scenario when they perceive themselves to be performing well or poorly.

Effects of Stress on Performance

Stress and Performance in the Clinical Setting
Stress has been reported to impair technical and nontechnical performance in various clinical settings. Different stressors have been identified including interruptions, distractions, time factors, technical factors, equipment problems, unavailability of expected resources, teamwork issues, patient factors (such as unpredictable deterioration), personal issues, and environmental factors [65–70]. The nontechnical skills impaired by stress relate to leadership, decision-making, and communication [71–75]. Clinical studies have shown that experienced surgeons experienced lower stress levels (HR, HRV, SCL, self-report, and eye blinks) and performed better than novices for technical tasks [17, 76–79].

Stress and Performance in Simulation

Effects of Stress on Technical Skills in Simulation For technical skills, it would appear that the Yerkes–Dodson law holds true. For example, moderate exam stress leads to improvements on fundamental technical skills in surgical residents [79]. In medical students, a positive association between stress (sAA) and performance (European Resuscitation Council (ERC) guidelines) was reported during high-fidelity SBE [32]. However, excessive stress impairs technical performance in surgeons, as was shown in a recent systematic review [8]. Many studies have demonstrated impaired performance of surgical tasks with increasing stress levels during simulation. In SBE, laparoscopic surgery (technically more complex) was found to be more stressful and associated with poorer performance compared to open surgery [17]. Other SBE studies in laparoscopy showed that medical students experienced higher stress (HR, BP, STAI) when directly observed by their instructor (over the shoulder) versus being unaware of being observed by the instructor in the control room [80] and when experiencing time pressure or multitasking [81]. High stress levels (SC, HR, HRV) were associated with impaired performance (objective structured assessment of technical skills, OSATS) in surgeons during crisis simulations [82]. Likewise, army nurses experiencing higher stress (HR, BP, SC, sAA) had lower performance (triage and treatment) in immersive SBE scenarios [83].

Task Difficulty Technical performance varies with perceived task difficulty. At low levels of task difficulty, higher levels of stress provide motivation in order to induce optimal performance. At high levels of task difficulty, lower levels of stress facilitate concentration and lead to optimal performance.

Regardless of task difficulty, a very high degree of stress impairs performance.

Learner's Proficiency The impact of stress on technical performance also varies with the learner's proficiency. In simulated laparoscopy, trainees had different patterns of stress response, depending on their proficiency. Firstly, baseline measurements of stress markers were different between proficient trainees and novices. Proficient trainees anticipated the difficulty of the task and stress markers (SC, Holter) were elevated sooner. Secondly, for the same level of stress during simulation, proficient trainees had a significantly higher performance (McGill Inanimate System for Training and Evaluation of Laparoscopic Skills, MISTELS) compared to novices [84]. Thus, less-experienced clinicians may be particularly susceptible to the influence of stress [85].

Effects of Stress on Nontechnical Skills in Simulation Nontechnical skills refer to the cognitive and interpersonal skills that underlie effective teamwork, typically encompassing the five crisis resource management (CRM) principles: role clarity, communication, mutual support, utilization of resources, and situation awareness [86]. These nontechnical skills can be assessed during a simulation session by various evaluation scales. Very few studies report the stress–performance relationship for nontechnical skills. Most of these studies sought to evaluate the stress response during performance in a simulated situation. Simulated breaking bad news provided significant stress responses in medical students (HR, cardiac output (CO), STAI, VAS) [87] and physicians (HR, SCL) [88], but these studies lack measurement of performance. One study found an impairment in performance of paramedics in calculating drug dosages following stressful scenarios in a human patient simulator [89]. A recent systematic review describes the effects of stress on performance in terms of attention, memory, decision-making and group performance, and the implications of this in the education of health professionals [90].

Effects of Stress on Attention As stress level increases and attention becomes more selective, there is growing exclusion of information leading to tunnel vision and premature closure (a tendency to stop considering other possible alternatives). This phenomenon can have diverse effect on performance, depending on the relevance of the peripheral information on performance.

Effects of Stress on Memory The effects of stress on memory are considered in the section above.

Effects of Stress on Decision-Making With increasing levels of stress, there is an increasing tendency to replace *vigilant decision-making* (considered an optimal form of decision-making using systematic, organized information search, thorough consideration of all options, time to evaluate and review data), with *hypervigilant decision-making,* (considered an impulsive, disorganized form of decision-making consisting of nonsystematic, selective information search, consideration of limited options, rapid evaluation of data, and selection of solution without reappraisal).

Effects of Stress on Group Performance Excessive stress leads to attentional narrowing in individuals under stress, a centralization of team leader's authority (less receptive to input from other team members) ending up in a loss of team perspective, loss of shared mental model, and a subsequent decrease in team performance.

Differences Between Technical and Nontechnical Skills Training for technical skills differs from nontechnical skills, mainly because the assessment of performance is not identically developed. Despite their differences, performance in technical skills and nontechnical skills are related, mainly because both can be impaired by stress and improved by SBE [91].

Effect of Repetitive Simulations on Stress and Performance

Currently, limited studies on repetitive simulation training have yielded discordant results. However, one study showed that intensivists' clinical performance as well as nontechnical skills (Anesthetists' Nontechnical Skills, ANTS) improved after one day of simulator training and were associated with a decrease in sAA [7]. Repetition of simulation-based training was associated with increases in surgical performance (OSATS), coping skills, and reduction in stress levels (HRV) [92]. In contrast, repeated exposure to SBE over 3 weeks did not result in blunting the physiological stress response (HR, SC) despite an improvement in nontechnical performance [93]. The differences in stress response between studies may reflect the differences in the scheduling of repetitive training (hours vs. weeks), as well as differences in peak cortisol concentrations compared to peak sAA activity after stress exposure.

The Learning–Performance Paradox

Learning is a continuous process of mastering new skills and developing a greater understanding about a topic whereas performance is a goal, produced when required, that is achievable through learning. Performance is tangible and measurable, while learning is a process that is intangible. In addition, learning may not produce same performance levels

Fig. 1.4 Stress and performance in simulation

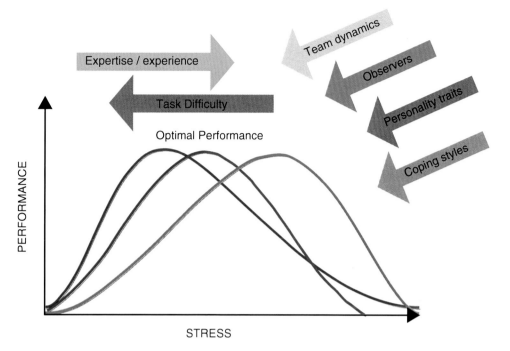

in all individuals. Learning is mandatory for medical competence. However, medical competence is not an achievement but rather a habit of contextual and developmental lifelong learning [85]. The trainee's performance assessed during a simulation session may predict the actual performance in a real-world situation. However, measurement of the performance of an individual during simulation does not necessarily give us information about his learning. SBE may thus be seen a series of successive short-term affective performances during a long-term learning process, with the ultimate aim of improving actual clinical performance (Fig. 1.4). See Table 1.2 for a summary of effects of stress on performance.

Managing Stress During Simulation

The manipulation of stress during medical simulation should be guided, in large part, by whether the objective of the simulation is assessing performance or ensuring learning. Throughout the chapter, we have discussed learning and performance separately in an attempt to tease out the multiple

levels at which stress can affect simulations, including the seemingly paradoxical effects of stress on learner outcomes. But this is an oversimplification because performance and learning interact on many levels. Similarly, many simulation programs are moving from a strictly educational focus to more of a clinical performance laboratory in which their findings during simulation inform organizational decision-making. Herein, we discuss some general stress-management strategies for medical simulations, but the reader will need to apply the principles based on their own program, learners, and objectives.

The Argument for Inclusion of Relevant Clinical Stressors

It has been suggested that stress during medical simulation increases the authenticity of the training by more closely matching that of the actual clinical environment (assumed to be more stressful). The resultant impairment of trainee's performance during SBE is more likely to parallel performance

Table 1.2 Summary of effects of stress on performance

Moderate stress increases performance, but excessive stress impairs performance
The optimal amount of stress for optimal performance is learner specific, task specific, and situation specific
The stress experienced and resulting performance vary with task difficulty. More difficult tasks evoke more stress and are more likely to result in poorer performance
The relationship between stress and performance varies with factors such as team dynamics, socio-evaluative factors like peer appraisal, presence of observers, the individual's personality traits and coping styles, etc.
With increasing expertise, stress decreases and performance increases
Repetitive simulation training increases performance, but its effect on stress response has not been sufficiently investigated

in clinical practice, thus providing the trainee a more accurate evaluation of their current proficiency and need for further training. Such authentic SBE might also provide a framework for teaching stress-management techniques to trainees in a learning environment, which may in turn help them manage stress in the clinical setting more effectively [80]. Additionally, the memory consolidating effects of stress are well established and are particularly effective when the stress coincides with highly arousing learning materials, as is the case in SBE [94]. Acute stress provides a learning opportunity by increasing memory consolidation but only if learning content, including stress, has not overloaded working memory resources.

Reducing Potential Sources of Extraneous Cognitive Load

Role of the Pre-scenario Briefing

While the role of debriefing has received widespread attention, the introduction of the learner to the simulation environment (i.e., pre-scenario briefing or otherwise known as pre-briefing) is potentially the most important opportunity to reduce stress for learners. The elements of an effective pre-scenario briefing are included in the Debriefing Assessment for Simulation in Healthcare (DASH) instrument [95] and are largely aimed at reducing stress reactions of students by openly discussing psychological safety, peer assessment, and evaluation. These recommended practices would theoretically enhance learning outcomes by minimizing the risk of stress impairing working memory. Similarly, briefing information such as the location of resources, mannequin findings, and learner expectations all require processing in working memory during simulations. Thus, routine and consistent briefing across successive simulations explaining the *rules of simulation* (e.g., the decision to push all drugs in real time vs. just verbalizing actions) will allow learners to construct schemata that they can store in long-term memory and access as needed, freeing up cognitive resources for simulation execution.

Reducing the Effects of Emotions and Stress

While activating learners' emotions and mimicking the real clinical environment are laudable goals, the resultant stress can be overwhelming to some learners. Increased emotional activation was related to increases in reported cognitive load in medical students participating during simulation sessions [96]. Students with the highest reported cognitive loads did not perform as well on testing administered 1 h after the teaching session, suggesting impaired learning outcomes from cognitive overload. In a subsequent randomized controlled trial, it was demonstrated that when final year medical students experienced the death of a simulated patient,

they reported more negative activating emotions [97] compared with students whose patient survived. The negatively affected students also reported higher cognitive loads and performed more poorly on objective testing administered 3 months later. These studies demonstrate that cognitive load caused by an increased emotional state can have a negative effect on learning during SBE. Patient death is an extreme event that activates emotions. In practice, the emotional reactions invoked during simulation training may be subtle, such as having an upset family member or an uncooperative patient. The decision to add such details should be made based on the relative importance of the emotional context for achieving learning objectives versus the risk that learning will not be successful if working memory limitations are surpassed.

Reducing Exposure to Extraneous Stress: Learning as Observers

Observers who are watching the simulation from the sidelines, but are not active participants of the scenario, appear to experience minimal stress during simulation training. However, their subsequent performance is equivalent to trainees in the *hot seat* during the scenarios, indicating that observers are able to learn despite not being subject to excessive stress during simulation training [93]. This has implications on reducing stress during simulation training as well as curriculum planning and resource allocation. On the other hand, the very presence of observers may affect the stress response of simulation participants in the *hot seat,* potentially having a negative impact on their learning and performance.

Role of the Debriefing

Debriefing is arguably the most important phase in simulation whereby learners are given the opportunity to recover from stress and emotions, make sense of the simulation experience, reflect on their performance, and consolidate their learning [98]. The elements and conduct of debriefing are covered in detail in Chap. 3. Simulation instructors should make full use of the debriefing phase to reduce stress in order to facilitate learning.

Titrating Stress and Cognitive Load to Enhance Learning and Performance

We have seen that during simulation training, it is important to balance the inclusion of relevant clinical stressors to enhance learning with those stressors that are extraneous to the objectives and can impair learning. The right amount of stress for optimal learning and performance is learner specific, task specific, and situation specific. Individuals seem to learn best when they are just outside their *comfort zone* [99]. In simulation language, this is to challenge individuals just beyond the *edge of their expertise*. By being cognizant of the various factors which contribute to intrinsic and extrinsic cognitive load, simulation trainers can consciously titrate the simulation experience for various learners, tasks and situations to achieve optimal learning and performance.

References

1. How to measure stress in humans? Centre for studies on Human stress. Fernand-Seguin Research Centre of Louis-H. Lafontaine Hospital Quebec, Canada. 2007. http://www.stresshumain.ca/documents/pdf/Mesures%20physiologiques/CESH_howMesureStress-MB.pdf.
2. Selye H. A syndrome produced by diverse nocuous agents. J Neuropsychiatr. 1998;10:230–1.
3. McGrath JE. Stress and behavior in organizations. In: Dunnette MD, editor. Handbook of industrial and organizational psychology. Chicago: McNally R; 1976. pp. 1351–95.
4. Tomaka J, Blascovich J, Kelsey RM, Leitten CL. Subjective, physiological, and behavioral effects of threat and challenge appraisal. J Pers Soc Psychol. 1993;65:248–60.
5. Mason JW. A review of psychoendocrine research on the pituitary-adrenal cortical system. Psychosom Med. 1968;30(suppl 5):576–607.
6. Bong C, Lightdale J, Fredette M, Weinstock P. Effects of simulation versus traditional tutorial-based training on physiologic stress levels among clinicians: a pilot study. Simul Healthc. 2010;5(5):272–8.
7. Müller MP, Hänsel M, Fichtner A, Hardt F, Weber S, Kirschbaum C, et al. Excellence in performance and stress reduction during two different full scale simulator training courses: a pilot study. Resuscitation. 2009;80:919–24.
8. Arora S, Sevdalis N, Nestel D, Woloshynowych M, Darzi A, Kneebone RL. The impact of stress on surgical performance: a systematic review of the literature. Surgery. 2010;147:318–30.
9. Speilberger CD, Gorsuch RL, Lushene R. STAI manual. Palo Alto: Consulting Psychologist Press; 1970.
10. Lovibond SH, Lovibond PF. Manual for the depression anxiety stress scales. 2nd ed. Sydney: Psychology Foundation; 1995. ISBN 7334-1423-0.
11. Antony MM, Bieling PJ, Cox BJ, Enns MW, Swinson RP. Psychometric properties of the 42-item and 21-item versions of the depression anxiety stress scales in clinical groups and a community sample. Psychol Assess. 1998;10(2):176–81.
12. Lesage FX, Berjot S, Deschamps F. Clinical stress assessment using a visual analogue scale. Occup Med (Lond). 2012;62:600–5.
13. Harvey A, Nathens AB, Bandiera G, LeBlanc VR. Threat and challenge: cognitive appraisal and stress responses in simulated trauma resuscitations. Med Educ. 2010;44:587–94.
14. Becker W, Ellis H, Goldsmith R, Kaye A. Heart rates of surgeons in theatre. Ergonomics. 1983;26:803–7.
15. Pagani M, Furlan R, Pizzinelli P, Crivellaro W, Cerutti S, Malliani A. Spectral analysis of R-R and arterial pressure variabilities to assess sympatho-vagal interaction during mental stress in humans. J Hypertens.1989;7:14–5.
16. Boucsein W. Electrodermal activity. New York: Plenum Press; 1992.
17. Smith WD, Chung YH, Berguer R. A virtual instrument ergonomics workstation for measuring the mental workload of performing video-endoscopic surgery. Stud Health Technol Inform. 2000;70:309–15.
18. Dorn LD, Lucke JF, Loucks TL, Berga SL. Salivary cortisol reflects serum cortisol: analysis of circadian profiles. Ann Clin Biochem. 2007;44:281–4.
19. Gozansky WS, Lynn JS, Laudenslager ML, Kohrt WM. Salivary cortisol determined by enzyme immunoassay is preferable to serum total cortisol for assessment of dynamic hypothalamic–pituitary–adrenal axis activity. Clin Endocrinol (Oxf). 2005;63(3):336–41.
20. Dickerson SS, Kemeny ME. Acute stressors and cortisol responses: a theoretical integration and synthesis of laboratory research. Psychol Bull. 2004;130:355–91.
21. Kudielka BM, Schommer NC, Hellhammer DH, Kirschbaum C, Acute HPA. Axis responses, heart rate, and mood changes to psychosocial stress (TSST) in humans at different times of day. Psychoneuroendocrinology. 2004;29:983–92.
22. Maheu FS, Collicutt P, Kornik R, Moszkowski R, Lupien SJ. The perfect time to be stressed: a differential modulation of human memory by stress applied in the morning or in the afternoon. Prog Neuropsychopharmacol Biol Psychiatr. 2005;29(8):1281–8.
23. Granger DA, Kivlighan KT, El-Shiekh M, Gordis EB, Stroud LR. Salivary alpha-amylase in biobehavioral research: recent developments and applications. Ann NY Acad Sci. 2007;1098:122–44.
24. Thoma MV, Kirschbaum C, Wolf JM, Rohleder N. Acute stress responses in salivary alpha-amylase predict increases of plasma norepinephrine. Biol Psychol. 91(3):342–8.
25. Takai N, Yamaguchi M, Aragaki T, Eto K, Uchihashi K, Nishikawa Y. Effect of psychological stress on the salivary cortisol and amylase levels in healthy young adults. Arch Oral Biol. 2004 Dec;49(12):963–8.
26. Nater UM, Rohleder N, Schlotz W, Ehlert U, Kirschbaum C. Determinants of the diurnal course of salivary alpha-amylase. Psychoneuroendocrinology. 2007;32:392–401.
27. Noto Y, Sato T, Kudo M, Kurata K, Hirota K. The relationship between salivary biomarkers and state-trait anxiety inventory score under mental arithmetic stress: a pilot study. Anesth Analg. 2005;101(6):1873–6.
28. Oldehinkel AJ, Ormel J, Bosch NM, Bouma EMC, Van Roon AM, Rosmalen JGM, et al. Stressed out? Associations between perceived and physiological stress responses in adolescents: the TRAILS study. Psychophysiology. 2011;48:441–52.
29. Arora S, Tierney T, Sevdalis N, Aggarwal, Nestel D, Woloshynowych M, et. al. The Imperial Stress Assessment Tool (ISAT): a feasible, reliable and valid approach to measuring stress in the operating room. World J Surg. 2010;34:1756–63.
30. Kharasch M, Aitchison P, Pettineo C, Pettineo L, Wang EE. Physiological stress responses of emergency medicine residents during an immersive medical simulation scenario. Dis Mon. 2011;57(11):700–5.
31. Girzadas DV, Delis S, Bose S, Rzechula K, Kulstad EB. Measures of stress and learning seem to be equally affected among all roles in a simulation scenario. Simul Healthc. 2009;4:149–54.
32. Keitel A, Ringleb M, Schwartges I, Weik U, Picker O, Stockhorst U, et al. Endocrine and psychological stress responses in a simulated emergency situation. Psychoneuroendocrinology. 2011;36:98–108.
33. Quilici AP, Pogetti RS, Fontes B, Zantut LFC, Chaves ET, Birolini D. Is the advanced trauma life support simulation exam more stressful for the surgeon than emergency department trauma care? Clinics. 2005;60(4):287–92.
34. Jones T, Goss S, Weeks B, Miura H, Bassandeh D, Cheek D. The effects of high-fidelity simulation on salivary cortisol levels in sRNA students: a pilot study. Sci World J. 2011;11:86–92.
35. Williams LJ. Cognitive load and the functional field of view. Hum Factors. 1982;24(6):683–92.
36. Lamble D, Kauranen T, Laakso M, Summala H. Cognitive load and detection thresholds in car following situations: safety implications for using mobile (cellular) telephones while driving. Accid Anal Prev. 1999;31(6):617–23.

37. Miller GA. The magical number seven, plus or minus two: some limits on our capacity for processing information. Psychol Rev. 1956;63:81–97.

38. Sweller J. Cognitive load during problem solving: effects on learning. Cogn Sci. 1988;12(2):257–85.

39. Sweller J, Ayres P, Kalyuga S. Cognitive load theory. New York: Springer; 2011.

40. Chandler P, Sweller J. Cognitive load theory and the format of instruction. Cogn Instr. 1991;8(4):293–332.

41. Van Merrienboer JJG, Sweller J. Cognitive load theory in health professional education: design principles and strategies. Med Educ. 2010;44(1):85–93.

42. Van Merrienboer JJG, Kirschner PA, Kester L. Taking the load off a learner's mind: instructional design for complex learning. Educ Psychol. 2003;38(1):5–13.

43. Ericcson K, Chase WG, Faloon S. Acquisition of a memory skill. Science. 1980;208(4448):1181–2.

44. Sweller J, Cooper GA. The use of worked examples as a substitute for problem solving in learning algebra. Cogn Instr. 1985;1:59–89.

45. Atkinson RK, Derry SJ, Renkl A, Wortham D. Learning from examples: instructional principles from the worked examples research. Rev Educ Res. 2000;70:181–214.

46. Vygotsky LS. Mind in society: the development of higher mental processes. Cambridge: Harvard University Press; 1978. (In: Cole M, John-Steiner V, Scribner S, Souberman E, editors)

47. Kalyuga S, Ayres P, Chandler P, Sweller J. The expertise reversal effect. Educ Psychol. 2003;38(1):23–31.

48. Paas F, Van Merrienboer J. The efficiency of instructional conditions: an approach to combine mental effort and performance measures. Hum Factors. 1993;35:737–43.

49. Paas FG. Training strategies for attaining transfer of problem-solving skill in statistics: a cognitive-load approach. J Educ Psychol. 1992;84(4):429.

50. Brünken R, Steinbacher S, Plass JL, Leutner D. Assessment of cognitive load in multimedia learning using dual-task methodology. Exp Psychol. 2002;49(2):109.

51. Paas FG, Van Merriënboer JJ. Variability of worked examples and transfer of geometrical problem-solving skills: a cognitive-load approach. J Educ Psychol. 1994;86(1):122.

52. Antonenko P, Paas F, Grabner R, van Gog T. Using electroencephalography to measure cognitive load. Educ Psychol Rev. 2010;22(4):425–38.

53. Van Gerven PW, Paas F, Van Merriënboer JJ, Schmidt HG. Memory load and the cognitive pupillary response in aging. Psychophysiology. 2004;41(2):167–74.

54. van Gog T, Scheiter K. Eye tracking as a tool to study and enhance multimedia learning. Learn Instr. 2010;20(2):95–9.

55. Paas F, Tuovinen JE, Tabbers H, Van Gerven PWM. Cognitive load measurement as a means to advance cognitive load theory. Educ Psychol. 2003;38(1):63–71.

56. Wolf OT. The influence of stress hormones on emotional memory: relevance for psychopathology. Acta Psychol. 2008;127(3):513–31.

57. Staal MA. Stress, cognition, and human performance: a literature review and conceptual framework. NASA technical memorandum, TM-2004-212824. Moffett Field: Ames Research Centre; 2004.

58. Cahill L, Gorski L, Le K. Enhanced human memory consolidation with post-learning stress: interaction with the degree of arousal at encoding. Learn Mem. 2003;10(4):270–4.

59. Kuhlmann S, Piel M, Wolf OT. Impaired memory retrieval after psychosocial stress in healthy young men. J Neurosci. 2005;25(11):2977–82.

60. Yerkes RM, Dodson JD. The relation of strength of stimulus to rapidity of habit-formation. J Comp Neurol Psychol. 1908;18:459–82.

61. Selye H. The stress of life. New York: McGraw-Hill; 1956.

62. Duffy E. The psychological significance of the concept of "arousal" or "activation." Psychol Rev. 1957;64:265–75.

63. Stokes AF, Kite K. On grasping a nettle and becoming emotional. In: Hancock PA, Desmond PA, editors. Stress, workload, and fatigue. Mahwah: Erlbaum; 2001.

64. Broadbent DE. Decision and Stress. London: Academic; 1971.

65. Mazur LM, Mosaly PR, Jackson M, Chang SX, Burkhardt KD, Adams RD, et al. Quantitative assessment of workload and stressors in clinical radiation oncology. Int J Radiat Oncol Biol Phys. 2012;83:e571–6.

66. Hassan I, Weyers P, Maschuw K, Dick B, Gerdes B, Rothmund M, et al. Negative stress-coping strategies among novices in surgery correlate with poor virtual laparoscopic performance. Br J Surg. 2006;93:1554–9.

67. Jezova D, Slezak V, Alexandrova M, Motovska Z, Jurankova E, Vigas M, et al. Professional stress in surgeons and artists as assessed by salivary cortisol. In: Stress Neuroendocrine and molecular approaches. Vols 1991, 1992. Philadelphia: Gordon & Breach Science Publishers; 1992. pp. 1953–62.

68. Yamamoto A, Hara T, Kikuchi K, Fujiwara T. Intraoperative stress experienced by surgeons and assistants. Ophthal Surg Lasers. 1999;30:27–30.

69. Sami A, Waseem H, Nourah A, Areej A, Afnan A, Ghadeer AS, et al. Real-time observations of stressful events in the operating room. Saudi J Anaesth. 2012;6:136–9.

70. Piquette D, Reeves S, LeBlanc VR. Stressful intensive care unit medical crises: how individual responses impact on team performance. Crit Care Med. 2009;37:1251–5.

71. Cumming SR, Harris LM. The impact of anxiety on the accuracy of diagnostic decision-making. Stress Health. 2001;17:281–6.

72. Arora S, Sevdalis N, Nestel D, Tierney T, Woloshynowych M, Kneebone R. Managing intraoperative stress: what do surgeons want from a crisis training program? Am J Surg. 2009;197:537–43.

73. Undre S, Koutantji M, Sevdalis N, Gautama S, Selvapatt N, Williams S, et al. Multidisciplinary crisis simulations: the way forward for training surgical teams. World J Surg. 2007;31:1843–53.

74. Wetzel CM, Kneebone RL, Woloshynowych M, Nestel D, Moorthy K, Kidd J, et al. The effects of stress on surgical performance. Am J Surg. 2006;191:5–10.

75. Hull F, Arora S, Kassab E, Kneebone R, Sevdalis N. Assessment of stress and teamwork in the operating room: an exploratory study. Am J Surg. 2011;201:24–30.

76. Berguer R, Smith WD, Chung YH. Performing laparoscopic surgery is significantly more stressful for the surgeon than open surgery. Surg Endosc. 2001;15:1204–7.

77. Bohm B, Rotting N, Schwenk W, Grebre S, Mansmann U. A prospective randomized trial on heart rate variability of the surgical team during laparoscopic and conventional sigmoid resection. Arch Surg. 2001;136:305–10.

78. Kikuchi K, Okuyama K, Yamamoto A, Hara T, Hara T. Intraoperative stress for surgeons and assistants. J Ophthal Nurs Technol. 1995;14:68–70.

79. Leblanc V, Woodrow S, Sidhu R, Dubrowski A. Moderate examination stress leads to improvements on fundamental technical skills in surgical residents. Am J Surg. 2008;196:114–9.

80. Andreatta PB, Hillard M, Krain LP. The impact of stress factors in simulation-based laparoscopic training. Surgery. 2010;147:631–9.

81. Poolton JM, Wilson MR, Malhotra N, Ngo K, Masters RSW. A comparison of evaluation, time pressure, and multitasking as stressors of psychomotor operative performance. Surgery. 2011;149:776–82.

82. Wetzel CM, Black SA, Hanna GB, Athanasiou T, Kneebone RL, Nestel D, et al. The effects of stress and coping on surgical performance during simulations. Ann Surg. 2010;251:171–6.

83. McGraw LK, Out D, Hammermeister JJ, Ohlson CJ, Pickering MA, Granger DA. Nature, correlates, and consequences of stress-related biological reactivity and regulation in Army nurses during combat casualty simulation. Psychoneuroendocrinology. 2013;38:135–44.

84. Ghazali A, Faure JP, Millet C, Brèque C, Scépi M, Oriot D. Patterns of stress response during simulated laparoscopy: preliminary results for novice and proficient participants. (In review).

85. Epstein RM. Assessment in medical education. N Engl J Med. 2007;356:387–96.

86. Weinstock P. Pediatric simulation instructor workshop. Boston: Harvard Medical School; 2013.

87. Hulsman RL, Pranger S, Koot S, Fabriek M, Karemaker JM, Smets EM. How stressful is doctor–patient communication? Physiological and psychological stress of medical students in simulated history taking and bad-news consultations. Int J Psychophys. 2010;77:26–34.

88. Shaw J, Brown R, Heinrich P, Dunn S. Doctors' experience of stress during simulated bad news consultations. Pat Educ Counsel. 2013;93:203–8.

89. LeBlanc VR, McArthur B, King K, MacDonald R, Lepine T. Paramedic performance in calculating drug dosages following stressful scenarios in a human patient simulator. Prehosp Emerg Care. 2005;9:439–44.

90. LeBlanc VR. The effects of acute stress on performance: implications for health professions education. Acad Med 2009;84(10):25–33.

91. Cook DA, Hatala R, Brydges R, Zendejas B, Szostek JH, Wang AT, et al. Technology-enhanced simulation for health professions education. JAMA. 2011;306:978–88.

92. Wetzel CM, George A, Hanna GB, Athanasiou T, Black SA, Kneebone RL, et al. Stress management training for surgeons-a randomized, controlled, intervention study. Ann Surg. 2011;253:488–94.

93. Bong C, Lee S, Allen J, Lim E, Goh ZQ, Kok C, Ng A. Effects of Stress on Observers and their subsequent performance during high fidelity simulation-based training. Oral presentation at IPSSW 2014. 2014. (In review)

94. Smeets T, Wolf OT, Giesbrecht T, Sijstermans K, Telgen S, Joëls M. Stress selectively and lastingly promotes learning of context-related high arousing information. Psychoneuroendocrinology. 2009;34:1152–61.

95. Brett-Fleegler M, Rudolph J, Eppich W, Monuteaux M, Fleegler E, Cheng A, et al. Debriefing assessment for simulation in healthcare: development and psychometric properties. Simul Healthc. 2012;7(5):288–94.

96. Fraser K, Ma I, Teteris E, Baxter H, Wright B, McLaughlin K. Emotion, cognitive load and learning outcomes during simulation training. Med Educ. 2012;46(11):1055–62.

97. Fraser K, Huffman J, Ma I, Sobczak M, McIlwrick J, Wright B, et al. The emotional and cognitive impact of unexpected simulated patient death: a randomized controlled trial. CHEST Journal [Internet]. 2013. http://dx.doi.org/10.1378/chest.13-0987.

98. Fanning RM, Gaba DM. The role of debriefing in simulation-based learning. Simul Healthc. 2007;2(2):115–25.

99. Yerkes R, Dodson J. The dancing mouse, a study in animal behavior. J Comp Neurol Psychol. 1907;18:459–82.

Essentials of Scenario Building for Simulation- Based Education

James L. Huffman, Gord McNeil, Zia Bismilla and Anita Lai

Simulation Pearls

1. Use a scenario-building process. Many simulation educators attempt scenario design in a haphazard fashion, which can lead to unintended and inconsistent learning outcomes. The process outlined in this chapter (although not the only one) is thorough and has proven useful to the authors through several years of use.

2. Consider which elements of engineering and psychological fidelity are most important to the curricular goals and target audience when designing the scenario. Be cognizant that higher fidelity does not always equate to improved learning.

3. Use distraction techniques wisely. The use of distraction can improve and ensure exposure to specific learning objectives and as such can add great value. However, when used inappropriately, they can also frustrate learners and detract from other potentially more important objectives.

4. Allow time to practice your scenario before full implementation. There are usually important considerations that did not come up in the early phases of the design process that will need to be accounted for prior to having learners participate in the scenario as part of their curriculum.

J. L. Huffman (✉)
Department of Emergency Medicine, University of Calgary, Alberta Health Services, Calgary, AB, Canada
e-mail: james.huffman@albertahealthservices.ca

G. McNeil
Department of Emergency Medicine, University of Calgary, Foothills Medical Centre and Alberta Children's Hospital, Calgary, AB, Canada
e-mail: gord.mcneil@albertahealthservices.ca

Z. Bismilla
Department of Paediatrics, University of Toronto, Toronto, ON, Canada
e-mail: zia.bismilla@sickkids.ca

A. Lai
Department of Emergency Medicine, University of Calgary, Calgary, AB, Canada
e-mail: anita.lai@albertahealthservices.ca

Introduction

Scenario design is a fundamental component of simulation-based education (SBE). Each simulation scenario is an event or situation that allows participants to apply and demonstrate their knowledge, technical skills, clinical skills and/or non-technical (teamwork) skills [1]. Effective scenario design provides the basis for educators to meet specific learning objectives and provide a meaningful learning experience for the participants.

This chapter is divided into two main sections. The first part provides the theory and rationale for a scenario design process as well as discussing some of the important considerations one should keep in mind during the design process. The second part of this chapter provides a practical approach to the scenario design process involving six main steps.

Taken as a whole, this chapter should provide not only an understanding of why the design process is important, but also rationale for making difficult design choices and a practical approach to designing scenarios applicable to educator and learner needs.

Objectives of the Chapter

The scope of SBE is broad. This chapter focuses primarily on designing scenarios for high-fidelity immersive simulation sessions, although many of the concepts explored can be applied to scenarios involving modalities ranging from low-fidelity task trainers to standardized patients. The principles of scenario design discussed here are important to consider regardless of the educational intervention being planned, whether it is low-stakes practice, high-stakes assessment or simulation-based research. The degree to which these theories are applied and the degree of rigor and standardization of scenario design will vary for these different contexts.

© Springer International Publishing Switzerland 2016
V. J. Grant, A. Cheng (eds.), *Comprehensive Healthcare Simulation: Pediatrics*,
Comprehensive Healthcare Simulation, DOI 10.1007/978-3-319-24187-6_2

Table 2.1 Dimensions of fidelity

Physical fidelity	Conceptual fidelity	Emotional fidelity
Environment (in situ or simulation lab)	Concerns theory, meaning, concepts, and relationships	The holistic experience of the situation
Mannequin (size, sex, capabilities, etc.)	Logical sequence (*If-Then* relationships)	Complexity/difficulty level of the scenario
Clinical equipment (pumps, IVs, carts, monitors, etc.)	Appropriate physiologic responses to changes	Appropriate addition of distractors and *stressors*
Moulage (wounds, fluids, smells, etc.)	Appropriate diagnostics available (and in their usual format)	Level of activation and feelings (pleasant or unpleasant feelings)
	Usual resources (human and equipment) available (or accounted for if unavailable)	

IV intravenous drip

Rationale for a Scenario Design Process

The perceived need for an educational intervention comes from many different triggers. It could be the result of a generalized approach to curriculum development or a specific identified gap in knowledge or procedural skills. While the use of simulation can be an effective technique to fill these needs, the approach in designing an effective scenario can be daunting. By using a structured process, a road map is created to define specific educational goals and to set the stage for the participants to suspend disbelief. It also allows for a recognizable format that can be more easily reproduced and followed by other educators. In our experience, a well-planned, structured, yet flexible scenario will be the springboard to a higher level of experiential learning.

Considerations and Theoretical Underpinnings

Simulation scenarios are designed for many purposes. They can be intended as tools to teach and train individuals or teams, to test systems in order to enhance efficiency or patient safety, to answer research questions, and to perform assessments [2]. The design of the scenario should reflect the intended purpose. For instance, when a scenario is used within a research study or for high-stakes assessments, the design should be specific, reproducible, and take into consideration all potential threats that may challenge the validity (or standardization) of the scenario for research or assessment purposes [3]. In this section, we will explore some additional considerations that should be taken into account when designing a scenario.

Curriculum and Scenario Design Within Simulation-Based Education

Simulation scenarios can be presented as isolated, one-time events; however, it is increasingly common for them to be integrated within a larger curriculum [4–6]. It is important to realize that each scenario's placement and purpose within that curriculum will influence its design. Specifically, the goals and objectives of the scenario(s) should be derived from the goals and objectives of the curriculum. The overall curriculum will also affect the time it will be possible to allot

to each scenario, the number of participants and facilitators required, and potentially what financial, human, and physical (space) resources will be needed to deliver the scenario.

It is important to identify which objectives are best met using simulation and which simulation modalities are the most appropriate (e.g., task trainer vs. high-fidelity mannequin, etc.) when designing a scenario [7–9]. Simulation should be reserved for those objectives which are most appropriate for its use and cannot be adequately addressed using other less resource-intensive educational modalities.

Scenario design, although one component of SBE, provides a foundation for the other components to build upon and provides a venue for participants to explore their learning objectives. An effective design allows the scenario to reliably address the stated learning objectives. The experiences from the scenario are then used as a jumping-off point during the debriefing to help learners identify learning issues and close gaps in knowledge and performance [10].

Fidelity/Realism

Another consideration in the scenario design process is the degree of fidelity that will be incorporated [11]. Fidelity is a measure of the realism of a simulation. It is an area of active research and debate. Our understanding of fidelity, particularly in the realm of SBE, has been greatly enhanced through the work of pioneers like Dieckmann and Rudolph [12, 13]. One of the most important developments is the realization that in order to engage our participants deeply in simulation, we need to recognize that humans think about fidelity in at least three dimensions: (1) the physical, (2) the conceptual and (3) the emotional (see Table 2.1) [13].

Physical fidelity refers to whether the simulation looks realistic [9, 13]. It concerns the mannequin itself, both its form and capabilities, as well as the surrounding environment and equipment. Conceptual fidelity concerns theory, meaning, concepts, and relationships. It is embodied in the *if-then* relationships such as "If there is significant hemorrhage, then the blood pressure will decrease"[13]. Finally, emotional fidelity concerns actions and relations of an emotional kind. These aspects of the simulation may relate to the participants' level of activation as well as how pleasant (or unpleasant) their experiences are perceived [13].

Historically, there has been a popular opinion that simulation experiences and outcomes improve as the precision of replication of the real world improves [9, 12, 14]. Specifically, assumptions have existed for some time that fidelity is the single critical determinant of transfer and that the higher the fidelity, the better the participants can transfer learning to real-life situations. However, this notion has recently been challenged [9, 12, 15]. When comparing the learning outcomes of high-fidelity to those obtained with low-fidelity simulations, the gains have only been found to be modest (in the range of 1–2%) and generally not statistically significant [9, 14]. Following in this vein, leading thinkers in the field have called for a reconceptualization of fidelity in terms of the primary concepts which underlay it, namely physical resemblance and functional task alignment [15]. In our opinion, thinking of fidelity in terms of the different subtypes described above can help to understand how tailoring different aspects of the scenario design may improve resemblance and alignment in order to enhance transfer, learner engagement, and suspension of disbelief.

When designing a scenario, you will still be required to make decisions regarding the degree of fidelity, weighing the potential benefits of increased physical resemblance, and/or functional task alignment against resource utilization and increased cognitive load. Important choices with respect to types of mannequins, use of confederates, etc. will need to be made. One needs to consider, for example, if transfer, learner engagement, or suspension of disbelief are optimized through the use of a high-fidelity mannequin or perhaps a low-fidelity version or even a task trainer that can suit the objectives equally well. Similarly, the location of the scenarios is another important consideration. A simulation lab is convenient and generally efficient but may not be as realistic as performing a scenario in the participants' natural working space (in situ) (see Chap. 12). If your objectives relate specifically to the environment in which the participants usually work or will be working, then the scenario should take place there. Otherwise, it may be reasonable to use the lab instead.

When choosing the mannequin you are going to use for your scenario, consider your learning objectives and which mannequin functions will be important to facilitate meeting those objectives (see Chap. 10). Examples include the need for eyes that open and close, accurate representation of the patient's physical size, accurate representation of a patient's airway, the ability to create difficult intubating conditions, accurate representations of heart and lung sounds, or the ability to make physiologic changes in real-time in response to the participants' actions (or lack thereof). Similar thought should be put into the other areas of physical fidelity listed earlier. Sometimes, the scenario will require high physical fidelity in order to maximize psychological fidelity and allow the participants to behave as if the situation were real (i.e., suspension of disbelief). Other times, maximizing certain aspects of fidelity may hinder you from addressing learning objectives at all (e.g., you are too busy operating a complex mannequin to hear what the participants are saying or, alternatively, your participants are overwhelmed by all they are seeing).

Some of the ways that conceptual and psychological fidelity are increased include having a well-written scenario which makes sense to the participants, having the mannequin respond physiologically the way a real patient would, having appropriate and typical diagnostics (radiographs, lab results, electrocardiograms (ECGs), etc.) and having the participants' usual resources (equipment, references, and people (i.e., consultants)) available to them.

Psychological and conceptual fidelity are arguably more important to learning than physical fidelity [9, 12]. However, this has not yet been demonstrated definitively in the literature. One study that specifically manipulated psychological fidelity showed a clear advantage for greater realism [16]. According to Dieckmann, "When learning is the focus, the flawless recreation of the real world is less important. It is necessary to find situations that help participants to learn, not necessarily the ones that exactly mimic any clinical counterparts" [12].

Teamwork

There are two related issues regarding teamwork that might influence the design process. First is the importance of including interprofessional and teamwork objectives in the design. Secondly, we also advocate strongly for the value of having actual interprofessional input into the scenario design process.

One of the main uses of SBE is to teach teamwork and interprofessional skills (see Chaps. 4 and 15 of this text) [17–19]. These objectives are sometimes overlooked in favor of those that focus specifically on clinical knowledge and technical skills. Although teaching clinical knowledge and technical skills are an important part of SBE, one of the values of simulation is the ability to promote team training and the development of interprofessional team skills. Thus, in the design process, the importance of including objectives related to interprofessional skills and teamwork (as well as higher order clinical skills) should not be underestimated [5, 20].

The development of a simulation scenario can be optimized by employing an interprofessional and collaborative strategy in scenario design. Through involving members of different healthcare professions in the design process, potential issues around the interprofessional objectives can be more easily predicted. In addition, the realism of the scenario as it relates to each individual profession will also be maximized. This approach will indirectly maximize the individual engagement of the participants who attend from the various healthcare professions. Similarly, we recommend involving not only healthcare providers, but where possible others such as educators and simulation operators/engineers/technicians. While there is no direct evidence that such an approach is beneficial in the design phase of SBE, there are examples from engineering and clinical medicine [21, 22].

When designing a scenario which includes teamwork-related objectives, there are many strategies which can be employed in order to maximize the opportunity to trigger teamwork issues [23]. One such method is challenging the team with multiple tasks/problems (e.g., hypoglycemia, seizure, hypotension, and respiratory arrest). Another strategy is called the *wave effect*. This is where team members are introduced sequentially into the scenario (e.g., nurses, then residents, then fellows, etc.). The benefit of this strategy is that each time a team member is introduced, there should be some sort of communication between new and existing team members. Other methods include (but are not limited to) introducing junior team members, introducing parents or team members who are distractors or who make mistakes, using phone calls, and providing fewer than normal team members [23].

The Use of Distraction

One commonly used element of scenario design is distraction, referring to elements either indirectly or tangentially related to the clinical material being presented, but which aim to add an element of complexity to the scenario. The general goal of distraction is to draw the attention of the caregivers away from the task at hand. Distractions generally come in the form of either personnel issues (e.g., anxious/distressed parent or caregiver, argumentative consultant, phone call with unexpected lab results, etc.), equipment issues (e.g., an endotracheal tube that has a faulty cuff or is plugged, a piece of equipment missing from the crash cart or that is not working properly, etc.), or environment issues (e.g., mass casualty incident (multiple patients), fire in the operating room, etc.).

Distraction can be a powerful tool for bringing particular learning objectives to light. These techniques can ensure that particular objectives are met when they may not arise spontaneously within a scenario. For example, if a learning objective for a scenario is to manage the chaotic environment of a resuscitation, adding a confederate (i.e., scripted actor) who plays the role of a distressed family member will ensure that there is at least some chaos to manage. Another example might involve a scenario where the primary objective is to manage a respiratory arrest, with a secondary objective to teach a systematic approach to managing hypoxia in an intubated patient. As such, a faulty endotracheal tube may be placed in the scenario to meet this purpose. In both of these examples, the use of distractors ensures the participants will encounter the situations that force them to deal with the stated learning objectives.

Some designs also employ distraction to increase the degree of difficulty in the scenario for more advanced participants. One example of this is to have a confederate playing a patient's caregiver be more distressed and difficult to calm down when a more skilled learner group is participating in the scenario. Similarly, a consultant might strongly (and more vehemently, based on the skill level of the learners) suggest an inappropriate course of action. However, distraction needs to be used very carefully and with specific objectives in mind. Distraction can also lead to the team becoming derailed and not meeting other important learning objectives because they become fixated on or even overwhelmed by the distracting issue/objective. The concept of cognitive load theory is extremely relevant to the use of distraction in scenario design (please see Chap. 1) [24–26]. These distractors increase the intrinsic cognitive load of the participants and have the potential to impair acquisition of the primary learning objectives. It is our experience that while early in their careers, many educators underestimate the difficulty of the scenarios they are developing, and subsequently plan on adding one or more distractors in order to make the scenario more appropriately challenging for their participants, while ultimately creating a scenario the learners find difficult and confusing. This is another reason why piloting of a scenario would be both appropriate and helpful.

Summary of Pediatric-Specific Scenario Design Issues

There are several elements unique to the design of pediatric scenarios. Since pediatrics spans many age groups and sizes, it is essential to have mannequins of an appropriate size to maximize realism for the age of the patient in the scenario. For example, it would be challenging for participants to effectively perform a realistic neonatal resuscitation on a toddler-sized mannequin or perform a scenario meant for an adolescent on an infant-sized mannequin. Ensuring the presence of age-appropriate clinical supplies is also important. This includes appropriate sizes of airway equipment, intravenous catheters, and defibrillator pads, among others. The availability of these adjuncts will enhance realism and lessen the frustration of the participants who may feel they were lead to be unprepared if given inappropriate materials to work with in the scenario. Quite often, the simple fact that the scenario is an acutely ill pediatric patient itself leads to more profound stress reactions in participants, as compared to those involving adult patients. Anticipating more profound emotional reactions when designing the pediatric scenario will allow one to design a scenario that does not overwhelm participants. Being cognizant of a higher performance anxiety in participants involved in pediatric scenarios will also help anticipate the debriefing approach (refer to Chap. 3).

Lastly, given the nature of pediatrics, a caregiver is a frequently used confederate in pediatric scenarios, independent of planned distraction. When used appropriately, confederates can give essential historical and physical findings to the participants and simulate the typical confounder of dealing with caregiver and patient simultaneously, especially if the patient in the scenario is pre-verbal and cannot answer questions themselves. The addition of a confederate into the scenario needs to be well-scripted and the confederate must thoroughly understand the case objectives [27]. If not, they may actually hinder your participants' achievement in the scenario by distracting them from the primary objectives, giving incorrect or poorly timed information or missing important aspects altogether.

The Scenario Design Process

Introduction

Designing a high-quality simulation scenario involves many different factors. The goal is to recognize the educational needs of the participants and, through a simulated environment, produce a realistic experience to maximize specific learning objectives within the confines of physical space, time, finances, and available resources. To help design and develop a high-quality simulation scenario, six key steps have been identified to assist in making the process more efficient and effective (see Table 2.2) [1].

Target Audience, Learning Objectives, and Simulator Modalities

The first step in designing a scenario is identifying the learner(s) and their educational needs. This will be the basis for writing objectives that are relevant to the level of the participant. Scenarios often skip this critical step and attempt to use a set of objectives that are inappropriate for the level of the learners. For example, designing learning objectives that are appropriate for an experienced healthcare team that involves complex resuscitation skills would be inappropriate for undergraduate students, and would likely lead to frustration for both the facilitator and the learners. Targeting the

Table 2.2 The six-step scenario design process

The six-step scenario design process
1. Target audience, learning objectives, and simulator modalities
2. Case description and scenario environment
3. Staging needs: equipment, moulage, confederates, and adjuncts
4. The script: scenario framework and stages
5. Computer pre-programming
6. Practice scenario

learner groups' needs and not the facilitators' wants is an important element of scenario design. Investing time to recognize the needs of the learners is essential in good scenario design. Sometimes, this information is available from an established curriculum, while other times this information requires a formal needs assessment of the learner group. Designing appropriate scenario objectives will also allow other facilitators to easily review the scenarios and decide whether the scenario written meets the educational needs of other groups.

As simulation scenario design is a dynamic process, there may be several layers present when writing objectives. It is important to have primary objectives, which are felt to be essential goals of participating in the simulation scenario. These objectives will inform the primary debriefing discussion and the *take home* learning messages. There may also be secondary objectives, which, while important, are not the critical message that is being delivered. For example, while a primary objective may be to teach medical students endotracheal intubation in an infant, the secondary objective may be discussion of different sedating agents to achieve sedation in the context of the intubation. Secondary objectives may be reviewed and discussed during the debriefing, but the primary objectives cover the areas that are designed to be taught in the scenario and should be covered during the debriefing. While it is essential to have objectives, the facilitator must also be flexible enough to teach about issues that the participants identify during debriefing. A successful scenario and debriefing will cover all the primary objectives and still have an opportunity to address any other specific learning needs of the participants.

One of the pitfalls of writing objectives for simulation scenarios is that it is easy to become overzealous or over-inclusive. Writing too many objectives can make the educational plan unachievable in the desired time allotted for both the scenario and the debriefing. The length and complexity of a scenario will help determine how many objectives to write. In general, a scenario may have 2–4 primary objectives that the facilitator feels are essential to teach and then several secondary objectives that may be covered. It should be remembered that in many scenarios, not every secondary objective is covered; however, a list of primary objectives will help ensure the most important educational material is not missed.

Another important pitfall of writing objectives is they are not modified with piloting or running through the scenarios. Sometimes, a scenario that has been run through several times may have the participants repeatedly identifying issues not initially identified as an objective. In this circumstance, the scenario design as written is likely highlighting different objectives and thus the original objectives should be re-examined to determine if these new issues should be added as new objectives or replace other objectives that are not being identified.

In general, objectives can also be subdivided into knowledge, skills (procedural or technical), and behaviors or teamwork (communication, roles, resource utilization, awareness, etc.). Some scenarios focus more on one area than others, but in general a mix of all three objective subgroups often forms a well-rounded and well-structured scenario. Once the objectives are written, the preferred simulation modality can be chosen. There are several considerations in choosing a simulation modality. The objectives will help direct which simulation modality is most appropriate for each scenario. In general, high-fidelity simulation sessions are most useful for complex clinical knowledge-based objectives and for practicing teamwork skills. Low-fidelity simulation sessions are often useful for practicing procedural or technical skills and less complex scenarios, especially when an appropriate team is not available. The level of realism required will also help determine the simulation modality needed. In situ high-fidelity simulation with diagnostic adjuncts (e.g., laboratory results, ECG, diagnostic imaging) may be necessary to achieve realism for certain participants seeking experiential learning. Other scenario objectives may dictate that this high-fidelity level of simulation and realism will actually be distracting and irrelevant to the learning objectives and a low-fidelity simulation may be the best option.

Case Description and Scenario Environment

The case summary describes the initial patient clinical presentation and gives details such as past medical history, allergies, and vital signs. It is the case vignette that the participants receive to start the scenario. It also gives the participant details of the location where the scenario is taking place, available resources, and the participant's role (e.g., a staff physician in a tertiary emergency department or a nursing student in the patient's room of a rural hospital). This element is essential as it sets the stage for the remainder of the scenario.

Scenario cases are typically either developed from the memory of actual cases or are completely invented in a prototypical fashion. Each method has its own advantages and disadvantages. Real-life cases are soundly based in the accuracy of the scenario and can include important subtleties of the clinical presentation, which enhances realism. This realism may allow for faster buy-in from participants. Also, participants often feel more truly prepared for a future critical event in their own working environment if they feel they have just been exposed to a real-life scenario. While a real case can often be easier to design because the adjuncts for the case (laboratory results, ECG, diagnostic imaging) are readily available, the overall access to these cases may be limited, particularly if these cases are rare. Furthermore, choosing which real-life adjuncts and details to include in the scenario is extremely important. Sometimes, real-life scenarios have details that are not as important during a simulation scenario and there is a risk of overloading the participants with too many of these details. While these scenarios are historically accurate, they might be confusing and distracting to the participant especially in the compressed time of a simulation scenario.

The prototypical case is an excellent option for the more routine types of cases that require fewer clinical details. A brief febrile seizure scenario for medical students often does not need to be steeped in all the details of a real case. If, however, the case has specific and important clinical details, the pitfall of the prototypical case is that the subtleties of the case may be missing and the scenario may become unrealistic. Rare presentations are also well-suited for prototypical scenarios since the initial need is to be exposed to the case prior to the true clinical exposure. Attention to detail is a critical component of these scenarios so that they are not misleading or inaccurate. Often, diagnostic adjuncts from other sources need to be used (such as the Internet) and careful attention to the specific details of these adjuncts needs to be given. For example, a chest X-ray of a patient with a right-sided pneumonia should match the physical findings outlined in the scenario. Giving participants a chest X-ray of an intubated patient, which has not yet occurred in the scenario, or using an ECG where the heart rate is significantly different from what the learners are seeing on the monitor causes confusion and contributes to a lack of realism.

Often a combination of real-life and prototypical case scenario designs can be very successful. Taking a real-life case and modifying some of the details to fit the desired educational objectives allows for a blend of realism and clinical accuracy while still meeting the specific learning needs of the participants. For example, while a clinical case of a seizure in a 5-year-old may be readily available, expanding on the initial presentation to include other clinical features of intracranial tumor (e.g., vomiting and headache) may be factitiously added to the scenario to form a new case that is uncommonly seen.

When using real-life scenarios, privacy must always be ensured. Specific consent must be obtained from the patient or family for use in this educational environment. Any patient identification from labs, ECG, and diagnostic imaging must be removed. Furthermore, the name given to the mannequin in the scenario should not reflect the actual patient's name (or any perceived association by the participants). It is imperative to be aware of the background of these real-life cases as your current staff members may have experienced the actual scenario firsthand and still have emotional concerns associated with the case. If prototypical cases are being used, the web has a large compository of clinical pictures, video, ECG, and diagnostic imaging. In these cases, avoiding copyright infringements is important and at a minimum the sources should be identified.

Staging Needs: Equipment, Moulage, Confederates, and Adjuncts

Equipment

The specific details of how to enhance the learning experience of the participants with equipment, moulage, confederates, and other adjuncts is the next appropriate step in scenario design. Using similar equipment to what the participants would actually use in their regular clinical practice enhances the realism of the scenario. It also allows the participants to more accurately practice the specific subtle physical skills related to the pieces of equipment in question and more confidently translate these physical skills to future clinical practice. For example, participants who use the same type of defibrillation unit in simulation as they do in actual practice will be quicker and more confident when they need to perform this action in a real-life defibrillation situation. In contrast, using equipment that is either outdated or not likely to be used by the participants in future experiences may frustrate participants because they may feel they are learning a skill not relevant to their practice. As an example, nurse participants who are required to use intravenous pumps not relevant to their usual clinical practice may make them feel confused and disconnected as they feel the scenario is not in touch with their own clinical needs. Furthermore, although not often a preplanned learning objective, participants often gain valuable experience reviewing the use of clinical equipment during simulation. For example, while the intent of the simulation scenario may not be to discuss application of defibrillation pads and their connections to the machine, the participants often highlight this as an important learning experience that would otherwise be missed without having appropriate similar equipment available. However, clinical equipment that requires significantly long set-up should be avoided, unless its use is a specific objective within the scenario.

Ensuring a complete and comprehensive list of all equipment and supplies needed for the scenario is essential for the environment to be adequately prepared for the scenario. This list should include the type of monitors to be used or displayed, intravenous fluids, lines and pumps, specific medications that may be requested by the team, typical medication resources, documentation records, and other ancillary clinical equipment that is commonly used (e.g., glucometer, otoscope, penlight, etc.). In some facilities, empty vials of medications or previously expired medications are collected and refilled with water in order to allow the teams to draw up and administer the medications in real time. When doing in situ simulations, great care must be taken to ensure the simulated medications are not mistaken for real medications and accidently mixed into the patient care clinical supplies. Some facilities label their medication as *simulation only* or *teaching use only*, while some facilities do not allow for the use of expired medications in active patient care areas.

Moulage

Moulage is another important consideration of scenario design that can enhance realism and provide actual physical cues to the patient's physical condition. Moulage may take many different and complex forms. A few simple examples would be a wig with long hair for a female patient, a red dye-soaked bandage applied to a forehead to simulate a traumatic laceration, a leg bandaged with gauze to simulate a fracture, an open bottle of nail polish remover to simulate ketotic smell of diabetic ketoacidosis. The more complex use of paints and gels from *moulage kits* can be used to create wounds, rashes, burns, etc. However, moulage can be extremely time-consuming. As such, the use of photographs and video can be as effective as more complicated moulage techniques. While complex moulage can significantly enhance the level of realism, this must be balanced with the time, effort, and finances (human resources) available for each simulation (Fig. 2.1a, b, c, d, e, f, g).

Confederates

Confederates are another useful adjunct to consider in scenario design. Confederates can be simulation staff or volunteers as well as trained actors depending on resources available. Confederates are particularly useful in pediatric simulation scenarios since young children will almost always have a caregiver by their side. The confederate can divulge important patient information as well as confirm physical characteristics that are difficult to simulate. For example, a confederate mother with her anaphylactic child may comment that she feels her child's swollen lips are progressively worsening (or improving) or that the urticaria seems to be spreading more. Adding this element can be a critical point in adding appropriate realism to a scenario. Confederates can also be a significant source of distraction. This distraction can be useful if their involvement enhances realism or the learning objective is to manage the child as well as an anxious parent. However, confederates need to have a specific script that does not distract from the scenario. Overacting or inappropriate drama may detract from the scenario and the learning objectives. Consider using the confederate only if it is truly felt to enhance the scenario's realism and support the learning objective. Additionally, the confederate should have only one role. It often gets confusing to participants if the confederate is the paramedic at the beginning of the scenario but then becomes the father later in the scenario.

Other Adjuncts

Other adjuncts can be added to the scenario design process depending on the level of the learner and the desired learning objectives. Laboratory results, diagnostic imaging, ECGs,

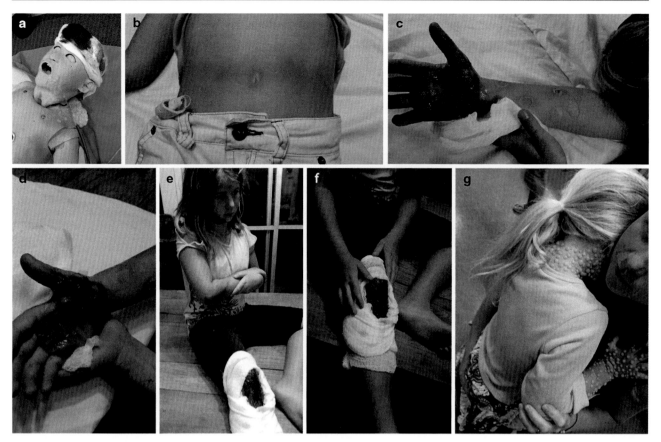

Fig. 2.1 a–g Moulage photos. (Photo with permission from James Huffman)

video clips, photos, patient charts, and nursing flow sheets can all be collected in advance and available to the facilitator. Photos and videos can be especially powerful adjuncts to engage the learners, especially for things such as rashes or seizures. The more advanced the learners or the more complex the scenario, the higher the demand for realistic and complete adjuncts. However, trying to anticipate in advance every adjunct the participants may want can be a challenge. Choose adjuncts that are most important to supporting the learning objectives rather than attempting to include every possible option. Reevaluation of the scenario design following piloting will help identify which adjuncts may need to be added or removed. As discussed earlier, all real-life patient adjuncts must have patient identifiers removed and any images or video accessed from the web should be acknowledged to avoid copyright infringement.

The Script: Scenario Framework and Stages

The next step in scenario design is deciding on how the flow of the scenario should ideally take place. The scenario is often divided into individual stages or frames. Each stage or frame often comprises either a key event or a change in the condition of the patient (Table 2.3). Building on the case

vignette, the first stage may represent the patient's initial vital signs and has an identifiable problem that the participants must address. For example, a child that presents with hypoxia and altered mental status requires the participants to effectively obtain a pertinent history and physical exam, treat the hypoxia, and address possible causes of the altered level of consciousness. The length of the stage will vary with the sophistication of the learners, but these issues need to be addressed before proceeding to the next stage. Once the participants have had an opportunity to manage their patient and address immediate concerns, the next stage may be advanced to continue with the scenario. For example, once the participants have addressed the issues of the aforementioned patient with hypoxia and altered mental status, the next key event will have the child experience a tonic–clonic seizure. This new event will require ongoing management by the participants. However, some groups may not get through even the first frame during the allocated time. Either way, significant learning points will be highlighted in the post-scenario debriefing. These stages continue with each key event or change in patient condition and should reflect the objectives outlined. Having defined objectives for each stage often makes the scenario flow more smoothly. In some scenarios, key events may occur regardless of the learners' actions, but they should give the participants time to respond

Table 2.3 An example of a scenario script of foreign body upper airway obstruction in a 4-year-old

Scenario transitions/patient parameters	Effective management	Consequences of ineffective management	Notes
1. Initial assessment: Child is sitting up with obvious distress. Intermittent stridor at rest especially when approached by medical staff **T**: 37.2 **HR**: 142 **RR**: 32 **SAO₂**: 98% RA **BP**: 90/62 **Resp**: No WOB Chest clear Stridor **CNS**: crying intermittently **CVS**: CRT 3 s **Rest of exam**: normal	Participants should recognize signs of impending airway compromise. Initiate patient monitoring including pulse oximetry Vital signs are available, but patient upset with IV attempt and drops O_2 sat (Oxygen Saturation) and drools. Keep the child comfortable and do not force him to wear a face mask. Consult ENT for rigid bronchoscopy in operating room Consult anesthesia		ENT and anesthesia will be available in 20 min
2. Patient develops progressive stridor and drooling and has periods of cyanosis	Participants should consider airway options and prepare. Best option in stable patient: await ENT but have double set up ready. (Oral intubation with ketamine and surgical circothyroidotomy ready and prepped) Participant may ask for CXR and lateral soft tissue neck Labs and ECG are unobtainable	Attempting to lie patient down will cause immediate cyanosis and bradycardia	Discussion of sedating meds Discussion of surgical circothroidotomy

ENT ear, nose, and throat specialist, *T* temperature, *HR* heart rate, *IV* intravenous drip, *RR* respiratory rate, *SAO₂* Oxygen Saturations, *RA* room air, *Resp* respiration, *WOB* work of breathing, *CNS* central nervous system, *CVS* cardiovascular system, *CRT* capillary refill time, *CXR* chest radiograph, *ECG* electrocardiogram

to the change in parameters as they progress through the stage.

In the framework presented, a list of other educational reminders for the facilitator can be added. For example, a reminder of a point-of-care serum glucose checked in a patient with an altered level of consciousness (whether hypoglycemia is the core element of the scenario or not) can be useful. This column should include the results of any similar tests in order for the facilitators to feed back this clinical information to the learners.

Computer Pre-programming

Depending on the simulation mannequin platform, varying degrees of pre-programming are available. Some facilitators like to pre-program the mannequin's computer to run a certain scenario regardless of the actions of the participants. These are typically designed for less complex scenarios (e.g., short advanced life support course scenarios) or scenarios that need to be standardized (e.g., research scenarios, testing scenarios). As an example, running a standardized pulseless ventricular tachycardia scenario that degenerates over 5 min to asystole may be pre-programmed and will be unchanged regardless of how the participants perform. These scenarios have the advantage of allowing the facilitator to focus on the

participants' behavior and not be distracted by the computer. The disadvantage of this approach is the lack of flexibility in participants' approach to patient care.

The next level of pre-programming allows the facilitator to pre-program each specific stage. In stage one, the computer will display the initial vital signs and other physical parameters pre-programmed for the baseline of the scenario but will not progress to the next stage until advanced by the facilitator. Once the facilitator feels it is the appropriate time in the scenario, the facilitator will advance the computer to the next stage of pre-programmed vital signs and other physical parameters. This allows the facilitator to control how quickly the scenario runs and is responsive to the actions of the participants. It does not, however, allow full flexibility when the participants perform actions clearly not anticipated by the facilitator in advance.

The next level of programming is to begin with initial vital signs and physical parameters but have no further pre-programming. This allows the facilitators to change the computer parameters with each of the participant's actions and allows for the most amount of flexibility. It is often the most realistic approach, especially in more complex patient scenarios, since participants often do not perform consistently in every scenario. The disadvantage of this approach is the challenge of managing the computer as well as trying to observe and analyze the actions of the participants in terms of

Table 2.4 Common issues with simulation and potential solutions in the scenario design phase. (Used with permission from Angèle Landriault)

Common issue	Solution
Learning objectives are rarely met/encountered by participants	Limit the number of learning objectives and design scenarios to specifically address predefined learning objectives
	Considerations when determining the reasonable number of objectives include Time Resources Realism Past training (level of the learner)
A confederate undermines the participants' learning or causes confusion during the scenario	Carefully script simple confederate roles designed to ensure that predefined learning objectives are attained
	Discuss the case and their role with the confederate ahead of time
The scenario design cannot accommodate a participant's actions (i.e., they ask for a reasonable resource you had not planned on providing)	An interprofessional design team will help predict more possible actions participants may make
	Ensure there is at least one practice run of the scenario prior to implementing it in your curriculum (may need more for high-stakes/research simulations)
Participants complain that the scenario is not realistic for them	Carefully consider all aspects of realism when designing your scenario
	Address known realism issues in the pre-briefing
Scenario is not proceeding as planned (recognized while ongoing)	Instructors adjust patient condition or direct confederates to provide hints in order to guide progress of simulation to address predefined learning objectives
Scenario adjuncts/AV materials not available when requested	Interprofessional design team and practice runs will help create a list of needed resources beforehand

AV audio-visual

preparing for the debriefing. While this is the most responsive and dynamic approach, it often requires an advanced facilitator, two co-facilitators or a facilitator and a computer programmer/simulation technician to be successful. A hybrid of both pre-programming and *on the fly* facilitation allows for the greatest amount of flexibility related to the actions of the participants (whether expected or unanticipated by the scenario creator), while reducing the amount of tasks needing to be performed simultaneously by the facilitator.

Practice Scenario

The final stage in scenario design is to pilot the scenario and perform a test run. Often, elements that were not considered when the scenario was first designed become blatantly apparent in the practice run. Participants often invest significant time and energy when agreeing to partake in a scenario and expect that the scenario will run smoothly. They may be confused and feel that they are being tricked if the scenario is missing important key elements. Ensure all necessary equipment, laboratory results, imaging, and other adjuncts are appropriate for your scenario. If confederates are part of the scenario, ensure that these roles are practiced and the scripts are adjusted accordingly. Review the scenario to ensure it unfolds in such a way that the participants' educational objectives are being met. It is tempting to avoid this step, particularly with experienced scenario designers, but we strongly advise to practice before you perform. Table 2.4 lists several common issues and offers possible solutions [1].

Conclusions

Scenario design is a complex but fundamental component of SBE. Time spent in consideration of each of the individual components will ensure the scenario is appropriate for the learners and will more likely meet their learning objectives. In addition, by following the six-step approach outlined in the second part of this chapter, the resulting scenario will contain all the necessary elements to ensure a high-quality scenario is being delivered to the learners.

References

1. Terrett L, Cardinal P, Landriault A, Cheng A, Clarke M. Simulation scenario development worksheet (Simulation Educator Training: course material). Ottawa: Royal College of Physicians and Surgeons of Canada; 2012.
2. McGaghie WC, Issenberg SB, Petrusa ER, Scalese RJ. A critical review of simulation-based medical education research: 2003–2009. Med Educ. 2010;44:50–63.
3. Holmboe E, Rizzolo MA, Sachdeva AK, Rosenberg M, Ziv A. Simulation-based assessment and the regulation of healthcare professionals. Simul Healthcare. 2011;6:S58–S62.
4. Khan K, Pattison T, Sherwood M. Simulation in medical education. Med Teach. 2011;33:1–3.
5. McGaghie WC, Siddall VJ, Mazmanian PE, Myers J. Lessons for continuing medical education from simulation research in undergraduate and graduate medical education: effectiveness of continuing medical education: American College of Chest Physicians Evidence-Based Educational Guidelines. Chest. 2009;135:62S–8S.
6. Cook DA, Brydges R, Zendejas B, Hamstra SJ, Hatala R. Technology-enhanced simulation to assess health professionals: a systematic review of validity evidence, research methods, and reporting quality. J Assoc Am Med Coll. 2013;88:872–83.

7. McGaghie WC, Issenberg SB, Cohen ER, Barsuk JH, Wayne DB. Does simulation-based medical education with deliberate practice yield better results than traditional clinical education? A meta-analytic comparative review of the evidence. J Assoc Am Med Coll. 2011;86:706–11.

8. Issenberg SB, McGaghie WC, Petrusa ER, Lee Gordon D, Scalese RJ. Features and uses of high-fidelity medical simulations that lead to effective learning: a BEME systematic review. Med Teach. 2005;27:10–28.

9. Norman G, Dore K, Grierson L. The minimal relationship between simulation fidelity and transfer of learning. Med Educ. 2012;46:636–47.

10. Lisko SA, ODell V. Integration of theory and practice: experiential learning theory and nursing education. Nurs Educ Perspect. 2010;31(2):106–8.

11. Maran NJ, Glavin RJ. Low- to high-fidelity simulation—a continuum of medical education? Med Educ. 2003;37:22–8.

12. Dieckmann P, Gaba D, Rall M. Deepening the theoretical foundations of patient simulation as social practice. Simul Healthc. 2007;2:183–93.

13. Rudolph JW, Simon R, Raemer DB. Which reality matters? Questions on the path to high engagement in healthcare simulation. Simul Healthc. 2007;2:161–3.

14. Cheng A, Lang TR, Starr SR, Pusic M, Cook DA. Technology-enhanced simulation and pediatric education: a meta-analysis. Pediatrics. 2014;133:e1313–23.

15. Hamstra SJ, Brydges R, Hatala R, Zendejas B, Cook DA. Reconsidering fidelity in simulation-based training. J Assoc Am Med Coll. 2014;89:387–92.

16. Brydges R, Carnahan H, Rose D, Rose L, Dubrowski A. Coordinating progressive levels of simulation fidelity to maximize educational benefit. 2010. J Assoc Am Med Coll. 2010;85:806–12.

17. Cooper SJ, Cant RP. Measuring non-technical skills of medical emergency teams: an update on the validity and reliability of the Team Emergency Assessment Measure (TEAM). Resuscitation. 2014;85:31–3.

18. Glavin RJ, Maran NJ. Integrating human factors into the medical curriculum. Med Educ. 2003;37:59–64.

19. Flin R. Identifying and training non-technical skills for teams in acute medicine. Qual Safe Health Care. 2004;13:i80–i4.

20. Rudolph JW, Simon R, Raemer DB, Eppich WJ. Debriefing as formative assessment: closing performance gaps in medical education. Acad Emerg Med. 2008;15:1010–16.

21. Hoffman DR. An overview of concurrent engineering. Reliability and maintainability symposium. 1998. doi:10.1109/RAMS.1998.653529.

22. Gilbert JHV, Yan J, Hoffman SJ. A WHO report: framework for action on interprofessional education and collaborative practice. J Allied Health. 2010;39(Suppl 1):196–7.

23. Cheng A, Donoghue A, Gilfoyle E, Eppich W. Simulation-based crisis resource management training for pediatric critical care medicine: a review for instructors. Pediatr Crit Care Med. 2012;13:197–203.

24. van Merriënboer JJG, Sweller J. Cognitive load theory in health professional education: design principles and strategies. Med Educ. 2010;44:85–93.

25. Paas F, Renkl A, Sweller J. Cognitive load theory and instructional design: recent developments. Educ Psychol. 2003;38:1–4.

26. Fraser K, Ma I, Teteris E, Baxter H, Wright B, McLaughlin K. Emotion, cognitive load and learning outcomes during simulation training. Med Educ. 2012;46:1055–62.

27. Cheng A, Auerbach M, Hunt EA, Chang TP, Pusic M, Nadkarni V, Kessler D. Designing and conducting simulation-based research. Pediatrics. 2014;133:1091–101.

Taylor Sawyer, Marisa Brett Fleegler and Walter J. Eppich

Simulation Pearls

1. Debriefing is a key component of the simulation experience and is essential to facilitate learning.
2. Limited evidence is available to guide the use of one framework or approach over any other. Some guidance is provided in terms of when certain approaches may be more useful and effective, but educators should pick the format and approach they are most comfortable with, and that they feel will be most beneficial to their learners based on the context and learning objectives of the training.
3. Creating a supportive learning environment is essential for effective debriefing. The use of co-debriefers, scripted debriefing and video-enhanced debriefing can also be utilized to augment the debriefing experience.

Introduction

> "Simulation is just an excuse to debrief"
> Author unknown

Debriefing is an essential component of simulation-based education (SBE). In this chapter, we offer pediatric simulation educators an overview of debriefing, provide several

frameworks to serve as a guide for debriefing practice, highlight the importance of creating psychological safety as a prerequisite for critical reflection, explore pediatric-specific considerations for debriefing, consider formal and informal approaches for educator faculty development simulation, and present methods of assessing debriefing quality.

Origin and Importance of Debriefing

Debriefing has been a critical part of healthcare simulation since its inception. Simulation and debriefing in healthcare education have expanded dramatically in recent decades, from the pioneering introduction of mannequin-based simulation to present-day applications, ranging from skills-based competencies to teamwork and behavioral objectives [1]. Mirroring the impact of aviation and the military on healthcare simulation as a whole, debriefing itself has its genesis in military after-action reviews (AARs) and aviation post-flight reviews, augmented by important contributions from fields such as business communication and psychology [2]. Debriefing in healthcare supports both clinical and behavioral learning objectives [3, 4]. Crew resource management programs in aviation debrief around issues of communication and leadership to specifically address the human factors that contribute to accidents [2]. These programs were the precursors to the domain of healthcare debriefing known as crisis resource management training in health care, which targets the human factors that contribute to medical errors [5]. The importance of this focus has expanded dramatically since the recognition of the role of human factors in medical errors in the 1999 report *To Err is Human* published by the Institute of Medicine [6].

The terms *debriefing* and *feedback* are sometimes used interchangeably; while they overlap, there are important distinctions. Feedback is typically understood as a "unidirectional communication about the recipient's behavior" [7] in which "specific information about the comparison between a trainee's observed performance and a standard, [is] given

T. Sawyer (✉)
Department of Pediatrics, University of Washington School of Medicine, Seattle Children's Hospital, Seattle, WA, USA
e-mail: tlsawyer@uw.edu

M. B. Fleegler
Department of Pediatrics, Division of Emergency Medicine, Harvard Medical School, Boston Children's Hospital, Boston, MA, USA
e-mail: marisa.brett@childrens.harvard.edu

W. J. Eppich
Departments of Pediatrics and Medical Education, Department of Pediatric Emergency Medicine, Northwestern University Feinberg School of Medicine, Ann & Robert H. Lurie Children's Hospital of Chicago, Chicago, IL, USA
e-mail: w-eppich@northwestern.edu

© Springer International Publishing Switzerland 2016
V. J. Grant, A. Cheng (eds.), *Comprehensive Healthcare Simulation: Pediatrics,*
Comprehensive Healthcare Simulation, DOI 10.1007/978-3-319-24187-6_3

Table 3.1 Comparison of debriefing and feedback

	Debriefing	Feedback
Purpose	To review events and explain, analyze and synthesize information	To explain or clarify learning points
Context	Learner-centered conversational format	Instructor-centered teaching
Direction of communication	Two-way communication between simulation instructor and participants	One-way communication, with instructor feeding information to student

with the intent to improve the trainee's performance" [8], whereas debriefing is a "bidirectional and reflective" discussion [7]. The definition of debriefing has been elaborated as "a facilitated or guided reflection in the experiential learning cycle that helps learners develop and integrate insights into later action" [9]. Table 3.1 provides a comparison of debriefing and feedback. Both debriefing and feedback play a role in healthcare simulation, depending upon the desired learning objectives. Debriefing has broad applications to simulation-based learning; its usefulness is paramount for multidisciplinary and interprofessional training, more sophisticated learners and more complex learning objectives. A straightforward procedural task and novice learners may benefit both from more direct feedback as well as the guided reflection that formal debriefing offers, depending on the learning objectives, the available time, and the instructor's preferences.

The critical role of debriefing in healthcare simulation is widely acknowledged. A widely attributed phrase in simulation education is that "simulation is just an excuse to debrief." This phrase captures the central role of debriefing in discussing and reflecting on experiences, central to the principles of adult learning theory and experiential learning theory [10]. Kolb's experiential learning cycle contains four phases: concrete experience, reflective observation, abstract conceptualization, and active experimentation [11] (Fig. 3.1). Simulated patient care provides a chance for active experimentation, while debriefing provides a facilitated and guided opportunity for reflection. Ultimately, Kolb frames this cycle as a learning spiral, with each iteration of experience and reflection deepening the learning.

The value of debriefing is also supported by empirical evidence. In a Best Evidence Medical Education (BEME) Collaboration review of the features of high-fidelity medical simulation that result in effective learning, feedback was identified as the most important element [12]. In particular, feedback was noted to allow learner self-assessment and progression to skill maintenance across a variety of feedback variables, including timing and types. The optimal debriefing strategies or methods for various types of SBE are not yet clearly defined by current research [7]. Utilizing debriefing in simulation offers the potential to bridge to an increased use of debriefing in real-life, daily clinical practice.

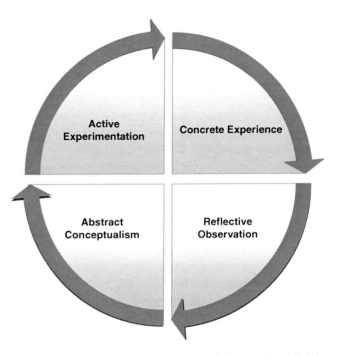

Fig. 3.1 Experiential learning cycle. (Adapted from Kolb and Kolb's *The Learning Way, Simulation Gaming*, 2009 [11])

Frameworks and Approaches for Debriefing in HealthCare Simulation

Although debriefing is often described as a fluid and dynamic process, a number of debriefing frameworks exist that help organize the process, particularly for the inexperienced debriefer. These overlapping, but distinct, strategies rely on a supportive environment to enhance a broad range of learning objectives from technical to nontechnical. An understanding of various frameworks and approaches to debriefing and feedback allows simulation educators to tailor debriefings to the learners' stage of training, the time allotted for the debriefing portion of a simulation event, and the particular learning objectives of a particular session, as different debriefing strategies may have advantages over others depending on the setting [13].

Lederman describes seven common structural elements of the debriefing process [14]. These elements include (a) the debriefer, (b) the participants, (c) the experience, (d) the

Fig. 3.2 Photograph of post-simulation facilitated debriefing conducted in situ in the intensive care unit. (Photograph courtesy of Taylor Sawyer)

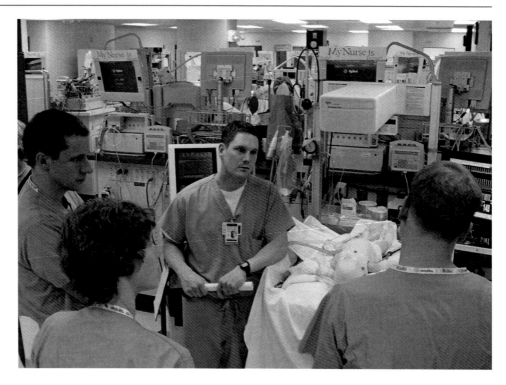

impact of the experience, (e) the recollection of the experience, (f) the mechanisms for reporting on the experience, and (g) the time to process it. Over the past three decades, several frameworks to conduct debriefing and approaches to facilitate the debriefing conversation have emerged. Many of these debriefing frameworks adhere to Lederman's basic elements and provide specific structure to the debriefing conversation in order to promote learning. However, some models such as learner-guided debriefing and intra-simulation debriefing diverge form Lederman's paradigm and offer novel approaches for simulation debriefing.

Regardless of the debriefing structure, the basic purpose remains the same—to allow those who have had an experience to reflect and discuss and analyze the experience and its meanings [14]. When facilitated effectively, the debriefing process provides a means of formative assessment by helping learners to identify, explore, and close performance "gaps" [9]. The goal is for learners to improve poor performance and maintain good performance in subsequent events, both simulated and in the actual clinical environment [9].

Debriefing Frameworks

Establishing a contextual framework within which the debriefing conversation unfolds helps both simulation participants and debriefers. When the debriefing conversation moves through defined phases, it promotes efficient use of time, keeps the discussion *on track*, and focuses on im-

portant topics. The frameworks are grouped based on the inclusion of a facilitator during the debriefing (facilitator-guided versus learner-guided) and the timing of the debriefing during the simulation session (post-simulation versus intra-simulation).

Facilitator-Guided Post-simulation Debriefing

The most common debriefing model used in SBE is for a single trained facilitator or debriefer or a small number of trained facilitators or debriefers to facilitate a conversation with simulation participants in order to discuss the events that occurred during the simulation scenario (Fig. 3.2). Several frameworks describe a *three-phase* model, in which the debriefing conversation progresses through three sequential phases of discussion, each of which is aimed at a separate, yet important goal. Other frameworks involve more than three phases. Regardless of the number of phases, or purpose of each phase, the goal of all of the frameworks is to answer three basic questions: what happened, what was the effect of the experience on participants, and what does it mean [15].

Three-Phase Models

The most well-known three-phase frameworks for SBE debriefing includes *reaction, analysis*, and *summary* phases [9, 16]. The first phase of this model *(reaction)* allows the debriefer and simulation participants to explore initial reactions, including emotional reactions, to the simulation experience. Participants can *blow off steam* prior to completing the remainder of the debriefing. In this first phase, a common opening question to the debriefing conversation is "How did that make you feel?" In addition, relevant facts of the case are clarified. During the second phase *(analysis)* of the debriefing, the focus is on what happened during the simulation and why participants performed the way they did. This phase can be further broken down into four steps, which include: (a) identification of a performance gap, (b) providing feedback on the performance gap, (c) investigating the basis for the performance gap, and (d) helping to close the performance gap through further discussion and teaching [9]. It should be noted that a performance gap could also be a positive decision or behavior that should be reinforced with the participants or that some participants may not have been aware of during the scenario. The third phase *(summary)* is dedicated to distilling lessons learned and codifying the insights gained during the analysis phase.

Another three-phase approach, which includes *gather, analyze,* and *summarize* phases, is known as the G.A.S. approach [17]. In this framework, the first phase *(gather)* allows the team leader to provide a narrative of the simulation events, with supplementation from the team. The second phase *(analyze)* is dedicated to learner-centered reflection and analysis of the actions during the simulation. During this phase, pointed questions are used to stimulate reflection and expose the learners' thinking processes. The final phase *(summary)* ensures that all the important learning objectives and teaching points were covered and to review lessons learned. The G.A.S. debriefing framework is described as a "structured and supported" format for post-simulation debriefing [17]. The structure is provided via the specific debriefing phases with related goals, actions, and time estimates. The support is provided by the inclusion of both interpersonal support, as well as the use of protocols, algorithms, and best evidence used to inform debriefing. The G.A.S. format for post-simulation debriefing has been adopted by American Heart Association (AHA) and has been incorporated in the pediatric advanced life support (PALS) course [18, 19, 25].

Multiphase Models

One multiphase approach to post-simulation debriefing is based on the US Army's AAR [20]. In this framework, the debriefing conversation progresses through seven distinct phases, which include: *D*efining the rules of the debriefing, *E*xplaining the learning objectives, *B*enchmarking performance, *R*eviewing expected actions during the simulation, *I*dentifying what happened, *E*xamining why things happened the way they did, and *F*ormalize learning. The acronym *DE-BRIEF* can be used to remember the seven steps. It should be noted that several steps in this multiphase model over-

lap with those of the three-phase models described above, for example, allowing the group to discuss what happened, why it happened, and how performance could be improved next time. However, the AAR format is unique in its explicit outlining of learning objectives, its reliance of clear performance benchmarks, and the disclosure of what the simulation instructor/facilitator explicitly expected to happen during the simulation [20]. The inclusion of these phases in the debriefing conversation ensures a shared mental model during the debriefing. It also allows participants to clearly understand the intended learning objectives of the training and provides an opportunity to objectively compare their performance against a known standard. Through the explicit review of expected actions during the scenario, the AAR format removes any ambiguity regarding the nature and intent of the simulation for the participants, prior to progressing on to the examination of what happened and why.

There is another multiphase model of debriefing in the debriefing framework, which is called "TeamGAINS" [21]. Using this framework, the facilitator guides the debriefing conversation through six sequential steps including:

1. Reactions of the participants, initiated with the question "How did that feel?"
2. Debriefing of the clinical component of the scenario
3. Transfer from simulation to reality
4. Discussion of behavioral skills and relation to clinical outcomes
5. Summarization of learning experience
6. Supervised practice of clinical skills, if needed

The TeamGAINS framework integrates several approaches to debriefing the simulation team, including *G*uided team self-correction, *A*dvocacy-*I*nquiry, and *S*ystemic-constructivist (GAINS), which are discussed later in this chapter. Use of the TeamGAINS format during debriefing has been associated with positive ratings of debriefing utility, psychological safety, and leader inclusivity [21]. The various approaches included in TeamGAINS can prove challenging for novice educators to master, but the approaches such as circular questions borrowed from systemic-constructivist approaches offer advanced debriefers additional tools for their repertoire [22].

The empiric evidence base for debriefing in healthcare simulation is limited [23]. As such, educators currently have little guidance to suggest that any one framework for post-simulation debriefing described above is better, or worse, than any other. A summary of the different facilitator-guided post-simulation debriefing formats is provided in Table 3.2. It is likely that any of the above frameworks can be effective, if used appropriately by well-trained and engaged simulation facilitators. In general, the various frameworks we have presented all share a structured format, which helps facilitators guide the debriefing conversation, make good use of the allotted time, and address the key learning objectives.

Table 3.2 Comparison of facilitator-guided post-simulation debriefing frameworks

Framework	Phases	Purpose of phase
Good judgment [9, 16]	Reactions	Exploration of feelings and a time to share emotions (i.e., "blow off steam")
	Analysis	Identify performance gaps, give feedback on performance gaps, investigate the basis for the performance gaps, engage in directed discussion and didactics
	Summary	Distill lessons learned and codify insights gained during the analysis phase
G.A.S. [17]	Gather	Team leader provides a narrative of event, with supplementation from the team
	Analyze	Pointed questions are used to stimulate reflection and shed light on the thinking process of the learners
	Summarize	Verify all important learning objectives and teaching points were covered and review lessons learned
AAR [20]	Define	Define the rules of the debriefing
	Explain	Explain the learning objectives
	Benchmark	Explain performance standards (benchmarks) that were evaluated, if any
	Review	Review expected actions during the simulation
	Identify	Identify what happened during the simulation
	Examine	Examine why things happened the way they did, and provide feedback on the performance gaps
	Formalize learning	Formalize learning with a focus on what went well, what did not, and what participants would do differently next time
TeamGAINS [21]	Reactions	Reactions of the participants, initiated with the question "How did that feel?"
	Clinical debriefing	Debriefing of the clinical component of the scenario
	Transfer	Transfer from simulation to reality
	Behavioral skills discussion	Discussion of behavioral skills and relation to clinical outcomes
	Summarization	Summarize the learning experience
	Repeated practice	Supervise practice of clinical skills, if needed

Facilitator-Guided Intra-simulation Debriefing

In order to maximize the time spent devoted to active and deliberate practice of key skills [24], recent reports describe methods for conducting debriefings during the simulation scenario—a debriefing method known as *intra-simulation debriefing*. Rather than waiting until the completion of the simulation case or scenario to debrief and provide feedback, intra-simulation debriefing occurs during the simulation scenario. This type of debriefing is provided through a series of short and highly focused, debriefing/feedback events, which occur any time when feedback or correction is required. One example is the combination of *stop action* debriefing with repeated practice on troublesome skills, named "rapid-cycle deliberate practice" (RCDP) [25]. RCDP focuses on the correction of errors in real time. Using RCDP, the facilitator stops the actions of the participants any time an error occurs and uses a "pause, rewind 10 s, and try it again" approach to allow the participants to redo that section of the scenario again after the facilitator provides corrective feedback. The debriefing/feedback episodes focus on coaching the participants to maximize performance in real time. The basic principles of RCDP include (a) maximization of time learners spend in simulation-based deliberate practice, (b) allow facilitators an efficient way to teach specific evidence-based approaches to medical care, and (c) foster psychological safety within the simulation environment [25]. RCDP has been shown to improve performance of pediatric residents during simulated pediatric cardiac arrest scenarios compared to historic controls trained using traditional post-simulation debriefings [25].

Learner-Guided Debriefing

A clear departure from the facilitator-led frameworks described above is a debriefing method in which there is no facilitator to lead or guide the debriefing discussion, otherwise known as learner-guided debriefing. In this framework, the individual learners or teams debrief themselves. This type of learner-guided debriefing has been referred to as "self-debriefing" for individuals, [26] or "within-team debriefing" when conducted by teams [27]. Reports of learner-guided debriefing describe the use of teamwork evaluation tools as a framework for reflection and formative self-assessment. During learner-guided debriefing the participants use these teamwork tools to guide their own debriefing and discussions.

There is some evidence that learner-guided debriefing may be as effective as facilitator-guided debriefing. One study compared learner-guided to facilitator-guided debriefing for anesthesiology residents managing intraoperative cardiac arrest [26]. Residents were randomized to either self-

debriefing using a behavioral assessment tool (anesthesia nontechnical skills tool) or traditional instructor-led facilitated debriefing. Both groups demonstrated improvements in performance from pre-test to post-test. There were no significant differences in the degree of improvement between self-debriefing and instructor-led debriefing groups. A follow-up study compared the effectiveness of learner-guided debriefing using the Ottawa Global Rating Scale as a framework compared to facilitator-guided debriefing on team performance during a simulated anesthesia crisis scenario and once again found similar, but not statistically different, improvement in both groups [27]. These results suggest that effective learning of nontechnical skills may be achieved equally through learner-guided debriefing without the aid of an instructor, which could improve resource utilization and the feasibility of team-based simulation at a program level [27].

Practically speaking, it is important to highlight that the debriefing framework may be less important than the simple act of debriefing itself. It is likely that any of the debriefing frameworks described would be more beneficial at improving performance over no debriefing.

Debriefing Approaches

There are several approaches to facilitate and optimize debriefing conversations that operate within the frameworks elaborated above. We define *approaches* to debriefing as particular methods and conversational techniques utilized during debriefings, which are aimed at optimizing the provision of information and maximizing the impact of the debriefing experience. These *approaches* are different to the *frameworks* discussed above, which describe the organizational context within which the debriefing unfolds and/or provides an outline for the conversational flow. Several published approaches to debriefing that can be used to facilitate the debriefing conversation and to engage pediatric learners are reviewed below.

Perhaps the best known approach to debriefing is the *debriefing with good judgment* approach [16]. The components of this approach include: (1) the conceptual model of *reflective practice*, which seeks to surface mental *frames of mind* that drove participants' actions during the simulation session; (2) a debriefing stance that encourages simulation instructors to share their viewpoint, while at the same time allowing the participants to share their unique insights (i.e., the *good judgment* approach); and (3) utilization of the conversational technique known as *advocacy-inquiry*, a technique adopted from the business and organizational behavior literature. When using advocacy-inquiry, instructors *advocate* their point of view and subjective judgment of an event that transpired during the simulation, then *inquire* about the participants frame of mind in relation to the event

[16]. Using the good judgment approach allows instructors to manage the tension between sharing honest feedback while still maintaining the trust of trainees [16]. *Debriefing with good judgment* requires formal training for effective implementation. This approach has been taught in courses and workshops around the world and is widely practiced by pediatric simulation instructors.

A blended approach to debriefing called "Promoting Excellence and Reflective Learning in Simulation" (PEARLS) integrates three specific approaches to the analysis phase of debriefing and provide guidance for their targeted use [28]. The three approaches are *learner self-assessment, focused facilitation*, and *directive feedback* or focused teaching. During learner self-assessment, the debriefing facilitator guides a discussion in which the participants self-assess their performance. This is typically accomplished via the *plus/delta* method: The facilitator asks open-ended questions regarding "what went well?" *(plus)* and "what could be changed?" *(delta)*. Benefits of learner self-assessment via the plus/delta approach include the ease of use and the ability to identify multiple issues quickly. Disadvantages include the potential to overlook the rationale, or reason, for observed performance gaps, not being able to debrief all the identified issues on the list that has been generated, and the possibility for the debriefing to go offtrack. In terms of focused facilitation, debriefers can use any number of strategies to facilitate focused discussion surrounding key learning points. These include advocacy-inquiry [16], circular questioning [21, 22], self-guided team correction [29], or alternatives and their pros and cons [30]. The main advantage to this approach is that the rationale/frames of the participants are fully identified; however, the disadvantages are that it is a more difficult skill to master and the technique requires more debriefing time to be successful. Finally, directive feedback is the focused information that the debriefer provides to participants in order to correct perceived performance gaps, without engaging in discussion to identify the underlying rationale for action. Directive feedback is a well-known and efficient method to modify performance [31]. The disadvantages include the pure instructor-driven nature of the approach and lack of group discussion, as well as a potential risky assumption on behalf of the debriefer that they know the rationale for the performance gap. In addition, the debriefer must provide the context for why they are correcting technique/behavior in order for learning to be achieved.

When using the PEARLS approach, significant consideration is given to the available time for debriefing and whether or not a clear rationale is evident for the participants' action to help determine the specific method used. When there is limited time and the rationale for simulation participant actions is clear, directive feedback and teaching are used to close performance gaps. In situations where there is a limited time and the rationale is unclear, learner self-assessment is used to identify performance gaps and then either the learners or the instructor close the performance gap. If there is ample time and/or the rationale for actions is unclear then focused facilitation is used to identify and analyze individual performance gaps and the gaps are closed through a reflective practice approach.

The TeamGAINS framework specifically incorporates several facilitative approaches to post-simulation debriefing and also provides specific guidance for their use. The approaches include the conversational technique of *advocacy-inquiry*, as well as *guided team self-correction* and *systemic-constructivist* debriefing. Guided team self-correction provides structure and a technique for simulation participants to correct their own actions [29]. Using this approach, the debriefing conversation is supported by a pre-specified model of teamwork against which the simulation team is asked to compare their performance against, both positively and negatively. The debriefing facilitator guides the participants to reflect on specific components of the teamwork model (e.g., "Give me an example of when priorities were clearly and appropriately stated"), and then waits for the team to offer their input prior to sharing their own opinion and observations [21]. Systemic-constructivist debriefing is a theory of debriefing founded in systemic therapy, a form of psychotherapy [22]. Within this theory of debriefing, a specific approach that has been applied to medical debriefing is *circular questioning* [21]. As opposed to direct questions, the facilitator asks a third person to describe the relationship between the other two people while in their presence. For example, the facilitator could ask a nurse to comment on what the senior physician did upon walking into the room and how the resident physicians reacted. In this approach, the participants are asked to *circle back* and comment from an outside perspective on the interaction of the other team members.

An important point to consider when comparing the approaches reviewed here is that the success of a specific debriefing approach is highly dependent on both the experience and expertise of the debriefer, as well as the experience and expertise of the learner group in regards to the specific simulation scenario and learning objectives. Novice learners, and those with limited experience with the case depicted in the simulation scenario, will likely require significantly more instructor-centered methods of debriefing, including direct feedback and teaching. More experienced learner groups will likely need less direct feedback, and the debriefing conversation will progress well using learner-centered techniques including learner self-assessment and team self-correction. Systemic-constructivist methods such as circular questioning and the *debriefing with good judgment* approach may work well with either type of learner, depending on the context and content of the simulation and the level of insight of the individual learners.

Application of these Frameworks and Approaches to Pediatric Simulation

While the frameworks and approaches to debriefing described in this chapter were not specifically developed for pediatric SBE, many have been applied to pediatric SBE. Specific examples of this include: (1) the use of the *intra-simulation debriefing* during PALS training for pediatric residents [25], (2) the use of the three-phase model of debriefing during neonatal resuscitation simulation training [32], and (3) the use of the G.A.S. format for post-simulation debriefing during the PALS course [18, 19].

Strategies to Optimize Debriefing in HealthCare Simulation

The previous sections have provided an overview of conceptual frameworks and specific debriefing approaches to help guide debriefing practice. One significant challenge is how to create the right environment for debriefing. Several factors have great potential to optimize the effectiveness of debriefing in healthcare simulation: (a) an emphasis on a safe learning environment for honest reflection and feedback (i.e., psychological safety); (b) an understanding of aspects unique to pediatric simulation; (c) knowledge and experience of the interplay of additional debriefing strategies such as co-debriefing, scripted debriefing, and video-assisted debriefing; (d) the importance of both formal and informal faculty development strategies, including evaluation of the debriefer.

Creating Supportive Learning Environments for Debriefing

A challenging, yet supportive, learning environment is an essential prerequisite for SBE [9, 33], not only for allowing learners to engage fully in the simulation experience but also to promote honest and critical reflection about performance during the debriefing. Psychological safety is a sense of confidence that a participant will not feel rejected, embarrassed, or punished for speaking up regarding both their personal performance, as well as the performance of the team. Mutual respect and trust within the educator and learner group are essential to promote individual risk-taking [34, 35] and help learners to accept challenge [36]. In order to engender feelings of psychological safety, trust, and respect that form the foundation for receiving critical performance feedback and for the open discussion of mistakes, educators can take several key steps [35].

- Introductions: Educators and learners should introduce themselves to the group, share expectations for the ses-

sion, and build rapport [37]. Educators should learn and use learners' names to demonstrate authentic interest in their learning and promote a flattened hierarchy between educators and learners depending on cultural and language customs [38].

- Expectations: Educators should provide a session overview in order to ensure that expectations are clear, including ground rules for working together and potentially including goals and learning objectives. Establish confidentiality around the learners' performance during the simulation sessions. Remind learners that the goal of the session is not to be perfect from the start, but to be challenged, learn from mistakes, and improve [44].

- Debriefing and Feedback: Educators should be explicit about how and when learners will receive feedback [39] and how the debriefing process will unfold. It can be helpful to highlight the significance of specific, honest yet nonthreatening feedback [40] in helping everyone improve their performance. If the simulation is paused to discuss relevant points or identify errors, disclose to the learners that they may be interrupted at various times during the simulated case so that they can receive feedback.

- Orientation to space/equipment/resources: Educators should take the time to orient learners to the simulated learning environment, including available resources, engaging with the simulator or other embedded simulated persons, such as parents, caregivers, or other care providers such as nurses. It can also be helpful to review specific physical findings on the simulation manikin being used, and how to get other relevant clinical information (e.g., general appearance, capillary refill time, muscle tone, and so on) in order for the team to work through the case [38].

Unique Aspects of Pediatric Simulation Relevant for the Debriefing

Pediatric simulation educators must consider several pediatric-specific factors and challenges when planning, implementing, and debriefing simulated pediatric illness, especially for infants and toddlers. In contrast to simulation representing adolescents and adults, simulated infants and toddlers do not speak. Much as in clinical practice, this provides an added layer of complexity to pediatric care, and integrating simulated parents or caregivers can address several issues simultaneously. For example, simulated parents can provide relevant history or relay important physical findings essential to manage the case. These are worth mentioning here since how adequately (or inadequately) educators attend to these details for the simulation scenario can have significant downstream impact during the debriefing and help prevent learner frustration related to perceived realism. Of course, the primary learning objective of a case could be related to interacting with a simulated parent or caregiver. With planning and coaching, simulated parents can also participate in the subsequent debriefing and even provide learners' with critical performance feedback from a different perspective [41].

Key considerations for integrating simulated parents into a debriefing:

- The simulated parents can use learners' initial reactions during the opening of the debriefing to guide their comments.
- In general, simulated parents can be coached to specifically address issues related to how the learner(s) introduced themselves, how well they listened, how they used or attended to nonverbal communication, and how well they used language that parents can understand [42]. Additional specific areas can be tailored the learning objectives of the case, for example, how to deal with family member presence during a critical event or how to deal with a distracting family member. In addition, a simulated parent can comment on how well the team communicated with the child.
- During the debriefing, simulated parents should be encouraged to speak from the first-person perspective (e.g., "When you used a lot of medical terms, it was confusing for me") [42]. In this context, it is important to remember that the actual simulation has ended and that comments and feedback to learners should be offered without any emotional overlay that contributes to enhanced realism during the simulation. In this way, great care should be taken as to the actual value of having the simulated parent participate in the debriefing, especially with inexperienced learners.

The Interplay of Additional Debriefing Strategies

Specific debriefing strategies, such as co-debriefing with more than one debriefing facilitator, the use of video to enhance debriefing, and scripted debriefing are additional strategies that may play important roles in enhancing the debriefing experience.

Co-debriefing involves the co-facilitation of the debriefing by more than one person. Various combinations exist, including a more experienced facilitator with a less experienced one, as well as co-facilitators from different healthcare professions or disciplines. If co-debriefers use strategies to proactively coordinate their efforts seamlessly and react appropriately to the unique nature of two or more facilitators providing feedback simultaneously, the varied perspectives from co-debriefers can be advantageous. In addition, while one debriefer pursues a specific line of questioning, a co-debriefer can monitor learners' reactions and act to support a lead debriefer should difficulties arise. However, if the co-

debriefers are not on the same page regarding debriefing philosophy, preferred debriefing framework or reactive strategies for events that occur during the debriefing, the potential for disagreement between facilitators exists, which have the potential to negatively impact the debriefing and associated learning.

The use of video to enhance debriefing is widespread, although the evidence to support its use is unclear [43, 44]. For video to be used appropriately and effectively, we recommend short clips that are presented with a clear purpose that make the visual replay of the event more critical than a simple discussion of the event without video. Video review can potentially be time-consuming, both in cueing the correct video sequence and allowing enough time for the video sequence to be shown and discussed. In addition, video review should not be used in a punitive fashion to demonstrate a specific individual's lack of skill or inappropriate management. However, use of video can be a powerful way to demonstrate team performance during a scenario [45].

Scripted debriefing may play an important role in the debriefing experience, particularly for novice instructors trying to learn the specific language and flow of debriefing. There is some evidence that the use of a debriefing script can lead to better learning outcomes in both knowledge and team behaviors [46]. In 2010, debriefing tools were incorporated into the instructor training materials of both the PALS and advanced cardiac life support (ACLS) courses of the AHA in an effort to standardize the method of debriefing across training centers [19]. Additionally, the PEARLS-blended debriefing approach includes a debriefing script to promote adherence to debriefing structure as well as a guide to formulate specific questions using the various debriefing approaches [28]. The use of a debriefing script also has the potential to serve as a faculty development aid.

Debriefing is a skill usually acquired through participation in a variety of faculty development opportunities but further enhanced through on-going debriefing practice. Little is known as to the frequency or number of debriefing experiences needed to achieve competence or proficiency. Some faculty development opportunities are formal, such as participation in simulation educator courses and workshops, as well as graduate degrees in simulation. Others opportunities are informal, occurring during authentic teaching activities while under the supervision of more experienced simulation educators. Ideally, a blended approach to simulation faculty development involves formalized, structured experiences with ongoing support in the form of role modeling and peer coaching from trusted colleagues. Engaging in co-debriefing with a supportive, more experienced colleague who provides scaffolding can play a powerful role in enhancing debriefing skill development. To promote peer feedback, a shared understanding of behaviors that promote debriefing effectiveness can serve to set standards for a simulation program.

Assessing the Effectiveness of Debriefing

Healthcare simulation has evolved since its inception from a reliance on face validity to an evidence-based assessment of its effectiveness on educational and clinical outcomes [47–50]. Similarly, while debriefing has long been relied on as the *sine qua non* of healthcare simulation and a critical link to its experiential aspect for the adult learner [13], recognition of the importance of debriefing quality and the formal assessment of debriefing represents the next phase in the growth of simulation-based debriefing [3].

Evaluating the effectiveness of debriefing is a burgeoning area of simulation research. Amongst the increasing number of published debriefing assessment tools [21, 33, 40, 49–55], relatively few psychometrically rigorous tools have been developed. These tools vary in their complexity and generalizability but all share the basic framework of a quantitative assessment of the essential components of debriefing. Here, we will specifically examine two published tools used to evaluate the effectiveness of debriefing: the Debriefing Assessment for Simulation in Healthcare (DASH) and the Objective Structured Assessment of Debriefing (OSAD), which has versions developed for both surgical and pediatric applications [40, 49, 55].

The DASH tool is a criterion-referenced behaviorally anchored rating scale that examines concrete behaviors in order to evaluate strategies and techniques used to conduct debriefings. The DASH is designed to allow assessment of debriefings from a variety of disciplines (including pediatrics), small or large groups of participants, various educational objectives, and different physical and time constraints. The DASH examines the simulation instructor's abilities in debriefing across six elements: (1) establishing an engaging learning environment, (2) maintaining an engaging learning environment, (3) structuring the debriefing in an organized way, (4) provoking engaging discussion, (5) identifying and exploring performance gaps, and (6) helping trainees achieve or sustain future performance [55]. Performance in each element is rated on a 7-point Likert-type scale from "extremely ineffective/detrimental" to "extremely effective/outstanding" [55]. There are versions of the DASH available for use by trained raters, students, and for instructor self-assessment. In an evaluation of its psychometric properties, the DASH tool showed good evidence of reliability and preliminary evidence of validity [33]. The assessment of specific behaviors offers the opportunity for formative as well as summative evaluation, supporting debriefing skills development.

The OSAD is an assessment tool initially designed to assess surgical debriefing practices [40]. It consists of eight categories related to debriefing: approach, environment, engagement, reaction, reflection, analysis, diagnosis, and application. It has been demonstrated to have strong inter-rater reliability and internal consistency and has been used to demonstrate an improvement in both frequency and quality of debriefing after an educational intervention [40, 50]. Each dimension of the OSAD is scored on a 5-point Likert-type scale containing defined anchors for scores 1, 3, and 5 to aid scoring and consistency. The pediatric-specific OSAD tool was developed after a literature review and interviews with pediatric debriefing facilitators and learners [49]. It relies on the same eight dimensions as the original OSAD tool. No literature currently exists on the reliability or validity of the pediatric OSAD.

Valid debriefing assessment tools will offer the opportunity to evaluate debriefers and provide them with formative assessment, as well as to assess educational interventions in debriefing. The tools themselves are in effective road maps for high-quality debriefings.

The Future of Debriefing

Given the importance of debriefing in pediatric simulation and the current paucity of evidence regarding the relative effectiveness of different debriefing methodologies, future research in debriefing assessment is required in order to optimize the methods used in pediatric simulation debriefing [23]. Furthermore, research comparing the effectiveness of different approaches to debriefing (in various contexts) will help to better define the best approach to use in specific situations. Particular attention needs to be paid to the importance of various factors inherent to debriefing practice (timing of debriefing, length of debriefing, etc.), as well as various factors that can enhance or affect debriefing (video debriefing, co-debriefing, and scripted debriefing). Additionally, work should continue to provide ongoing education and faculty development in the art and science of debriefing methodologies for pediatric simulation educators. The availability of validated tools to assess the effectiveness of debriefing may provide important information to improve individual debriefer skills.

References

1. Abrahamson S, Denson JS, Wolf RM. Effectiveness of a simulator in training anesthesiology residents. J Med Educ. 1969;44(6):515–9.
2. Gardner R. Introduction to debriefing. Semin Perinatol. 2013;37(3):166–74.
3. Fanning RM, Gaba DM. The role of debriefing in simulation-based learning. Simul Healthc. 2007;2(2):115–25.
4. Mackinnon R, Gough S. What can we learn about debriefing from other high-risk/high-stakes industries? Cureus 6(4): e174.
5. Howard SK, Gaba DM, Fish KJ, Yang G, Sarnquist FH. Anesthesia crisis resource management training: teaching anesthesiologists to handle critical incidents. Aviat Space Environ Med. 1992;63(9):763–70.

6. Institute of Medicine (IOM). To err is human. In: Kohn LT, Corrigan JM, Donaldson MS, editors. Building a safer health system. Washington, D.C: National Academy Press; 1999.

7. Cheng A, Eppich W, Grant V, Sherbino J, Zendejas B, Cook DA. Debriefing for technology-enhanced simulation: a systematic review and meta-analysis. Med Educ. 2014;48(7):657–66.

8. van de Ridder JM, Stokking KM, McGaghie WC, ten Cate OT. What is feedback in clinical education? Med Educ. 2008;42(2):189–97.

9. Rudolph JW, Simon R, Raemer DB, Eppich WJ. Debriefing as formative assessment: closing performance gaps in medical education. Acad Emerg Med. 2008;15(11):1010–6.

10. Kolb DA. Experiential learning: experience as the source of learning and development. Englewood Cliffs: Prentice Hall; 1984.

11. Kolb AY, Kolb DA. The learning way: meta-cognitive aspects of experiential learning. Simul Gaming. 2009;40(3):297–327.

12. Issenberg SB, McGaghie WC, Petrusa ER, Lee Gordon D, Scalese RJ. Features and uses of high-fidelity medical simulations that lead to effective learning: a BEME systematic review. Med Teach. 2005;27(1):10–28.

13. Dismukes RK, Gaba DM, Howard SK. So many roads: facilitated debriefing in healthcare. Simul Healthc. 2006;1(1):23–5.

14. Lederman LC. Debriefing: toward a systematic assessment of theory and practice. Simul Gaming. 1992;23:145–60.

15. Pearson M, Smith D. Debriefing in experience-based Learning. Simul Game Learn. 1986;16(4):155–172.

16. Rudolph J, Simon R, Dufresne R, Raemer D, There's N. Such thing as "Nonjudgmental" debriefing: a theory and method for debriefing with good judgment. Simul Healthc. 2006;1(1):49–55.

17. Phrampus P, O'Donnell J. [internet] Debriefing in simulation education—using a structured and supported model. [updateditor 2009 Jan; cited 2014 Sep 25]. 2014. http://www.google.com/url?sa=t&rct=j&q=&esrc=s&source=web&cd=1&cad=rja&uact=8&ved=0CB4QFjAA&url=http%3A%2F%2Fwww.wiser.pitt.edu%2Fsites%2Fwiser%2Fns08%2Fday1_PP_JOD_DebriefingInSimEdu.pdf&ei=YKkZVKWwD-jXiwLd4IDYCA&usg=AFQjCNFCYMxW7Fpny4pusB53SoF7bFruKQ&sig2=IXegi9GhXfL2sFWD0X-W9QA.

18. Pediatric Advanced Life Support Provider Manual editor. Dallas: American Heart Association; 2011.

19. Cheng A, Rodgers D, Van Der Jagt E, Eppich W, O'Donnell J. Evolution of the pediatric advanced life support course: enhanced learning with a new debriefing tool and web-based module for pediatric advanced life support instructors. Pediatr Crit Care Med. 2012;13(5):589–95.

20. Sawyer T, Deering S. Adaptation of the U.S., Army's after-action review (AAR) to simulation debriefing in healthcare. Simul Healthc. 2013;8(6):388–97.

21. Kolbe M, Weiss M, Grote G, Knauth A, Dambach M, Spahn DR, et al. TeamGAINS: a tool for structured debriefings for simulation-based team trainings. BMJ Qual Saf. 2013;22(7):541–53.

22. Kriz WC. A systemic-constructivist approach to the facilitation and debriefing of simulations and games. Simul Gaming. 2010;41:663–80.

23. Raemer D, Anderson M, Cheng A, Fanning R, Nadkarni V, Savoldelli G. Research regarding debriefing as part of the learning process. Simul Healthc. 2011;6(7):52–7.

24. Ericsson KA. Deliberate practice and acquisition of expert performance: a general overview. Acad Emerg Med. 2008;15(11):988–94.

25. Hunt EA, Duval-Arnould JM, Nelson-McMillan KL, Bradshaw JH, Diener-West M, Perretta JS, et al. Pediatric resident resuscitation skills improve after "rapid cycle deliberate practice" training. Resuscitation. 2014;85(7):945–51.

26. Boet S, Bould D, Bruppacher H, Desjardins F, Chandra D, Naik V. Looking in the mirror: self-debriefing versus instructor debriefing for simulated crises. Crit Care Med. 2011;39(6):1377–81.

27. Boet S, Bould D, Sharma B, Revees S, Naik V, Triby E, et al. Within-Team debriefing versus instructor-led debriefing for simulation-based education: a randomized controlled trial. Ann Surg. 2013;258(1):53–8.

28. Eppich W, Cheng A. Promoting excellence and reflective learning in simulation (PEARLS): development and rationale for a blended approach to healthcare simulation debriefing. Simul Healthc. 2014. (Submitted for Publication).

29. Smith-Jentsch KA, Cannon-Bowers JA, Tannenbaum S, Salas E. Guided team self-correction: impacts on team mental models, processes, and effectiveness. Small Group Res. 2008;39:303–29.

30. Fanning RM, Gaba DM. Debriefing. In: Gaba DM, Fish KJ, Howard SK, Burden AR, editors. Crisis management in anesthesiology. 2nd ed. Philadelphia: Elsevier Saunders; 2015. p. 65–78.

31. Archer JC. State of the science in health professional education: effective feedback. Med Educ. 2010;44(1):101–8.

32. Sawyer T, Sierocka-Casteneda A, Chan D, Berg B, Lustik M, Thompson M. Deliberate practice using simulation improves neonatal resuscitation performance. Simul Healthc. 2011;6(6):327–36.

33. Brett-Fleegler M, Rudolph J, Eppich W, Monuteaux M, Fleegler E, Cheng A, et al. Debriefing assessment for simulatn in healthcare: development and psychometric properties. Simul Healthc. 2012;7(5):288–94.

34. Edmondson AC. Psychological safety and learning behavior in work teams. Adm Sci Q. 1999;44:350–83.

35. Rudolph JW, Raemer DB, Simon R. Establishing a safe container for learning in simulation: the role of presimulation briefing. Simul Healthc. 2014. Epub Sep 3.

36. Edmondson AC. The competitive imperative of learning. Harv Bus Rev. 2008;86(7–8):60–7.

37. Buskist W, Saville BK. Rapport-building: creating positive emotional contexts for enhancing learning and teaching.[internet] Teaching tips. 2014. http://www.psychologicalscience.org/teaching/tips/tips_0301.cfm. Accessed 22 Oct 2014.

38. Eppich WJ, O'Connor L, Adler MD. Providing effective simulation activities. In: Forrest K, McKimm J, Edgar S, editors. Essential simulation in clinical education. Chichester: Wiley-Blackwell; 2013. p. 213–234.

39. Molloy E, Boud D. Changing conceptions of feedback. In: Boud D, Molloy E, editors. Feedback in higher and professional education: understanding it and doing it well. London: Routledge; 2013. p. 11–33.

40. Arora S, Ahmed M, Paige J, Nestel D, Runnacles J, Hull L, et al. Objective structured assessment of debriefing (OSAD): bringing science to the art of debriefing in surgery. Ann Surg. 2012;256(6):982–8.

41. Cleland JA, Abe K, Rethans JJ. The use of simulated patients in medical education: AMEE guide No 42. Med Teach. 2009;32:477–86.

42. Pascucci RC, Weinstock PH, O'Connor BE, Fancy KM, Meyer EC. Integrating actors into a simulation program: a primer. Simul Healthc. 2014;9(2):120–6.

43. Savoldelli GL, Naik VN, Park J, Joo HS, Chow R, Hamstra SJ. Value of debriefing during simulated crisis management: oral versus video-assisted oral feedback. Anesthesiology. 2006;105(2):279–85.

44. Sawyer T, Sierocka-Casteneda A, Chan D, Berg B, Lustik M, Thompson M. The effectiveness of video-assisted debriefing versus oral debriefing alone at improving neonatal resuscitation performance: a randomized trial. Simul Healthc. 2012;7(4):213–21.

45. Cheng A, Donoghue A, Gilfoyle E, Eppich W. Simulation-based crisis resource management training for pediatric critical care medicine: a review for instructors. Pediatr Crit Care Med. 2012;13(2):197–203.

46. Cheng A, Hunt E, Donoghue A, Nelson-McMillan K, Nishisaki A, LeFlore J, et al. Examining pediatric resuscitation education using simulation and scripted debriefing: a multicenter randomized trial. JAMA Pediatrics. 2013;167(6):528–36.

47. McGaghie W, Draycott T, Dunn W, Lopez C, Stefanidis D. Evaluating the impact of simulation on translational patient outcomes. Simul Healthc. 2011;6(Suppl):S42–7.

48. Cook DA, Hatala R, Brydges R, et al. Technology-enhanced simulation for health professions education: a systematic review and meta-analysis. JAMA. 2011;306:978–88.

49. Brydges R, Hatala R, Zendejas B, Erwin P, Cook D. Linking simulation-based educational assessments and patient-related outcomes: a systematic review and meta-analysis. Acad Med. 2014 Nov 4. [Epub ahead of print] (Runnacles J, Thomas L, Sevdalis N, Kneebone R, Arora S. Development of a tool to improve performance debriefing and learning: the paediatric objective structured assessment of debriefing (OSAD) tool. Postgrad Med J. 2014. Epub Sep 8).

50. Ahmed M, Arora S, Russ S, Darzi A, Vincent C, Sevdalis N. Operation debrief: a SHARP improvement in performance feedback in the operating room. Ann Surg. 2013;258(6):958–63.

51. Gururaja RP, Yang T, Paige JT, et al. Examining the effectiveness of debriefing at the point of care in simulation-based operating room team training. In: Henriksen K, Battles JB, Keyes MA et al., editors. Advances in patient safety: new directions and alternative approaches (Vol 3: performance and tools). Rockville: Agency for Healthcare Research and Quality (US); 2008.

52. Reed SJ. Debriefing experience scale; development of a tool to evaluate the student learning experience in debriefing. Clin Simul Nurs. 2012;8:e211–e7.

53. Dreifuerst KT. Using debriefing for meaningful learning to foster development of clinical reasoning in simulation. J Nurs Educ. 2012;51(6):326–33.

54. Dias Coutinho VR, Amado Martins JC, Fátima Carneiro Ribeiro Pereira M. Construction and validation of the simulation debriefing assessment scale. Revista de Enfermagem Referência. 2014;4(2):41–50.

55. Simon R, Raemer D, Rudolph J. Debriefing assessment for simulation in healthcare©—student version, short form. Cambridge: Center for Medical Simulation; 2010. https://www.harvardmedsim.org/debriefing-assesment-simulation-healthcare.php.

Simulation-Based Team Training

4

Elaine Gilfoyle, Elaine Ng and Ronald D. Gottesman

Simulation Pearls

- Human factors are a major source of error in healthcare and should be the focus of specific training in the simulated clinical environment.
- Simulation-based education has been effectively utilized for pediatric acute care team training with demonstrated improvements in confidence, knowledge, skills, teamwork behaviors, and patient outcomes.
- There are many teamwork assessment tools available. Some tools are developed to assess the entire team versus the leader alone, while others are developed as a standalone teamwork tool versus embedded in a tool used for resuscitation performance overall.
- Developing simulation-based team training must include consideration of the purpose of such training, understanding the needs of the participants and careful planning of the learning environment.

E. Gilfoyle (✉)
Department of Pediatrics, Department of Critical Care, University of Calgary, Alberta Children's Hospital, Calgary, AB, Canada
e-mail: elaine.gilfoyle@albertahealthservices.ca

E. Ng
Department of Anesthesia, Department of Anesthesia and Pain Medicine, University of Toronto, Hospital for Sick Children, Toronto, ON, Canada
e-mail: Elaine.ng@sickkids.ca

R. D. Gottesman
Department of Pediatrics, Department of Pediatric Critical Care, McGill University, Montreal Children's Hospital/McGill University Health Center, Montreal, QC, Canada
e-mail: ronald.gottesman@mcgill.ca

Team Training: Burden of Medical Error and the Role of Teamwork

Human error is common across all areas of healthcare, and those errors result in significantly increased patient morbidity and mortality [1, 2]. Errors are more likely to occur in complex environments such as the intensive care unit and emergency department [3, 4]. This is due to several factors: the higher number of interventions performed per patient [5]; the need for multiple care providers to interact with each other to achieve common goals [6, 7]; and the provision of care in a high-stakes, high-stress environment, which may further impair healthcare providers' performance [8, 9]. Resuscitation events are at particularly high risk of error [10, 11]. Errors usually relate to either not adhering to established resuscitation guidelines or medication errors, with the underlying reason being healthcare providers not working effectively as a team [12, 13].

Team training for pediatric resuscitation team members has become a common component of medical, nursing, and allied health professional education (Fig. 4.1). A significant volume of simulation-based research has been published recently, suggesting that simulation-based team training (SBTT) has a positive effect on healthcare provider performance [14]. Research linking team training with real-life performance and actual patient outcome is more difficult to conduct; therefore, there are fewer published studies examining these outcomes. However, a recent study demonstrated that hospital-wide adoption of team training (among other changes to how resuscitation teams are educated) improved survival from cardiac arrest at an American pediatric hospital compared to historical outcome data [15]. Hopefully, we will see more studies examining the impact of team training on real-life patient outcomes published in the near future.

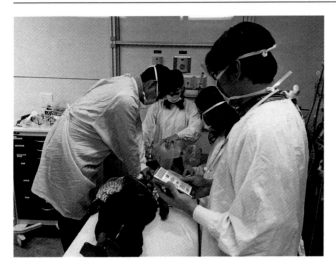

Fig. 4.1 Team photo. (Photograph courtesy of KidSIM Pediatric Simulation Program)

Team Training: A Competency Framework

As described above and in other sections of this book, human factors play a significant role in terms of healthcare provider performance. The errors that clinicians make are more often related to human factors, rather than lack of knowledge or technical issues with medical equipment. Formalized team training has been developed in many areas of healthcare in order to address these types of errors, including pediatrics [16, 17]. Each group of educators uses their own set of learning objectives or list of competencies [18]; however, there is substantial overlap among those that are published. The section below describes a user-friendly framework, which organizes educational content under four main teamwork competencies: role responsibility, communication, situational awareness, and decision-making (Table 4.1) . This framework fits nicely with a teamwork performance assessment tool developed in obstetrics but is also applicable to any area of acute care, including pediatrics [19].

Role Responsibility

Acute care teams consist of several members from different clinical professions, most commonly medicine, nursing, and respiratory therapy, among others. These team members take on different roles (leader, airway person, medication person, documenter, etc.). These roles must be assigned but are often assumed based on the profession of the team member. For example, the team leader is usually a physician and the medication person is usually a nurse. The leader is ultimately responsible for assigning roles. Furthermore, all tasks (i.e., workload) required during the resuscitation must be assigned and distributed, so that team members take own-

ership of tasks to ensure completion. Tasks ordered into thin air are not as likely to be completed since this ownership is lacking. Finally, team members must recognize and verbalize their performance limitations so that tasks are assigned to the most appropriate member. For example, if some of them have not been trained in how to operate the defibrillator, then they are not the best person to be assigned this important task.

Communication

There are many different aspects to good communication during an acute situation, ten of which will be discussed here (Table 4.1). Communication of both clinical observation and orders must be handled very carefully, so that they are not missed or misunderstood. There are three important overarching aspects to the proper communication of orders: (1) Team members must *direct their communication* by using names or other ways (e.g., tap on the shoulder) of

Table 4.1 Teamwork competency and behavior framework

Teamwork competency	Teamwork behavior
Role responsibility	Assign roles
	Distribute workload
	Recognize and verbalize performance limitation
	Verbalize overload
	Cross-monitor roles
Communication	Use directed communication
	Give clear and concise orders
	Use closed communication loop
	Think out loud
	Leader seeks input from team members
	Team members suggest ideas/plans to leader
	Orient new members, if required
	Give all information to leader
	Speak with calm voice
	Resolve conflicts and deal with distractions quickly and effectively
Situational awareness	Quickly develop a shared mental model
	Conduct frequent re-assessment and re-evaluation of patient
	Prioritize attention effectively as situation requires
	Avoid fixation errors
	Anticipate and plan
	Allocate resources (human and equipment) effectively
	Call for help when needed
Decision-making	Team members receive orders only from leader
	Use all available relevant information
	Set priorities dynamically

identifying the specific recipients of their communication (i.e., eye contact alone is not enough given that people sometimes are not listening even when they are looking directly at someone talking to them). (2) Team leaders must give *clear and concise orders* (miscommunication occurs when orders are incomplete, short forms or abbreviations are used, or assumptions are made that the person receiving the order understands some unsaid detail of the order—this is especially true for medication orders). (3) Team members must use a *closed communication loop* when sharing information or giving/receiving orders. A proper closed communication loop includes the following steps: team member shares information with another team member or leader gives order, person receiving information/order repeats it back to ensure accuracy, and (in the case of an order) person carrying out order lets leader know when task is complete.

In order to ensure that all team members have shared situational awareness (see below), free sharing of ideas must occur. This is accomplished by team members *thinking aloud* when ideas come to them, with the *leader asking for input* from team members, and when *team members share their ideas* with the leader for consideration. Since leaders are receiving all information and trying to process it quickly in real time in order to formulate a management plan, it is not uncommon for them to miss clinical information or to not consider possible diagnoses or plans for management. Team members may think of an idea that has not yet occurred to the leader. These ideas should be shared, so that all ideas are considered before a final plan is proposed by the leader. The challenge, though, is that while it is desirable to share ideas and important information, one should be strategic and avoid distraction or disruption at crucial moments during a resuscitation event. Finally, when a new member joins the team, then they must be oriented to what is happening with the patient, so that they can be most helpful in accomplishing tasks, as well as offer useful ideas.

The *leader must receive all relevant information* about the status of the patient so that they are in the best position possible to make informed decisions about ongoing patient management (see below).

Finally, establishing a collegial and collaborative team environment is essential to good team functioning. This is accomplished by *speaking with a calm voice* (so that other team members do not misinterpret a raised tone of voice to be anger), as well as *resolving all conflicts and dealing with all distractions* (volume of noise in the room, number of people at the bedside, etc.) as quickly as possible.

information, and the ability to project future events based on this understanding" [20]. It is vital that all team members maintain as much SA as possible but recognizing that there are certain times where team members must pay full attention to performing a task, which will result in temporarily losing SA for a short period of time.

A shared understanding of the diagnosis and overall treatment plan, called *sharing a mental model,* will ensure that team members can all be as helpful and efficient as possible in carrying out their duties. Ensuring that a shared mental model exists is accomplished by some of the communication behaviors listed above, such as thinking aloud and sharing ideas. Ensuring that the correct mental model is shared is accomplished by *conducting frequent reassessments and re-evaluations* of the patient. This will ensure that changes to the patient's status will not go unrecognized by the team. These reassessments are best done: (a) after a clinical deterioration, (b) after an intervention, (c) during a pause in the action, and (d) when there is uncertainty to the cause of events. In addition, team members must *prioritize their attention effectively,* since people are only capable of holding a small number of pieces of information in our short-term memory at any one time. It would be easy for a key change in patient status to be missed if no one is paying attention at the time when the change happened. A concrete example of this is the suggestion that the leader remains hands off and does not participate in performing procedures directly on the patient. In addition, it is essential that team members *avoid making fixation errors,* which are defined as a "persistent failure to revise a diagnosis or plan in the face of readily available evidence suggesting that a revision is necessary" [21].

High-functioning teams can *anticipate and plan,* whenever possible, so that future tasks can be completed in a shorter period of time. For example, nurses in charge of the drug cart often draw up multiple doses of a medication, in anticipation that they will be needed, since it is more efficient to calculate the dose and volume only once, instead of repeating the calculation again in a few minutes.

Finally, the *resources required (both human and equipment)* for a team to complete their tasks may need to be considered. New equipment may have been brought to the patient's bedside, or the team might need to *call for help* (for advice or for someone to attend in person to help perform all necessary tasks). All these must be coordinated, typically by the leader. If there are not enough people on the team to perform all the tasks required at any given time, then the leader may have to prioritize the tasks.

Situational Awareness

Situational awareness (SA) is defined as "a person's perception of elements in the environment, comprehension of that

Decision-Making

Decisions regarding patient diagnosis and treatment must be made at several points during an acute situation such as a resuscitation. It is important that *all orders come from the leader* because they are in the best position to make the most informed decision. The leader is the person least likely to make a fixation error or miss important information because he/she should not have had their attention diverted at any time during the event. The leader (and other team members) should *use all available information* in order to come up with the best diagnosis and treatment plan, since not including certain information can lead to misdiagnosis and fixation errors. Finally, priorities may need to change at different points during the event, with changes in patient status, the incorporation of new information, or response to previous interventions. Therefore, the team should be ready and willing to *set their priorities dynamically*, so that they can quickly change course with minimal delays in providing optimal care to the patient.

Team Training: The Evidence

SBTT began in earnest in 1992 when the concepts of crisis resource management (CRM) were first introduced in anesthesiology practice [22]. Over the past 2 decades, SBTT has been extensively adopted by many healthcare professionals with the view of improving patient care and avoiding errors. With the exponential creation of simulation centers and the increasing allocation of scarce resources to SBTT, it has become imperative to review the merits and outcomes of these activities. A systematic review of published studies up until November 2012 was conducted, looking at the effect of SBTT on patient safety outcomes. Despite study variability, there was evidence that simulation training improved technical performance of individuals and teams during critical events and complex procedures [23]. Furthermore, limited evidence also supported improvements in patient outcome at the healthsystem level [15].

Another critical synthesis and literature review demonstrated significant gaps in the literature, with the need for a specific research framework to advance the ability to relate patient outcomes to SBTT, or at a minimum, risk mitigation [24]. Rigorous attention to the evidence-based development, implementation and assessment of SBTT will be needed to properly affect knowledge transfer. A similar systematic review of the transfer of learning and patient outcomes using simulated CRM management has also been conducted [25]. The authors included studies that demonstrated evidence of Kirkpatrick's levels 3 (behavior: transfer of learning to the workplace) and 4 (results: patient outcome) [26]. A total of 9 out of 7455 eligible simulation studies (up to September 2012) met those criteria. Of the nine selected studies, four showed measurable transfer of CRM learning into the clinical environment. Five studies

measured patient outcomes, with one demonstrating significantly improved patient mortality by 37% [27]. This systematic review also highlights how few CRM studies assess outcomes in the real clinical environment. Finally, a review of multiple studies in neonatal, pediatric, and adult resuscitation simulation training showed evidence of improvement in the performance of CRM team skills (e.g., leadership, interpersonal skills, distribution of workload, communication, and professional behavior), further supporting the effectiveness of CRM training in improving team functioning and dynamics [23].

A *sine qua non* of highstakes, highacuity teams is that they are interprofessional and multidisciplinary by necessity. The added complexity of team dynamics is especially true in the operating room with team members representing various surgical specialties, anesthesiology, nursing, and respiratory therapy, with a inherent historical hierarchy amongst surgical teams. A systematic review of simulation for interprofessional and multidisciplinary teams in the operating room included 18 studies from ten centers [28]. All scenarios were conducted in situ and utilized computerized mannequins and/or partial task trainers. The variable nature of technical and nontechnical (CRM) outcomes prevented direct comparisons between studies. Common barriers to implementation were reported including difficulties with recruitment, lack of surgical model fidelity, and costs. Another significant and commonly reported barrier was the challenge of providing time for in situ team training in a busy operating room environment. Contributors to success included pre-briefing, allowing adequate time for learning, and creating a safe environment of equality between nurses and physicians.

Another systematic review of interprofessional and multidisciplinary teams in the operating room included 26 studies published from 1990 to 2012 [29]. About half of the studies were conducted off-site in simulated operating rooms with an emphasis on technical skills. Two of the studies involved new procedure acquisition and led to the creation of novel safety checklists that were incorporated into clinical practice. The other point-of-care (in situ) studies were noted to be more psychologically engaging, enhanced interprofessional communication, and helped to identify and solve problems within the actual work environment.

Trauma resuscitation also requires high-functioning teams who practice excellent CRM principles. A systematic review of the trauma literature for the efficacy of simulation-based trauma team training of nontechnical skills reveals a total of 13 studies that were included for final review [30]. Seven studies were subcategorized per Kirkpatrick's levels of learning [26]. Only two studies were at the patient outcome level (level 4). One study demonstrated an improvement in time from arrival to computed tomography scanning, endotracheal intubation and final disposition to the operating room [31]. The second study found an improvement in task completion and timing to definitive treatment [32]. Neither study had an overall effect on the duration of ICU/hospital stay, morbidity, or mortality.

Finally, a systematic review of 29 articles analyzed in situ simulation for continuing healthcare professions education [33]. The salient conclusions were that appropriate needs assessments were rarely used, instructors were rarely provided with specialized assessment and feedback skills, scenarios frequently inappropriately mixed multiple levels of performance, outcome measures were informal, and evaluation methods were poor. Studies could not be properly cross–analyzed. This really reflects the current ad hoc nature of in situ professional development training for healthcare practitioners. Overall, there appears to be a lag in the appropriate development of quality continuous professional development simulation-based team training compared to curriculum-driven simulation-based team training in undergraduate and postgraduate professions' education.

Taken as a whole, the current body of evidence suggests a need to move towards more meaningful research that utilizes evidence-based best practices in developing validated tools of SBTT instruction and assessment. Very little is known about the potential impact on organizations and practice. Future studies assessing patient outcomes will help in the quest for ultimately mitigating errors and improving patient safety.

Team Training: Incorporation into Established Curricula

Simulation has been used extensively in pediatric acute care team training and assessment including resuscitation, pediatric medicine, anesthesia, critical care medicine, and trauma care.

Resuscitation

The pediatric advanced life support (PALS) course developed and offered by the American Heart Association offers the fundamentals of resuscitation education for those involved in providing pediatric acute care. PALS is a 2-day, 14-h course that provides guidelines and protocols for identification and acute management of airway, respiratory and cardiac problems [34]. Use of mannequins and task trainers has always been a feature of these courses. Over the years, there has been a transition away from didactic presentations to video-based discussions and small-group learning using simulation and hands-on practice. The most recent editions have placed an additional emphasis on teamwork skills,

with the integration of video-based discussion. Scripted debriefing to aid in the debriefing of simulation scenarios has also been incorporated into the most recent iterations of the course [35]. One of the challenges in the delivery of these courses is that frequently the participants are from diverse backgrounds and professional designations with variable education needs. Many of these courses also take place outside of the participants' home institution and are likely not in the context of the participants' usual clinical environment. Some learners are placed in leadership roles, even though they may never assume a similar position in their normal work environment. Many institutions require their employees to have active certification in these courses as a minimal requirement to participate on pediatric acute care teams. PALS is meant to be part of a larger continuing education program [36], but there is a historical reliance on PALS training itself and its recertification every 2 years to maintain essential competencies. It has been demonstrated that PALS knowledge is actually insufficient for in-hospital resuscitation and is not sustained over time [37]. Simulation-based studies have revealed inadequate training for leadership and equipment use leading to delays in treatment [38].

Pediatrics

Limitations with the PALS model suggest that it is necessary to provide an ongoing practice for acute resuscitation with hospital-based care providers. The knowledge and skills that are used in everyday practice may not be sufficient to deal with the variety of medical issues that may be encountered during cardiopulmonary arrest situations. A number of studies have demonstrated the effectiveness of mock code programs in terms of self-perception of confidence and preparedness and a decrease in anxiety [39]. Incorporation of team training and human error curriculum into a Neonatal Resuscitation Program has led to an increase in team behavior, including information sharing, inquiry and assertion, evaluation of plan, vigilance, and workload management. Simulated resuscitation practices were completed in a shorter time. The effect on team behaviors persisted for at least 6 months after the initial training [40, 41]. Impact on clinical outcome was demonstrated in a study that observed increased survival rates that correlated with increased number of mock codes [42]. In a modular, standardized, simulation-based resuscitation curriculum for pediatric residents, objective assessment demonstrated correlation of increased training with higher performance scores in medical management and teamwork skills [43]. Other innovative teaching methods, such as just-in-time training [44], PALS reconstructed [45], and rapid cycle deliberate practice [46] have been developed to improve the learning outcomes of pediatric acute care providers.

Anesthesia

The principles of anesthesia management are generally translatable for patients of all ages; however, the practice of pediatric anesthesia requires specific knowledge and skills, which can be incorporated into context-specific team training exercises. The operating room (OR) is generally thought of as the main site where acute care team training should take place for anesthesiologists and anesthesia trainees. In fact, interprofessional team training for three main healthcare professions in the OR (anesthesiologists, nursing staff, and surgeons) would be more valuable overall than the uniprofessional training of one group. Team leadership is normally assumed by the anesthesiologists for medical crises, but there are other situations where there are conflicting priorities such that each professional group may wish to lead and/or direct team members to manage their own primary concern. In order to recreate these complex situations, task trainers that are familiar to surgeons or equipment that is normally managed by nursing staff can be incorporated into the setup of a traditional simulation mannequin with a vital signs monitor in order to increase the cognitive load on the participants. As an example, a laparoscopic nephrectomy model can be placed on top of a simulation mannequin, and the usual drapes and equipment will recreate a typical OR set-up. During a crisis, such as hypovolemic shock, the surgeons may require additional equipment to control the bleeding and the anesthesiologists may require additional resuscitation medications and fluids. Nursing resources may be limited. Perfection of teamwork skills would be essential to expertly manage such complex events. One limiting factor is that pediatric-sized surgical models are not always readily available commercially and may need to be innovatively created at the local sites.

In situ simulation that involves real teams in the real-work environment may add realism and increased engagement in the simulation. Clinical decision-making skills and teamwork were effectively taught in a series of in situ simulations for otolaryngology teams that consisted of surgical trainees, anesthesia trainees, nurse anesthetists, and OR nurses [47]. At the Hospital for Sick Children, a series of in situ simulation sessions in the operating room uncovered system problems, which posed as latent safety threats. For example, a few medications that were requested for resuscitation were not immediately available on the arrest cart, and it was assumed their storage location was well known. Another example was difficulty in locating the code switches which was later reported to OR administration for follow-up.

A large proportion of procedural sedation and general anesthetic administration for children are actually provided outside of the OR (such as the endoscopy unit, the burn unit, oncology wards, intensive care units, and emergency departments) for various procedures such as lumbar punctures, bone marrow aspirates, and closed fracture reductions, among many others. Other off-site sedation locations include diagnostic imaging (for use in magnetic resonance imaging, interventional radiology, and cardiac intervention units). In situ simulation can certainly be used to determine system issues and processes in all these environments where expertise and resources may not be as readily available as in the operating room.

Team Training: Incorporating Teamwork Principles into a Simulation Scenario

Most SBTT currently occurs in either university- or hospital-based simulation centers or increasingly in the in situ context-enhanced simulation training environment.

Irrespective of the site of training, the four major elements of the framework for SBTT remain constant: role responsibility, communication, situational awareness, and decision-making. Simulation exercise setup is discussed in more detail in Chap. 2.

The first elements to consider are the *purpose* and *aims* of simulation activity. Although this seems intuitive, clearly defined learning outcomes that align with the curriculum are often poorly considered, misaligned, or too many goals are created for a single SBTT activity. The type of knowledge, skills, and attitudes or behaviors addressed in simulation refers to the various learning domains that need to be considered in SBTT. Learning outcomes should be developed and aligned to the level of expertise required within each domain.

The unit of participation in the simulation refers to the *individuals or teams* where focus is required for SBTT: both as individuals with defined roles and as part of the functional team as a unit. The experience level of simulation participants requires targeting the learning to the experience and capabilities of the participants. This is both a challenge and an opportunity in SBTT due to the heterogeneous makeup of interprofessional teams. Teamwork principles are mostly devoid of technical skills or medical expertise and the team dynamics of common goal setting take precedence. Occasionally, novice healthcare providers are integrated into experienced teams for SBTT. This can be used as an excellent opportunity to highlight the importance of recognizing role limitations, asking for help, and speaking-up.

The healthcare domain in which the simulation is applied provides context for SBTT. Various examples include surgical care, pediatric critical care, neonatal intensive care, and emergency care, among others. The healthcare disciplines of personnel participating in the simulation also intersect with the previous elements. Personnel may not be limited to physicians, nurses, and respiratory therapists but should include all usual team member roles, depending on the context. SBTT may even include non-direct patient healthcare

Table 4.2 How to incorporate teamwork learning objectives into a simulation scenario. (Reprinted with permission from Cheng et al. [48])

Crisis resource management principles	Strategy to incorporate crisis management principle into the scenario
Leadership	Wave effect[a]—introduce team members in a sequential fashion (e.g., nurses → residents → fellow)
	Introduce a new team member
	Introduce a potential, new team leader (e.g., critical care physician, anesthesiologist)
Communication	Take people out of their comfort zone (e.g., start scenarios without nurse/without doctors)
	Introduce *handover*, for example, paramedic handing over to emergency team; nursing handover at shift change
	Introduce a scripted medication error
	Withhold information (e.g., relevant medical history)
	Give critical information to a team member (e.g., blood glucose) during critical point in scenario (e.g., cardiac arrest)
	Introduce a parent or caregiver as a potential distractor
Teamwork (human resources)	Challenge team with multiple tasks/problems (e.g., hypoglycemia, seizure, hypotension, respiratory arrest)
	Wave effect[a]—introduce team members in a sequential fashion (e.g., nurses → residents → fellows)
	Introduce a junior team member (e.g., medical student)
	Introduce parents or team members who are distractors
	Introduce a team member who makes some mistakes
	Use phone calls
	Provide fewer team members
Resource use	Withhold critical equipment (e.g., defibrillator)
	Provide broken or improperly sized equipment (e.g., rupture endotracheal tube cuff)
	Provide an abundance of resources (e.g., scatter multiple endotracheal tubes on top of crash cart)
	Use a phone call to introduce the case and allow time for team to prepare for resuscitation (e.g., trauma arriving to emergency department)
Situational awareness	Design challenging scenario with more frequent physiological changes
	Design scenario history, physical or case progression to promote fixation error (e.g., cardiogenic shock from myocarditis presenting as vomiting and diarrhea)
	Challenge team leader to prioritize by providing laboratory and radiology results or introducing team members during critical points in scenario (e.g., during intubation)
	Introduce a team member who makes mistakes

[a] Wave effect is defined as the sequential introduction of team members during a simulated resuscitation. The benefit of this strategy is that each time a team member is introduced, there should be some sort of communication between new and existing team members. This strategy also provides the initial one or two providers the opportunity to manage the patient directly, often desirable for more junior learners

providers such as unit clerks, administrative staff and housekeeping staff.

A useful conceptual framework in SBTT scenario design is based on utilizing the naturalist approach versus the pre-scripted approach [48]. The naturalist approach relies on real-time chance opportunities to elicit and observe CRM behaviors from team members. Even if the scenario was primarily designed to teach non-CRM skills such as technical skills, SBTT inevitably leads to many time points where CRM principles can be highlighted. This constructivist approach requires significant instructor skill in capturing these points for discussion during debriefing. Although this approach has the potential advantage of less preparation time and perhaps lower resource utilization, there is a real risk of failing to elicit important CRM principles. The naturalist approach may be best reserved for highly skilled teams that have the opportunity for frequent practice. The behaviorist-based pre-scripted approach relies on purposeful scenario design crafted to elicit specific CRM behaviors. Case deve-

lopment and progression; the use of standardized patients as confederates or distractors; careful control of the simulated environment with the addition or withholding of data—all must be carefully pre-scripted. Triggers need to be embedded [49]. Multiple strategies for linking CRM principles to scenario design are described in Table 4.2. Scenario designers should avoid *over pre-scripting* whereby participants can become overwhelmed with information overload and stress and ultimately disengage from the case. Trickery, and overacting should be avoided.

The pre-scripted approach allows for the alignment of the participants' prior experience, the learning objectives, and the debriefing methods. This framework is appropriate for all learners and is especially useful when specific CRM principles need to be addressed. This approach also works well for isolated learning events and longitudinaltiered learning. The potential disadvantages of longer preparation time, higher resource utilization, and perhaps higher costs are outweighed by the increased ability to tailor SBTT learning.

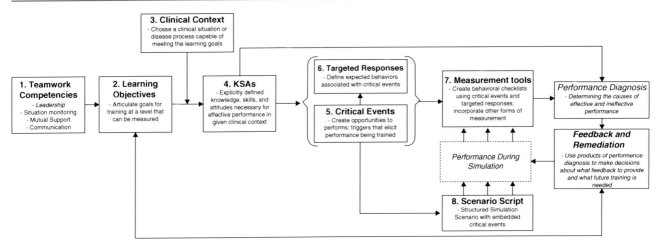

Fig. 4.2 Event-based approach to training (EBAT). (With permission from Rosen et al. [49])

The feedback method(s) accompanying simulation is essential to create learning and should be predetermined as part of the planning process. Various models of feedback and methodologies are described in greater detail in Chap. 3.

The event-based approach to training (EBAT) utilizes a methodology that links critical events with targeted responses in the domains of knowledge, skills, and attitudes (Fig. 4.2) [49]. These sequential steps create a set of targeted competencies that link the specific learning outcomes to specific performance metrics and facilitate enhanced longitudinal curriculum development in SBTT.

Another useful evidence-based framework for creating learning in SBTT (although not unique to SBTT) was developed in which specific elements of SBTT training were included [50]: focus training content on critical teamwork competencies; emphasize teamwork and team processes over task work; guide training based on desired team-based learning outcomes and organizational resources; incorporate hands-on, guided practice; match similar on-the-job mental processes and simulation-based training content to augment training relevance and transfer to practice; provide both outcome and behavior-based feedback; evaluate training impact through clinical outcomes and work behaviors and reinforce desired teamwork behaviors through coaching and performance evaluation [50]. A useful framework of best practices for evaluating team training in healthcare was created through the Joint Commission in the USA (2011) [51] These best practices include recommendations on sources of information to be used when designing evaluation plans, consideration of the organizational context of teams, variance of performance to be expected, timeframe to be used, and dissemination plans [51]. We are only starting to evaluate work-based outcomes and transfer to practice. Ultimately SBTT should have a positive impact on clinical processes, clinical outcomes, and enhanced patient safety, but it will need to be measured objectively.

Debriefing Considerations

Effective debriefing is an essential aspect of SBTT. Reflection on the scenario experience and self-assessment is a powerful tool to anchor learning and to improve team functioning. Issues of the specificity, the diagnostic nature, and the timing of the feedback have tremendous influence on the learning outcomes [24]. Likewise, the *debriefer* must be trained and skilled in the use of effective debriefing.

The various methods of debriefing with their indications and limitations are presented elsewhere in this book (see Chap. 3).

Assessment Tools for Team Training

In order to create a link between SBTT and clinical outcomes and patient safety, the first challenge is to create reliable and valid tools that support the assessment of SBTT. Many assessment tools have been created that show excellent reliability and face validity but lack the robust ability to predict improved performance in the clinical setting and improved patient outcomes. There have been many tools published over the past 20 years, each focusing on different target groups and in different clinical environments (Table 4.3). Each tool incorporates different teamwork behaviors, although the content overlaps substantially, since one can argue that good teamwork should look the same, no matter what acute care clinical environment it is developed for. Some are developed as part of an overall assessment of performance during acute care/resuscitation, and some others focus on teamwork alone (see Chap. 7).

There are two broad categories that describe the target of each assessment tool: those targeted at assessing the leader and those targeted at assessing the entire team. Table 4.3 describes this breakdown. It may be easier to assess the

Table 4.3 Teamwork assessment tools for acute care medicine

Tool	Clinical environment or target of assessment	Leader versus entire team	Embedded within resuscitation assessment or stand-alone teamwork assessment	Teamwork domains included
Brett-Fleegler et al. [52]	Pediatric resident	Leader	Embedded	Professionalism Leadership Management
Cooper et al. [53, 54]	Resuscitation teams	Entire team	Stand-alone	Teamwork Leadership Task management
Fletcher et al. [55]	Consultant anesthetist	Leader	Stand-alone	Task management Team working Situation awareness Decision-making
Frankel et al. [56]	Multiple: obstetrics, operating room, and multidisciplinary rounds	Entire team	Stand-alone	Coordination Cooperation Situational awareness Communication
Gaba et al. [57]	Anesthesia	Entire team	Stand-alone	Orientation Inquiry/Advocacy/Assertion Communication Feedback Leadership/followership Group climate
Grant et al. [58]	Pediatric resident	Leader	Embedded	Leadership Communication skills
Guise et al. [19]	Obstetric teams	Entire team	Stand-alone	Role responsibility Communication Situational awareness Decision-making
Kim et al. [59]	ICU residents	Leader	Stand-alone	Leadership Situational awareness Communication skills Problem-solving Resource utilization
Lambden et al. [60]	Pediatric resident	Leader	Embedded	Communication and interaction Cooperation and team skills Leadership and managerial skills Decision-making
Mishra et al. [61]	Operating room teams	Entire team	Stand-alone	Leadership and management Teamwork and cooperation Problem-solving and decision-making Situation awareness
Reid et al. [62]	Pediatric resuscitation teams	Entire team	Embedded	Leadership Management
Sevdalis et al. [63]	Operating room teams	Entire team	Stand-alone	Communication Coordination Leadership Monitoring Cooperation
Thomas et al. [64]	Neonatal resuscitation teams	Entire team	Stand-alone	Information sharing, inquiry Assertion, intentions verbalized Teaching Evaluation of plans Workload management Vigilance/environmental awareness

Table 4.3 (continued)

Tool	Clinical environment or target of assessment	Leader versus entire team	Embedded within resuscitation assessment or stand-alone teamwork assessment	Teamwork domains included
Weller et al. [65]	Critical care unit teams	Entire team	Stand-alone	Leadership and team coordination
				Mutual performance monitoring
				Verbalizing situational information
Wright et al. [66]	Medical student teams	Team members scored individually, then averaged	Stand-alone	Appropriate assertiveness
				Decision-making
				Situation assessment
				Leadership
				Communication

performance of one individual within the team, therefore potentially improving the reliability of the tool. However, the validity of these leader-only tools may be called into question, since some elements of good teamwork behavior specifically allow for other team members to improve the overall performance of the team, despite potential limitations of the leader's performance.

Conclusions

Research in team training has greatly expanded our understanding of the importance of this type of educational opportunity in changing healthcare provider's behavior in the simulation environment. We now know what are the key elements of team training, how to incorporate specific objectives into a scenario, and how to modify this for different learners. What we do not know yet is whether this training improves learner's performance in real life, and whether this translates into improvement in patient outcome. This training is time and resource consuming; so, we must determine if it is worth the effort by linking this training to real patient outcomes. If there is a positive link, then consideration should be made to having this training offered to all healthcare providers on an ongoing basis.

References

1. Kohn L, Corrigan J, Donaldson M. To err is human: building a safer health system. Washington, DC: Institute of Medicine; 2000.
2. Brennan TA, Leape LL, Laird NM, Hebert L, Localio AR, Lawthers AG, et al. Incidence of adverse events and negligence in hospitalized patients. Results of the Harvard Medical Practice Study I. N Engl J Med. 1991;324(6):370–6.
3. Bracco D, Favre JB, Bissonnette B, Wasserfallen JB, Revelly JP, Ravussin P, et al. Human errors in a multidisciplinary intensive care unit: a 1-year prospective study. Intensive Care Med. 2001;27(1):137–45.
4. Rothschild JM, Landrigan CP, Cronin JW, Kaushal R, Lockley SW, Burdick E, et al. The critical care safety study: the incidence and nature of adverse events and serious medical errors in intensive care. Crit Care Med. 2005;33(8):1694–700.
5. Donchin Y, Gopher D, Olin M, Badihi Y, Biesky M, Sprung CL, et al. A look into the nature and causes of human errors in the intensive care unit. Crit Care Med. 1995;23(2):294–300.
6. Barrett J, Gifford C, Morey J, Risser D, Salisbury M. Enhancing patient safety through teamwork training. J Healthc Risk Manag. 2001;21(4):57–65.
7. Bergs EA, Rutten FL, Tadros T, Krijnen P, Schipper IB. Communication during trauma resuscitation: do we know what is happening? Injury. 2005;36(8):905–11.
8. Pierre M St, Hofinger G, Buerschaper C, editors. Crisis management in acute care settings: human factors and team psychology in a high stakes environment. 2nd ed. Berlin: Springer; 2013.
9. Hunziker S, Laschinger L, Portmann-Schwarz S, Semmer NK, Tschan F, Marsch S. Perceived stress and team performance during a simulated resuscitation. Intensive Care Med. 2011;37(9):1473–9.
10. Risser DT, Rice MM, Salisbury ML, Simon R, Jay GD, Berns SD. The potential for improved teamwork to reduce medical errors in the emergency department. The MedTeams Research Consortium. Ann Emerg Med. 1999;34(3):373–83.
11. Lammers RL, Willoughby-Byrwa M, Fales WD. Errors and error-producing conditions during a simulated, prehospital, pediatric cardiopulmonary arrest. Simul Healthc. 2014;9(3):174–83.
12. Hoff WS, Reilly PM, Rotondo MF, DiGiacomo JC, Schwab CW. The importance of the command-physician in trauma resuscitation. J Trauma. 1997;43(5):772–7.
13. Yeung JH, Ong GJ, Davies RP, Gao F, Perkins GD. Factors affecting team leadership skills and their relationship with quality of cardiopulmonary resuscitation*. Crit Care Med. 2012;40(9):2617–21.
14. Fernandez Castelao E, Russo SG, Cremer S, Strack M, Kaminski L, Eich C, et al. Positive impact of crisis resource management training on no-flow time and team member verbalisations during simulated cardiopulmonary resuscitation: a randomised controlled trial. Resuscitation. 2011;82(10):1338–43.
15. Knight LJ, Gabhart JM, Earnest KS, Leong KM, Anglemyer A, Franzon D. Improving code team performance and survival outcomes: implementation of pediatric resuscitation team training. Crit Care Med. 2014;42(2):243–51.
16. Gilfoyle E, Gottesman R, Razack S. Development of a leadership skills workshop in paediatric advanced resuscitation. Med Teach. 2007;29(9):e276–83.
17. Falcone RA Jr, Daugherty M, Schweer L, Patterson M, Brown RL, Garcia VF. Multidisciplinary pediatric trauma team training using high-fidelity trauma simulation. J Pediatr Surg. 2008;43(6):1065–71.
18. Clay-Williams R, Braithwaite J. Determination of healthcare teamwork training competencies: a Delphi study. Int J Qual Health Care. 2009;21(6):433–40.

19. Guise JM, Deering SH, Kanki BG, Osterweil P, Li H, Mori M, et al. Validation of a tool to measure and promote clinical teamwork. Simul Healthc. 2008;3(4):217–23.
20. Wright MC, Taekman JM, Endsley MR. Objective measures of situation awareness in a simulated medical environment. Qual Saf Health Care. 2004;13(Suppl 1):i65–71.
21. Gaba DM, Fish KJ, Howard S. Crisis management in anesthesiology. New York: Churchill Livingstone; 1994.
22. Gaba DM. Improving anesthesiologists' performance by simulating reality. Anesthesiology. 1992;76(4):491–4.
23. Schmidt E, Goldhaber-Fiebert SN, Ho LA, McDonald KM. Simulation exercises as a patient safety strategy: a systematic review. Ann Intern Med. 2013;158(5 Pt 2):426–32.
24. Eppich W, Howard V, Vozenilek J, Curran I. Simulation-based team training in healthcare. Simul Healthc. 2011;6(Suppl):S14–9.
25. Boet S, Bould MD, Fung L, Qosa H, Perrier L, et al. Transfer of learning and patient outcome in simulated crisis resource management: a systematic review. Can J Anesth. 2014;61:571–82.
26. Kirkpatrick DLKJ. Evaluating training programs—the Four Levels. 3rd ed. San Francisco: Berrett-Koehler; 2006.
27. Riley W, Davis S, Miller K, Hansen H, Sainfort F, Sweet R. Didactic and simulation nontechnical skills team training to improve perinatal patient outcomes in a community hospital. Jt Comm J Qual Patient Saf/Jt Comm Resour. 2011;37(8):357–64.
28. Cumin D, Boyd MJ, Webster CS, Weller JM. A systematic review of simulation for multidisciplinary team training in operating rooms. Simul Healthc. 2013;8(3):171–9.
29. Tan SB, Pena G, Altree M, Maddern GJ. Multidisciplinary team simulation for the operating theatre: a review of the literature. ANZ J Surg. 2014;84(7–8):515–22.
30. Gjeraa K, Moller TP, Ostergaard D. Efficacy of simulation-based trauma team training of non-technical skills. A systematic review. Acta Anaesthesiol Scand. 2014;58(7):775–87.
31. Capella J, Smith S, Philp A, Putnam T, Gilbert C, Fry W, et al. Teamwork training improves the clinical care of trauma patients. J Surg Educ. 2010;67(6):439–43.
32. Steinemann S, Berg B, Skinner A, DiTulio A, Anzelon K, Terada K, et al. In situ, multidisciplinary, simulation-based teamwork training improves early trauma care. J Surg Educ. 2011;68(6):472–7.
33. Rosen MA, Hunt EA, Pronovost PJ, Federowicz MA, Weaver SJ. In situ simulation in continuing education for the healthcare professions: a systematic review. J Contin Educ Health Prof. 2012;32(4):243–54.
34. Kleinman ME, Chameides L, Schexnayder SM, Samson RA, Hazinski MF, Atkins DL, et al. Part 14: pediatric advanced life support: 2010 American Heart Association Guidelines for Cardiopulmonary Resuscitation and Emergency Cardiovascular Care. Circulation. 2010;122(18 Suppl 3):S876–908.
35. Cheng A, Rodgers DL, van der Jagt E, Eppich W, O'Donnell J. Evolution of the Pediatric Advanced Life Support course: enhanced learning with a new debriefing tool and Web-based module for Pediatric Advanced Life Support instructors. Pediatr Crit Care Med. 2012;13(5):589–95.
36. Bhanji F, Mancini ME, Sinz E, Rodgers DL, McNeil MA, Hoadley TA, et al. Part 16: education, implementation, and teams: 2010 American Heart Association Guidelines for Cardiopulmonary Resuscitation and Emergency Cardiovascular Care. Circulation. 2010;122(18 Suppl 3):S920–33.
37. Grant EC, Marczinski CA, Menon K. Using pediatric advanced life support in pediatric residency training: does the curriculum need resuscitation? Pediatr Crit Care Med. 2007;8(5):433–9.
38. Hunt EA, Walker AR, Shaffner DH, Miller MR, Pronovost PJ. Simulation of in-hospital pediatric medical emergencies and cardiopulmonary arrests: highlighting the importance of the first 5 min. Pediatrics. 2008;121(1):e34–43.
39. Allan CK, Thiagarajan RR, Beke D, Imprescia A, Kappus LJ, Garden A, et al. Simulation-based training delivered directly to the pediatric cardiac intensive care unit engenders preparedness, comfort, and decreased anxiety among multidisciplinary resuscitation teams. J Thorac Cardiovasc Surg. 2010;140(3):646–52.
40. Thomas EJ, Taggart B, Crandell S, Lasky RE, Williams AL, Love LJ, et al. Teaching teamwork during the Neonatal Resuscitation Program: a randomized trial. J Perinatol. 2007;27(7):409–14.
41. Thomas EJ, Williams AL, Reichman EF, Lasky RE, Crandell S, Taggart WR. Team training in the neonatal resuscitation program for interns: teamwork and quality of resuscitations. Pediatrics. 2010;125(3):539–46.
42. Andreatta P, Saxton E, Thompson M, Annich G. Simulation-based mock codes significantly correlate with improved pediatric patient cardiopulmonary arrest survival rates. Pediatr Crit Care Med. 2011;12(1):33–8.
43. Stone K, Reid J, Caglar D, Christensen A, Strelitz B, Zhou L, et al. Increasing pediatric resident simulated resuscitation performance: a standardized simulation-based curriculum. Resuscitation. 2014;85(8):1099–105.
44. Sam J, Pierse M, Al-Qahtani A, Cheng A. Implementation and evaluation of a simulation curriculum for paediatric residency programs including just-in-time in situ mock codes. Paediatr Child Health. 2012;17(2):e16.
45. Kurosawa H, Ikeyama T, Achuff P, Perkel M, Watson C, Monachino A, et al. A randomized, controlled trial of in situ pediatric advanced life support recertification ("pediatric advanced life support reconstructed") compared with standard pediatric advanced life support recertification for ICU frontline providers*. Crit Care Med. 2014;42(3):610–8.
46. Hunt EA, Duval-Arnould JM, Nelson-McMillan KL, Bradshaw JH, Diener-West M, Perretta JS, et al. Pediatric resident resuscitation skills improve after "rapid cycle deliberate practice" training. Resuscitation. 2014;85(7):945–51.
47. Volk MS, Ward J, Irias N, Navedo A, Pollart J, Weinstock PH. Using medical simulation to teach crisis resource management and decision-making skills to otolaryngology housestaff. Otolaryngol Head Neck Surg. 2011;145(1):35–42.
48. Cheng A, Donoghue A, Gilfoyle E, Eppich W. Simulation-based crisis resource management training for pediatric critical care medicine: a review for instructors. Pediatr Crit Care Med. 2012;13(2):197–203.
49. Rosen MA, Salas E, Wu TS, Silvestri S, Lazzara EH, Lyons R, et al. Promoting teamwork: an event-based approach to simulation-based teamwork training for emergency medicine residents. Acad Emerg Med. 2008;15(11):1190–8.
50. Salas E, DiazGranados D, Weaver SJ, King H. Does team training work? Principles for healthcare. Acad Emerg Med. 2008;15(11):1002–9.
51. Weaver SJ, Salas E, King HB. Twelve best practices for team training evaluation in healthcare. Jt Comm J Qual Patient Saf. 2011;37(8):341–9.
52. Brett-Fleegler MB, Vinci RJ, Weiner DL, Harris SK, Shih M-C, Kleinman MEA. Simulator-based tool that assesses pediatric resident resuscitation competency. Pediatrics. 2008;121(3):e597–603.
53. Cooper SJ, Cant RP. Measuring non-technical skills of medical emergency teams: an update on the validity and reliability of the Team Emergency Assessment Measure (TEAM). Resuscitation. 2014;85(1):31–3.
54. Cooper S, Cant R, Porter J, Sellick K, Somers G, Kinsman L, et al. Rating medical emergency teamwork performance: development of the Team Emergency Assessment Measure (TEAM). Resuscitation. 2010;81(4):446–52.
55. Fletcher G, Flin R, McGeorge P, Glavin R, Maran N, Patey R. Anaesthetists' Non-Technical Skills (ANTS): evaluation of a behavioural marker system. Br J Anaesth. 2003;90(5):580–8.

56. Frankel A, Gardner R, Maynard L, Kelly A. Using the Communication and Teamwork Skills (CATS) assessment to measure healthcare team performance. Jt Comm J Qual Patient Saf. 2007;33(9):549–58.

57. Gaba DM, Howard SK, Flanagan B, Smith BE, Fish KJ, Botney R. Assessment of clinical performance during simulated crises using both technical and behavioral ratings. Anesthesiology. 1998;89(1):8–18.

58. Grant EC. The development of a valid and reliable evaluation tool for assessment of pediatric resident competence in leading simulated pediatric resuscitations: University of Calgary; 2008.

59. Kim J, Neilipovitz D, Cardinal P, Chiu M, Clinch J. A pilot study using high-fidelity simulation to formally evaluate performance in the resuscitation of critically ill patients: the University of Ottawa Critical Care Medicine, High-Fidelity Simulation, and Crisis Resource Management I Study. Crit Care Med. 2006;34(8):2167–74.

60. Lambden S, DeMunter C, Dowson A, Cooper M, Gautama S, Sevdalis N. The Imperial Paediatric Emergency Training Toolkit (IPETT) for use in paediatric emergency training: development and evaluation of feasibility and validity. Resuscitation. 2013;84(6):831–6.

61. Mishra A, Catchpole K, McCulloch P. The Oxford NOTECHS System: reliability and validity of a tool for measuring teamwork behaviour in the operating theatre. Qual Saf Health Care. 2009;18(2):104–8.

62. Reid J, Stone K, Brown J, Caglar D, Kobayashi A, Lewis-Newby M, et al. The Simulation Team Assessment Tool (STAT): development, reliability and validation. Resuscitation. 2012;83(7):879–86.

63. Sevdalis N, Lyons M, Healey AN, Undre S, Darzi A, Vincent CA. Observational teamwork assessment for surgery: construct validation with expert versus novice raters. Ann Surg. 2009;249(6):1047–51.

64. Thomas EJ, Sexton JB, Helmreich RL. Translating teamwork behaviours from aviation to healthcare: development of behavioural markers for neonatal resuscitation. Qual Saf Health Care. 2004;13(Suppl 1):i57–64.

65. Weller J, Frengley R, Torrie J, Shulruf B, Jolly B, Hopley L, et al. Evaluation of an instrument to measure teamwork in multidisciplinary critical care teams. BMJ Qual Saf. 2011;20(3):216–22.

66. Wright MC, Phillips-Bute BG, Petrusa ER, Griffin KL, Hobbs GW, Taekman JM. Assessing teamwork in medical education and practice: relating behavioural teamwork ratings and clinical performance. Med Teach. 2009;31(1):30–8.

The Role of Simulation in Improving Patient Safety

Marc Auerbach, Kimberly P. Stone and Mary D. Patterson

Simulation Pearls

1. The role of pediatric simulation in improving patient safety is evolving and has tremendous potential.
2. Simulation is increasingly being used to evaluate systems and processes in both a retrospective and prospective fashion.
3. Simulation is a powerful bridge between existing safety initiatives and frontline providers.
4. The integration of simulation into ongoing patient safety, risk reduction, and quality initiatives has great potential to demonstrate the return on investment of simulation and to improve patient outcomes.

Background

Pediatric simulation practitioners often conduct their work to improve proximal outcomes such as provider skills and teamwork. In addition, simulation can be used within the broader context of the practice and improvement of patient safety as it allows for an individual-provider and/or team-based and/or systems-based approach to patient safety. Simulation activities can be focused on a single individual (knowledge, skills, and attitudes), individuals interacting with other individuals (teamwork, communication), and

M. Auerbach (✉)
Department of Pediatrics, Section of Emergency Medicine, Yale University School of Medicine, New Haven, CT, USA
e-mail: marc.auerbach@yale.edu

K. P. Stone
Department of Pediatrics, Division of Emergency Medicine, University of Washington School of Medicine, Seattle Children's Hospital, Seattle, WA, USA
e-mail: Kimberly.stone@seattlechildrens.org

M. D. Patterson
Department of Pediatrics, Northeast Ohio Medical University, Rootstown, OH, USA
e-mail: Marydpatterson84@gmail.com

individuals interacting with systems (in situ simulation). Collaborations between simulation practitioners and safety scientists from other disciplines such as systems/industrial engineering, human factors, health-outcomes research, and the behavioral sciences are critical to future innovations in our field. The application of theory and processes from these domains has great potential to maximize the impact of simulation on improving the safety behaviors of healthcare providers/teams, technologies/devices, and the performance of the system itself.

Pediatric-specific reviews on the role of simulation in patient safety have been published and largely discuss microsystem applications of simulation including routine training for emergencies, training for teamwork, testing new procedures for safety, evaluating competence, testing device usability, investigating human performance, and providing skills training outside of the production environment [1, 2]. A number of recent publications point to the value of simulation in improving the safety of pediatric patients through translational outcomes [3–7]. Many pediatric institutions are at the cutting edge of innovation in the development of a systems-based approach to patient safety with simulation-based activities integrated into their quality, risk, and safety initiatives (see Table 5.1 for examples).

This chapter will begin with patient safety terminology; discuss the role of simulation to enhance patient safety at the provider, team, and systems level; outline the importance of systems and simulation integration in a robust patient safety program; and conclude with future directions for simulation and patient safety.

Definitions

The elements of patient safety and how it is practiced are the subject of multiple perspectives and domains, and it is important that common language be applied to the various characteristics and activities of patient safety. It is only by

© Springer International Publishing Switzerland 2016
V. J. Grant, A. Cheng (eds.), *Comprehensive Healthcare Simulation: Pediatrics*,
Comprehensive Healthcare Simulation, DOI 10.1007/978-3-319-24187-6_5

Table 5.1 Applications of simulation for patient safety

Level	Institution	Application
Provider *for example, active errors leading to complications (technical, psychomotor, cognitive)*	Multiple institutions—see INSPIRE network [60]	Skills development—bench-top task trainers in simulation labs
	Yale-New Haven Children's Hospital, New Haven, CT, USA	Skills assessment/retention—requirement to demonstrate simulation competency before performing an infant lumbar puncture
	Multiple institutions—see INSPIRE network [60]	
	Alberta Children's Hospital, Calgary, AB, Canada	Skills assessment/development—inclusion of a patient safety scenario (handover, line confusion, etc.) in annual pediatric nursing update and pediatric resident academic curriculum
	Seattle Children's Hospital, Seattle, WA, USA	Skills assessment/development—inclusion of patient safety cases (handover issues, medical error, etc.) in pediatric academic curriculum
Teams *for example, lack of shared mental model leading to drug-dosing error*	Yale-New Haven Children's Hospital, New Haven, CT, USA	Requirement to attend team-training simulations annually
	Cincinnati Children's Hospital, Cincinnati, OH, USA	
	Seattle Children's Hospital, Seattle, WA, USA	
	Cincinnati Children's Hospital, Cincinnati, OH, USA	Scenarios/debriefing on safety culture topics: flattening authority gradient, normalization of deviance
Micro-system *for example, EMR design, RCA, LST, development of new processes*	Tulane University Hospital, New Orleans, LA, USA [43, 44]	Application of simulation to improve traditional RCA methods in surgery
	Cincinnati Children's Hospital, Cincinnati, OH, USA [47]	In situ simulations to LSTs
	Cincinnati Children's Hospital, Cincinnati, OH, USA [50]	New difficult airway process developed using simulation improved the airway response system and decreased response time
	Yale-New Haven Children's Hospital, New Haven, CT, USA Seattle Children's Hospital, Seattle, WA, USA	New massive bleeding emergency protocol with iterative simulations resulted in a reliable process and decreased lab turnaround time
	Seattle Children's Hospital, Seattle, WA, USA	Usability testing in simulated environment
	Bristol Medical Simulation Centre, Bristol, UK	Creation and testing of a new child abduction policy
	McMaster Children's Hospital, Hamilton, Ontario, Canada [59]	New equipment (flow-inflating bags) tested and selected based on use in simulation
	McMaster Children's Hospital, Hamilton, Ontario, Canada [59]	Testing and implementing a new cardiac death protocol in the ICU
Macro-system *for example, patient flow, facility design/testing*	University of California at Davis Medical Center, Sacramento, CA, USA [58]	Discrete event simulations to models for ED flow
	Seattle Children's Hospital, Seattle, WA, USA	Cardboard mock-ups while designing new ED-identified inadequate room design to accommodate resuscitation team and equipment
	Children's Hospital Colorado, Aurora, CO, USA [51] Children's Hospital Philadelphia, Philadelphia, PA, USA Cincinnati Children's Hospital, Cincinnati, OH, USA Columbia University, New York, NY, USA University of Alabama, Birmingham, AL, USA McMaster Children's Hospital, Hamilton, ON, Canada Seattle Children's Hospital, Seattle, WA, USA Texas Children's Hospital, Houston, TX, USA	Testing new departments prior to opening to identify environmental and systems threats
	Alberta Children's Hospital, Calgary, AB, Canada	Formal iterative loop from formal patient safety reports to simulation program to creation and implementation of identified curriculum for providers

ED emergency department, *EMR* electronic medical record, *INSPIRE* International Network for Simulation-Based Pediatric Research, Innovation, & Education, *RCA* root cause analysis, *LST* latent safety threat assuring that there are similar concepts relative to the language and terms used in describing patient safety that programs can move forward with some confidence in work that utilizes simulation as a means to develop and enhance patient safety. Therefore, the first requirements are to define and develop common understanding of basic terms and concepts in patient safety.

Patient safety refers to *"freedom from accidental or preventable injuries produced by medical care"* [8]. Thus, practices or interventions that improve patient safety are those that reduce the occurrence of preventable adverse events. Patient safety is often described as a characteristic or something that an organization possesses or achieves. Moreover, the usual definitions of patient safety describe it in terms of what patient safety is not (i.e., the events that constitute an absence of patient safety) [9]. More realistically, patient safety is dynamic; it is something that an organization and most importantly the people in the organization think about and practice [10]. When an organization believes it has achieved *safety*, the organization may have *lost it*.

A number of frameworks exist to describe **patient safety domains**. Donabedian provided one of the earliest frameworks to describe quality of care that included three domains: (1) structure of care, (2) process of care, and (3) outcomes of care [11]. In this model, **structure** includes those things external to the patient: the environment, organizational and human resources, and the regulations and policies affecting patient care. The **process** includes what actually occurred in the care of the patient and includes the patients' and providers' activities. One might think of it as the actual work

performed in caring for the patient. Finally, the **outcome** describes the effect of the care on the individual patient as well as the population as a whole [11].

More recent safety frameworks provide more detail, specifically describing the patient, healthcare providers, and system factors that affect patient safety. For example, the Systems Engineering Initiative for Patient Safety (SEIPS) model describes patient safety in terms of the interactions, relationships, and influences of various system components, including the individuals that are part of the system [12] (see Fig. 5.1). This more sophisticated and multifactorial model allows for a more nuanced view of the various elements that affect patient care.

The terms *quality* and *safety* in healthcare are sometimes confused or used interchangeably. In order to clarify this confusion, the Institute of Medicine describes six elements of high-quality patient care. High-quality care is safe, effective, efficient, patient-centered, timely, and equitable [13]. In this model, safety is described as only one element of quality healthcare. An alternative way to think about the relationship between safety and quality is to envision safety as the floor or threshold of care and quality as the ceiling or goal [14]. Healthcare may be safe but not meet the other six targets for quality of care established by the Institute of Medicine. However, safe care is a requisite element of high-quality healthcare.

High-reliability organizations (HROs) manage to conduct operations in high-risk environments in a remarkably safe fashion. HROs are defined as organizations that operate in high-risk environments or are engaged in high-risk

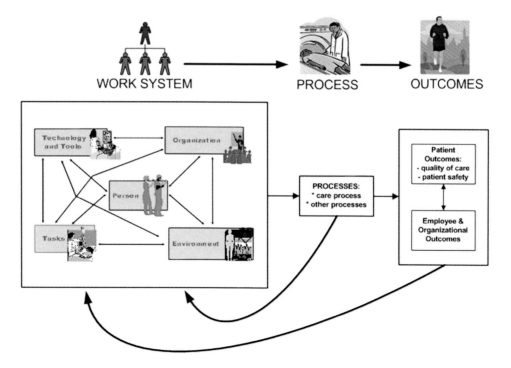

Fig. 5.1 Systems Engineering Initiative for Patient Safety model of work system and patient safety. (Reproduced with permission from [12] (BMJ Publishing Group))

activities but suffer fewer than expected adverse events. Some examples of industries with HROs include commercial aviation, military (aircraft carriers), and nuclear power. HROs have five specific characteristics that have been described: (1) reluctance to simplify, (2) sensitivity to operations, (3) deference to expertise, (4) preoccupation with failure, and (5) commitment to resilience [15]. In recent years, a number of healthcare organizations have attempted to develop an HRO culture and practice HRO behaviors. Of interest, many of the types of organizations that are exemplars of an HRO utilize simulation and/or regular training as a tool to develop and maintain an HRO culture and HRO behaviors [16]. For example, licensed civilian nuclear power plants in the USA require their operators to participate in ongoing simulation-based training approximately 25% of the time that they are working. The Nuclear Regulatory Commission sets standards for the fidelity of the nuclear simulators, the types of training, and scenarios that should occur as well as standards for simulation instructors [17].

Simulation-Based Patient Safety Activities at the Provider Level

At the core of patient safety are healthcare providers equipped with the knowledge and skills necessary to safely diagnose and treat patients and their varied, often complex, medical concerns. This applies to both trainees and frontline providers in all healthcare fields—medicine, nursing, pharmacy, respiratory therapy, etc. Herein lies one of the fundamental tensions in healthcare provider education—providing trainees the opportunities to learn while at the same time providing safe care to patients. Since its introduction into healthcare, simulation has been used successfully to improve providers' knowledge, skills, behaviors, and attitudes. A large systematic review reported that simulation-based training was associated with large effects for outcomes of confidence, knowledge, skills, attitudes, and behaviors [18]. A review conducted specifically in pediatrics noted large effects on knowledge, skills, and behaviors in 57 studies [19]. Further discussion of this evidence can be found in this book, Chaps. 7 ("Assessment"), 13 ("Simulation along the healthcare education continuum"), and 15 ("Interprofessional Education"). Through simulation, the apprenticeship paradigm of *"do one, see one, teach one"* is giving way to a thoughtful competency-based approach with graded levels of supervision and independence or entrustment assigned to the trainee based (in part) on performance in a simulated setting. These efforts will continue to ensure that providers at all levels and in all disciplines work in an environment in which they can develop and maintain their skills while keeping patients safe.

With the increasing focus on competency and the rapid pace at which new equipment, technologies, procedures, and processes are incorporated into healthcare, simulation can provide a means by which providers can continually train, practice, and be assessed in an ongoing manner. In some institutions, healthcare providers are being required to demonstrate competency with new equipment, technology, and processes in order to receive and/or maintain clinical privileges. At a national level, anesthesia leads the medical field and has included simulation as part of the maintenance of professional certification of physicians through the American Board of Anesthesiology since 2010. All physicians seeking recertification are required to participate in 6 h of simulations and structured debriefs and to identify areas of improvement in their own practices [20, 21]. Since 2009, residents completing surgical residencies in the USA have been required to successfully complete a Fundamentals of Laparoscopic Surgery course. While other specialty boards (e.g., family medicine) utilize computer-based simulations, no other medical boards require full-body or haptic-type simulations for initial certification or recertification [21]. Currently, simulation is not part of the pediatric board examination process; however, many institutions have started to implement simulation as a requirement at the local level (examples in Table 5.1). The application of simulation for summative assessment has been limited by the availability of robust assessment tools that are sufficiently valid to inform these high-stakes decisions (see also Chap. 7 "Assessment").

Recent studies have taken the important step of translating improvements in knowledge and skill into improved patient outcomes. A systematic review noted 50 studies reporting patient outcomes and that simulation was associated with small to moderate benefits on patient outcomes [22]. In fields outside of pediatrics, significant effects have been noted for central-line placement [23], obstetrical-neonatal outcomes [4], and laproscopic surgery [24]. Unfortunately, of the 50 studies included in this review, only 4 were in pediatrics [22]. One such pediatric study showed improved cardiopulmonary arrest survival rates for pediatric patients following the implementation of simulation-based *mock code* resident resuscitation training [3]. Additional pediatric studies have demonstrated a positive effect of simulation on acquisition of procedural skills (see also Chap. 11).

Simulation also has a role in advancing providers' adherence to established patient safety tools, such as the use of care bundles. For example, evidence-based practice to decrease central-line infections have been well studied with the result being an effective bundle of practices that, when performed together, have a significant impact on the rate of central-line-associated bloodstream infections. What was unclear was the best way to ensure that staff were trained and followed the recommended procedures. A simulation-based intervention reduced central-line infections by 74% compared with a unit in which residents were not required to undergo training [25]. Additionally, this intervention was noted to be highly cost-effective with a net annual savings of US$700,000 per US$100,000 allocated [26]. Unfortunately, cost-benefit analyses are infrequent and incomplete in most simulation studies [27].

Simulation-Based Patient Safety Activities at the Team Level

The role of teamwork and communication in improving patient safety is well established, with studies demonstrating deficiencies in these domains contributing to an estimated 70% of medical errors [28]. Interprofessional simulation provides a training ground for teams to practice and improve their teamwork and communication skills. Numerous studies have incorporated simulation-based teamwork training modules and identified improvement in teamwork behaviors. [29–34]. An example of a well-developed and widely disseminated team-training program is the Agency for Healthcare Research and Quality (AHRQ) TeamSTEPPS program [35]. Compared to a didactic-only TeamSTEPPS program, a simulation-based TeamSTEPPS program was associated with 37% decrease in adverse outcomes. [29]. Likewise, a systematic review noted that in nine studies, simulation-based crisis resource management training translated to improved patient outcomes and decreased mortality [36].

Simulation affords the opportunity to embed key behaviors in high-risk clinical endeavors. For example, the concept of a shared mental model was introduced and practiced in simulation-based training in a pediatric emergency department. This term is common to safety science and refers to the team members being "on the same page" [37]. In practice, sharing a mental model involves four elements: "this is what I think is going on," "this is what we have done," "this is what we need to do," and "does anyone have any other ideas" or "what am I missing." We encourage team leaders to share a mental model in the first 3–5 min of any crisis situation and to update it frequently. Alternatively, any team member can ask for the mental model or that the mental model be updated when the situation is not progressing as expected or the situation is confusing. The introduction of this concept was viewed as so helpful by emergency nurses in one study that they incorporated it as a required item in a resuscitation flow sheet. If the team leader had not shared a mental model in the first 3–5 min of caring for a patient, the nursing team leader would request it [6].

Handoffs between providers are another example of key safety behaviors ripe for simulation-based process improvement and research [38]. One institution incorporated simulation-based handoff training into teamwork and communication training following a serious event investigation that identified lack of handoff standardization as a root cause of the serious event. Observations after the training demonstrated an increase in the communication of crucial information between nurses during handoffs [39]. Another group used simulated patient cases to study patient handoffs as a first step in creating an effective, standardized handoff process [40].

Simulation-Based Patient Safety Activities at the System Level

The preceding paragraphs focus on the potential to improve providers' and team performance in order to reduce patient harm. Newer approaches to patient safety involve a systems-based approach with the view that errors or safety threats reflect the risks and hazards that providers and patients face in the context of a poorly designed system [41, 42]. Instead of focusing on individual failings, this approach identifies the components of the system that contribute to harm and involves the implementation of systemic changes that minimize the likelihood of these events. A robust simulation-based patient safety program involves identification of system threats using both retrospective reviews of adverse events and near misses as well as prospective efforts to identify and mitigate risk before an actual patient incident occurs (examples are provided in Table 5.1).

Retrospective Approach to Safety at the System Level

Simulation can be used to retrospectively examine why an error occurred (e.g., simulation-informed root cause analysis (RCA)). Simulation of adverse outcomes (SAO) has been used in the surgical arena as a method of conducting investigations of the causality of adverse surgical outcomes [43, 44]. This process involved conducting each simulation up to seven times (with debriefings) to identify sources of errors in order to augment traditional RCA processes. The addition of simulation and re-creation of adverse events identified an increased number of systems issues compared to a traditional RCA. The debriefings allowed for a greater understanding of *why* and *how* decisions leading to the adverse event were made. By re-creating the adverse event, it became possible to understand what the individual team members were seeing and hearing that made the actions seem logical at the time of the event. These types of simulations can also identify periods of heavy workload, possible task fixation, and loss of situation awareness.

Prospective Approach to Safety at the System Level

Prospective risk reduction applies methods developed in the engineering community (e.g., human factors or ergonomics, systems engineering, probabilistic risk assessment, cognitive task analysis) and used in other HROs combined with simulation techniques to optimize the safety of the system. A good example was the use of simulation during implementation of a new electronic medical record. When Yale-New Haven Children's Hospital implemented a new electronic medical record, simulation was used for provider training. The program collaborated with human factors engineers and informatics experts to provide feedback on the usability of the system in the clinical environment from providers during in situ simulations prior to formal implementation in the clinical environment. One specific example from this work was a group of simulations that provided information on the implications of nurses working with a new electronic medical record while concurrently caring for a severely injured trauma patient in the actual clinical environment. This work identified that it was difficult for the documenting nurse to see the vital signs on the monitor while working on the electronic record. The documenting nurse also reported multiple challenges with the usability of the graphic user interface. This work resulted in a requirement for an additional nurse in trauma resuscitations due to the increased workload during the first months of implementation (Marc Auerbach, written communication, October 2014).

Another familiar use of simulation to prospectively improve safety is through the use of in situ simulation to identify potential latent safety threats (LSTs). LSTs have been defined as systems-based threats to patient safety that can materialize at any time and are previously unrecognized by healthcare providers [45]. In situ simulation in a pediatric emergency department (ED) proved a practical method for the detection of LSTs as well as reinforcing team training [46–49]. In its most effective form, in situ simulation can become a routine expectation of staff that positively influences operations and the safety climate in high risk-clinical settings [6]. In situ simulation can also be used to monitor the impact of other risk reduction strategies (new processes and procedures) through on-demand measurement and is discussed in more detail in Chap. 12 (examples are provided in Table 12.1). The authors encourage simulation practitioners to collaborate with content experts as they embark on these types of systems-level simulation-based initiatives.

Simulation for Improving the Safety of New Processes

Incorporating simulation into process development offers an opportunity to *road test* the process and revise it before clinical implementation. In one institution, a new process for response to critical airways was developed and tested using simulation [50]. Six simulations were conducted at baseline, and six simulations were conducted to test the new critical airway response. While two of the six simulated patients "died" in the original airway response system, no simulated patients "died" in the new airway response system. In addition, there was a significant decrease in the otolaryngologist's response time to the emergency department. In another experience, five iterative simulations were used in the development of a massive bleeding emergency protocol. The final protocol was more pragmatic and reliable for staff and resulted in marked reductions in laboratory turnaround times for crucial bleeding labs (Kimberly Stone, written communication, October 2014).

Simulation to Improve the Safety of New Environments

Simulation has been used to test the staffing model and safety of a new pediatric ED [5], a new general ED [6], and a children's hospital's obstetrical unit [51]. In the case of the new pediatric ED, in situ simulation prior to clinical occupancy resulted in changes to team members' roles and responsibilities as well as identifying latent threats in the new clinical space. Several hospitals have successfully utilized in situ simulation prior to opening new hospital units to identify and mitigate LSTs identified before caring for patients as documented in Table 5.1 [51].

Systems Integration: Simulation–Patient Safety–Quality

Simulation programs can maximize their impact on safety through systems integration. Systems integration is defined by the Society for Simulation in Healthcare (SSH) as "consistent, planned, collaborative, integrated and iterative application of simulation-based assessment and teaching activities with systems engineering and risk management principles to achieve excellent bedside clinical care, enhanced patient safety, and improved metrics across the healthcare system" [52]. An institution's simulation activities should be

Table 5.2 Opportunities to integrate simulation within existing patient safety initiatives

Patient safety initiative	Simulation *value added*
Quality improvement—event reporting	Simulation-based in situ events reported in system
Quality improvement—PDSA	Simulation integrated into PDSA
Risk management (incident or safety reports including those that do not meet the criteria for a serious safety event)	Simulation to re-create patient safety events for RCA or to re-create potential adverse events or near misses that do not meet the criteria of a serious safety event
Guidelines/committees	Testing new processes/policies/procedures
Human resources	Simulation in interview process
Biomedical engineering	Testing/training for new products
Systems engineering	Studying/improving flow of patients
Architecture/facilities	Testing new spaces/redesigning existing spaces
Performance improvement	Lean, Six Sigma integrated with simulations

PDSA plan, do, study, act, *RCA* root cause analysis, *FMEA* failure mode effects analysis

integrated into ongoing safety programs. Examples of opportunities for integration are listed in Table 5.2. This integration should result in regular bi-directional flow of information between these groups. For example, the goals and objectives of simulation-based exercises are created based on perceived risk, adverse events, and near misses identified from realpatient databases. Subsequently, the simulations and debriefings inform the analysis of how to reduce risk. Optimally, simulations and debriefings identify and bring attention to risks that may not have been otherwise recognized and help organizations to anticipate and mitigate harm to patients. In Fig. 5.2, we provide an example of how simulation can be integrated into ongoing patient safety activities after a serious event (see also Chap. 6 "Systems Integration").

In an integrated system, simulation-based activities are a part of everyday activities of an institution that is expected by staff as part of their daily work. Additionally, in some established programs, errors or threats identified in simulation are reported in the hospital event reporting system in the same manner that a real patient event is reported (e.g., Yale-New Haven Children's Hospital, Seattle Children's Hospital). This provides a clear reporting structure, allows for prioritization and tracking of actionable findings, and applies the accepted quality and safety nomenclature to simulation-based events (near miss, serious safety event, etc.). Formal reporting of simulation-identified threats also removes the responsibility of the mitigation of identified risks from the simulation team as, typically, the simulation team or program will not have the ability to influence the multiple factors often involved in systems issues. The risk is when providers participate in simulations, but do not believe that feedback from those sessions will be heard or lead to change, they come to believe that the organization is building safety only on the backs of the increased vigilance of providers rather than by addressing system issues[45]. An effective simulation *culture* exists when there is *buy-in* from the highest level of leadership

(top-down) and from the frontline providers (bottom-up) across multiple disciplines.

Barriers/Challenges to Simulation in Patient Safety

In order to fully realize the potential of simulation to improve the practice of patient safety, it will be critical to develop tools that are able to link simulation practices to improvement in patient outcomes. It will also be necessary to leverage the expertise of those working in various fields of safety sciences in domains external to healthcare. Terry Fairbanks, human factors expert and emergency physician, has stated that when airlines wanted to become safer, they did not ask pilots and flight attendants how to become safer, they involved engineers, cognitive psychologists, and human factors experts (Terry Fairbanks, written communication, June 2013).

The cost of implementing simulation in terms of provider time, instructor time, and equipment/resources can be balanced through savings related to improved quality of care, avoidance of adverse events, reduction in malpractice and liability insurance, and decreased litigation costs. Additional study is needed to understand the cost avoidance associated with simulation-based safety activities.

Future Directions

Though simulation has historically been utilized to assess individual and team competencies, in recent years simulation is increasingly being used to assess system competencies and to evaluate new facilities, new teams, and new processes [5, 6, 50, 51]. Historically, healthcare providers have not embraced expertise that originated outside of healthcare;

Fig. 5.2 Example of simulation integration into patient safety. *IV* intravenous, *IO* intraosseous, *RN* registered nurse, *RCA* root cause analysis, *EMR* electronic medical record

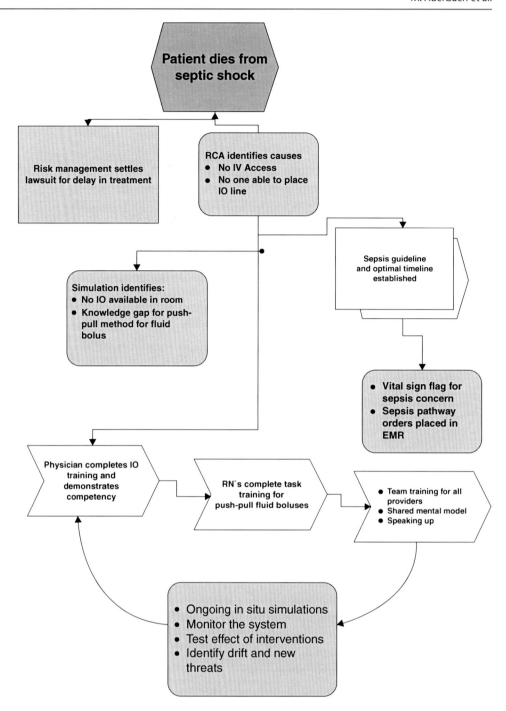

however, increasingly, there is a recognition of relevant expertise in fields outside of healthcare and a willingness to incorporate this expertise in healthcare simulation and safety work. This includes recognition of the value of human factors, cognitive task analysis, and engineering (cognitive, industrial, and systems) in addressing some of the major issues facing healthcare today.

In recent years, resident work hours in the USA have been reduced. Though the hours and length of shifts for residents have substantially decreased from the typical number of hours worked by residents a decade ago, there has not been a corresponding increase in the length of postgraduate medical training [53, 54]. It is well described that expertise in any domain is related to the hours spent in deliberate practice and coaching [55]. A significant issue for those in medical education is how to assure competence with a decreased number of hours devoted to training and an ever-increasing knowledge base. The question of whether simulation can accelerate the development of expertise is beginning to be explored but is yet unanswered [56]. It is clear that simulation-based deliberate practice in laparoscopic surgery or central line placement results in improved performance in an actual clinical environment [22–26]. However, it is less clear that non-procedural expertise, for example, recognition of the patient with sepsis, is sensitive to simulation-based training. To understand the effect of simulation on the development of this type of medical expertise will require collaboration with experts in the development of expertise, naturalistic decision-making, and cognitive bias and de-biasing.

Another area of safety that is suitable for simulation is the exploration of the adaptive capacity of systems and teams relative to unexpected disturbances. This is related to the safety science of resilience engineering. While resilience engineering is employed in other industries, it has only recently surfaced in healthcare. Often, resilience engineering is concerned with retrospective evaluation of systems that have failed or succeeded spectacularly such as the space shuttle Columbia and Challenger disasters [57]. Though still theoretical, simulation offers a prospective way to evaluate systems' adaptive responses, tolerance for disturbance, and ability to recover from disruptions to the system. In healthcare, this could mean evaluation of existing and proposed systems relative to normal function and the ability to adapt to and recover from unexpected events in healthcare. Simulation also offers a method to evaluate the effect of proposed changes in the system relative to adaptive capacity and the brittleness of a system in the face of changing resources, for example, staffing, team configuration, and institution of an electronic health record.

In the future, as a simulation community, we will need to demonstrate that integrated simulation-based patient safety programs lead to measurable improvements in the healthcare that is delivered, a financial return on investment, and improved health outcomes.

Conclusions

Simulation is a natural partner for ongoing patient safety activities at the individual, team, and systems levels of organizations. A growing number of simulation-based training programs are linking their program improvements in knowledge, skills, and teamwork to patient outcomes. Increasingly, simulation is being used at the systems level to identify and mitigate patient safety risks. Simulation can facilitate the discovery of error-producing conditions before those conditions affect patients and a deeper understanding of these conditions when they have affected patients. Safety science and simulation experts will need to integrate and coordinate their activities within existing and new programs in order to achieve maximum patient safety.

References

1. Griswold S, Ponnuru S, Nishisaki A, Szyld D, Davenport M, Deutsch ES, et al. The emerging role of simulation education to achieve patient safety: translating deliberate practice and debriefing to save lives. Pediatr Clin North Am. 2012;59(6):1329–40.
2. Nishisaki A, Keren R, Nadkarni V. Does simulation improve patient safety? Self-efficacy, competence, operational performance, and patient safety. Anesthesiol Clin. 2007;25(2):225–36.
3. Andreatta P, Saxton E, Thompson M, Annich G. Simulation-based mock codes significantly correlate with improved pediatric patient cardiopulmonary arrest survival rates. Pediatr Crit Care Med. 2011;12(1):33–8.
4. Draycott T, Sibanda T, Owen L, Akande V, Winter C, Reading S, et al. Does training in obstetric emergencies improve neonatal outcome? BJOG. 2006;113(2):177–82.
5. Geis GL, Pio B, Pendergrass TL, Moyer MR, Patterson MD. Simulation to assess the safety of new healthcare teams and new facilities. Simul Healthc. 2011;6(3):125–33.
6. Patterson MD, Geis GL, Falcone RA, LeMaster T, Wears RL. In situ simulation: detection of safety threats and teamwork training in a high risk emergency department. BMJ Qual Saf. 2013;22(6):468–77.
7. Patterson MD, Geis GL, LeMaster T, Wears RL. Impact of multidisciplinary simulation-based training on patient safety in a paediatric emergency department. BMJ Qual Saf. 2013;22(5):383–93.
8. http://www.psnet.ahrq.gov/popup_glossary.aspx?name=patientsafety. Accessed 9 Jan 2014.
9. Lawton R, Taylor N, Clay-Williams R, Braithwaite J. Positive deviance: a different approach to achieving patient safety. BMJ Qual Saf. 2014;23:880–3.
10. Frankel AS, Leonard MW, Denham CR. Fair and just culture, team behavior, and leadership engagement: the tools to achieve high reliability. Health Serv Res. 2006;41(4 Pt 2):1690–709.
11. Donabedian A. The quality of care. How can it be assessed? JAMA. 1988;260(12):1743–8.
12. Carayon P, Schoofs Hundt A, Karsh BT, Gurses AP, Alvarado CJ, Smith M, et al. Work system design for patient safety: the SEIPS model. Qual Saf Health Care. 2006;15(Suppl 1):50–8.
13. Institute of Medicine (U.S.). Committee on Quality of Health Care in America editor. Crossing the quality chasm: a new health system for the 21st century. Vol. xx. Washington, D.C.: National Academy Press; 2001. p. 337.
14. Stevens P, Matlow A, Laxer R. Building from the blueprint for patient safety at the hospital for sick children. Healthc Quart. 2005;8:132–9.
15. Weick KE, Sutcliffe KM. Managing the unexpected: assuring high performance in an age of complexity. 1st ed. Vol. xvi. San Francisco: Jossey-Bass; 2001. p. 200.
16. Chassin MR, Loeb JM. High-reliability healthcare: getting there from here. Milbank Q. 2013;91(3):459–90.
17. International Atomic Energy Agency. Use of control room simulators for training of nuclear power plant personnel Vienna. Austria: Nuclear Power Engineering Section, International Atomic Energy Agency; 2004. p. 101. http://www-pub.iaea.org/MTCD/publications/PDF/te_1411_web.pdf.
18. Cook DA, Hatala R, Brydges R, Zendejas B, Szostek JH, Wang AT, et al. Technology-enhanced simulation for health professions education: a systematic review and meta-analysis. JAMA. 2011;306(9):978–88.
19. Cheng A, Lang TR, Starr SR, Pusic M, Cook DA. Technology-enhanced simulation and pediatric education: a meta-analysis. Pediatrics. 2014;133:1313–23. (?rest of journal citation)

20. Levine AI, Flynn BC, Bryson EO, Demaria S Jr. Simulation-based maintenance of certification in anesthesiology (MOCA) course optimization: use of multi-modality educational activities. J Clin Anesth. 2012;24(1):68–74.

21. Levine AI, Schwartz AD, Bryson EO, Demaria S Jr. Role of simulation in U.S. physician licensure and certification. Mount Sinai J Med NY. 2012;79(1):140–53.

22. Zendejas B, Brydges R, Wang AT, Cook DA. Patient outcomes in simulation-based medical education: a systematic review. J Gen Intern Med. 2013;28(8):1078–89.

23. Barsuk JH, Cohen ER, Feinglass J, McGaghie WC, Wayne DB. Use of simulation-based education to reduce catheter-related bloodstream infections. Arch Intern Med. 2009;169(15):1420–3.

24. Sroka G, Feldman LS, Vassiliou MC, Kaneva PA, Fayez R, Fried GM. Fundamentals of laparoscopic surgery simulator training to proficiency improves laparoscopic performance in the operating room-a randomized controlled trial. Am J Surg. 2010;199(1):115–20.

25. Barsuk JH, Cohen ER, Potts S, Demo H, Gupta S, Feinglass J, et al. Dissemination of a simulation-based mastery learning intervention reduces central line-associated bloodstream infections. BMJ Qual Saf. 2014;23(9):749–56.

26. Cohen ER, Feinglass J, Barsuk JH, Barnard C, O'Donnell A, McGaghie WC, et al. Cost savings from reduced catheter-related bloodstream infection after simulation-based education for residents in a medical intensive care unit. Simul Healthc. 2010;5(2):98–102.

27. Zendejas B, Wang AT, Brydges R, Hamstra SJ, Cook DA. Cost: the missing outcome in simulation-based medical education research: a systematic review. Surgery. 2013;153(2):160–76.

28. Smith IJ. The Joint Commission guide to improving staff communication. 2nd ed. Oakbrook Terrace: Joint Commission Resources; 2009. p. x, 142.

29. Riley W, Davis S, Miller K, Hansen H, Sainfort F, Sweet R. Didactic and simulation nontechnical skills team training to improve perinatal patient outcomes in a community hospital. Jt Comm J Qual Patient Saf. 2011;37(8):357–64.

30. Salas E, DiazGranados D, Weaver SJ, King H. Does team training work? Principles for healthcare. Acad Emerg Med. 2008;15(11):1002–9.

31. Weaver SJ, Dy SM, Rosen MA. Team-training in healthcare: a narrative synthesis of the literature. BMJ Qual Saf. 2014;23(5):359–72.

32. Sigalet EL, Donnon TL, Grant V. Insight into team competence in medical, nursing and respiratory therapy students. J Interprof Care. 2014;22:1–6. [Epub ahead of print].

33. Sigalet E, Donnon T, Cheng A, Cooke S, Robinson T, Bissett W, Grant V. Development of a team performance scale to assess undergraduate health professionals. Acad Med. 2013;88(7):989–96.

34. Sigalet E, Donnon T, Grant V. Undergraduate students' perceptions of and attitudes toward a simulation-based interprofessional curriculum; the KidSIM ATTITUDES questionnaire. Simul Healthc. 2012;7(6):353–8.

35. Kyriacou DN, Ricketts V, Dyne PL, McCollough MD, Talan DA. A 5-year time study analysis of emergency department patient care efficiency. Ann Emerg Med. 1999;34(3):326–35.

36. Boet S, Bould MD, Fung L, Qosa H, Perrier L, Tavares W, et al. Transfer of learning and patient outcome in simulated crisis resource management: a systematic review. Can J Anaesth. 2014;61(6):571–82.

37. Mathieu JE, Heffner TS, Goodwin GF, Salas E, Cannon-Bowers JA. The influence of shared mental models on team process and performance. J Appl Psychol. 2000;85(2):273–83.

38. Cooper JB. Using simulation to teach and study healthcare handoffs. Simul Healthc. 2010;5(4):191–2.

39. Berkenstadt H, Haviv Y, Tuval A, Shemesh Y, Megrill A, Perry A, et al. Improving handoff communications in critical care: utilizing simulation-based training toward process improvement in managing patient risk. Chest. 2008;134(1):158–62.

40. Kendall L, Klasnja P, Iwasaki J, Best JA, White AA, Khalaj S, et al. Use of simulated physician handoffs to study cross-cover chart biopsy in the electronic medical record. AMIA Annu Symp Proc. 2013;2013:766–75.

41. Russ AL, Fairbanks RJ, Karsh BT, Militello LG, Saleem JJ, Wears RL. The science of human factors: separating fact from fiction. BMJ Qual Saf. 2013;22(10):802–8.

42. Carayon P, Xie A, Kianfar S. Human factors and ergonomics as a patient safety practice. BMJ Qual Saf. 2014;23(3):196–205.

43. Simms ER, Slakey DP, Garstka ME, Tersigni SA, Korndorffer JR. Can simulation improve the traditional method of root cause analysis: a preliminary investigation. Surgery. 2012;152(3):489–97.

44. Slakey DP, Simms ER, Rennie KV, Garstka ME, Korndorffer JR Jr. Using simulation to improve root cause analysis of adverse surgical outcomes. Int J Qual Health Care. 2014;26(2):144–50.

45. Alfredsdottir H, Bjornsdottir K. Nursing and patient safety in the operating room. J Adv Nurs. 2008;61(1):29–37.

46. Patterson MD, Blike GT, Nadkarni VM. In situ simulation: challenges and results. In: Henriksen K, Battles JB, Keyes MA, Grady ML, editors Advances in patient safety: new directions and alternative approaches (Vol 3: performance and tools). Advances in Patient Safety, Rockville; 2008.

47. Wetzel EA, Lang TR, Pendergrass TL, Taylor RG, Geis GL. Identification of latent safety threats using high-fidelity simulation-based training with multidisciplinary neonatology teams. Jt Comm J Qual Patient Saf. 2013;39(6):268–73.

48. Burton KS, Pendergrass TL, Byczkowski TL, Taylor RG, Moyer MR, Falcone RA, et al. Impact of simulation-based extracorporeal membrane oxygenation training in the simulation laboratory and clinical environment. Simul Healthc. 2011;6(5):284–91.

49. Wheeler DS, Geis G, Mack EH, LeMaster T, Patterson MD. High-reliability emergency response teams in the hospital: improving quality and safety using in situ simulation training. BMJ Qual Saf. 2013;22(6):507–14.

50. Johnson KGG, Oehler J, Houlton J, Tabangin M, Myer C, Kerrey B. High fidelity simulation to design a novel system of care for pediatric critical airway obstruction.(The American Society of Pediatric Otolaryngology April 2012; San Diego, CA2012 (? should this be Johnson K, Geis G, Oehler J, Meinzen-Derr J, Bauer J, Myer C et al. Simulation to implement a novel system of care for pediatric critical airway obstruction). Arch Otolaryngol Head Neck Surg. 2012;138(10):907–11.

51. Ventre KM, Barry JS, Davis D, Baiamonte VL, Wentworth AC, Pietras M, et al. Using in situ simulation to evaluate operational readiness of a children's hospital-based obstetrics unit. Simul Healthc. 2014;9(2):102–11.

52. http://www.ssih.org/Portals/48/Accreditation/Provisional_Docs/2013_ProvisionalAccreditationStandards.pdf. Accessed 12 Mar 2014.

53. Desai SV, Feldman L, Brown L, Dezube R, Yeh HC, Punjabi N, et al. Effect of the 2011 vs 2003 duty hour regulation-compliant models on sleep duration, trainee education, and continuity of patient care among internal medicine house staff: a randomized trial. JAMA Intern Med. 2013;173(8):649–55.

54. Ahmed N, Devitt KS, Keshet I, Spicer J, Imrie K, Feldman L, et al. A systematic review of the effects of resident duty hour restrictions in surgery: impact on resident wellness, training, and patient outcomes. Ann Surg. 2014;259(6):1041–53.

55. Ericsson KA. Deliberate practice and the acquisition and maintenance of expert performance in medicine and related domains. Acad Med. 2004;79(Suppl 10):70–81.

56. Phillips JK, Klein G, Sieck WR. Expertise in judgment and decision making: a case for training intuitive decision skills. In: Harvey DJKN, editor. Blackwell handbook of judgment and decision making. Malden: Blackwell Publishing Ltd; 2004.

57. Nemeth C, Wears R, Woods D, Hollnagel E, Cook R. Minding the gaps: creating resilience in healthcare. In: Henriksen K, Battles JB, Keyes MA, Grady ML, editors Advances in patient safety: new directions and alternative approaches (Vol 3: performance and tools). Rockville: Advances in Patient Safety; 2008.

58. Connelly LG, Bair AE. Discrete event simulation of emergency department activity: a platform for system-level operations research. Acad Emerg Med. 2004;11(11):1177–85.

59. Huang L, Norman D, Chen R. Addressing hospital-wide patient safety initiatives with high-fidelity simulation. Phys Executive J. 2010:36 (4):34–39.

60. INSPIRE Network. 2014. http://inspiresim.com/. Accessed 12 April 2014.

Systems Integration, Human Factors, and Simulation

Kimberly P. Stone, Lennox Huang, Jennifer R. Reid and Ellen S. Deutsch

Simulation Pearls

1. Health care is a complex, interconnected system with interrelationships. A systems approach seeks to understand both the components and the whole, and their interactions.
2. Simulation can focus on identifying systems properties that are problematic, contributing to defects or problems, or properties such as resilience, which contribute to safe, effective, and efficient healthcare delivery.
3. Lean, Six Sigma, Safety I and Safety II principles provide different frameworks and perspectives for understanding and improving healthcare delivery systems.
4. The integration of simulation into efforts to improve organizational safety and communication infrastructure can optimize change.

K. P. Stone (✉) · J. R. Reid
Department of Pediatrics, Division of Emergency Medicine, University of Washington School of Medicine, Seattle Children's Hospital, Seattle, WA, USA
e-mail: Kimberly.stone@seattlechildrens.org

J. R. Reid
e-mail: Jennifer.reid@seattlechildrens.org

E. S. Deutsch
Department of Anesthesiology, Department of Critical Care Medicine, The Children's Hospital of Philadelphia, Philadelphia, PA, USA
e-mail: edeutsch@ecri.org

E. S. Deutsch
Pennsylvania Patient Safety Authority, Plymouth Meeting, PA, USA
e-mail: edeutsch@ecri.org

L. Huang
Department of Pediatrics, McMaster University, McMaster Children's Hospital, Hamilton, ON, Canada
e-mail: lennoxhuang@yahoo.com

A Systems-Based Approach to Health Care

Consider what might happen if you are a member of a code team called to an emergent resuscitation: a child with anaphylaxis. Each team member, including you, has great knowledge and technical skills. The team has practiced together and quickly establishes the leader and support roles, the correct diagnosis, a shared mental model, and closed-loop communication. You resuscitate the child, start the appropriate treatments, and the child improves. You are not just a team of experts, but an expert team!

Now consider an alternate scenario with the same team: Someone is sent to get the code cart, but does not return for a prolonged period of time. After three failed attempts to establish intravenous access, the drill is retrieved to place an intraosseous line, but the drill does not work. Once the code cart arrives, the team struggles to calculate how to dilute the contents of the 1:1000 vial of epinephrine to achieve the desired weight-based dose. The team is still a team of experts, but without effective systems to support them, they are not functioning as an expert team.

Each of these problems likely has many contributory factors. Attempts to correct or resolve these problems may well identify other problems. A systems approach recognizes that systems—such as our complex care processes—are consisted of many components, with interrelationships between the components and the whole. Definitions of systems vary, with an underlying common thread: A system is a collection of parts forming a greater whole. The International Council of Systems Engineering (INCOSE) offers the following definition of a system:

> A construct or collection of different elements that together, produce results not obtainable by the elements alone. The elements, or parts, can include people, hardware, software, facilities, policies, and documents; all things required to produce systems-level results. Results include system level qualities, properties, characteristics, functions, behavior and performance. The value added by the system as a whole, beyond that contributed independently by the parts, is created by the relationship among the parts; how they are interconnected [1].

© Springer International Publishing Switzerland 2016
V. J. Grant, A. Cheng (eds.), *Comprehensive Healthcare Simulation: Pediatrics*,
Comprehensive Healthcare Simulation, DOI 10.1007/978-3-319-24187-6_6

A systems approach recognizes that there must be integration between the components and the whole. In health care, this integration is dynamic, complex, and not always predictable. One way to conceptualize the complex relationships between the user, tool, task, environment, and processes is illustrated in Fig. 6.1.

In our case example above, the task could be resuscitating the patient, with subtasks of assembling the appropriate team, making an accurate diagnosis, retrieving necessary equipment, administering the correct medications, and so on. Our users are the physicians, nurses, and respiratory therapists who provide direct care, as well as social workers, security personnel, pharmacists, radiology technicians, unit clerks, environmental service personnel, and others who provide support services. The patient is also the *user*, as the system is intended to function for his/her benefit, but in this particular case his/her participation is mostly passive; actions are done *to* or *for* him/her. Our tools are broadly defined, including supplies and medications, and equipment, such as the intraosseous drill. Tools could also include knowledge and past experiences.

The environment in which our resuscitation occurs is, in its simplest form, the physical space that we are working within. In our example, the code cart is located too far away, interfering with timely retrieval of equipment. Changing the physical environment, such as moving the code cart closer, could improve the team's ability to provide timely care. Our working environments are more than the physical spaces we inhabit; our activities are impacted by the availability of all resources: equipment, supplies, information, and people. There are also less tangible components, including interpersonal interactions and organizational culture.

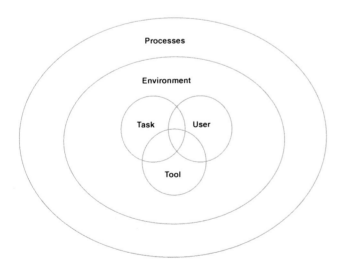

Fig. 6.1 Systems integration: a schematic representation depicting the independence, overlap, and dependence of different systems elements (task, tool, user, environment, and processes) related to the overall system

Processes surround and underpin the environment and its contents. Processes may be codified and formal (e.g., policies, procedures, clinical care pathways, and checklists) or informal (e.g., learning what works by trial and error). For example, scarcity of supplies may stimulate hoarding. Previous experiences with success—or with pushback—may stimulate looking for alternative paths to obtain resources such as equipment or even knowledge. We learn who or where to ask for equipment, supplies, and information, and sometimes seek these resources outside of formalized pathways.

Patient care activities can be divided conceptually (see Fig. 6.1), but the interactions between those components are important and unavoidable. A system is a set of interrelated components functioning together toward some common objective(s) or purpose(s). Systems are composed of components, attributes, and relationships [2]. A systems approach involves understanding the whole, the parts, and their interrelationships. Health care can be characterized as a diverse collection of multiple imperfect systems with complicated, dynamic interactions. Components include people, tools, resources, and the environment. The products of these systems include direct and indirect patient care, documents, behavior and performance of healthcare professionals, errors, and adverse events. These systems exist at all levels: from individual clinics all the way up to complex organizations coordinating care across the spectrum of health and illness.

Applying a systems approach to health care creates a framework for understanding and changing behaviors and clinical outcomes. This approach is especially important in the area of patient safety as noted in the 1999 Institute of Medicine report To Err is Human:

> Preventing errors and improving safety for patients require a systems approach in order to modify the conditions that contribute to errors. People working in health care are among the most educated and dedicated work force in any industry. The problem is not bad people; the problem is that the system needs to be made safer [3].

In our example, we do not really know why the intraosseous drill failed. One possibility is that the user was deficient. A systems approach challenges us to look deeper. Training may contribute to earlier recognition of problems with the tool, prompting a request for another drill. But no amount of individual or team training, practice or experience, will directly contribute to making the drill work. Potential contributors to tool failure include tool factors (e.g., limited durability and battery failure), environmental or organizational factors (e.g., limitations in funding priorities, oversight, protocols, staffing, or training), and process factors (e.g., insufficient testing or maintenance and lack of availability of replacement units) [4].

Similarly, we do not really know why it was difficult to calculate the correct dose of epinephrine. Potential contributory causes could be ergonomic (e.g., the contents of the vial are listed in a microscopic font) or cognitive (e.g., it is difficult, particularly under stress, to calculate correctly and tenfold calculation errors are common; epinephrine is a *scary* drug to make a mistake with).

Human factors expertise can help. *Human factors* is sometimes misunderstood as "the weaknesses of humans" contributing to system failures. Since all healthcare systems have been created by humans:

> The search for a human in the path of a failure is bound to succeed. If not directly at the sharp end—as a 'human error' or unsafe act—one can usually be found a few steps back. The assumption that humans have failed therefore always vindicates itself [5].

Human factors addresses characteristics of human beings that are applicable to the design of systems and devices [6]. Human factors design takes into account the capabilities of people (physical, cognitive, or other) to create a work system that takes advantage of our capabilities and, conversely, builds in support where our capabilities are limited. The science of human factors uses knowledge of human functions and capabilities to maximize compatibility in the design of interactive systems of people, machines, and environments: ensuring their effectiveness, safety and ease of performance [6]. Human factors expertise encompasses science and exploration related to perception and performance, augmented cognition, decision-making, communication, product design, virtual environments, aging, macroergonomics, and other areas [7].

Role of Simulation in Systems Integration

If we look at Fig. 6.1 again, from the perspective of a simulation educator or researcher, rather than a healthcare provider, we can make similar analogies. Our tools include the mannequins, task trainers, virtual simulators, standardized patients, even our knowledge of simulation and healthcare content. Our users are the learners or assessees, who participate in the simulation. Our task is to help individuals, teams, or organizations learn, or demonstrate competence or skills proficiency. Our environment could be a simulation center, in situ simulation location, or spaces such as conference rooms, or outdoor environments in which simulations can occur. Processes may include equipment management, protocol development, informational interface with potential simulation users, etc. Each of these components is an interrelated component of our simulation program.

The anaphylaxis case example at the start of the chapter can be replicated as a simulation scenario. The responses of simulation participants and problems encountered may not be exactly the same, but, if we conduct our simulation with real teams, in real settings, using real equipment, we will have the opportunity to better understand and improve the real systems. Debriefing can focus on understanding the context in which we provide patient care. Focused questions can intentionally and explicitly seek to better understand system capacities and constraints.

Specific variations can be made, altering the age of the patient or the clinical location, to identify systems issues that prevent optimal resuscitation of different types of patients in different settings. Simulated intentional probes create an opportunity to identify real-world challenges before there is a near miss or patient harm event. Pediatric simulations in North Carolina EDs were performed to assess the quality of pediatric trauma resuscitations. Although the goal of the simulations was to identify educational interventions, systems issues were identified that would need to be addressed before any educational intervention would be successful, such as the lack of child-sized cervical collars in many of the EDs and the inability to identify IO needles due to mislabeling [8].

In situ simulation, using care team members, existing equipment, resources, and patient care sites, offers the opportunity to evaluate the system of care and identify latent safety threats (LSTs) that could predispose to medical error. LSTs have been defined as systems-based threats to patient safety that can materialize at any time and are previously unrecognized by healthcare providers [9]. Categorizations of LSTs have included medication, equipment, resource, and knowledge gaps. A greater number of LSTs were identified per scenario during simulations conducted in situ versus in a simulation lab (1.8 vs. 0.8, respectively) [10]. Identification of LSTs in simulation allows for system-level fixes before patient harm as demonstrated in the pediatric emergency department [11], obstetrical unit [12], and with ECMO (Extracorporeal Membrane Oxygenation) simulations [13]. Simulation incorporates an opportunity to debrief to understand the rationales for observed behaviors and the context in which care is provided, a luxury not often available in real patient care. Whether the goal of the simulation is identification of LSTs or not, a structured debrief often elicits underlying systems constraints that contribute to observed behaviors. Thus, identification of LSTs may be intentional or serendipitous. And asking participants to identify and consider LSTs is one way to take the focus off the individual (user) performance. Some programs have embedded simulation LSTs into their formal organizational safety reporting systems.

The same anaphylaxis simulation case can be replicated with a variety of *ages* of infant, pediatric and adolescent mannequins in different hospital locations, yielding new and distinct systems issues in dealing with pediatric patients across the age spectrum, or identifying challenges that span larger systems. Skilled simulation educators or researchers may pause the action, restart, repeat, and rework scenarios to stress the system and understand capabilities and constraints. Team members can observe parts of the care continuum they may not generally have the opportunity to witness, adding to the larger team's understanding of vital processes and ultimately, breaking down silos in which healthcare providers often work.

Because simulation provides opportunities to bring stakeholders together, repeat scenarios as needed and observe potentially infrequent events, simulation is a natural partner in the Plan-Do-Study-Act (PDSA) cycle of improvement. Simulation can be incorporated in the planning phase, in the application of learnings, and then processes can be tested and retested iteratively using simulation. Figure 6.2 provides an example of how simulation can be used throughout the PDSA cycle to address identified systems issues.

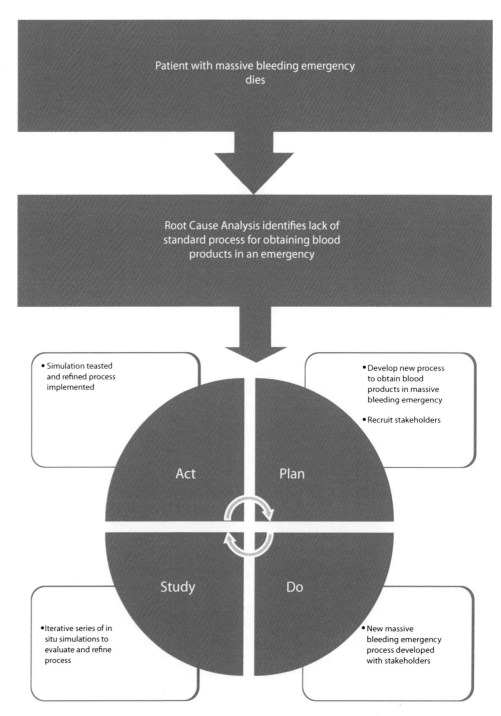

Fig. 6.2 Example of simulation integration with the PDSA cycle. Also incorporates a combined Safety I and Safety II application

Frameworks

Lean

There are several approaches to taking a closer look at systems-related issues. Lean methodology offers a collection of tools and principles that may assist in identifying and solving problems related to process and environment. Lean is a management strategy with the goal of minimizing waste and maximizing efficiency, with the assumption that this will also improve safety and quality. The origin of Lean can be traced to the Toyota Production System developed in the 1950s–1970s by Taiichi Ohno and Shigeo Shingo. James Womack's 1990 book *The Machine That Changed the World* is largely credited with the popularizing Lean terminology and production principles [14]. In Lean, value is always defined from the customer's (patient's) perspective. Any step or activity that helps a patient achieve their ultimate goal is considered valuable. Waste is anything that consumes resources or time but does not help a patient achieve their desired goal or outcome. A key goal of Lean is to eliminate nonessential waste and maximize value. The eight types of waste and examples are provided in Table 6.1. While debriefing a simulation, asking participants to identify and consider sources of waste is one way to take the focus off the individual (user) and begin to consider the task, tool, environment, and processes that define the system of care.

One of the basic workplace organization tools in Lean is termed 5S or 6S. The name derives from a list of five Japanese words used as a guide to organizing the work environment. The original 5S tool has been modified in health to include an important sixth *S*—safety. The 6S framework can be integrated with simulation activities to examine and change the clinical environment (see Table 6.2)

In our opening example, the 6S tool provides a systematic framework for examining issues. *Sort* challenges us to

Table 6.1 Eight types of waste [20]

Type of waste	Example
Inventory	Excess stocked equipment that is not used regularly
Waiting or delays	Waiting to be treated in a clinic
Overproduction	Drawing up extra doses of medications that are not used
Transportation	Patients needing to go to geographically distant areas of a hospital for tests/procedures during a single clinic visit
Motion	Excessive movement of team members in a clinical care area during a resuscitation
Errors/mistakes	Having to repeat or redo a task because of an error
Over-processing	Unnecessarily repeating tests/documentation
Underutilized human capacity	High-skilled individuals performing low-skill activities

Table 6.2 Lean Healthcare 6S tool [20]

6S	
Sort	Useful from necessary
Set in order (straighten)	Everything in its place, with visual cues
Sweep/shine	"Spring cleaning"
Standardize	Make cleaning, inspection, safety part of the routine job
Sustain	Establish an environment including audits/cues to ensure 6S sticks
Safety	Proactively look for potential safety issues, make the environment safe

determine whether the most relevant tools are easily accessible and identifiable, such as whether the code cart is cluttered with non-emergent equipment. *Set in order* challenges us to ask whether the code cart should be in a different location and whether there are clear visual cues to efficiently guide people to critical equipment. *Sweep or Shine* questions whether there are older pieces of equipment, materials or even protocols that need to be removed. *Standardize* challenges us to ask if there are routines around who, when and how the drill and equipment are inspected and whether all carts and rooms have similar organization. *Sustain* challenges us to ask what is in place to ensure changes from the previous *4S* are maintained, guaranteeing the drill is always findable and functional. *Safety* challenges us to ask what additional LSTs are present, but have yet to be uncovered and mitigated. In addition to the drill, is there another piece of equipment at risk for failure? Each element in the 6S tool can assist teams to examine issues, whether in real patient care or in simulation, from a systems perspective.

Six Sigma

Six Sigma offers another framework, consisting of principles and tools, for examining systems and improving quality [15, 16]. Six Sigma and its primary tool, define, measure, analyze, improve, and control (DMAIC), are used to improve the quality of processes by identifying and removing defects (errors) and minimizing variability. Six Sigma was developed in the 1980s by Motorola and became central to General Electric's business strategy in the 1990s [16]. In Six Sigma, quality is always defined from the customer (patient) perspective. A key goal is to eliminate defects (errors) and develop processes that function error free 99.99966 % of the time.

DMAIC is the acronym for a five-phase, data-driven quality tool used to improve processes: define, measure, analyze, improve, and control. In our opening example, DMAIC provides a systematic approach for examining our anaphylaxis case examples. *Define* challenges us to specify the problem or the goal: an error-filled resuscitation, with the opportunity to decrease the number or errors and delays. *Measure* challenges us to evaluate the current resuscitation process, such as quantifying current times for code cart acquisition and medication preparation, or whether participants accomplish specific tasks. *Analyze* challenges us to identify root causes: inadequate signage for code cart location, reliance on memory and mental math for medication reconstitution and dosage determination. *Improve* challenges us to eliminate these causes: develop new signage, and provide prepackaged equipment and medication or job aids that eliminate relying on individual performance. *Control* challenges us to develop a sustainable system: create simulation training and audits to monitor the process.

Six Sigma is based on the assumption that a best process is known, or knowable; this is true for many but not all healthcare delivery processes.

Safety I and Safety II

In contrast to Lean and DMAIC, which provide concrete frameworks for process improvement and presume that best processes are known, or knowable, Safety I and II offer different perspectives of patient safety. *Safety I* focuses on what goes wrong, to retroactively identify root causes, develop plans to avoid those risks and prevent the repetition of errors [17]. Within health care, for every error, there are still a large number of processes which go "right." A Safety I perspective focuses on the error, even if it is a rare event. In our anaphylaxis case example, the malfunctioning drill could be a rare and unexpected event. Simulation could re-create the scenario, in the same location and with the same team members. Root cause analysis could clarify whether participants knew how to use the drill correctly, whether there was some aspect of storage that damaged the drill, whether participants knew how to access spare batteries, whether spare batteries were in stock, or any additional components of the process that did not function in a desirable manner.

An alternate view of patient safety focuses on what goes right, Safety II: what happens during the error-free times, which comprise the vast majority of patient care interactions. Safety II assumes that systems are complex and incompletely understood. Human variability is essential to make necessary adjustments, preventing errors in varying conditions. The Safety II framework shifts the analytic perspective from a reactive to a proactive approach [17]. Safety II also recognizes that what may seem to be slack or even excess, may in fact be the margin which becomes a valuable resource when the system is stressed.

In our anaphylaxis case example, a simulation with a Safety II approach could examine multiple clinical settings with different teams (e.g., the emergency department, operating room, pediatric floor, and primary care clinic) varying

barriers (e.g., variable staffing, missing equipment, and patient language barrier) to understand how teams overcome these barriers. Discoveries could lead to the development of job aids with dilution instructions, doses that are "ready to go" and a process to delegate calculation tasks to additional team members. Insight into each team's adjustments sheds light on systematic changes that could reinforce success. Simulation complements both Safety I and Safety II, providing the opportunity to examine how participants overcome inherent challenges.

Integration of Simulation Program and Hospital Infrastructure

We have illustrated how simulation can be used from a systems approach, to identify user, tool, task, environment, and process issues that either place our patients at risk or prevent harm. These discoveries can be serendipitous or intentionally sought out. Regardless of how the discoveries are made, and whether they are based on a Safety I or Safety II perspective, creating change that improves health care for our patients is the ultimate goal.

To maximize change, uncovered issues need to be directed to people and components in the system that can create and sustain change. In our anaphylaxis case example, facilities may need to create new signs, which maintenance staff installs. Clinical and supply staff may need to collaborate to identify, price and test drills in order to make a purchasing recommendation. Education leaders may need to develop a program to establish and periodically refresh correct drill techniques. Representatives from medicine, nursing, pharmacy, and supply chain, may need to identify the most reliable process for epinephrine preparation and standardize it throughout the institution. Researchers, using quality improvement or traditional research techniques, could examine performance over time. How solutions to systems issues are integrated into the change management system of an organization will determine their impact. Issues identified in one clinical area, such as the ineffective drill, but not shared with other clinical areas, limits learning to silos. Increasingly, systems issues identified in simulation are being escalated in the same hospital error-reporting structures as real patient cases [Marc Auerbach, written communication, August 2014; Kimberly Stone, written communication, August 2014]. In these error-reporting systems, issues are reviewed, and distributed to leadership responsible for user, tool, task, environment, or process changes in the same manner as concerns which were identified based on actual patient care events. Engaging all areas of the organization which contribute to specific patient care processes supports system-wide change, breaking down silos often associated with healthcare organizations.

Conclusions

Health care is a complex adaptive system; components of the system learn and adjust their behavior or responses, contributing to increasing complexity; the results of these interactions can be unpredictable. Healthcare systems exhibit complex behaviors that emerge out of the complexity of the large number of procedural, biologic, and sociotechnical rules—whether understood and articulated or not—that drive the system and impact the interdependent interactions between components [18]. It is not possible to completely understand, let alone control, all of these interactions. However, it is possible to use simulation to learn more about, and improve, these interactions and our capabilities to provide the safest, highest quality health care to our patients.

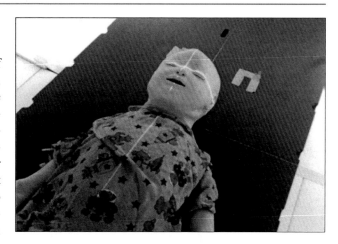

Fig. 6.3 Pediatric simulator in a proton therapy bed. (Image courtesy of Dr. Ellen S Deutsch, Center for Simulation, Advanced Education and Innovation, the Children's Hospital of Philadelphia)

Example 1: Application of a Systems Approach for Identifying Patient Safety Risks in a Proton Therapy Unit

A proton therapy unit, previously only treating adults, planned to begin providing services to pediatric patients. Simulated emergencies for pediatric patients (see Fig. 6.3) identified systems issues related to users (clarification of whether the pharmacist or the anesthesia technician would provide medications, to avoid duplication of efforts), tools (the nearest pediatric resuscitation cart was too far away; an additional cart was obtained), and environment (providers accustomed to working in a pediatric facility identified that the need for a pediatric (vs. adult) team must be specified during the activation of an emergency response).

Example 2: Application of Lean Framework to Systems-Focused Simulation for Redesign of an Existing Resuscitation Room Delays in care (e.g., applying monitors, administering medications, obtaining equipment) led to a series of simulations to examine user, tool, environment, and processes in an existing resuscitation room. Issues were identified and addressed using the 6S tool. Figure 6.4 shows the resuscitation room prior to the 6S exercise. Areas of clutter, a headwall with respiratory equipment, monitoring equipment, reference guides, etc., were *sorted* and outdated equipment discarded. *Straightening* led to co-locating task-based supplies. Airway equipment for physicians (oxygen attachments, bag mask, suction, and intubation materials) was placed together in an airway cart on the patient's right. Monitoring equipment for nurses (heart rate monitors, temperature probes, blood pressure cuffs, etc.) was placed together on the patient's left side. To *standardize* the new

environment, ensuring routine cleaning and inspection, a room setup check-list included photographs. To *sustain* the changes, visual cues were placed throughout the room (blue bordered labels and photographs). Recognizing that *safety* issues could have been created or remain, a feedback box was added to collect ongoing issues. Figures 6.5 and 6.6 show the resuscitation room after the 6S exercise.

Example 3: Application of Six Sigma, DMAIC, and Simulation to Improve Handoff Communication Handoffs between providers are a risk factor for adverse events. The Six Sigma DMAIC methodology was applied to improve the postoperative handoff process for children with heart disease. *Define* identified 18 essential handoff elements. *Measure* identified a mean of 5.6 errors per handoff event concentrated in medical history and current surgical intervention. *Analyze* identified three factors negatively affecting the handoff process: lack of standardization, inconsistent participation by clinicians recently involved in the patient's care and interruptions/distractions during the handoff process. *Intervention* and *control* phases included creating a standardized handoff model and training to that model using simulation. Researchers found that using this methodology resulted in reduced time to obtain clinically important diagnostic information [19].

Example 4: Application of Both a Safety I and Safety II Perspective to Simulation for a New Process Patients are at risk for profound hemorrhage as a postsurgical complication or secondary to trauma or illness. Delivering the appropriate blood products, equipment, and personnel, safely and efficiently, is a complex process. In order to design a new massive bleeding emergency protocol, a series of simulations were conducted with multiple teams in multiple different clinical areas: Pediatric Intensive Care, Cardiac

Fig. 6.4 Existing resuscitation room prior to 6S exercise. (Image courtesy of Drs. Kimberly Stone and Jennifer Reid of the Pediatric Emergency Medicine Simulation Program at Seattle Children's Hospital 2014c)

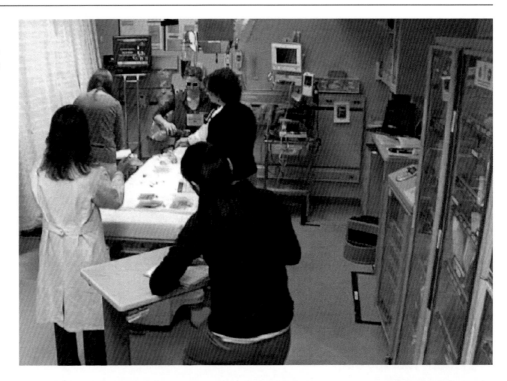

Fig. 6.5 Same resuscitation room after 6S exercise. (Image courtesy of Drs. Kimberly Stone and Jennifer Reid of the Pediatric Emergency Medicine Simulation Program at Seattle Children's Hospital 2014c)

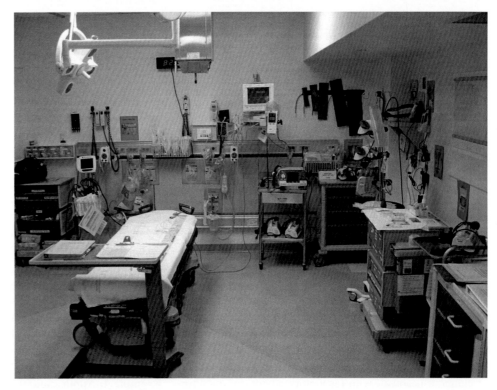

Intensive Care, Neonatal Intensive Care, Operating Room, and Emergency Department. During each scenario, observers identified how different teams overcame barriers to safe and efficient care, developing a new massive bleeding emergency protocol that incorporated best practices from throughout the institution. Figure 6.2 outlines the process using the PDSA cycle.

Example 5: Integration of Simulation Issue Identification into Hospital Infrastructure Creating a system for identifying, prioritizing, and disseminating issues, requiring accountability, tracking mitigation strategies and communicating progress, can leverage simulation's ability to create change. Prior to opening several new clinical units, we conducted simulation testing to identify safety issues. All safety

Fig. 6.6 Visual cues identified after 6S exercise to *standardize* and *sustain* change. (Image courtesy of Drs. Kimberly Stone and Jennifer Reid of the Pediatric Emergency Medicine Simulation Program at Seattle Children's Hospital 2014c)

issues were reviewed by a clinical and facilities expert. Each was designated as critical, high, medium, or low priority based on the significance and time sensitivity. Critical issues, such as a non-functional code alarms, could place a patient at risk of death or significant injury, and needed to be resolved prior to staff training. Broad leadership (e.g., directors of construction, clinical engineering, demand flow, information technology, environmental services, telecommunications, and patient care units) was required to attend a "daily huddle" addressing identified issues. Critical issues were discussed with the entire group to facilitate collaborative problem solving between interdependent teams. Huddles occurred every morning, with updates on issue resolution, until the new units opened for patient care.

References

1. INCOSE, A brief history of systems engineering. 2012. http://www.incose.org/mediarelations/briefhistory.aspx. Accessed 27 Sept 2012.
2. Systems science and engineering. In: Blanchard BS, Fabrycky WJ, editors. Systems engineering and analysis, 5th edn. New Jersey: Prentice Hall; 2011. p. 3.
3. Institute of Medicine Committee on Quality of Health Care in America. Why do errors happen? In: Kohn LT, Corrigan JM, Donaldson MS, editors. To Err is Human. Washington, DC: National Academies Press; 2000. p. 49.
4. Chang A, Schye PM, Croteau RJ, O'Leary DS, Loeb JM. The JCAHO patient safety event taxonomy: a standardized terminology and classification schema for near misses and adverse events. Intl J Qual in Health Care. 2005;17(2):95–105.
5. The driving forces. In: Hollnagel E, Woods DD, editors. Joint cognitive systems foundations of cognitive systems engineering. Florida: CRC Press; 2005. p. 9.
6. Human Factors and Ergonomics Society. https://www.hfes.org//Web/AboutHFES/about.html. Accessed 8 Aug 2014.
7. Human Factors and Ergonomics Society. https://www.hfes.org/Web/TechnicalGroups/descriptions.html. Accessed 22 Aug 2014.
8. Hunt EA, Hohenhaus SM, Luo X, Frush KS. Simulation of pediatric trauma stabilization in 35 North Carolina emergency departments: identification of targets for performance improvement. Pediatrics. 2006;117(3):641–8.
9. Alfredsdottir H, Bjornsdottir K. Nursing and patient safety in the operating room. J Adv Nurs. 2007;61(1):29–37.
10. Wetzel EA, Lang TR, Pendergrass TL, Taylor RG, Geis GL. Identification of latent safety threats using high-fidelity simulation-based training with multidisciplinary neonatology teams. Jt Comm J Qual Patient Saf. 2013;39(6):268–73.
11. Patterson MD, Geis GL, Falcone RA, LeMaster T, Wears RL. In situ simulation: detection of safety threats and teamwork training in a high risk emergency department. BMJ Qual Saf. 2013;22(6):468–77.
12. Guise JM, Lowe NK, Deering S, Lewis PO, O'Haire C, Irwin LK, et al. Mobile in situ obstetric emergency simulation and teamwork training to improve maternal-fetal safety in hospitals. Jt Comm J Qual Patient Saf. 2010;36(10):443–53.
13. Burton KS, Pendergrass T, Byczkowski TL, Taylor RG, Moyer MR, Falcone RA, et al. Impact of simulation-based extracorporeal membrane oxygenation training in the simulation laboratory and clinical environment. Simul Healthc. 2011;6(5):284–91.
14. Womack JP, Jones DT, Roos D. The machine that changed the world. New York: Scribner; 1990.
15. Borror CM, editor. The certified quality engineer handbook. Third edn. Wisconsin: ASQ Quality Press; 2009. p. 321–32.
16. Tennant G. Six Sigma: SPC and TQM in manufacturing and services. Vermont: Gower Publishing; 2001. p. 7–36.
17. Hollnagel E. A tale of two safeties. Nucl Saf Simul. 2013;4(1) 1–9.
18. Karwowski W. A review of human factors challenges of complex adaptive systems: discovering and understanding chaos in human performance. Hum Factors. 2012;54(6):983–95.
19. Mistry KP, Jaggers J, Lodge AJ, Alton M, Mericle JM, Frush KS, et al. Using Six Sigma methodology to improve handoff communication in high-risk patients. In: Henriksen K, Battles JB, Keyes MA, Grady ML, editors. Advances in patient safety: new directions and alternative approaches (Vol 3: performance and tools). Maryland: Agency for Healthcare Research and Quality; 2008.
20. Graban M. Lean hospitals: improving quality, patient safety, and employee engagement. New York: Productivity Press; 2011. p. 37–44, 89–96.

Assessment in Pediatric Simulation

Aaron William Calhoun, Aaron Donoghue and Mark Adler

Simulation Pearls

1. Assessment is a form of measurement, allowing simulation-based medical educators to make meaningful inferences about their learners' potential performance in the real world.
2. Validity is an argument supported by data from a number of complementary data sources.
3. Validity is a characteristic of the assessment data obtained from specific learners in specific environments and is not inherent in the instrument itself.
4. A substantial array of assessment instruments germane to pediatric simulation exist, many of which are readily available for use.

Introduction

Assessment is an expansive topic that impinges upon many fields. Given that whole textbooks have been devoted to this subject, we will, by necessity, provide an overview of this topic only as it specifically pertains to simulation. One distinction to consider is the use of *simulation itself* as a comprehensive tool by which to assess learners—such as the Objective Standardized Clinical Exam (OSCE) component of the United States Medical Licensing Exam (USMLE)—versus the use of *standard assessment methodologies* (surveys, checklists, etc.) within the context of the simulated environment. In the companion textbook to this volume [1], the former subject has been addressed in great detail. We perceive, however, a growing interest in the simulation community for information regarding the latter and thus have chosen to direct the chapter toward this question.

Why Assess?

What do we hope to accomplish through the use of formal assessment of our simulations? A fundamental observation is that we perform assessment continually as we engage in our educational activities. From the beginning of the case to the conclusion of each debriefing, faculty engaged in simulation-based educational activities are constantly rendering judgments, both verbally and internally, regarding the quality of care given, the knowledge level of participants, the communication skills of the team as a whole, and a myriad of other issues. Without this ongoing process, we indeed would have nothing of significance to offer our learners during the debriefing process. There is a vast difference, however, between these ongoing personal judgments and the rigorous process needed to form assessments that are consistent and meaningful. Though the primary act of assessment may be similar, a number of additional facets of the process must be considered and systematically examined if we are to have any confidence that our judgments truly represent a learner's actual skill in the area assessed. The degree to which one is held accountable for demonstrating the validity of assessment data is linked to the stakes of the assessment as it is unfair to learners to report scores that could affect their future

A. W. Calhoun (✉)
Department of Pediatrics, Division of Critical Care, University of Louisville School of Medicine, Kosair Children's Hospital, Louisville, KY, USA
e-mail: Aaron.calhoun@louisville.edu

A. Donoghue
Department of Pediatrics and Critical Care Medicine, Department of Emergency Medicine and Critical Care Medicine, Perelman School of Medicine of the University of Pennsylvania, Children's Hospital of Philadelphia, Philadelphia, PA, USA
e-mail: donoghue@email.chop.edu

M. Adler
Department of Pediatrics and Medical Education, Northwestern University Feinberg School of Medicine, Chicago, IL, USA
e-mail: m-adler@northwestern.edu

Department of Pediatrics, Ann & Robert H. Lurie Children's Hospital of Chicago, Chicago, IL, USA

© Springer International Publishing Switzerland 2016
V. J. Grant, A. Cheng (eds.), *Comprehensive Healthcare Simulation: Pediatrics*,
Comprehensive Healthcare Simulation, DOI 10.1007/978-3-319-24187-6_7

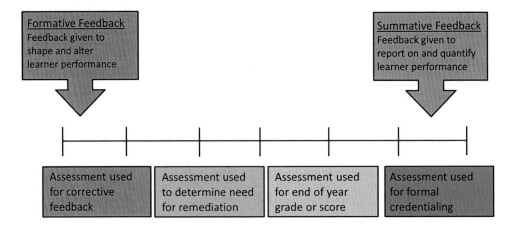

Fig. 7.1 The spectrum of assessment: formative versus summative

practice or careers without having subjected the tools used to generate those scores to rigorous study.

This naturally leads to a second question: If we agree that assessment forms part of the underpinning of all simulation-based education, what is the intended use of these assessments or judgments? In general, we either seek to assess learners or learner groups or assess educational interventions or curricula. When assessing learners or learner groups, this process spans a spectrum from learner-directed feedback that provides information intended to enhance current performance (*formative assessment*), to assessments used to provide a pass/fail *grade* of a learner's ultimate performance in a given area or to provide a certification or other formal qualification that the learner can then display as proof of their abilities (*summative assessment*) [2, 3]. This spectrum is delineated in Fig. 7.1. A number of possibilities also lie between these extremes, such as the use of assessment for the identification of those in need of remedial training. While information gained from these *hybrid* types of assessment might not form a part of their ongoing educational record, it is doing more than simply informing the learner as to their current performance in a given area.

When using assessment to study programmatic impact, many of the same validity and reliability considerations that will be discussed in the body of the chapter apply. This topic is discussed more thoroughly in subsequent chapters dedicated to simulation research (see Chap. 30).

Definition of Terms

Thus far, we have been discussing assessment without developing a proper definition. Simply put, assessment is a form of *measurement,* in this case the measurement of knowledge, skill, or performance level with respect to a specific educational construct. This may be skill at performing a lumbar puncture (LP), knowledge regarding a particular resuscitation algorithm, or ability to communicate within a team structure. The purpose of this measurement is to allow the educator to make inferences regarding a subject's knowledge, skill, or attitudes in the real-world situation recreated by the simulation [4, 5].

As in any other field of scientific inquiry, the performance of these measurements further required the use of *calibrated instruments* or *tools* in order to be reproducible and precise. Therefore, just as the measurement of length requires a ruler, the measurement of performance in a simulation requires some sort of rating scale representative of the concept being assessed. In the case of length, the calibration of this ruler is performed by comparing individual rulers to a specific formalized standard. Similarly, assessment possesses a formalized, evidence-based process used to determine the validity of the data it produces. *Validity* is, as Downing and Haladyna state, the "single most important characteristic of assessment data," and concerns the degree to which the assessment data arising from the use a specific assessment for a particular learner group in a particular environment is meaningful, useable, and corresponds to the construct or concept that we are actually intending to measure [6]. *Reliability*, although often considered a distinct construct, is formally a subset of validity and concerns the extent to which measurements are consistent across raters, settings, and time. It is important to note that validity is a characteristic of the data and not a characteristic of the instrument.

This chapter will address the above issues by:

1. Describing the *structure of assessment and assessment instruments* by discussing the different subjects to which assessment instruments can be applied as well as addressing the most frequent question and response types.

2. Outlining the currently accepted *hypothesis-driven research approach to instrument validation*. This will include an in-depth discussion of the current conception

of validity that draws from the work of Kane and others [7–10].

3. Describing the *practical use of assessment tools,* drawing attention to implementation strategies and the timing of tool use within individual simulation sessions.

4. *Reviewing the existing assessment literature* in an effort to highlight a number of different instruments for which reliability and validity data have been provided (Table 7.1).

It is our hope that this chapter will enable the reader to more rigorously assess and evaluate their learners.

The Structure of Assessment and Assessment Instruments

The structure of assessment addresses two categories: the *subject* and the *observed process.* Considerations of these categories then are used to refine the data collection strategy, rater selection and preparation, and the specific question design of the tool.

The Subject of Assessment

Assessment of individual simulation participants has been heavily relied on for the demonstration of knowledge and skill (cognitive or psychomotor), particularly with respect to procedural performance. Simulations constructed for individual assessment can be designed to address specific learning objectives and areas of knowledge based on the projected subject's level of experience and clinical discipline. Historically, there are far more examples of assessment at this individual level than at the higher, but potentially more important, level of the team.

A team has been defined as "two or more individuals with specialized knowledge and skills who perform specific roles and complete interdependent tasks to achieve a common goal or outcome" [11]. In simulations conducted with a team of healthcare providers, the opportunity exists to assess dynamic and interpersonal phenomena in the realm of crisis resource management such as communication, teamwork, leadership and followership, and role clarity in a way that cannot be done with individual learners. Team assessments also have the potential to enhance the realism of simulated scenarios when a cross section of multidisciplinary personnel are involved, allowing the team to function in a more representative manner. While the importance of assessing and improving these phenomena is desirable, their complexity and qualitative nature make them challenging to express in an interpretable and reportable way, and rigorous evidence for effectiveness is still lacking in published literature [12, 13].

The Observed Process

Here a distinction should be drawn between *explicit* processes (behaviors that can be directly observed) and *implicit* processes (judgments or thought processes that cannot directly be seen but must instead be inferred based on actions). For example, in a cardiac arrest scenario, the task "recognize pulselessness" is implicit as it is primarily mental in nature and thus must be inferred from verbal statements such as a directive to begin chest compressions. Determining this requires some degree of judgment on the part of the rater, which can be subject to bias. In contrast, the tasks "palpate pulse" and "start chest compressions" are explicit and readily appreciable by observation alone. While the explicit tasks may have been performed, however, it may or may not follow that the learner in question performed them with an appropriate understanding or cognitive context (e.g., appropriately checking a pulse but failing to start compressions). Thus, both types of processes are essential and complementary components of assessment and may both be included in a given assessment instrument.

A further distinction should be made between *objective* versus *subjective* measurement. Objective measurement refers to either discrete, analytical rubrics with correct answers or to specific task performance and is suited to a more granular analysis of the simulation. By contrast, subjective measurement can be used to rate more complex behavioral constructs and generally requires the judgment of expert raters [14]. Data on OSCEs have demonstrated that checklists alone (objective measures) do a poor job of measuring expertise in trainees, suggesting that subjective measurements, though more challenging from a validity standpoint, are essential [15].

Within these two categorical frameworks lies a further distinction between assessments that focus on clinical skills and actions, and those that focus on interpersonal dynamics/relationships. Clinical skills and actions refer to psychomotor, verbal, or cognitive tasks of varying degrees of complexity and are typically scored based on whether they were or were not completed (dichotomous scoring), whether they were done correctly, whether they were done in an appropriate amount of time, or whether they were done in the appropriate sequence. These tasks can be either explicit or implicit and can be assessed either objectively or subjectively depending on the specific skill's level of complexity. Assessments focusing on interpersonal dynamics and relationships typically focus on various elements of crisis resource management such as communication, leadership, and professionalism [16–23]. Constructs in this category can be either explicit or implicit but are often more subjective than objective.

Table 7.1 Tools suitable for use in a pediatric simulation environment with published psychometric data

Primary question	Name of tool	Subjects assessed	Question type	Length
Teamwork and leadership skills	Team dimensions rating form [64]	Multidisciplinary critical care teams	7-point Likert scale and global rating	23 items in 4 domains followed by global rating
	TEAM [65]	Emergency department code teams	4-point anchored observational scale and global rating	11 items in 3 domains followed by global rating
	EM Physician Non-Technical Skill Assessment [66]	Emergency department clinicians	9-point anchored Likert scale	12 items in 4 domains
	T-NOTECHS [67]	Emergency department trauma teams	5-point anchored Likert scale	27 items in 5 domains
	CRM Self-Efficacy Instrument [68]	Resident resuscitation teams	5-point Likert scale	24 items in 4 domains
	The Mayo High Performance Teamwork Scale [69]	Resident and nurse resuscitation teams	3-point behavioral checklist	16 items
	CATS [70]	Nonspecific	3-point checklist (weighted)	21 items in 4 domains
	OSCAR [71]	Nonspecific	6-point Likert scale	48 items in 6 domains
	TFAT [72, 73]	Hospitalist resuscitation teams	7-point Likert scale	11 items in 3 domains
	Resuscitation team leader evaluation [74]	Pediatric resuscitation teams	3-point anchored Likert scale	26 items in 2 domains
	IPETT [75]	Pediatric resuscitation teams	7-point anchored Likert scale	14 items (of 32) in 4 domains
	STAT [76]	Multidisciplinary pediatric resuscitation teams	3-point behavioral checklist (weighted)	26 items (of 95 total)
	TPDSCI[a] [20]	Multidisciplinary pediatric resuscitation teams	5-point anchored Likert scale	5 items in 5 domains
	EMT-TEAMWORK-long form/short form [77]	Two-person emergency medical technician teams	7-point Likert scale	45-item long form with a 30-item short form
	Pediatric advanced resuscitation leadership checklist [78]	Pediatric resuscitation teams	Dichotomous and 3-point behavioral checklist	17 items
	TRACS [79]	Pediatric residents	Dichotomous behavioral checklist (weighted)	5 items (of 72 total) in 1 domain
	KTPS [23]	Undergraduate medical, nursing, and respiratory therapy students	5-point behaviorally anchored rubric	12 items
Clinical skills and behavioral checklists	GPAT [80]	Emergency medicine residents	7-point anchored Likert scale	3 scenario-specific checklists (7 items per scenario)
	Clinical Performance Tool [26, 41]	Pediatric residents	3-point behavioral checklist	4 scenario-specific checklists (5–7 items per scenario)
	TRACS [79]	Pediatric residents	Dichotomous behavioral checklist (weighted)	67 items (of 72 total) in 3 domains
	Neonatal Resuscitation Skills Scoring Instrument [81]	Pediatric residents	Dichotomous behavioral checklist (weighted)	44 items in 8 domains
	STAT [76]	Multidisciplinary pediatric resuscitation teams	3-point behavioral checklist (weighed)	59 items (of 95 total) in 3 domains
	IPETT [75]	Pediatric resuscitation teams	6-point anchored Likert scale	18 items (of 32) in 4 domains
	NRP Megacode Assessment [82]	Multidisciplinary teams	3-point behavioral checklist	20 items
	Pediatric Anesthesia Checklists [83]	Pediatric anesthesia trainees	Dichotomous behavioral checklist	10 scenario-specific checklists (8–10 items per scenario)
	Neonatal Resuscitation Skills Scoring Instrument—Modified [84]	Pediatric and family medicine residents	Dichotomous behavioral checklist and time to event	30 items in 7 domains followed by 7 time-to-event questions

Table 7.1 (continued)

Primary question	Name of tool	Subjects assessed	Question type	Length
Procedural skills	Performance Assessment Scale for Simulated Intraosseous Access [85]	Pediatric residents	3-point and dichotomous behavioral checklist (weighted) and time to event questions	12 items followed by 3 time time-to-event questions
	JIT-PAPPS Version 3 [40]	Pediatric ICU staff	Dichotomous behavioral checklist (weighted) and global rating	34 items in 2 domains followed by 2 global ratings
	Central Line Checklist [86]	Pediatric residents	3-point behavioral checklist and visual analog global rating	24 checklist items followed by 1 global score
	Internal Jugular and Subclavian Central Venous Cannula Insertion Checklist [87]	Medicine residents	Dichotomous behavioral checklist	27 items
	Infant LP checklist[b] [88–91]	Pediatric residents	Dichotomous behavioral checklist	15 items
Communication skills	Gap-Kalamazoo Assessment Form[a] [30, 34, 36]	Multidisciplinary clinician teams or single learners	5-point Likert scale and Forced-Choice Rating Scale	11 items in 9 domains
	The Four Habits Model [36, 92]	Single physician learners	4-point and 5-point Likert scale	23 items in 4 domains followed by 24 additional items
	Common Ground Assessment Instrument [36, 93]	Multidisciplinary clinician teams or single learners	3-point to 6-point Likert scale and dichotomous behavioral checklist	27 items in 7 domains
	Calgary–Cambridge Guide [36, 94]	Multidisciplinary clinician teams or single learners	3-point and dichotomous behavioral checklist	70 core process skills[c]
	Patient Perception of Patient-Centeredness Questionnaire [36, 95]	Single physician learners	4-point Likert scale	9-item physician form and 9-item patient forms
	Communication Assessment Tool [36, 96]	Multidisciplinary clinician teams or single learners	5-point Likert scale	15-item physician form and 16-item team form
	Macy Communication Checklist [36, 97]	Multidisciplinary clinician teams or single learners	3-point behaviorally anchored rubric	18 items in 6 domains
	Five-Step Patient-Centered Interviewing Evaluation Tool [36, 98]	Single learners	Dichotomous behavioral checklist	21 items in 5 domains
	American Board of Internal Medicine Patient Assessment for Continuous Professional Development[a] [35, 36]	Single physician learners	5-point Likert scale	10 items
	SEGUE Framework and Instrument [36, 99]	Single physician learners	Dichotomous behavioral checklist	32 items in 6 domains
	C3 instrument [36, 100]	Single physician learners	7-point Likert scale	29 items in 5 domains

TEAM Team Emergency Assessment Measure, *EM* emergency medicine, *T-NOTECHS* Modified nontechnical skills scale for trauma, *CRM* crisis resource medicine, *CATS* Communication and Teamwork Skills Assessment, *OSCAR* Observational Skill-Based Clinical Assessment Tool for Resuscitation, *TFAT* Team Functioning Assessment Tool, *IPETT* Imperial Pediatric Emergency Training Toolkit, *STAT* Simulation Team Assessment Tool, *TPDSCI* Team Performance During Simulated Crises Instrument, *EMT* emergency medical technician, *TRACS* Tool for Resuscitation Assessment using Computerized Simulation, *KTPS* KidSIM Team Performance Scale, *GPAT* Global Performance Assessment Tool, *NRP* Neonatal Resuscitation Program, *JIT-PAPPS* Just-In-Time Pediatric Airway Provider Performance Scale, *LP* lumbar puncture, *ICU* intensive care unit, *SEGUE* Set the stage, Elicit information, Give information, Understand the patient's perspective, and End the encounter

[a] Tools explicitly designed and studied for 360°/multi-rater use

[b] All validity data were collected among adult practitioners. At present, no published pediatric validation data exist

[c] The Calgary–Cambridge Guide is a communication skill assessment development methodology, not a single instrument

Data Collection Strategies

Two basic strategies for data collection exist: *real-time observation* and *post hoc analysis* using video-recorded data. Obtaining data from simulations in real time by live observers is advantageous in that recall bias and the inability to see or hear events due to recording limitations are curbed. Live observers also have the opportunity to clarify or explore implicit processes with subjects as they are happening or in the context of debriefing. For post hoc analysis, conclusions about these processes must often be reached inferentially. Disadvantages of live observers include considerations of time and personnel.

The use of video recording during training sessions has been reported in a variety of modes of simulation training. Video recording provides direct and unbiased information regarding events during a simulation and offers the benefit of one or more raters being able to retrospectively review events as often as is necessary for data abstraction. Data availability during video-recorded encounters, however, does depend on measured tasks being visible and/or audible to a reviewer, a limitation when implicit processes are assessed. Video recording also involves a significant burden of cost and equipment, informed consent, and a secure means of storage and retention of videos. Multiple camera angles may also be necessary to assess interpersonal dynamics and other more complex skills to assure that enough data are present in the recording to generate a complete assessment, a frequent issue in the literature [24–26].

Rater Selection and Preparation

Assessment by raters requires time and personnel with knowledge bases commensurate with the constructs being assessed. For simulations designed to assess more complex subjective and/or implicit phenomena, this means that raters must be content experts with sufficient experience to permit accurate and objective judgment. Common threats to rater validity include the avoidance of extreme ratings (*central tendency* or *leniency*), generalizing isolated performance elements to an entire scale (*halo error* or *recency effect*), or scoring based on relative or generalized contexts (*stereotype* or *contrast* effect) [27]. Training is frequently used to mitigate these biases. Examples include rater error training, where raters are taught to recognize and avoid frequent rating errors; performance dimension training, where raters are given definitions and examples to become familiar with underlying constructs; frame of reference training, where examples are used to assist raters in discriminating between levels of performance; and behavioral observation training, where raters undergo training to improve their observational and perception skills [27–29].

While many assessment tools are intended for raters of a single discipline, 360° assessment strategies exist that can gather a wealth of additional information by collecting data from intra- and interdisciplinary peer sources as well as from faculty raters [30–33]. For simulations involving standardized patients (SPs), their impressions can also be solicited. This approach yields a more robust measure of learner performance as it is experienced by the entire team [31–33]. Ideally all participating in the session are involved, but this can be quite resource intensive, and thus many educators opt for a reduced dataset derived from a few individual assessors only. In order to preserve the holistic implications of 360° assessment, this reduced application is best denoted as multi-rater assessment. Multi-rater and 360° assessment methodologies have been successfully applied in the simulated environment for the assessment of teamwork and communication skills, and a number of instruments calibrated to use this technique exist in the literature (Table 7.1) [20, 30, 32, 34–36].

Self-assessment has the advantage of being universally applicable and relatively easy to perform. Its obvious shortcomings relate to the potential degree of bias in subjects making qualitative judgments about their own performance, and the inaccuracy of self-assessment has been repeatedly demonstrated in the literature [37, 38]. One means for overcoming this issue is the use of *gap analysis,* a technique derived from the business literature. By making the assumption that the results of an assessment validated for the particular environment in which it is used constitute a reproducible measure of learner skill, gap analysis can then be used to generate additional information regarding learner self-appraisal, the degree to which they accurately understand their current skill level [20, 30, 34]. The mathematical approach for performing gap analysis is straightforward, namely subtracting the learner self-rating from the composite rating generated during the multi-rater assessment process. This can be performed as a global calculation or, for individual subdomains, within an assessment [20]. By focusing on the difference between self-rating and the overall assessment, specific domains in which the learner has overestimated their performance *(self-over-appraisal)* or underestimated their performance *(self-under-appraisal)* can be highlighted. These gaps can be further correlated with areas noted by the faculty raters as meeting or exceeding expectations and those identified as needing improvement [20, 30, 34]. A schema for interpreting these correlations is displayed in Fig. 7.2.

Question Design

Question design begins by determining the tasks to be assessed, followed by the creation and prioritization of items, addressing sequencing of items, preliminary testing, and revision and finalizing [39]. Weighting of items permits a greater degree of precision in evaluating performance when compared to a simple checklist of dichotomous items. This

Fig. 7.2 Interpretation of gap analysis data. Interpretation first involves determining the gap range which represents *accurate self-appraisal*. A number of ranges have been proposed, typically -0.5 to $+0.5$ or -1 to 1 [34]. Once gaps have been calculated and the presence of *self-under-appraisal* or *self-over-appraisal* has been determined, these findings can be correlated with the absolute scores using the interpretative grid presented here

	Over-rating of Performance (Gap of -0.5 to -1 or less)	Under-rating of Performance (Gap of 0.5 to 1 or greater)
Domain Scored as a "Meeting or Exceeding Expectations"	<u>Known strengths</u> of the learner team. Only brief attention should be focused here.	<u>Unrecognized Strengths</u> of the learner team. These areas should receive focused attention during debriefing. Attention can be focused on these areas to improve learner's sense of their own abilities.
Domain Scored as a "Needing Improvement"	<u>Unrecognized Weaknesses</u> of the learner team. These areas should receive focused attention during debriefing as they may represent "blind spots" in the learner's self perception	<u>Known weaknesses</u> of the learner team. Only brief attention should be focused here.

is accomplished by having tasks assigned a greater or lesser number of points that contribute to a total score. Alternately, tasks can carry multiple ordinal values which reflect increments of improved performance. Additional potential sources of item weighting may include the results of a specific needs assessment or failure mode analysis determining which tasks are more contributory to good or bad outcomes [40]. Specific tasks associated with a given process, without which a desired clinical change or outcome would be impossible or implausible (such as insertion of an endotracheal tube), can also be selected a priori as fundamental to a given scenario, such that their omission or incorrect performance constitutes a failure. Few clinical scenarios can be said to have a gold standard with regard to the weighting of tasks and thus this process often relies heavily on expert consensus or Delphi methodology [41, 42]. Any weighting schema should be explained clearly to allow others to judge its value for themselves.

Finally, these questions need to be anchored by means of a rating scale. Five common types exist: Likert scales, the Dreyfus conceptual framework, Behaviorally Anchored Rating Scales (BARS), time-to-event measurements, and Global Rating Scales (Table 7.2).

- *Likert scales* are the most commonly used form of response items in qualitative research and permit the translation of subjective responses to items into a numerical score. Advantages of the use of Likert scales include their ease of use and (theoretically) negligible need for rater training if items are well written and defined. Challenges include several novel sources of bias in responses, such as the tendency by raters to avoid the extreme values of a given scaled item (central tendency bias) and the influence of wording variations on response (acquiescence bias).

- The *Dreyfus conceptual framework* is a variant of the Likert scale that defines a series of five stages in the acquisition of a specific skill by a trainee beginning with novice and ending with mastery [43]. The underpinnings of the model involve the evolution of a learner's understanding and performance from the rote application of rules and guidelines to a deeper, more holistic grasp of the concepts.

- *BARS* use scaled responses to items that examine dimensions of behavior specifically pertinent to a given scenario or set of scenarios. BARS are most often developed through an iterative process where critical behaviors are identified (usually by some form of needs assessment, critical incident analysis, or task analysis) and are then converted by experts into scaled responses. Shortcomings of BARS include a tendency toward overrating of the learner's level of mastery by faculty (leniency bias), halo effect, and poor discriminatory capacity [44].

- *Time to event* is a frequent metric in resuscitation algorithms, and many published examples of time-to-event metrics used as outcomes in pediatric simulation have been modeled to reflect these guidelines-based gold standards. Explicit processes are much more likely to be assessed in an unbiased fashion using a time-to-event approach. Depending on the scenario design, these data can often be obtained from the time stamps generated within the simulation log, reducing the need for additional faculty devoted specifically to assessment. Differences in the physical fidelity of the simulated environment, however, can lead to issues when time to event scores are compared between alternative simulation modalities [45].

- *Global rating scales*, or *holistic* scales, allow raters to provide an overall assessment of a subject's performance.

Table 7.2 A taxonomy of assessment tool response types

Scale type	Likert scale	Dreyfus Scale	BARS	Time to event	Global Rating Scale
Focus of data collection	Rates learner's general performance of a procedure or technique	Rates learner's progress (with view to mastery) in a procedure or technique	Rates learner's ability to perform a discrete task	Measures the time needed to initiate key interventions	Raters learner's performance in a global area of practice
Example question	Please rate the learner's ability to perform effective CPR	Please rate the learner's progress in the skill of intubation	Please rate the learner's ability to initiate CPR	Please record the elapsed time (in seconds) between the onset of PEA and the initiation of effective CPR	Please assess the learner's ability to diagnose and manage shock:
	1. Poor	1. Novice	1. No CPR initiated		1. Improper sequence or never performed
	2. Fair	2. Competent	2. Delayed initiation		2. Too late to be effective and incomplete
	3. Good	3. Proficient	3. Timely initiation		3. Late but possibly effective, including a minimum of needed steps
	4. Very good	4. Expert			4. Delayed request for needed steps but all included
	5. Excellent	5. Master			5. Timely request for needed steps
					6. Expeditious request for needed steps with additional laboratory analyses considered

BARS Behaviorally Anchored Rating Scale, *CPR* cardiopulmonary resuscitation, *PEA* pulseless electrical activity

The main advantage of these scales is their ability to incorporate a theoretically limitless set of performance components into a single-scaled metric, reducing the need for quantifying more elusive elements. Unfortunately, this translates into a corresponding need for significant rater expertise and judgment about the construct being assessed in order to provide a reproducible score. In healthcare simulation, this typically means that only experienced clinicians can effectively use global scales. Additionally, it can be difficult to predict and/or account for biases specific to a given reviewer.

Understanding Validation: A Hypothesis-Driven Approach

Before considering this topic, it must be emphasized that assessment instruments are not of universal applicability. Rather, specific tools are constructed to measure specific constructs in specific environments with specific learner groups for a specific purpose. Given this understanding, *validity* refers to our ability to argue that a specific instrument actually measures what we think it does. The data to support this are obtained by the process of *validation,* in which research is conducted in an effort to support a preconceived hypothesis regarding the performance of an assessment tool designed

to measure the intended construct with a specific group of learners. Figure 7.3 illustrates the above relationships.

When developing or choosing an assessment, one has to demonstrate sufficient evidence to meet the intended use, which can be challenging and resource intensive. The demonstration or argument for validity can be supported by variety of sources. Current literature identifies five common categories in which these sources can be placed: content, response process, internal structure, relationship to other variables and evidence of impact or consequences resulting from use [10, 46]. Downing provided a set of examples of evidence in each category, which are included in Table 7.3 [7].

Content evidence seeks to link the assessment to the construct being measured and is typically demonstrated by reference to external models or theoretical constructs and methods that were used to guide tool development. *Response process* relates to aspects of data quality and tool usability and requires the demonstration of a thoughtful tool development process, and the vetting of the tool for usability, and appropriate question design. A number of questions should be addressed that pertain to this process:

- What makes each item sufficiently important to be on the checklist? Conversely, do the items provide sufficient information to illuminate the construct assessed or are more needed?

Fig. 7.3 Conceptual representation of validity. This figure depicts the relationship between the learner and learning environment, the construct being assessed, and the assessment instrument. *Educational environments* are built to allow *specific learner groups* to interact with a construct being taught or assessed. *Evaluators* use *assessment instruments* to quantify this interaction for formative or summative purposes. Validity is the degree to which the assessment instrument accurately and reliably captures this interaction

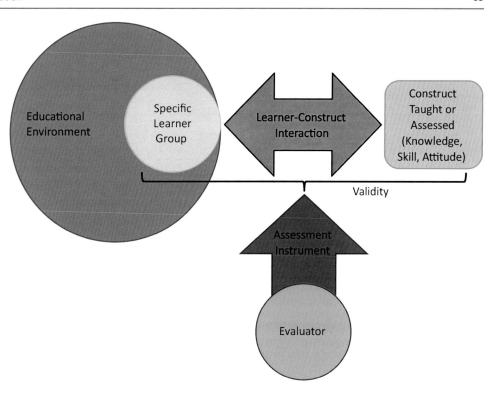

Table 7.3 Some sources of validity evidence for proposed score interpretations and examples of some types of evidence. (Table reproduced with permission from [7])

Content	Response process	Internal structure	Relationship to other variables	Consequences
• Examination blueprint • Representativeness of test blueprint to achievement domain • Test specifications • Match of item content to test specifications • Representativeness of items to domain • Logical/empirical relationship of content tested to achievement domain • Quality of test questions • Item writer qualifications • Sensitivity review	• Student format familiarity • Quality control of electronic scanning/scoring • Key validation of preliminary scores • Accuracy in combining different formats scores • Quality control/accuracy of final scores/marks/grades • Subscore/subscale analyses • Accuracy of applying pass/fail decision rules to scores • Quality control of score reporting to students/faculty • Understandable/accurate descriptions/interpretations of scores for students	• Item analysis data: 1. Item difficulty/discrimination 2. ICCs/TCCs 3. Inter-item correlations 4. Item-total correlations • Score scale reliability • SEM 1. Generalizability 2. Dimensionality 3. Item factor analysis 4. Differential Item Functioning (DIF) 5. Psychometric model	• Correlation with other relevant variables • Convergent correlations—internal/external: 1. Similar tests • Divergent correlations—internal/external 1. Dissimilar measures • Test-criterion correlations • Generalizability of evidence	• Impact of test scores/results on students/society • Consequences on learners/future learning • Positive consequences outweigh unintended negative consequences? • Reasonableness of method of establishing pass/fail (cut) score • Pass/fail consequences: 1. Pass/fail decision reliability-Classification accuracy 2. CSEM at pass score 3. False positives/negatives 4. Instructional/learner consequences

ICCs/TCCs item/test characteristic curves, *SEM* standard errors of measurement, *DIF* differential item functioning, *CSEM* conditional standard error of measurement

• How important are the items in relation to one another?
• Can the rater observe each item in a manner that permits it to be scored?
• Is there consensus by the design group that the items are appropriate for the population evaluated?
• What is the planned mode of analysis, and does the scoring framework collect data in the proper manner to permit that analysis (e.g., how might a response of "not done" be scored)?
• Is the creation of an overall aggregate score intended or justified? Would separate domains with an assessment make more sense?

Internal structure relates to psychometric assessments and encompasses the *reliability* of the instrument. It is important

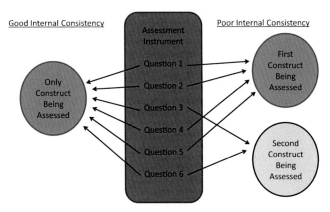

Fig. 7.4 Conceptual representation of internal consistency. This figure depicts the concept of internal consistency. Instruments are said to have good internal consistency if each item or question corresponds to one overarching construct. Instruments are said to have poor internal consistency if items or questions correspond to multiple constructs. Please note that many instruments are specifically designed to have multiple subdomains intended to represent separate but complementary constructs. In this case, it is not appropriate to assess overall internal consistency (as opposed to subdomain-specific internal consistency) as in this circumstance the global value is expected to be low

here to emphasize that reliability is only one part of an overall argument that must be made and does not stand on its own [7]. Common metrics used to describe data in simulation include *internal consistency, inter-rater, and intra-rater reliability. Generalizability analysis* is also included in this category. Internal consistency measures the degree to which individual items correlate as evidence that the tool (or a domain within a tool) is measuring a relatively unified construct (Fig. 7.4). By way of example, imagine a hypothetical checklist addressing a specific procedure that contains 20 items, of which six are procedural, five relate to consent, and nine are about sterility and other ancillary processes. We might find that there is poor consistency between the sterility and the specific procedural steps. The interpretation of this information then depends on the nature of the construct we are assessing as we would not necessarily expect all subdomains of *procedural competence* to correlate (a learner may be meticulous about sterility but unskilled with regard to the actual procedure). Internal consistency should be used to support the argument only when we believe there should be consistency based on the nature of the construct being assessed.

In contrast, inter-rater reliability measures how well scores generated by different raters using the tool correlate (Fig. 7.5). Low inter-rater reliability implies that different raters perceive the content of the tool differently and thus are contributing significant variability to the score. Intra-rater simply measures how well an individual rater is consistent across time. *Generalizability analysis* is an analytical method used to quantify the degree by that a variety of sources

(often raters, cases, and sessions) lead to score variation beyond the individual's performance. It further allows one to understand the impact of changing the number of raters or cases [47]. Alternatively, internal consistency and inter-rater reliability can be assessed using classical psychometric statistical metrics such as Cronbach's alpha, Cohen's kappa, or correlation metrics (Pearson's, Spearman's, or Intraclass).

Relationship to other variables examines the association between scores obtained on the assessment and other learner characteristics that might result in similar stratification (learner experience level or previous educational exposure are common variables examined). Note that this portion of the argument is particularly susceptible to statistical power as an underpowered study may not detect a meaningful difference when one exists in reality [48]. Typical statistical tests used to compare mean or median scores (Student's *t*-test, Wilcoxon rank-sum test, etc.) are often used.

Consequence relates to the impact of testing or the effect of pass/fail decisions that are made based on the assessment instrument. The burden of proof required of an assessment is directly related to the impact it will have on subjects, curricula, or larger processes. A formative assessment might require a modest evidence base while the burden on a national assessment such as the Step 2 Clinical Skills is substantial (and ongoing) [7]. In the middle are the smaller efforts that might lead to remediation or performance assessments that become part of the permanent record.

The recent past has seen a substantial amount of scholarly activity regarding assessment tools, with variation in the amount of information provided regarding these instruments' performance characteristics. In some cases, studies have insufficient evidence to support the use of instruments described or lack a hypothesis-driven approach from the outset. The theoretical underpinnings of validity have undergone substantial changes over the past century [9, 49]. The current approach to instrument validation has been described in a number of scholarly works and is summarized below in three steps [8, 9, 49, 50]:

1. *Proposal of a hypothesis:* This hypothesis should explicitly state the *what, who,* and *why* of the validation study. Formally, this represents the creation of an interpretive argument that addresses what meaning will be drawn from the score, over what conditions the information can be generalized, if and how the data can be extrapolated to the construct in question, and how the resulting data will affect decisions made regarding the learner. By way of example, consider a study examining a novel tool to assess pediatric LP performance. A possible hypothesis for this study would be "The Lumbar Puncture (LP) Checklist will produce valid data to discriminate amongst pediatric residents for the purpose of providing formative feedback at the end of the first year of training."

Fig. 7.5 Conceptual representation of inter-rater reliability. This figure depicts the concept of inter-rater reliability. Instruments are said to have good inter-rater reliability if different raters assessing the same learners performing a given task generate similar scores using the instrument. Instruments are said to have poor inter-rater reliability if those same raters generate scores using the instrument that significantly differ

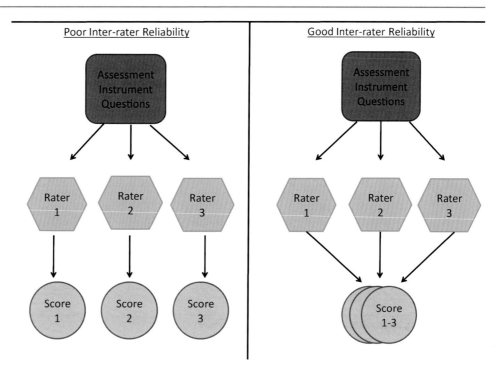

2. *Hypothesis-driven generation of study design:* In this step, the researcher must consider possible confounders that may differ between potential subjects. To build on the above example, pediatric residents would be expected to have ongoing clinical experiences in performing LPs that would need to be controlled for in a way that would likely be unnecessary if medical students were the target population. This step is also sensitive to the ultimate goal of the tool's use, as a greater degree of rigor (possibly including the adoption of a mastery learning model) is needed to support its use for summative assessment purposes such as promotion and grading. Finally, the study should be deliberately designed to produce data regarding as many different types of validity evidence as possible.

3. *Argument-driven analysis:* Once assessment data have been obtained, the resultant data must be organized in a validity argument that supports the tool's use in a particular population for a specific purpose [7–9, 51]. It is important to remember that validity is not portable; one cannot assume that an instrument can be used for a new purpose or audience based on evidence supporting its use in a different situation. Nor is a validity argument binary (the test is valid or not) but rather represents an aggregation of evidence giving relative support to validity in the study context [52].

Given that many readers will not be engaged in the act of validation, but rather the interpretation of studies that claim to support the validity of a tool, we have provided an example of a validity argument using the LP checklist referenced in the process above in Table 7.4. As should be apparent from the discussion, validation can be a difficult process to successfully complete. Fortunately, a large number of tools currently exist in the literature, and so it is often not necessary to generate and validate an additional instrument for most uses (Table 7.1). This outlined process of triangulating multiple streams of evidence should be used by simulation educators to critically assess the evidence for any tool that they wish to adopt. Educators should take care to use tools only in the manner in which and for the populations in whom they have been validated.

Implementation of Assessment Tools and Delivery of Feedback

When considering implementation and delivery of feedback, the intended goal of the assessment process must first be considered. Specifically, is the assessment meant to provide *formative* feedback intended to impact learner behavior, or is it intended to provide a *summative* report of the learner's abilities for use as a grade or as research data (Fig. 7.1)? In all cases, the immediate concern is the timing of the assessment process and its effect on the data obtained. While we recognize that, in many cases, assessments are intended to accomplish both purposes, it is helpful to consider both separately in order to highlight important distinctions.

Implementing Formative Assessment

Debriefing, the process in which verbal feedback to learners is provided based on the real-time assessments of the

Table 7.4 Elements of a validity argument with exemplars

Source of validity	Exemplar of appropriate argument using validation of LP checklist study
Content	An expert panel of clinicians who perform LPs as well as educational and assessment experts were convened. They were informed of our purpose and our subject population. Items were generated by this group according to a literature-based checklist development model [101]
Response process	Data were acquired via a web-based form pilot tested and revised prior to the validation study. Raters were trained using examples of good and poor performance recorded in exemplar videos
Internal structure	The rater reliability and impact of testing across sessions and item of the tools were assessed statistically using a generalizability study to provide information on the sources of variability in the scores, including a rater reliability metric [47]
Relationship to other variables	Performance of our target audience, as well as more advanced subjects (fellows and attendings), was assessed using the tool and compared using repeated measures ANOVA. This comparison demonstrated a statistically significant difference in score between these groups, with fellows and attendings scoring meaningfully and significantly higher than junior trainees. Care should be taken to consider whether your comparison groups make sense (e.g., would faculty do better than fellows?), and pilot testing should be done to assure this is so. An alternative outcome might be to measure real-world clinical LP performance. This is substantially more resource intensive but would represent stronger evidence and may be needed if the checklist is intended for summative assessment
Consequences	Our proposed use of the LP tool is for formative feedback only, and so we might argue that additional evidence is not needed above what has been provided to support its use. Alternatively, we could ask what the impact of the assessment on learners might be, such as the creation of overconfident practitioners who decline potentially necessary supervision based on their experience

LP lumbar puncture, *ANOVA* analysis of variance

facilitators, has rightly been noted as the most important component of the simulation-based learning environment [53, 54]. If, as was asserted at the beginning of the chapter, all simulations involve an ongoing informal process of assessment, then debriefing represents the primary feedback delivery mechanism for that ongoing assessment and the point at which the learners are most open to self-reflection [55]. This allows the implementation and delivery of formalized formative assessment to be conceptualized as a means of augmenting the information delivered by the debriefing and encouraging learners to continue the reflective learning process post debriefing [55]. For simple assessment data, such as the time to event, a number of the existing simulation software platforms have built-in modules that allow this information to be presented during or immediately after the debriefing process [56–58]. Assessments of greater complexity, however, require more labor to perform and analyze, which raises the question of how this process should relate to the debriefing. Specifically, it must be asked whether and how the imposition of the formalized assessment process between the case and the debriefing affects the content of the debriefing [59]. Research data in this area are lacking, and so we cannot be absolutely proscriptive, but we suggest, if the desire of course faculty is to use the assessment data in a formative manner, that strong consideration be given to implementing the assessment after the debriefing in order to preserve the core educational flow of the session as failure to do this may well compromise the reflective process that the assessment is intended to promote.

Once the assessment data have been obtained, it is necessary to consider how it should be delivered. Here, it should be noted that this question affects formative feedback only, as pure summative feedback is not intended for learner education. Although real time delivery of feedback during or shortly after debriefing represents the ideal, this real-time delivery strategy can be a challenge for more complex tools given the need to collate the information obtained by the assessment process. In situations such as this, post hoc written feedback may be the best option. When considering how to structure such a feedback report, several questions should be asked. First, how should the data best be represented (written vs graphical) to maximally impact learners? Second, what mechanisms should be put into place to highlight significant data points that require more in-depth review and consideration? Though literature on these questions is scant, some guidance can be derived from the business world. One review of feedback delivery mechanisms suggested several strategies that are applicable to simulation, including comparing scores to accepted norms or an ideal, visually highlighting the areas of greatest concern and greatest strength, and listing specific behavioral changes indicated by the assessment [60]. These are not mutually exclusive, and feedback mechanisms using a number of the above approaches can be used. For all the above strategies, provision of narrative feedback in parallel with quantitative data can add an additional level of depth [60, 61]. If feedback is delivered via email or another other impersonal route, it is also vital to offer the possibility of one-on-one contact with the instructor to review the information if the learner desires.

Implementing Summative Assessment

For summative assessment, the same basic consideration pertains, namely the appropriate time to implement the assessment process in relationship to the session as a whole and the debriefing in particular. In this case, however, increased value must be placed on maintaining the purity of the data obtained from that process. By definition, debriefing involves a faculty facilitated process of active self-reflection by learners and thus cannot help but compromise the independence of rater observations, potentially causing faculty scores and learner self-scores to artificially converge [53, 54, 62]. While this effect may not be meaningful in the context of formative assessment, it becomes a significant issue for summative assessment and is especially troublesome in assessment performed for research purposes (particularly in validation studies, as the inter-rater reliability can be artificially inflated by this phenomenon). Indeed, for many assessments performed for purely summative means, such as the OSCEs conducted as part of the USMLE, no debriefing is offered at all [63]. Regardless of how (or whether) the debriefing is performed, it is clear that summative assessment data should be obtained in a manner that assures independence of observation. This can be accomplished by gathering assessment data at the close of the simulation itself prior to the debriefing or, if this is not possible, at a later date based on a review of session video recordings by faculty assessors uninvolved with the session. This latter approach may be best for research purposes.

While the differences between formative and summative assessment implementation have been highlighted, we recognize that in many contexts simulation educators may well desire to assess their learners for both formative and summative purposes simultaneously. In situations such as this, the summative purposes should prevail with regard to assessment timing. Once the debriefing is complete, the assessment data can subsequently be compiled into a formative report.

Available Pediatric Assessment Tools

Over the past decade, the literature regarding assessment tools germane to pediatrics has steadily grown. Many of these tools have been investigated thoroughly and have evidence supporting their use. We present in Table 7.1 a collection of those tools known to the authors that have been used in real and simulated pediatric environments or in adult environments readily translatable to simulation-based pediatric education. Given the difficulties inherent in the creation and validation of new assessment tools, we hope that this list will enable pediatric simulation educators to find an existing assessment modality suited to their needs.

Conclusions

Assessment is an inherent part of simulation-based medical education, and the methods we choose to perform those assessments can profoundly impact the feedback given to our learners. By giving attention to assessment as a measurement process requiring tools shown to be valid to address the specific learners, situations, and constructs we wish to assess, we can be sure that the information we provide our learners is as accurate and useful as possible. Simulation-based medical educators are encouraged to use the principles outlined above in their selection and implementation of assessment methodologies. It is our hope that the list of current tools will encourage their use and further development.

References

1. Scalese R, Hatala R. Competency assessment. In: Levine AI, DeMaria S, Schwartz AD, Sim AJ, editors. The comprehensive textbook of healthcare simulation. New York: Springer; 2013. pp. 135–60.
2. Harlen W, James M. Assessment and learning: differences and relationships between formative and summative feedback. Assess Educ Princ Policy Pract. 2006;4(3):365–79.
3. Williams D, Black P. Meanings and consequences: a basis for distinguishing formative and summative functions of assessment? Br Educ Res J. 1996;22(5):537–48.
4. Mislevy R, Steinberg L, Almond R. Focus article: on the structure of educational assessments. Meas Interdisc Res Perspect. 2003;1(1):3–62.
5. Pellegrino J. Knowing what students know. Issue Sci Technol. 2002–2003;19(2):48–52.
6. Downing S, Haladyna T. Validity threats: overcoming interference with proposed interpretations of assessment data. Med Educ. 2004;38(3):327–33.
7. Downing S. Validity: on meaningful interpretation of assessment data. Med Educ. 2003;37(9):830–7.
8. Kane M. Validation as a pragmatic, scientific activity. J Educ Meas. 2013;50(1):115–22.
9. Kane M. Validating the interpretations and uses of test scores. J Educ Meas. 2013;50(1):1–73.
10. American Educational Research Association, American Psychological Association, & National Council on Measurement in Education. Standards for educational and psychological testing. Washington, DC: American Educational Research Association; 1999.
11. Baker D, Gustafson S, Beaubien J, Salas E, Barach P. Medical team training programs in healthcare. In: Henrikson K, Battles JB, Marks ES, Lewin DI, editors. Advances in patient safety: from research to implementation (Vol 4: Programs, Tools, and Products). Rockville: Agency for Healthcare Research and Quality (US); 2005. pp. 253–67.
12. Buljac-Samardzic M, Dekker-van Doorn C, van Wijngaarden J, van Wijk K. Interventions to improve team effectiveness: a systematic review. Health Policy (Amsterdam, Netherlands). 2010;94(3):183–95.
13. Eppich W, Howard V, Vozenilek J, Curran I. Simulation-based team training in healthcare. Simul Healthc. 2011;6:14–9.
14. Boulet J, Murray D. Review article: assessment in anesthesiology education. Can J Anaesth (Journal canadien d'anesthesie). 2012;59(2):182–92.

15. Hodges B, Regehr G, McNaughton N, Tiberius R, Hanson M. OSCE checklists do not capture increasing levels of expertise. Acad Med. 1999;74(10):1129–34.

16. Abdelshehid C, Quach S, Nelson C, Graversen J, Lusch A, Zarraga J, et al. High-fidelity simulation-based team training in urology: evaluation of technical and nontechnical skills of urology residents during laparoscopic partial nephrectomy. J Surg Educ. 2013;70(5):588–95.

17. Boon W, McAllister J, Attar M, Chapman R, Mullan P, Haftel H. Evaluation of heart rate assessment timing, communication, accuracy, and clinical decision-making during high fidelity simulation of neonatal resuscitation. Int J Pediatr. 2014;2014:927430.

18. Spanager L, Beier-Holgersen R, Dieckmann P, Konge L, Rosenberg J, Oestergaard D. Reliable assessment of general surgeons' non-technical skills based on video-recordings of patient simulated scenarios. Am J Surg. 2013;206(5):810–7.

19. Tobler K, Grant E, Marczinski C. Evaluation of the Impact of a simulation-enhanced breaking bad news workshop in pediatrics. Simul Healthc. 2014;9(4):213–9.

20. Calhoun A, Boone M, Miller K, Taulbee R, Montgomery V, Boland K. A multirater instrument for the assessment of simulated pediatric crises. J Grad Med Educ. 2011;3(1):88–94.

21. McEvoy M, Butler B, MacCarrick G. Teaching professionalism through virtual means. Clin Teach. 2012;9(1):32–6.

22. Ponton-Carss A, Hutchison C, Violato C. Assessment of communication, professionalism, and surgical skills in an objective structured performance-related examination (OSPRE): a psychometric study. Am J Surg. 2011;202(4):433–40.

23. Sigalet E, Donnon T, Cheng A, Cooke S, Robinson T, Bissett W, et al. Development of a team performance scale to assess undergraduate health professionals. Acad Med. 2013;88(7):989–96.

24. Cheng A, Auerbach M, Hunt E, Chang T, Pusic M, Nadkarni V, et al. Designing and conducting simulation-based research. Pediatrics. 2014;133(6):1091–101.

25. Cheng A, Hunt E, Donoghue A, Nelson-McMillan K, Nishisaki A, Leflore J, et al. Examining pediatric resuscitation education using simulation and scripted debriefing: a multicenter randomized trial. JAMA Pediatr. 2013;167(6):528–36.

26. Donoghue A, Ventre K, Boulet J, Brett-Fleegler M, Nishisaki A, Overly F, et al. Design, implementation, and psychometric analysis of a scoring instrument for simulated pediatric resuscitation: a report from the EXPRESS pediatric investigators. Simul Healthc. 2011;6(2):71–7.

27. Feldman M, Lazzara E, Vanderbilt A, DiazGranados D. Rater training to support high-stakes simulation-based assessments. J Contin Educ Health Prof. 2012;32(4):279–86.

28. Gorman C, Rentsch J. Evaluating frame-of-reference rater training effectiveness using performance schema accuracy. J Appl Psychol. 2009;94(5):1336–44.

29. Holmboe E, Ward D, Reznick R, Katsufrakis P, Leslie K, Patel V, et al. Faculty development in assessment: the missing link in competency-based medical education. Acad Med. 2011;86(4):460–7.

30. Calhoun A, Rider E, Meyer E, Lamiani G, Truog R. Assessment of communication skills and self-appraisal in the simulated environment: feasibility of multirater feedback with gap analysis. Simul Healthc. 2009;4(1):22–9.

31. Foster C, Law M. How many perspectives provide a compass? Differentiating 360-degree and multi-source feedback. Int J Select Assess. 2006;14(3):288–91.

32. Lockyer J. Multisource feedback in the assessment of physician competencies. J Contin Educ Health Prof. 2003;23(1):4–12.

33. Violato C, Marini A, Toews J, Lockyer J, Fidler H. Feasibility and psychometric properties of using peers, consulting physicians, coworkers, and patients to assess physicians. Acad Med. 1997;72(10 Suppl 1):S82–4.

34. Calhoun A, Rider E, Peterson E, Meyer E. Multi-rater feedback with gap analysis: an innovative means to assess communication skill and self-insight. Patient Educ Couns. 2010;80(3):321–6.

35. Lipner R, Blank L, Leas B, Fortna G. The value of patient and peer ratings in recertification. Acad Med. 2002;77(Suppl 10):S64–6.

36. Rider E, Nawotniak R. A practical guide to teaching and assessing the ACGME core competencies. 2nd ed. Marblehead: HC pro; 2010.

37. Eva K, Regehr G. Self-assessment in the health professions: a reformulation and research agenda. Acad Med. 2005;80(Suppl 10):S46–54.

38. Eva K, Regehr G. Knowing when to look it up: a new conception of self-assessment ability. Acad Med. 2007;82(Suppl 10):S81–4.

39. Stufflebeam D. Guidelines for developing evaluation checklists: the checklists development checklist (CDC). 2000. http://www. wmich.edu/evalctr/archive_checklists/guidelines_cdc.pdf. Accessed 20 June 2014.

40. Nishisaki A, Donoghue A, Colborn S, Watson C, Meyer A, Niles D, et al. Development of an instrument for a primary airway provider's performance with an ICU multidisciplinary team in pediatric respiratory failure using simulation. Respir Care. 2012;57(7):1121–8.

41. Donoghue A, Nishisaki A, Sutton R, Hales R, Boulet J. Reliability and validity of a scoring instrument for clinical performance during pediatric advanced life support simulation scenarios. Resuscitation. 2010;81(3):331–6.

42. Ventre K, Collingridge D, DeCarlo D. End-user evaluations of a personal computer-based pediatric advanced life support simulator. Simul Healthc. 2011;6(3):134–42.

43. Pena A. The Dreyfus model of clinical problem-solving skills acquisition: a critical perspective. Med Educ Online. 2010;15. doi:10.3402/meo.v15i0.4846.

44. Kingstrom P, Bass A. A critical analysis of studies comparing behaviorally anchored rating scales and other rating formats. Pers Psychol. 1981;34(2):263–89.

45. Donoghue A, Durbin D, Nadel F, Stryjewski G, Kost S, Nadkarni V. Effect of high-fidelity simulation on pediatric advanced life support training in pediatric house staff: a randomized trial. Pediatr Emerg Care. 2009;25(3):139–44.

46. Messick S. Meaning and values in test validation: the science and ethics of assessment. Educ Res. 1989;18(2):5–11.

47. Shavelson R, Webb N. Generalizability theory: a primer. Newbury Park: Sage Publications; 1991.

48. Cook D, Hatala R. Got power? A systematic review of sample size adequacy in health professions education research. Adv Health Sci Educ. 2014.

49. Brennan R. Commentary on "validating the interpretations and uses of test scores". J Educ Meas. 2013;50(1):74–83.

50. Downing S, Yudkowski R. Assessment in health professions education. New York: Routledge; 2009.

51. Novack D, Dube C, Goldstein M. Teaching medical interviewing: a basic course on interviewing and the physician-patient relationship. Arch Intern Med. 1992;152(9):1814–20.

52. Cook D, Beckman T. Current concepts in validity and reliability for psychometric instruments: theory and application. Am J Med. 2006;119(2):166.e7–16.

53. Fanning R, Gaba D. The role of debriefing in simulation-based learning. Simul Healthc. 2007;2(2):115–25.

54. Issenberg S, McGaghie W, Petrusa E. Features and uses of high-fidelity medical simulations that lead to effective learning: a BEME systematic review. Med Teach. 2005;27(1):10–28.

55. Rudolph J, Simon R, Dufresne R, Raemer D. There's no such thing as "nonjudgmental" debriefing: a theory and method for debriefing with good judgment. Simul Healthc. 2006;1(1):49–55.

56. Group SB. Studiocode solutions for healthcare 2014. 2014. http://www.studiocodegroup.com/solutions/healthcare/highlights/.

57. Healthcare C. Metivision 2013. 2013. http://www.caehealthcare.com/eng/center-management/metivision. Accessed 2 June 2014.

58. Medical L. Laerdal 2014. 2014. http://www.laerdal.com/us/. Accessed 1 June 2014.

59. Raemer D, Anderson M, Cheng, Fanning R, Nadkarni V, Savoldelli G. Research regarding debriefing as part of the learning process. Simul Healthc. 2011;6(7):S52–7.

60. Leslie J, Fleenor J. Feedback to managers: a review and comparison of multi-rater instruments for management development. 3rd ed. Greensboro: Center for Creative Leadershio; 1998.

61. Overeem K, Lombarts K, Arah O, Klazinga N, Grol R, Wollersheim H. Three methods of multi-source feedback compared: a plea for narrative comments and coworkers' perspectives. Med Teach. 2010;32(2):141–7.

62. Bell B, Cowie B. Formative assessment and science education. Dordrecht: Kluwer Academic Publishers; 2001.

63. Examiners NBoM. Step 2 clinical skills (CS) content description and general information. 2014. http://www.usmle.org/pdfs/step-2-cs/cs-info-manual.pdf. Accessed 21 Oct 2014.

64. Weller J, Frengley R, Torrie J, Shulruf B, Jolly B, Hopley L, et al. Evaluation of an instrument to measure teamwork in multidisciplinary critical care teams. BMJ Qual Saf. 2011;20(3):216–22.

65. Cooper S, Cant R, Porter J, Sellick K, Somers G, Kinsman L, et al. Rating medical emergency teamwork performance: development of the team emergency assessment measure (TEAM). Resuscitation. 2010;81(4):446–52.

66. Flowerdew L, Brown R, Vincent C, Woloshynowych M. Development and validation of a tool to assess emergency physicians' nontechnical skills. Ann Emerg Med. 2012;59(5):376–85.e4.

67. Steinemann S, Berg B, DiTullio A, Skinner A, Terada K, Anzelon K, et al. Assessing teamwork in the trauma bay: introduction of a modified "NOTECHS" scale for trauma. Am J Surg. 2012;203(1):69–75.

68. Plant J, van Schaik S, Sliwka D, Boscardin C, O'Sullivan P. Validation of a self-efficacy instrument and its relationship to performance of crisis resource management skills. Adv Health Sci Educ Theory Pract. 2011;16(5):579–90.

69. Malec J, Torsher L, Dunn W, Wiegmann D, Arnold J, Brown D, et al. The mayo high performance teamwork scale: reliability and validity for evaluating key crew resource management skills. Simul Healthc. 2007;2(1):4–10.

70. Frankel A, Gardner R, Maynard L, Kelly A. Using the communication and teamwork skills (CATS) assessment to measure health care team performance. Jt Comm J Qual Patient Saf. 2007;33(9):549–58.

71. Walker S, Brett S, McKay A, Lambden S, Vincent C, Sevdalis N. Observational skill-based clinical assessment tool for resuscitation (OSCAR): development and validation. Resuscitation. 2011;82(7):835–44.

72. Sutton G, Liao J, Jimmieson N, Restubog S. Measuring multidisciplinary team effectiveness in a ward-based healthcare setting: development of the team functioning assessment tool. J Healthc Qual. 2011;33(3):10–23. quiz–4.

73. Sutton G, Liao J, Jimmieson N, Restubog S. Measuring ward-based multidisciplinary healthcare team functioning: a validation study of the team functioning assessment tool (TFAT). J Healthc Qual. 2013;35(4):36–49.

74. Grant E, Grant V, Bhanji F, Duff J, Cheng A, Lockyer J. The development and assessment of an evaluation tool for pediatric resident competence in leading simulated pediatric resuscitations. Resuscitation. 2012;83(7):887–93.

75. Lambden S, DeMunter C, Dowson A, Cooper M, Gautama S, Sevdalis N. The imperial paediatric emergency training toolkit (IPETT) for use in paediatric emergency training: development and evaluation of feasibility and validity. Resuscitation. 2013;84(6):831–6.

76. Reid J, Stone K, Brown J, Caglar D, Kobayashi A, Lewis-Newby M, et al. The simulation team assessment tool (STAT): development, reliability and validation. Resuscitation. 2012;83(7):879–86.

77. Patterson P, Weaver M, Weaver S, Rosen M, Todorova G, Weingart L, et al. Measuring teamwork and conflict among emergency medical technician personnel. Prehosp Emerg Care. 2012;16(1):98–108.

78. Gilfoyle E, Gottesman R, Razack S. Development of a leadership skills workshop in paediatric advanced resuscitation. Med Teach. 2007;29(9):e276–83.

79. Brett-Fleegler M, Vinci R, Weiner DA. A simulator-based tool that assesses pediatric resident resuscitation competency. Pediatrics. 2008;121(3):e597–603.

80. Adler M, Vozenilek J, Trainor J, Eppich W, Wang E, Beaumont J, et al. Comparison of checklist and anchored global rating instruments for performance rating of simulated pediatric emergencies. Simul Healthc. 2011;6(1):18–24.

81. van der Heide P, van Toledo-Eppinga L, van der Heide M, van der Lee J. Assessment of neonatal resuscitation skills: a reliable and valid scoring system. Resuscitation. 2006;71(2):212–21.

82. Lockyer J, Singhal N, Fidler H, Weiner G, Aziz K, Curran V. The development and testing of a performance checklist to assess neonatal resuscitation megacode skill. Pediatrics. 2006;118(6):e1739–44.

83. Fehr J, Boulet J, Waldrop W, Snider R, Brockel M, Murray D. Simulation-based assessment of pediatric anesthesia skills. Anesthesiology. 2011;115(6):1308–15.

84. Sawyer T, Sierocka-Castaneda A, Chan D, Berg B, Lustik M, Thompson M. Deliberate practice using simulation improves neonatal resuscitation performance. Simul Healthc. 2011;6(6):327–36.

85. Oriot D, Darrieux E, Boureau-Voultoury A, Ragot S, Scepi M. Validation of a performance assessment scale for simulated intraosseous access. Simul Healthc. 2012;7(3):171–5.

86. Thomas S, Burch W, Kuehnle S, Flood R, Scalzo A, Gerard J. Simulation training for pediatric residents on central venous catheter placement: a pilot study. Pediatr Crit Care Med. 2013;14(9):e416–23.

87. Barsuk J, McGaghie W, Cohen E, Jayshankar S, Wayne D. Use of simulation-based mastery learning to improve the quality of central venous catheter placement in a medical intensive care unit. J Hosp Med. 2009;4(7):397–403.

88. Kessler D, Auerbach M, Pusic M, Tunik M, Foltin J. A randomized trial of simulation-based deliberate practice for infant lumbar puncture skills. Simul Healthc. 2011;6(4):197–203.

89. Gaies M, Morris S, Hafler J, Graham D, Capraro A, Zhou J, et al. Reforming procedural skills training for pediatric residents: a randomized, interventional trial. Pediatrics. 2009;124(2):610–9.

90. Kilbane B, Adler M, Trainor J. Pediatric residents' ability to perform a lumbar puncture: evaluation of an educational intervention. Pediatr Emerg Care. 2010;26(8):558–62.

91. Lammers R, Temple K, Wagner M, Ray D. Competence of new emergency medicine residents in the performance of lumbar punctures. Acad Emerg Med. 2005;12(7):622–8.

92. Stein T, Frankel R, Krupat E. Enhancing clinician communication skills in a large healthcare organization: a longitudinal case study. Patient Educ Couns. 2005;58(1):4–12.

93. Lang F, McCord R, Harvill L, Anderson D. Communication assessment using the common ground instrument: psychometric properties. Fam Med. 2004;36(3):189–98.

94. Kurtz S. Teaching and learning communication in veterinary medicine. J Vet Med Educ. 2006;33(1):11–9.

95. Stewart M, Brown J, Weston W, McWhinney I, MCWilliam C, Freeman T. Patient-centered medicine: transforming the clinical method. 2nd ed. Oxford: Radcliffe Medical Press; 2003.

96. Makoul G, Krupat E, Chang C. Measuring patient views of physician communication skills: development and testing of the communication assessment tool. Patient Educ Couns. 2007;67(3):333–42.

97. Stevens D, King D, Laponis R, Hanley K, Zabar S, Kalet A, et al. Medical students retain pain assessment and management skills long after an experiential curriculum: a controlled study. Pain. 2009;145(3):319–24.

98. Smith R. Patient centered interviewing: an evidence based method. 2nd ed. Philadelphia: Lippincott Williams & Wilkins; 2002.

99. Makoul G. The SEGUE Framework for teaching and assessing communication skills. Patient Educ Couns. 2001;45(1):23–34.

100. Haidet P, Kelly P, Chou C, Curriculum ftC, Group CS. Characterizing the patient-centeredness of hidden curricula in medical schools: development and validation of a new measure. Acad Med. 2005;80(1):44–50.

101. Shmutz J, Eppich W, Hoffman F, Heimberg E, Manser T. Five steps to develop checklists for evaluating clinical performance: an integrative approach. Acad Med. 2014;89(7):1–10.

Standardized Patients

Dawn Taylor Peterson

Simulation Pearls
- It is important to determine if a standardized patient or a simulated patient is necessary to accomplish the learning objectives of the scenario.
- The structure and type of training required for a standardized patient or (or family member) depends on the learning objectives of the case and whether or not the simulation is part of a high-stakes summative assessment or is simply designed for educational purposes.
- Careful considerations must be made, and safeguards must be put into place, when children and/or adolescents are used as standardized patients or simulated patients.
- Simulated patients and family members can be an effective tool for teaching communication skills as well as delivering bad news and facilitating difficult conversations.

Introduction

The use of standardized patients in medical education originated in 1964 [1] and has been growing in scope and impact over the past 60 years. While some educators believe that standardized patients are currently underused in healthcare education [2], the integration of standardized patients into the education and evaluation of healthcare professionals has increased dramatically over the past 20 years [3].

According to a 2012 survey distributed by the Council on Medical Student Education and Pediatrics, 35 % of pediatric clerkship directors surveyed reported using standardized patients with their students. These respondents also reported using children and adults as simulated patients 60 % of the time [4]. The use of standardized patients in medical education has also been determined to be a best practice for

teaching communication skills, interpersonal skills, and facilitating difficult conversations [5].

Historically, simulation centers and standardized patient programs have been divided geographically with separate operational structures under the university, academic, or hospital umbrella, resulting in two separate staffs and two distinctly different training programs. Recently, however, many simulation centers have combined programs under one umbrella, which integrates high-fidelity simulation programs along with standardized patient and simulated patient programs [6]. The result has proven to be an effective structure for training standardized patients and educating healthcare professionals from any area or discipline.

Common Terms and Definitions

Standardized patients are now considered a unique discipline [7] and are being recognized as a specific occupation in countries all over the world [8]. As the field of standardized patients becomes more robust and formalized, it is important to clarify common terms and definitions. The term SP is commonly used to make reference to a standardized patient, a standardized participant, or a simulated patient [9], and in some settings, it is intended to reference a simulated client or patient instructor [8]. However, recent studies have made a distinction between the two terms [10, 11]. In accordance with these studies, this chapter will refer to a standardized patient as one who has been rigorously trained to display symptoms in a consistent, sequential, and unchanging manner for multiple learners in a high-stakes summative assessment. Standardized patients are also trained to rate students and clinicians using rubrics and checklists and to deliver structured feedback based on performance.

Simulated patient are trained to portray a patient for formative assessment purposes and may or may not provide feedback to the learner. The focus of the simulated patient is not necessarily on the standardization of the symptoms but more on the authenticity and believability of the performance.

D. T. Peterson (✉)
Office of Interprofessional Simulation, Department of Medical Education, University of Alabama at Birmingham, School of Medicine, Birmingham, AL, USA
e-mail: dtpeterson@uab.edu

© Springer International Publishing Switzerland 2016
V. J. Grant, A. Cheng (eds.), *Comprehensive Healthcare Simulation: Pediatrics*,
Comprehensive Healthcare Simulation, DOI 10.1007/978-3-319-24187-6_8

Table 8.1 Common terms and definitions

Standard-ized patient or simulated patient	The terms standardized patient and simulated patient are often used interchangeably to refer to a non-clinician who has been trained to portray a patient with a specific set of symptoms or psychological issues [3, 9, 52]
Simulated family member	A person who is trained to act as the family member of a patient in a simulation scenario. Simulated family members can also be referred to as embedded simulation persons [52]
Simulated client or unan-nounced standardized patient	A person who is trained to present as a real patient in a health clinic setting in order to observe and assess the clinician's decision-making skills. Clinicians are unaware that they are being observed by the simulated client [25]. In the USA, these individuals are typically referred to as *unannounced standard-ized patients*
Hybrid simulation	When two or more modalities of simulation (i.e., task trainers, simulators, or standardized/simulated patients) are combined for a simulation session [9, 52]. In this chapter, a hybrid simulation refers to the combination of a high-fidelity simulator and a stan-dardized or simulated patient or family member
Formative assessment	Assessment for educational purposes; formative assessment includes observation of the learners and feedback based on their actions [52]
Summative assessment	Assessment for evaluation purposes; summa-tive assessments are measurements of a learner's proficiency and competency in a specific area; summative assessments are typically high-stakes evaluations [52]

Simulated patients typically spend more training time on character development, background stories, interpersonal relationships, and reactions to difficult conversations. One of the key challenges in the field is the lack of standardized terminology, which can often times cause misunderstanding or miscommunication in the training and implementation of these individuals into a simulation scenario [11]. For this reason, a list of common terms and definitions used through-out this chapter is provided in Table 8.1.

The Association of Standardized Patient Educators (ASPE) is an international organization committed to sup-porting best practices in the field of standardized patient edu-cation. This group of simulation educators aims to enhance the professional knowledge and skill set of its members as well as promote research and scholarship in standardized patient methodology and education. In 2014, ASPE drafted a document outlining best practices for standardized patient teaching and evaluation in six different areas. These areas include standardized patient safety, quality assurance, case design, standardized patient training, standardized patient feedback, and professional development. At the time of writing this chapter, these standards were still in draft form. However, the organization hopes to publish the standards by the end of 2015 [8].

Recruitment and Training

General Information

The integration of standardized patients and simulated pa-tients into simulation scenarios requires specific preparation, planning, and training. It is important that the SP enriches rather than disrupts the scenario and that the individual un-derstands not only his or her role in the simulation but also the overall purpose and objective for the educational session. Regardless of whether the SP is a trained or untrained actor, structured training is necessary [6]. The coaching required to train SPs has evolved over the past 20 years to include sce-narios that are not necessarily standardized but focused on difficult conversations and communication skills. Educators must recruit, audition, and select persons who will enable the learners to meet the learning objectives of the scenario [7].

Recruiting Standardized and Simulated Patients

Recruitment can be one of the most challenging aspects of securing SPs. It is important to cast the right individual to portray patient and family roles so that the realism of the case is not affected. Even experienced actors can have diffi-culty portraying certain patients, especially if they have had personal experience with medical problems in the past. It is also important to choose SPs who are able to control their emotions [12].

SPs can be recruited from a variety of places. Some simulation centers choose to pursue professional actors [7, 12, 13], while others look to volunteers to fill the role of SPs [14]. Outside agencies such as AARP (formerly known as the American Association of Retired Persons), newspa-pers, health-related support groups, volunteer organizations, schools of performing arts, and referrals from existing SPs are also resources for recruiting additional people to the pro-gram [7]. If volunteers or family members of actual patients are being utilized as SPs in hospital simulation programs, it is important to properly screen candidates before selecting the best one. While family members of actual patients can add to the authenticity of a simulation, it is very important to place them in scenarios that do not kindle emotionally trau-matizing events [14].

Regardless of how SPs are recruited, it is important to consider the ethnicity, gender, and age of the individual with respect to the learning objectives of the case. While the age of the SP does not have to be the exact age of the patient being portrayed, it is important that the SP closely resembles the age of the patient. Some cases may be acceptable for a male or a female to portray. However, allowing male and female SPs to portray the same case for a high-stakes sum-mative assessment could potentially cause variation for the learners due to the fact that gender differences can and often do impact patient and clinician interaction as well as history taking [7, 15].

As soon as potential SPs have been recruited, it may be necessary to hold an audition. It is helpful to hold multiple auditions on one day in order for simulation staff and clinicians who are involved in the scenario to be present [7, 13]. This also allows staff and clinicians to compare performances of potential SPs so the best selection can be made for the case [7]. The length of the audition will depend on the complexity of the case and on whether or not the SP is being trained for a high-stakes summative assessment with structured feedback or for a formative learning session focusing on an emotional experience or a difficult conversation. Wallace suggests a 1.5–2-h audition for standardized patients who will be involved in summative evaluation [7]. Video recording auditions allows simulation center staff to build a database so that candidates can be reviewed if necessary at a later date. Pascucci et. al suggest holding auditions in 15-min intervals where the potential SP is given a scenario to review and then 3–5 min to audition or interact in the scenario followed by a short debriefing [13]. This type of audition is ideal for SPs who will be involved in formative assessments. In addition to acting ability, it is necessary to determine the observation skills, self-reflection skills, and memory skills of anyone who is going to be recruited as a potential SP. These individuals must also be reliable and willing to focus on standardizing their performance along with other SPs if necessary [7, 12].

Training for Summative Versus Formative Assessments

There is a distinct difference in training a standardized patient for a summative assessment and training a simulated patient for a formative assessment. Before any training can begin, it is important to determine if the case is for evaluation (i.e., summative assessment) or for education (i.e., formative assessment). The goal in a summative assessment is to train the standardized patient with a focus in standardization and the ability to give structured feedback. Standardized patients must display symptoms in a consistent, sequential, and unchanging manner for multiple learners. In summative assessments, standardized patient performance is not about creativity. It is about consistency. All learners involved in the case must be presented with the same information with minimal or no variation [13]. If the simulation is designed to evaluate specific clinical objectives, standardization is a must. Intense training will be required for the standardized patients to systematically perform the same case for all learners [2].

On the contrary, if the simulation is purely for education and is considered a formative assessment, then standardization and consistency are secondary to the development of an authentic role where simulated patients can interact with learners in a realistic and unscripted manner. These types of educational scenarios require a significant amount of background information and social history in order for the simulated patient to develop his or her character [13]. The authenticity and believability of the performance is most important in training simulated patients. This does not mean that simulated patients choose the direction of the scenario. Some consistency and scripting are required to be sure that the scenario unfolds in a similar way for each learner.

Training Standardized Patients

True standardized patient training requires structured and specific training [7, 9, 12, 16, 17]. Wallace suggests a training model of four training sessions and one practice session in order for a standardized patient to deliver a consistent and effective simulation encounter with structured feedback [7]. If standardized patients work in high-stakes clinical exams, authentic and precise performances are required [2]. Depending on the complexity of the case and the amount of documentation and feedback required, training a standardized patient for a summative high-stakes assessment can take between 10 and 20 h [12]. Standardized patients can only be consistently accurate if they are well trained, regularly monitored, and given repeated feedback on their performance by a licensed clinician [7].

If multiple standardized patients are being trained to present the same case, it is most effective to conduct group training [7, 12]. This can aid in standardization of the case and also allows the standardized patients to ask questions and learn from one another. It is also helpful to provide a video which emphasizes appropriate nonverbal behavior and emotion. Giving explicit examples of good and poor learner performances is beneficial for standardized patients when they are learning to give feedback [12].

If the summative assessment includes feedback delivered by the standardized patient, specific rater training is imperative. Rater training should focus on observations, judgment, and proper documentation [12] and is necessary to enable the standardized patient to effectively give feedback [7]. If physical findings are part of the simulation, it is important that clinicians are involved to help train standardized patients on how to produce appropriate signs and symptoms. Clinicians should also be involved in the final practice session before the standardized patient presents the case to the learners [16].

A comprehensive discussion on how to recruit, select, and train standardized patients is beyond the scope of this chapter. For more detailed information on recruiting and training standardized patients for summative assessments, please see *Coaching Standardized Patients for Use in the Assessment of Clinical Competence* [7] and *Objective Structured Clinical Examinations: 10 Steps to Planning and Implementing OSCEs and Other Standardized Patient Exercises* [12].

Training Simulated Patients

When training simulated patients for formative assessments, typically, the authentic character and true-to-life reactions of the patient are more important than standardization. The focus of simulated patient training is on character development and not necessarily scripted reproducibility. However, it is still important to determine the minimum level of consistency required for the learner, and those elements can be emphasized during training [18]. For some simulation scenarios, variation in simulated patient performance will not derail the overall goal of the simulation, especially if the scenario is designed for formative assessment [2]. Zabar recommends a minimum of 2 h of training for a formative assessment, which may focus on content related to delivering bad news or engaging in difficult conversations [12]. Simulated patient training should focus on presenting a believable social history, accurate symptoms related to the case, and authentic reactions in order for learners to gain the most from the simulation session. If the simulated patient encounter is part of a research study, it may be helpful to provide a template or script during training to help specify the role of the simulated patient. Cue cards or notes can also be provided for the simulated patient to use during the scenario. Video recordings of appropriate behaviors and reactions, along with pilot sessions, can also be beneficial for training simulated patients [19]. See Table 8.2 for a summary of considerations for training SPs for summative versus formative assessments.

Children as Standardized and Simulated Patients

While not an extremely common practice, children have been used as standardized patients and simulated patients for the past 20 years [20–26]. In 1995, Woodward conducted a focus group of seven children aged 6–18 who were routinely used as standardized patients to determine how the experience had affected them [20]. Parents were present during the focus group and were asked to allow the children to talk as much as possible. The mother of a 6-year-old who participated in the group said one emergency department simulation had frightened her child because the child overheard discussions that she might die. Although her child reported

Table 8.2 Summary of considerations for training SPs for summative and formative assessments

	Summative assessment (high-stakes evaluation)	Formative assessment (educational experience)
Type of patient	Standardized patient	Simulated patient
Goal of training	Standardization: scripted reproducibility with consistent responses enabling every learner to receive the exact same experience	Authenticity: realistic responses enabling each learner to have an authentic encounter based on their actions
Length of training	10–20 h	Minimum of 2 h
Elements of training	Detailed script of responses, rater training for checklists and feedback, clinician oversight of practice sessions, video review, and pilot session	Description of role and character, cue cards, examples of authentic responses, video review, and pilot session

that the simulation was fun and enjoyable, she had never thought about someone her age dying. Other young children in Woodward's focus group reported needing additional time to sit and think before giving feedback to learners. After analyzing the results of the study, Woodward determined children are at an increased risk than adolescents and adults of having negative effects following the experience of being a standardized patient.

Tsai conducted a review of the literature in 2004 to determine the extent to which children were being used as standardized patients and simulated patients. He concluded that successful child SP programs are limited because of ethical concerns; however, child SPs can be successful and effective for clinical assessment if careful attention is paid to selection and training [26].

In 2005, Brown reported using children as simulated patients for complex cases such as attention-deficit hyperactivity disorder (ADHD), depression, and anorexia. Children who were trained for these cases were recruited from local community theater or were children of medical faculty. Cases were designed by a psychologist, a standardized patient educator, and a psychiatrist. Children attended two training sessions, each of which was 90-min long. In the first training session, children were provided with the details of the case and an explanation of the medical signs and symptoms they were to display. In the second training session, children were able to practice being the patient. The children in this study were able to realistically interpret psychiatric disorders and were able to separate the activity as role-playing. Brown concluded that child SPs can be a very effective tool for residents and medical students to learn communication skills surrounding pediatric psychiatric disorders [21].

Children can be used in some settings as unannounced SPs or simulated clients, but care must be taken to protect children who participate in such experiences [25]. Children under the age of 15 have also been used as simulated patients in a pediatric decontamination drill [22]. This specific drill was deemed successful, but it was noted that the children needed constant supervision and assistance. When anecdotal records were reviewed, the children's moods were described as happy (25%), cooperative (80%), consolable (35%), fearful (15%), and crying (10%). The authors did not suggest any strategies for dealing with children who were upset by participating in the simulation.

The most common recommendation among those who have used children as SPs is the importance of holding focus groups following a child SP encounter to determine the effect the simulation had on the child's well-being [20, 21, 24, 25]. It is also important for educators and simulation staff to have a process in place to monitor the effects of simulation on small children [20]. Children should be carefully selected, and the roles they are asked to play should be developmentally appropriate. Any program involving child SPs should have adequately trained, licensed, and credentialed support staff to deal with children if sensitive issues arise because of the simulation experience [21]. It has also been recommended to only use children as SPs when absolutely necessary, paying careful attention to the number of hours that children are required to spend in a scenario [21, 26].

Adolescents as Standardized and Simulated Patients

Over the past 15 years, the use of adolescents as SPs has increased with respect to assessing clinicians' ability to have effective conversations regarding depression, suicide risk, sexuality, birth control, and other mental health issues [10, 27–37]. Similar to the utilization of child SPs, it is important to consider the psychological ramifications of using adolescents as SPs. Some adolescents report difficulty in totally immersing themselves in the case when sensitive issues such as self-harm are involved [31]. If adolescents are unable to be totally immersed in the case, it is likely that learners will find the simulation to be unrealistic and unbelievable. For this reason, some simulation centers choose to use young adults to portray adolescent patients [30].

However, some centers have found adolescents as young as 13–15 years old to be able to be successfully trained to portray patients with medical illness and give feedback to clinicians following a simulation experience [27]. Several studies have also shown 16- to 18-year old SPs to be effective in cases involving oral contraceptives, pregnancy concerns, and sexually transmitted diseases. Adolescent SPs of this age can be trained to give structured feedback and are able to do so, yet sometimes giving feedback to junior physicians can be difficult [10, 37].

If true adolescents are going to be trained and used as SPs, careful considerations should be made when recruiting, selecting, training, and debriefing the adolescents who take part in the simulation. It is necessary to determine why the adolescents are interested in portraying certain roles and also to be sure they are able to detach themselves from roles that could potentially cause psychological harm. Training for adolescent SPs should include developing coping strategies to get out of a role or out of character before debriefing. It is also important to remember that the context of the simulation, including the behavior and attitude of the clinicians in the simulation, can have an effect on the standardized patient's emotional well-being [36].

With good reason, some researchers have devoted much time studying the impact of playing a patient role on adolescents' emotional stress levels, with particular emphasis on depression and suicide contagion [32–34]. Suicide contagion refers to the association between an adolescent's contact with a suicide stimulus and future risk of suicide attempts. Typically, suicide contagion is observed in vulnerable adolescents within 2 weeks after contact with a suicide stimulus [38]. Because of the reality of this phenomenon, specific screening is suggested for all adolescents before involving them in any scenario that deals with suicide risk or attempted suicide [32, 33]. If properly screened and trained, vulnerable adolescents are able to participate as standardized patients in scenarios dealing with suicide attempts. However, it is recommended that a mental health specialist participates in case writing and in SP training and debriefing [34]. These precautions can and should apply to all adolescent standardized patient training involving sensitive topics such as sexuality, depression, and self-harm.

Current Trends in Pediatric Simulation

The use of standardized patients and simulated patients in pediatric clerkships, pediatric residencies, and pediatric nursing has become quite common [13, 14, 21–24, 30, 31, 35, 37, 39–47]. Whether SPs are used for objective structured clinical exams (OSCEs), group objective structured clinical exams (GOSCEs), communication scenarios, delivering bad news, or even hybrid simulations, the utilization of SPs has proven to be an effective means of educating pediatric healthcare providers. In the field of pediatric anesthesiology, SPs have been used in simulations that focus on the disclosure of medical error, dealing with angry family members, limitations of care, and *do not resuscitate* decisions [43]. Residents typically rate educational sessions with SPs as very effective in helping them to identify areas of improvement [5]. The use of SPs in simulations in addition to lectures was also found to be an effective tool for improving the management of chronic diseases such as asthma [48].

Communication and Interpersonal Skills

Communication is a fundamental skill necessary for clinical competence. Communication skills should not be viewed as an optional skill set for clinicians but rather viewed as one of the four necessary components required for good clinical practice (i.e., knowledge, problem solving, physical exam, and communication) (see Chap. 23). These skills should be developed in clinicians and healthcare professionals just as diligently as assessment skills, physical examination skills, and medical management skills. Good communication requires practice since it is often more complex than basic procedural skills [17], and simulation centers have proven to be an ideal location for that practice to occur.

Simulated patients are increasingly being used in simulation centers and by healthcare educators to focus on communication and interpersonal skills [5, 17, 21, 37, 39, 40, 43–49]. Simulated patients provide a safe learning environment where clinicians can practice verbal communication as well as nonverbal communication skills. Standardized patients can also be used to rate and give feedback to clinicians regarding their interpersonal and communication skills as long as expectations are clearly defined and appropriate rater training has taken place [17]. The use of standardized patients or simulated patients can also be beneficial in helping clinicians to practice patient education skills.

Difficult Conversations

Over the past 10 years, SPs have been frequently utilized in pediatric resident education as a psychologically safe way to practice conveying difficult news [21, 37, 39, 43, 45–47, 49]. Pediatric residents rotating in emergency medicine, anesthesiology, adolescent medicine, and general pediatrics are commonly interacting with SPs to practice communication skills related to sensitive discussions (e.g., oral contraceptives and sexuality) and delivering bad news. Practicing these types of conversations in the simulation center can help learners gain experience and confidence without practicing the skills on real patients [40]. Using an SP for these types of conversations allows for realistic reactions and feedback to clinicians on nonverbal skills and tone of voice. See Fig. 8.1 for a list of case examples involving difficult conversations.

Hybrid Simulations

Hybrid simulations, including a high-fidelity mannequin and a simulated family member, are commonly used in pediatric cases requiring clinical management of a patient as well as communication with a family member. Combining high-fidelity mannequins and standardized patients or simulated

- Childhood or Adolescent Depression
- ADHD
- Oral Contraceptives
- Sexual History
- Suicide Risk
- Substance Abuse
- Non-Accidental Trauma
- Domestic Violence
- Disclosure of a Medical Error
- Angry Family Members
- Do not resuscitate/Do not intubate (DNR/DNI)
- Sudden Infant Death
- Traumatic Brain Injury
- Genetic Test Results
- Terminal Diagnosis
- Life-Altering Diagnosis
- Limitations of Care
- Painful Diagnostic Procedures
- Concerning Physical Exam
- Expected Death of a Child
- Post Cardiac Arrest

Fig. 8.1 Case examples involving difficult conversations

patients provides an interactive method of simulation education that has been shown to be effective in teaching pediatric residents and subspecialties. The use of hybrid simulations has been documented with pharmacy students, pharmacy residents, nursing students, pediatric residents, medical students as well as hospital staff in a children's hospital [9, 13, 40, 50]. The primary benefit of a hybrid simulation is that it allows learners to perform basic clinical assessments and procedures on a mannequin while practicing their communication skills with an additional simulated patient or simulated family member, which is a more realistic parallel to what the learners will experience in their actual clinical practice in pediatrics. Incorporating simulated patients and simulated family members into high-fidelity simulation scenarios can also add an extra layer of complexity to the case and can increase the authenticity and applicability of the educational experience [9].

Figure 8.2 shows a hybrid simulation with a simulated patient who is portraying the mother of the infant mannequin. The case involves a bus accident where the mother and child are both injured. The mother is extremely anxious and is hesitant to allow the healthcare team to take the infant to begin their assessment. In this case, including a simulated patient as the mother provides for the expression of realistic reactions and emotions while hospital staff work on the injured infant who is struggling to breathe and needs significant airway management.

Hybrid simulations are also ideal for sensitive topics such as abuse, suicidal thinking, terminal illness, and sexuality that could potentially be upsetting if a child were to be used

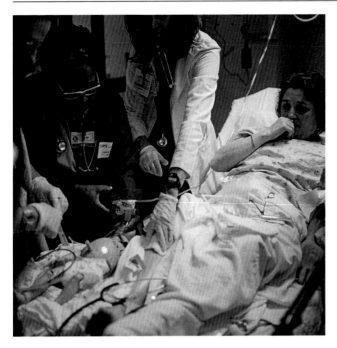

Fig. 8.2 Hybrid simulation with simulated patient and infant mannequin. (Photo by Charlie Prince, used with permission)

as the simulated patient. With content of this nature, it can
be effective to use a child mannequin and a simulated family member to focus on difficult conversations with learners
[40]. The use of simulated family members has become common practice in many hospital-based pediatric simulation
centers. In April 2014, Boston Children's Hospital reported
incorporating simulated family members into a third of their
mannequin-based scenarios [13].

Advantages and Challenges

There are several advantages to using SPs to train healthcare professionals, the main advantage being that SPs allow
learners the opportunity to practice in a psychologically safe
environment without encountering the risk of causing harm
to a real patient. SPs provide a means for healthcare professionals to rehearse difficult conversations and try new ways
of communicating with patients and their families. SPs can
also be scheduled at the convenience of the learner and made
available at certain points throughout a trainee's program to
help facilitate their learning goals. Standardized patients can
be arranged for extended periods of time providing standardized assessment and constructive feedback in addition to
that of clinical faculty [9]. Both standardized patients and
simulated patients can also provide specific insight into the
nuances of the learner's communication style such as body
language, tone, and eye contact [17].

Expense and administrative time are among the many
challenges of recruiting, training, and utilizing standardized

patients and simulated patients. The entire process of scheduling and training requires significant allocation of resources
including personnel, facilities, and finances [2]. Case development time, as well as the time it takes for the case to
be vetted by clinical faculty, can be a limitation [17]. Many
simulation centers are functioning at their maximum capacity, and hiring additional staff to schedule and train SPs can
prove challenging. Management and leadership can also be
a challenge for simulation programs [11]. It is important to
consider who will oversee the program and how it will be
funded.

Unannounced Standardized Patients

Unannounced SPs are standardized patients or simulated patients who are embedded into the regular clinic schedule or
hospital ward and act as real patients. The goal of using unannounced SPs is to gain an authentic assessment of a practitioner who is unaware that the patient is simulated [9]. The use
of unannounced SPs to assess pediatric resident competencies is not very common. However, Ozuah and Resnik conducted a study where unannounced SPs were used to assess
the impact of an educational intervention on the ability of pediatric residents to accurately classify asthma severity [35].
Rowe used six healthy children as unannounced SPs, also
referred to as simulated clients, to assess healthcare worker
practices during consultations in the country of Benin [25].
This study concluded that the use of unannounced SPs was
effective for assessing healthcare workers' performance of
basic clinical tasks and decision-making.

Arranging for unannounced SPs requires a great deal of
training and planning to protect the identity of the SP and to
maintain the fidelity of the patient role. Unannounced SPs
must be rigorously trained so they do not give away their
identity during the actual clinic visit. When unannounced
SPs are used, clinicians consent in advance and are not aware
of when the actual encounter with the SP will occur. The
biggest advantage of the unannounced SP is the ability to
capture difficult conversations and clinical encounters without having to consider the bias that might exist should the
clinician know the patient is a simulated person [51].

Conclusions

It has been well established that the use of standardized patients and simulated patients is an effective educational tool
as well as a best practice in teaching adults to become more
effective communicators and clinicians [5]. However, the
effective use of SPs in healthcare education requires careful consideration. SP educators and simulation center staff
should take the integration of standardized patients and

simulated patients into the curriculum very seriously. Students and clinicians participating in summative assessment simulations with standardized patients can potentially face huge consequences for poor performance. Of similar importance, the authenticity of simulated patients in formative assessments is critical if we are to expect learners to improve their communication and interpersonal skills. Although there are distinct challenges to using SPs in clinical education, the realism and authenticity they bring to the scenario is remarkable and can have a significant positive impact on the quality of care offered by current and future clinicians.

References

1. Barrows HS, Abrahamson S. The programmed patient: a technique for appraising student performance in clinical neurology. J Med Educ. 1964;39:802–5.
2. Weaver M, Erby L. Standardized patients: a promising tool for health education and health promotion. Health Promot Pract. 2012;13(2):169–74.
3. Levine AI, Swartz MH. Standardized patients: the "other" simulation. J Crit Care. 2008;23(2):179–84.
4. Vukin E, Greenberg R, Auerbach M, Chang L, Scotten M, Tenney-Soeiro R, et al. Use of simulation-based education: a national survey of pediatric clerkship directors. Acad Pediatr. 2014;14(4):369–74.
5. Reed S, Shell R, Kassis K, Tartaglia K, Wallihan R, Smith K, et al. Applying adult learning practices in medical education. Curr Probl Pediatr Adolesc Health Care. 2014;44(6):170–81.
6. Szauter K. Adding the human dimension to simulation scenarios. Simul Healthc. 2014;9(2):79–80.
7. Wallace P. Coaching standardized patients for use in the assessment of clinical competence. New York: Springer; 2007.
8. Association of Standardized Patient Educators. Standards of Practice (draft). 2014.
9. Howley LD. Standardized patients. In: Levine AI, DeMaria S, Schwartz AD, Sim AJ, editors. The comprehensive textbook of healthcare simulation. New York: Springer; 2013. p. 173–90.
10. Bokken L, van Dalen J, Rethans J-J. The case of "Miss Jacobs": adolescent simulated patients and the quality of their role playing, feedback, and personal impact. Simul Healthc. 2010;5(6):315–9.
11. Nestel D, Tabak D, Tierney T, Layat-Burn C, Robb A, Clark S, et al. Key challenges in simulated patient programs: an international comparative case study. BMC Med Educ. 2011;11:69.
12. Zabar S, Kachur E, Kalet A, Hanley K. Objective structured clinical examinations: 10 steps to planning and implementing OSCEs and other standardized patient exercises. New York: Springer; 2012.
13. Pascucci RC, Weinstock PH, O'Connor BE, Fancy KM, Meyer EC. Integrating actors into a simulation program: a primer. Simul Healthc. 2014;9(2):120–6.
14. Crow KM. Families and patients as actors in simulation: adding unique perspectives to enhance nursing education. J Pediatr Nurs. 2012;27(6):765–6.
15. Carson JA, Peets A, Grant V, McLaughlin K. The effect of gender interactions on students' physical examination ratings in objective structured clinical examination stations. Acad Med. 2010;85(11):1772–6.
16. Barrows HS. Training standardized patients to have physical findings. Springfield: Southern Illinois University, School of Medicine; 1999.
17. Kurtz SM, Silverman DJ, Draper J, van Dalen J, Platt FW. Teaching and learning communication skills in medicine. 2nd ed. United Kingdom: Radcliffe Publishing; 2005.
18. Erby LA, Roter DL, Biesecker BB. Examination of standardized patient performance: accuracy and consistency of six standardized patients over time. Patient Educ Couns. 2011;85(2):194–200.
19. Cheng A, Auerbach M, Hunt EA, Chang TP, Pusic M, Nadkarni V, et al. Designing and conducting simulation-based research. Pediatrics. 2014;133(6):1091–101.
20. Woodward CA, Gliva-McConvey G. Children as standardized patients: initial assessment of effects. Teach Learn Med Int J. 1995;7(3):188–91.
21. Brown R, Doonan S, Shellenberger S. Using children as simulated patients in communication training for residents and medical students: a pilot program. Acad Med. 2005;80(12):1114–20.
22. Fertel BS, Kohlhoff SA, Roblin PM, Arquilla B. Lessons from the "Clean Baby 2007" pediatric decontamination drill. Am J Disaster Med. 2009;4(2):77–85.
23. Holland B, Landry K, Mountain A, Middlebrooks MA, Heim D, Missildine K. Weaving the tapestry of learning: simulation, standardized patients, and virtual communities. Nurse Educ. 2013;38(6):269–72.
24. Lane JL, Ziv A, Boulet JR. A pediatric clinical skills assessment using children as standardized patients. Arch Pediatr Adolesc Med. 1999;153(6):637–44.
25. Rowe AK, Onikpo F, Lama M, Deming MS. Evaluating health worker performance in Benin using the simulated client method with real children. Implement Sci. 2012;7(1):95.
26. Tsai TC. Using children as standardised patients for assessing clinical competence in paediatrics. Arch Dis Child. 2004;89(12):1117–20.
27. Blake K, Greaven S. Adolescent girls as simulators of medical illness. Med Educ. 1999;33(9):702–3.
28. Blake KD, Gusella J, Greaven S, Wakefield S. The risks and benefits of being a young female adolescent standardised patient. Med Educ. 2006;40(1):26–35.
29. Fallucco EM, Conlon MK, Gale G, Constantino JN, Glowinski AL. Use of a standardized patient paradigm to enhance proficiency in risk assessment for adolescent depression and suicide. J Adolesc Health. 2012;51(1):66–72.
30. Fallucco EM, Hanson MD, Glowinski AL. Teaching pediatric residents to assess adolescent suicide risk with a standardized patient module. Pediatrics. 2010;125(5):953–9.
31. Felton A, Holliday L, Ritchie D, Langmack G, Conquer A. Simulation: a shared learning experience for child and mental health pre-registration nursing students. Nurse Educ Pract. 2013;13(6):536–40.
32. Hanson M, Tiberius R, Hodges B, Mackay S, McNaughton N, Dickens S, et al. Implications of suicide contagion for the selection of adolescent standardized patients. Acad Med. 2002;77(Suppl 10):S100–2.
33. Hanson M, Tiberius R, Hodges B, MacKay S, McNaughton N, Dickens S, et al. Adolescent standardized patients: method of selection and assessment of benefits and risks. Teach Learn Med. 2002;14(2):104–13.
34. Hanson MD, Niec A, Pietrantonio AM, Johnson S, Young M, High B, et al. Effects associated with adolescent standardized patient simulation of depression and suicidal ideation. Acad Med. 2007;82(Suppl 10):S61–4.
35. Ozuah PO, Reznik M. Using unannounced standardized patients to assess residents' competency in asthma severity classification. Ambul Pediatr. 2008;8(2):139–42.
36. Spencer J, Dales J. Meeting the needs of simulated patients and caring for the person behind them? Med Educ. 2006;40(1):3–5.

37. Woods JL, Pasold TL, Boateng BA, Hensel DJ. Adolescent health care and the trainee: roles of self-efficacy, standardized patients, and an adolescent medicine rotation. Simul Healthc. 2013;8(6):359–67.

38. Shaffer D, Hicks R. Suicide. In: Pless B, editor. Epidemiology of childhood disorders. New York: Oxford University Press; 1994. p. 339–65.

39. Peterson EB, Porter MB, Calhoun AW. A simulation-based curriculum to address relational crises in medicine. J Grad Med Educ. 2012;4(3):351–6.

40. Marken PA, Zimmerman C, Kennedy C, Schremmer R, Smith KV. Human simulators and standardized patients to teach difficult conversations to interprofessional health care teams. Am J Pharm Educ. 2010;74(7):120.

41. Gillett B, Peckler B, Sinert R, Onkst C, Nabors S, Issley S, et al. Simulation in a disaster drill: comparison of high-fidelity simulators versus trained actors. Acad Emerg Med. 2008;15(11):1144–51.

42. Wallace D, Gillett B, Wright B, Stetz J, Arquilla B. Randomized controlled trial of high fidelity patient simulators compared to actor patients in a pandemic influenza drill scenario. Resuscitation. 2010;81(7):872–6.

43. Fehr JJ, Honkanen A, Murray DJ. Simulation in pediatric anesthesiology. Paediatr Anaesth. 2012;22(10):988–94.

44. Konopasek L, Kelly KV, Bylund CL, Wenderoth S, Storey-Johnson C. The group objective structured clinical experience: building communication skills in the clinical reasoning context. Patient Educ Couns. 2014;96(1):79–85.

45. Overly FL, Sudikoff SN, Duffy S, Anderson A, Kobayashi L. Three scenarios to teach difficult discussions in pediatric emergency medicine: sudden infant death, child abuse with domestic violence, and medication error. Simul Healthc. 2009;4(2):114–30.

46. Tobler K, Grant E, Marczinski C. Evaluation of the impact of a simulation-enhanced breaking bad news workshop in pediatrics. Simul Healthc. 2014;9:213–9.

47. Ten Eyck RP. Simulation in emergency medicine training. Pediatr Emerg Care. 2011;27(4):333–41 (quiz 42-4).

48. Cohen AG, Kitai E, David SB, Ziv A. Standardized patient-based simulation training as a tool to improve the management of chronic disease. Simul Healthc. 2014;9(1):40–7.

49. Greenberg LW, Ochsenschlager D, O'Donnell R, Mastruserio J, Cohen GJ. Communicating bad news: a pediatric department's evaluation of a simulated intervention. Pediatrics. 1999;103(6 Pt 1):1210–7.

50. Kennedy JL, Jones SM, Porter N, White ML, Gephardt G, Hill T, et al. High-fidelity hybrid simulation of allergic emergencies demonstrates improved preparedness for office emergencies in pediatric allergy clinics. J Allergy Clin Immunol Pract. 2013;1(6):608–17. e1–14.

51. Siminoff LA, Rogers HL, Waller AC, Harris-Haywood S, Esptein RM, Carrio FB, et al. The advantages and challenges of unannounced standardized patient methodology to assess healthcare communication. Patient Educ Couns. 2011;82(3):318–24.

52. Palaganas J, Maxworthy J, Epps CA, Mancini MB, editors Defining excellence in simulation programs. New York: Lippincott, Williams, and Wilkins; 2014.

Screen-Based Simulation, Virtual Reality, and Haptic Simulators

Todd P. Chang, James Gerard and Martin V. Pusic

Simulation Pearls

1. Screen-based simulation (SBS) has inherent advantages of replicability, portability, asynchrony, distribution, and data tracking compared to most other forms of simulation.
2. SBS has substantial up-front financial and labor costs, is less appropriate for team-based education, and has limitations in its functional fidelity when compared to other forms of simulation.
3. SBS development requires early and continued collaboration between programmers, designers, clinical subject matter experts, and experts in education.

Introduction

Screen-based simulation (SBS) in health care education is a form of simulation in which a clinical scenario with one or more patients is presented through a digital screen surface [1, 2]. As with other forms of simulation, SBS provides the learner with a cognitively realistic and experiential setting without danger of actual patient or population harm [3]. It is best used when instruction is required for a wide audience of learners separated by space and time and the learning

objectives match a cognitive or psychomotor task that can be portrayed using simulation. Current technologies using flat-screen computers, wireless Internet, and mobile connectivity, as well as access to tablets and smartphones have created a ready-made infrastructure for SBS that is not possible with mannequin-based simulation (MBS). Depending on the knowledge, skills, behaviors, and attitudes being taught through SBS, the type of SBS may vary.

Types of Screen-Based Simulation

Virtual Patients

Within SBS, there are many different types of simulations, each with unique features and capabilities. One of the most common types is Virtual Patients (VPs). VPs use a rendering of a single patient to replicate a physician–patient encounter, often to teach and assess diagnostic skills. This method is favored by primary care specialties like pediatrics, and pediatric subspecialties such as hospital pediatrics or pediatric emergency medicine, as it emphasizes data gathering skills and interaction with the patient or family [4]. Pediatric VPs are particularly useful in demonstrating rare or subtle findings and pathologies that are otherwise difficult or unethical to convey in MBS or in real patients. National organizations such as the Committee for Student Education in Pediatrics (COMSEP) have coordinated interinstitutional collaboratives such as the Computer-assisted Learning in Pediatrics Program (CLIPP) cases, available to students at more than 80 US institutions [5]. The more robust VP simulators allow for naturalistic conversations using a keyboard or even voice recognition. Image and case banks allow for the deliberate practice with feedback on large numbers of virtual cases [6].

A large systematic review of VPs identified 45 quantitative, comparative studies and four qualitative studies [7, 8]. VPs as an educational intervention, in general, tend to have large effects in knowledge, clinical reasoning, and other skills when compared to no intervention; however, VPs have

T. P. Chang (✉)
Department of Pediatrics, Division of Emergency Medicine & Transport, University of Southern California Keck School of Medicine, Children's Hospital Los Angeles, Los Angeles, CA, USA
e-mail: Dr.toddchang@gmail.com

J. Gerard
Department of Pediatrics, Division of Emergency Medicine, Saint Louis University School of Medicine, SSM Cardinal Glennon Children's Medical Center, St. Louis, MO, USA
e-mail: gerardjm@slu.edu

M. V. Pusic
Department of Emergency Medicine, New York University School of Medicine, New York, NY, USA
e-mail: mpusic@gmail.com

© Springer International Publishing Switzerland 2016
V. J. Grant, A. Cheng (eds.), *Comprehensive Healthcare Simulation: Pediatrics*,
Comprehensive Healthcare Simulation, DOI 10.1007/978-3-319-24187-6_9

not shown improved outcome measures compared to other modes of teaching such as traditional lectures [7].

Virtual Worlds

Virtual worlds (VWs) are different from VPs. VWs immerse the learner within a virtual world through a controllable avatar and can present multiple patients, austere environments, and social interaction; Second Life is a common example [9, 10]. VWs are typically portrayed on the screen and use principles and technologies of virtual reality (VR). The ability to render three-dimensional graphics and rotate freely within the virtual space is now commonplace in many VW games and training programs and can be done on a screen. For example, a pediatric disaster triage simulation that would focus on triaging many patients quickly rather than focusing on the details of one patient would be best represented in a VW format. At some institutions, including military, aviation, and civilian simulation centers, VR technology has advanced such that a learner can be immersed within a large warehouse-like enclosure environment with multiple floor-to-ceiling screens to provide a total immersive experience. Such a custom-designed physical space may not be necessary using newer tools like *Oculus Rift* that instead use immersive, personal VR [11].

Virtual Task Trainers

Surgical and procedural subspecialties tend to use virtual task trainers (VTs), which are distinct from other SBSs; these focus on developing hand–eye coordination and psychomotor skills. Medical procedures that would normally use a screen—for example, laparoscopies, bronchoscopies—are commonly simulated using SBS and a haptic simulator, a handheld device that approximates the actual device used in the procedure. Haptic simulators are devices that simulate the weight, movement, and feel of handheld devices common in pediatric procedures and borrow principles and technologies from mannequins. Commercial procedural and surgical simulators are now widely available for a variety of procedures in adult and pediatric patients.

Resource Management Simulators Resource management simulators are a unique class of simulators often designed to demonstrate large population patterns; these simulations are used often at operational levels, by hospital or public health officials to simulate discrete events or mass casualty scenarios to look at municipal or global trends in resource allocation. Examples in pediatrics include disaster training, in which an entire ward, battlefield, or city ruins are portrayed in SBS. However, as panel management becomes increasingly relevant to primary care practitioners, resource management simulators could become more prevalent in pediatric education [12].

Advantages of Screen-Based Simulation

The inherent differences between SBS and MBS are found in its advantages and disadvantages. Notably, SBS has an edge over MBS because of five facets: replicability/standardization, portability, asynchrony, distribution, and data tracking.

Replicability/Standardization

The first and foremost advantage of SBS is its *replicability* or *standardization*. In MBS, a facilitator is running the simulation session. Although much of MBS can be programmed—for example, changing patient physiologies in response to correct and incorrect actions—the facilitator is free to change or add to the scenario depending on the learner needs and on other factors (e.g., not enough time). Facilitators, debriefers, and the course of MBS scenarios can vary from session to session, adding an element of variation when repeating MBS sessions across time or space. Often the variation is inconsequential, but it may mean differences in the way learners enjoy or learn from MBS. Controlling for variation between sessions in MBS is particularly troublesome in simulation-based research, as standardizing the scenarios is one of the requirements of preserving internal validity [13]. SBS, on the other hand, does not have problems with unintended variation.

Because the root of SBS is a digital coded program, it is inherently *replicable*. In other words, students using a virtual-reality SBS on an iPad in California are using the same program as those in Australia. Although the scenario may unfold differently depending on the user, the actual setup and SBS are identical, and the degree of variation can be controlled by the SBS developer as needed for training or for research. It is important to understand that despite this easy replicability and standardization, SBS is not used in isolation; SBS is integrated within the educational context, curricular pathway, or the learning resources provided for the student. Institutional differences may have substantial effect even with the identical SBS because of different contexts [14].

Portability

In addition, SBS is *portable*. Given the ubiquity of smart phones, tablets, and computers, SBS can be brought to the learner to their own device with only a download or active Internet connection. Most SBSs require only electricity or battery power, with no heavy mannequin parts to transport, repair, or safeguard, and no consumable parts that require replacing. *Portability* also refers to the lack of setup in SBS, particularly in contrast to complex high-fidelity MBS that often requires associated equipment and materials to create a highly realistic environment. Some higher-technology SBS requiring a large virtual space may require dedicated locations and dedicated VR equipment or haptic equipment, but the program itself on the screen is quite portable. SBS that only requires a tablet can be taken anywhere, allowing employees and healthcare workers to train and practice in the immediate healthcare arena or in the privacy of their own home. It can also be a useful training adjunct in areas of the world in which space is at a premium, for example, war zones or in commercial airplanes.

Asynchrony

Portability also leads to *asynchrony,* a major strength of SBS. Although just-in-time training and self-guided learning [15, 16] requires some facilitator or instructor to supervise the training process, SBS-based education can be done at any time without a facilitator immediately available. Most learners are unable to create, run, and debrief MBS scenarios on their own—at least, effectively, using best practices that a simulation-trained facilitator can. Facilitation time can be costly in MBS. With SBS, however, much of the simulation can be done at the learner's own discretion and time. Often, computer-based SBS and e-learning tend to occur during the evenings when personnel are sparse.

Distribution

Distribution also lies at the heart of the digital code of SBS. SBS can be distributed to large groups of people and devices across the world with a simple Internet connection or exchanging of disks, drives, and other solid-state media. With MBS, a scenario guide may be distributed, but multiple mannequins would be required. An Advanced Cardiac Life Support session using MBS cannot be distributed widely without incurring large costs for multiple mannequins, whereas an SBS-based session can be distributed to multiple devices instantly using file sharing or even an application store.

Data Collection

Finally, SBS can facilitate live *data collection* that can be utilized for learning, assessment, or research purposes. For most MBS sessions, video recordings, audio recordings, and a complex array of sensors within the MBS can record learner actions and errors well. All of these are naturally encompassed within the SBS programming, and a detailed score or report is much easier to derive than from MBS sessions. Some SBS can continuously collect data as the session is running (e.g., data such as latency—the time during which no active action is taking place). SBS is superior to MBS in collecting interaction data as long as its programming is designed to record that data; often, the decision on what not to track is more important than what to track, given the almost infinite possibilities within the software. Data about the learner is a trickier problem, but heart rate monitors [17], gaze-tracking software [18], and other add-ons allow data collection about the learner specifically. Even metadata such as how often and for how long a user participated within an SBS can be automatically collected.

Disadvantages of Screen-Based Simulation

However, the problems with SBS are not trivial, and the aforementioned advantages do not mean that all simulation scenarios should use SBS rather than MBS. The three most significant problems: high front-end costs, technological limitations, and screen limitations and fidelity, are detailed here.

High Front-End Costs

SBS are not trivial, and the aforementioned advantages do not mean that all simulation scenarios should use SBS rather than MBS. The three most significant problems are detailed here. SBS has much higher front-end costs and development time. Although MBS requires the actual mannequin, once the mannequin and equipment are procured, a low-fidelity scenario can be led by a skilled facilitator quickly. With SBS, without completing all of the design, development, piloting, and distribution, there is nothing to work with at all. Skilled facilitators can manage a scenario with missing equipment or occasional glitches with a mannequin simulator. For SBS, the core programming must be completed before use. Furthermore, as the technology to provide greater fidelity and realism is available to programmers, the skill level and staff needed to develop an SBS from scratch is prohibitive to those who do not have a background in coding or game development. Educators, teachers, and researchers must work with programmers and software developers to get through this first bar, which leads to large front-end costs. The highest proportion of this cost is usually programming or graphic design labor, with a smaller proportion on physical server space, distribution plans, and subject matter expert (SME) fees. Keep in mind that all of the advantages listed above depend on the programming; appropriate data collection in an analyzable form to an instructor or a researcher requires considerable preparation and programming. Often this high cost of admission is enough to dissuade many SBS-based projects. Furthermore, high *front-end costs* also mean that a developer that undertakes the SBS development also takes on much of the time costs. Most developers or firms are interested in recouping costs in the commercial application and development of SBS products. Early alignment between the healthcare workforce, educator, and researcher interests with the developers and programmers is necessary to get past this obstacle.

Technological Limitations

As with all computing technology, the occasional technical problem is inevitable. This can have mild effects during MBS but can single-handedly shut down SBS. Technical problems are particularly prone in synchronous SBS, when multiple learners are present from different geographic locales. When it works, the SBS is extremely powerful. However, one is dependent on appropriate power, stable Internet bandwidth and connectivity, adequate processing speeds on all devices, and all audiovisual add-ons and hardware working cross-platform. SBS requires considering different devices, operating systems, and input methods. Even well-funded massive multiplayer online role-playing games such as World of Warcraft require a minimum set of resources and requirements for a pleasant playing experience, and most SBS development has a fraction of the funding and support staff to maintain that atmosphere. Therefore, SBS needs some level of back-up or contingency plan to rapidly fix unanticipated issues in execution.

Screen Limitations and Fidelity

Finally, we come to the inherent limitation of the screen in SBS. The use of a two-dimensional screen means SBS must work harder to match the functional fidelity that can be replicated by MBS. This is in contrast to physical fidelity, defined as the raw audiovisual realism that SBS can do quite well—with well-financed programming. Functional fidelity, also termed functional task alignment [19], is arguably the most important for SBS [19–21]. Functional fidelity refers to the realism of outputs in response to inputs as part of cognitive fidelity—does the method of interaction feel authentic [21,22]? There are some that argue that functional fidelity is more important for learning in MBS than physical fidelity; this is likely true with SBS [21, 23].

Because SBS is experiential learning, the learner must experience the SBS in as natural and logical a context to the real setting [24]. For example, suppose a colonoscopy simu-

lator has rich graphics that looks exactly like a real patient's colon, there may even be a timer and audiovisual cues to improve psychological fidelity and engagement. Psychological fidelity is the immersive property of the simulation to invoke realistic emotions from the participant—anxiety, relief, or a sense of challenge. But if the simulator does not simulate the haptic or visual feedback of bumping into and stretching a colonic wall, the SBS feels fake. Devices portrayed by VTs should function like real colonoscopes, bronchoscopes, and laryngoscopes; if a scope bumps into a colon wall, there should be consequences: the tactile feedback to the learner, perhaps bleeding, and even a negative score [25]. Without this fidelity, learners could easily learn incorrect psychomotor habits. SBS has an inherent barrier to functional fidelity—the two-dimensional screen—and psychomotor functions, particularly for VTs, feel awkward and unrealistic when simple gestures on a tablet or keyboard entries do not match what is done in reality. As a result, SBS for psychomotor tasks often use haptic devices that simulate the feel, weight, and function of the handheld device.

Therefore, the limitations on functional fidelity for SBS is high enough that certain applications such as psychomotor skills requiring three-dimensional tactile skills (e.g., palpating a vein) are more realistically constructed using MBS. When an activity inherently requires a screen—a cardiopulmonary monitor, a laparoscopy monitor, a simulated telemedicine encounter—this limitation is minimized, since the screen is the actual device. When scenarios require significant team communication using both verbal and nonverbal cues, SBS can be a poorer construct than MBS. Scenarios requiring rapid, successive actions on a patient can be very difficult to convey if a complex array of menus and options is the featured user interface of the SBS. Even when learners prefer menus, it has minimal functional fidelity to the real-world setting [7]. Similarly, the concepts of team-based care are difficult to convey through SBS. SBSs that use multiple learners do exist; they require a level of collaboration to diagnose or treat a VP successfully [7]. However, the interactions afforded by the SBS and online technologies do not yet match the realities of how the majority of healthcare teams behave.

Screen-Based Simulation and Ideal Uses

That being said, SBS is more efficient than MBS for the following: screen-based task trainers, long narrative-based scenarios, and mass casualty or large resource-management scenarios. Screen-based task trainers are uniquely fit to use simulation that replicates the screen, as mentioned earlier. Narratives and storylines are particularly germane to SBS and the video game world [26] and is more poorly defined in a MBS session. This may mean a series of different encounters with a growing patient avatar for a primary care practitioner—which would require multiple different mannequins if using MBS—and encounters in which patient–provider communication is replicated using powerful speech engines and computerized facial expressions. For mass casualties or resource-management scenarios, SBS is ideal as the addition of another patient has minimal resource requirements whereas running a mass casualty scenario using MBS is very costly, and using human volunteers can be cost- or time-prohibitive. Resource-management scenarios require a more macro view of a clinic, ward, hospital, or city, which is almost impossible to simulate effectively using MBS.

Selected Examples of Screen-Based Simulation in the Medical Literature

Virtual Patients VPs are often used with medical students and in other disciplines in which communication and differential diagnoses are prevalent topics (Fig. 9.1). Psychiatric residents have demonstrated diagnostic skills using VPs portraying psychiatric disease and a system to navigate through history-taking and branching custom conversations [27, 28]. Even in the early 2000s, VPs with voice recognition were

successfully used to teach and assess communication skills [29]. We anticipate improvements in the ability of VPs to simulate nuanced emotional responses and recognize users' facial gestures that could further SBS in this arena. In the physical exam portrayals, VPs can portray limited exam findings for disaster triage [30]—which requires very minimal information—to more complex emergency medicine diagnoses [31]. A very realistic VP was developed simulating obesity's effects on respiratory physiology; anesthesiology residents correctly diagnosed obstructive sleep apnea more often with VPs than with hired standardized patient actors who otherwise provided identical histories [32]. In this way, SBS was able to better simulate a needed exam finding that was unethical or uncomfortable (i.e., unable to be done any other way); as a result, VPs can reinforce and even assess the learner's ability to come to diagnoses and management plans.

Virtual Worlds VWs in the twenty-first-century literature often use Second Life (Linden Lab, San Francisco, CA) or other similar three-dimensional avatar software in which the learner can move freely in a virtual environment to interact with other avatars. This SBS lends itself to having live instructors within the environment that can give customized feedback and coaching. Second Life was used for emergency medicine residents to practice mock oral boards skills in a

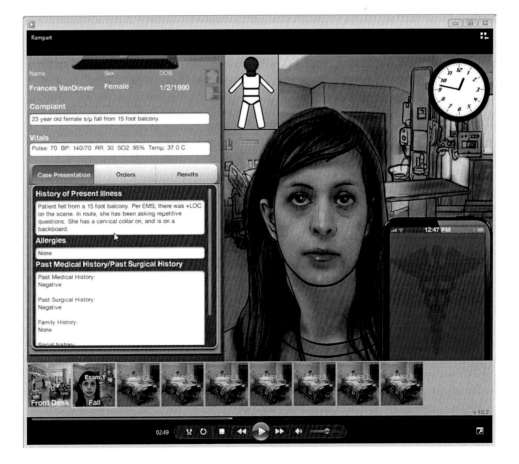

Fig. 9.1 Screenshot of a *virtual patient* encounter in a two-dimensional manner patient simulator. (Courtesy of BreakAway, Ltd., Hunt Valley, Maryland, USA. Reproduced with permission)

less-threatening setting, ideal for the generation of residents accustomed to this technology [9]. The literature supports the use of live communication in SBS as a method to draw out those who would otherwise be silent or introverted in live conversation [33]. VWs are extensively used in tactical military teaching as well, where this live coaching has been demonstrated as a method of deliberate practice [34]. Live instructors play actual combat soldiers (on either side) to provide guidance or additional challenge as needed. In particular, their exercise emphasized communication skills in an austere environment, and the live coaching technique can be replicated to many different healthcare scenarios in which teamwork communication is vital.

Virtual Task Trainers Evaluations of VTs are numerous. Most are attempts to validate a particular SBS VT with advanced haptic devices that operate in a similar manner to real instruments [25, 35–39] or to provide feasibility data on lower-cost VTs without a screen (e.g., box trainers) [40] (Fig. 9.2). We highlight a few studies exemplifying best educational practices. Improved effects have been demonstrated using a deliberate practice model in internal medicine residents [35]. Deliberate practice is a learning method particularly favored for psychomotor skills [41, 42] and procedures [43, 44], and it lends itself to simulation as learners are required to continually practice until a set level of mastery is achieved [43, 45, 46]. The video game concept of incremental challenge has been used in colonoscopy SBS [47, 48], in which progressively more difficult colon anatomical models are presented. As expected from the study, more expert colonoscopists performed better on the most difficult model [25] though data on serial improvements from the novices were not presented. The success of VTs as a SBS for healthcare professionals lies not only in the physical fidelity afforded by excellent graphics but also in the method in which learn-

ers are given formative and summative debriefing while using instructional concepts such as deliberate practice and incremental challenge (see Table 9.1).

Development of Screen-Based Simulation

When planning to develop an SBS, the scope of a project, including budgetary issues, the intended learner audience, specific learning objectives and implementation should all be taken into consideration. A careful evaluation of these factors prior to the start of development will help to ensure that educational objectives will be met and done so in the most cost-effective manner. Depending on the project's complexity, the time, personnel, and financial costs to develop a screen-based or virtual simulator will vary greatly. For example, an e-learning platform for simple factual knowledge will typically require less time, technical expertise, and money compared to a project to develop a serious game designed to teach procedural knowledge and higher-order reasoning skills.

At minimum, a SME that provides a clinical perspective on the fidelity and realism of the VP and interaction is required. This may be the primary case author for academic physicians, but it may be one or more clinicians brought in for clinical expertise. For example, a VP case of multiple children in wartime climate may require an SME in pediatrics, global medicine, and military medicine.

Excellent guidelines for developing VP cases have been published [50, 51]. In addition, an international consortium, *MedBiquitous,* provides guidelines on VP authoring that allows for more uniformity, simpler access, and distribution [52]. The development process is typically broken down into three phases: (1) preparation, (2) design and development, and (3) implementation.

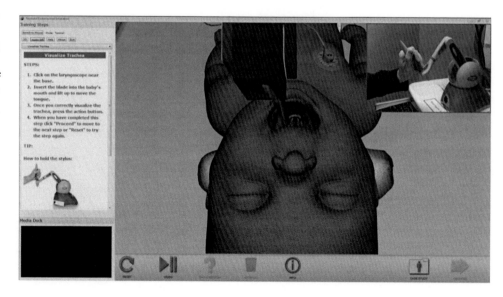

Fig. 9.2 Screenshot of a *virtual task trainer*. It depicts a virtual intubation device for infants and allows the user to grip an actual handle much like a laryngoscope would be gripped for intubation. (Used with permission of Marc Auerbach, Yale University, New Haven, Connecticut, USA, and mySmartSimulations, Inc.)

Table 9.1 Selected examples of screen-based simulation genres

Genre	Manuscript author	Synopsis
Virtual patient	Surgical patient evaluation	This feasibility study demonstrated how life-sized VPs provided teaching context for communication skills
	Stevens [29]	
	Obesity and OSA	OSA was diagnosed more correctly in VPs than in standardized patients due to portrayed obesity
	Wendling [32]	
	Psychiatric evaluation	Communication skills in nuanced fields such as psychiatry are feasible compared to standardized patients
	Williams [28]	
	Pataki [27]	
	Emergency room patient evaluation	Subjects in a virtual trauma ED with live communication improved team skills similarly to subjects in mannequin-based simulation drills
	Youngblood [31]	
	Disaster triage algorithm	VPs in large-scale disaster scenarios did not demonstrate learning effect
	Andreatta [30]	
Virtual world	Diabetes education in Second Life	Physicians enjoyed the novelty of learning diabetes care from colleagues in Second Life
	Wiecha [10]	
	Mock oral board examination in second life	Mock oral exams in Second Life were preferred over traditional mock oral exams by residents
	Schwaab [9]	
	Military tactical operations	Debriefers who participate in VWs with students enhance the coaching cycle during debriefing
	Alklind Taylor [34]	
Virtual task trainer	Bronchoscopy	Competency on bronchoscopy was similar in VT-trained junior residents and senior residents. Davoudi et al. demonstrate reliability and validity of a bronchoscopy VT assessment tool
	Blum [36]	
	Davoudi [38]	
	Colonoscopy	The GI Mentor II and Olympus simulators both have discriminant validity in colonoscopy. Simulator practice improved clinical skill over no simulator practice
	Fayez [25]	
	Koch [37]	
	Cohen [48]	
	Laparoscopy	The LapMentor improves basic animate skills over no training. Procedicus MIST improves technical skills differently than a low-fidelity box simulator
	Andreatta [39]	
	Tanoue [40]	
	Endoscopy	GI Mentor training improved clinical skill over no simulator practice
	Ferlitsch [35]	
	Percutaneous spinal fixation	Virtual needle insertion improves second attempt but no control group
	Luciano [49]	

VP *virtual patient*, OSA *obstructive sleep apnea*, ED *emergency department*, VW *virtual world*, VT *virtual task trainer*

Preparation

During the preparation phase, the specific learning objectives and target audience are defined. Costs can be cut significantly by exploring existing VPs or infrastructure that may reduce additional programming (i.e., code reuse) and still meet the learning objectives. In addition, during the preparation phase, technologic capabilities for the target audience are assessed. Some control or at least knowledge regarding the type of computer or mobile hardware, operating system, web browser software (including plug-ins), and connection access speed is mandatory.

There are a growing number of authoring applications available to medical educators interested in authoring VP cases [53]. Factors to consider when selecting a case authoring application include (a) whether the user interface is intuitive and functional; (b) what functionality is available to the author, and whether the feature sets included in the authoring application permit integration of content, media, documents and hyperlinks, design templates, and further complexity; (c) whether the application can integrate assessment, feedback, and data tracking to case completion; (d) how much the author controls participation, collaboration, and interactivity; (e) how easily it allows design and modification of the interface; and (f) whether the underlying system structure is robust and extensible.

Design and Development

During the design and development phase, a pedagogical model is selected on the basis of the goals of the project and how use of the VP will be incorporated into existing educational curricula. Examples of pedagogical models include solitary open learning, a structured linear learning style, or formation of learning communities [54]. The use of pediatric patients instead of adult patients should not necessarily change the pedagogical model, as the model is reflective of the interactions of the learner with the SBS. Once a pedagogical model is chosen, the narrative for the story, rules and expectations for the learner, and how feedback will be provided are then developed. During case development, the author should:

1. *Determine case content and choose a flow model:* The case content should be appropriate for the level of the intended learner. The design model can be linear, exploratory, or branching.
2. *Organize and storyboard the case before starting:* The specific stages and the connections between each stage are determined a priori. Storyboarding allows both the educator and programmer a visual framework within which to develop the SBS.
3. *Manage case complexity and match it to the case objectives:* Authors should ensure that the case complexity is customized and appropriate for the target learners.
4. *Include assessment and feedback:* Depending upon the type of VP being developed and the level of learners, feedback may be provided during the case in real time or may only occur at the completion of the case.
5. *Support an individualized approach to learning:* Authors can support individualized learning by permitting learner control over components of the case environment, as appropriate to the case's learning objectives, by allowing learners to self-pace, make active choices, and preview and review at their discretion.
6. *Maximize interactivity:* Interactivity increases engagement, heightening a learner's sense of participation, which in turn can facilitate the meaningful learning that is associated with active cognitive processing.
7. *Make navigation easy:* Intuitive and logical site navigation permits the learner to focus on the narrative content, associated learning objectives, and effective exploration of the clinical scenario. Even rich, compelling and relevant cases can be undone by confusing and obtuse user interfaces.
8. *Pilot test the case:* When enough of the case content is developed, the author should pilot test the case on several representative learners. Frameworks for assessing VR, such as the one developed by Moreno-Ger, can be used for formal end-user testing [55]. These frameworks take into consideration both content and user-interface issues.

Implementation

During the preparation and design phases, initial consideration regarding how the VP will be implemented and incorporated into existing training curricula should be given. Once the VP has been developed, the implementation phase takes place. It is important to note that a VP's relative novelty can attract students initially but wanes unless a strong perception of value is established from the first case onward. Educational value comes from having a high-quality engaging case that achieves its learning outcomes. To this end, an effective VP should tell a compelling story with valid clinical events that occur in response to the learner's decisions. Authors should refine their cases based on testing prior to release and from observing student's reactions and performances after implementation [14].

Creating a high-quality VP is a significant scholarly activity; therefore, academicians should consider peer review publication in *MedEdPortal* (http://www.mededportal.org/) through the American Academy of Medical Colleges and sharing the case using the MedBiquitous VP (MVP) data standard (www.medbiq.org) [52]. A VP authoring program can facilitate this process by exporting the case using this international ANSI-approved standard (www.ansi.org) which then can be imported into any MVP-compliant VP software application for reuse and repurposing.

Conclusion Screen-based Simulation has unique advantages and challenges compared to other forms of simulation and its different forms should be approached in the context of larger educational or training goal and objectives. A close working relationship with programmers and educators is essential for successful design, development, and implementation of SBS.

References

1. Ilgen J, Sherbino J, Cook DA. Technology-enhanced simulation in emergency medicine: a systematic review and meta-analysis. Acad Emerg Med. 2013;20:117–27.
2. Graafland M, Schraagen JM, Schijven MP. Systematic review of serious games for medical education and surgical skills training. Br J Surg. 2012;99:1322–30.
3. Kolb D. Experiential learning: experience as the source of learning and development. Englewood Cliffs: Prentice-Hall; 1984.
4. Feinberg R, Swygert KA, Haist SA, Dillon GF, Murray CT. The impact of postgraduate training on USMLE® Step 3® and its computer-based case simulation component. J Gen Intern Med. 2011;27(1):65–70.
5. Fall LH, Berman NB, Smith S, White CB, Woodhead JC, Olson AL. Multi-institutional development and utilization of a computer-assisted learning program for the pediatrics clerkship: the CLIPP Project. Acad Med. 2005;80(9):847–55. Epub 2005/08/27.

6. Pusic M, Andrews JS, Kessler DO, Teng DG, Pecaric MR, Ruzal-Shapiro C, Boutis K. Prevalence of abnormal cases in an image bank affects the learning of radiograph interpretation. Med Educ. 2012;46:289–98.

7. Cook D, Erwin PJ, Triola MM. Computerized virtual patients in health professions education: a systematic review and meta-analysis. Acad Med. 2010;85(10):1589–602.

8. Cook DA, Mark TM. Virtual patients: a critical literature review and proposed next steps. Med Educ. 2009;43(4):303–11.

9. Schwaab J, Kman N, Nagel R, Bahner D, Martin DR, Khandelwal S, Vozenilek J, Danforth DR, Nelson R. Using second life virtual simulation environment for mock oral emergency medicine examination. Acad Emerg Med. 2011;18:559–62.

10. Wiecha J HR, Sternthal E, Merialdi M. Learning in a virtual world: experience with using second life for medical education. J Med Internet Res. 2010;12(1):e1.

11. Yao R, Heath T, Davies A, Forsyth T, Mitchell N, Hoberman P. Oculus VR Best Practices Guide. 2014. http://mediagoblin.tami.org.il/mgoblin_media/media_entries/657/OculusBestPractices.pdf. Accessed 30 Aug 2014.

12. Bodenheimer T. The future of primary care: transforming practice. N Engl J Med. 2008;359(20):2086, 9. Epub 2008/11/14.

13. Cheng A, Auerbach M, Hunt EA, Chang TP, Pusic M, Nadkarni V, Kessler D. Designing and conducting simulation-based research. Pediatrics. 2014;133(6):1091–101.

14. Ellaway RH, Pusic M, Yavner S, Kalet AL. Context matters: emergent variability in an effectiveness trial of online teaching modules. Med Educ. 2014;48(4):386–96. Epub 2014/03/13.

15. Brydges R, Dubrowski A, Regehr G. A new concept of unsupervised learning: directed self-guided learning in the health professions. Acad Med. 2010;85(10):S49–55.

16. Brydges R, Carnahan H, Safir O, Dubrowski A. How effective is self-guided learning of clinical technical skills? It's all about process. Med Educ. 2009;43(5):507–15.

17. Jorna PGAM. Heart rate and workload variations in actual and simulated flight. Ergonomics. 1993;36(9):1043–54.

18. Tourassi G, Voisin S, Paguit V, Krupinski E. Investigating the link between radiologists' gaze, diagnostic decision, and image content. J Am Med Inform Assoc. 2013;20(6):1067–75. Epub 2013 Jun 20.

19. Hamstra S, Brydges R, Hatala R, Zendejas B, Cook DA. Reconsidering fidelity in simulation-based training. Acad Med. 2014;89(3)387–92.

20. Norman G, Dore K, Grierson L. The minimal relationship between simulation fidelity and transfer of learning. Med Educ. 2012;46(7):636–47.

21. Rudolph J, Simon R, Raemer DB. Which reality matters? Questions on the path to high engagement in healthcare simulation. Simul Healthc. 2007;2(3):161–3.

22. Dieckmann P, Gaba D, Rall M. Deepening the theoretical foundations of patient simulation as social practice. Simul Healthc. 2007;2(3):183–93.

23. Maran N, Glavin RJ. Low- to high-fidelity simulation—a continuum of medical education? Med Educ. 2003;37(Suppl 1):22–8.

24. Pezzulo G, Barsalou LW, Cangelosi A, Fischer MH, McRae K, Spivey MJ. Computational grounded cognition: a new alliance between grounded cognition and computational modeling. Front Psychol. 2013;3(612):1–11.

25. Fayez R FL, Kaneva P, Fried GM. Testing the construct validity of the Simbionix GI Mentor II virtual reality colonoscopy simulator metrics: module matters. Surg Endosc. 2010;24(5):1060–5.

26. Bedwell WL, Pavlas D, Heyne K, Lazzara EH, Salas E. Toward a taxonomy linking game attributes to learning: an empirical study. Simul Gaming. 2012;43(6):729–60.

27. Pataki C, Pato MT, Sugar J, Rizzo AS, Parsons TD, St George C, Kenny P. Virtual patients as novel teaching tools in psychiatry. Acad Psychiatry. 2012;36:398–400.

28. Williams K, Wryobeck J, Edinger W, McGrady A, Fors U, Zary N. Assessment of competencies by use of virtual patient technology. Acad Psychiatry. 2011;35(5):328–30.

29. Stevens A, Hernandez J, Johnsen K, Dickerson R, Raij A, Harrison C, DiPietro M, Allen B, Ferdig R, Foti S, Jackson J, Shin M, Cendan J, Watson R, Duerson M, Lok B, Cohen M, Wagner P, Lind DS. The use of virtual patients to teach medical students history taking and communication skills. Am J Surg. 2006;191(6):806–11.

30. Andreatta P, Maslowski E, Petty S, Shim W, Marsh M, Hall T, Stern S, Frankel J. Virtual reality triage training provides a viable solution for disaster-preparedness. Acad Emerg Med. 2010;17(8):870–6.

31. Youngblood P, Harter PM, Srivastava S, Moffett S, Heinrichs WL, Dev P. Design, development, and evaluation of an online virtual emergency department for training trauma teams. Simul Healthc. 2008;3(3):146–53.

32. Wendling A, Halan S, Tighe P, Le L, Euliano T, Lok B. Virtual humans versus standardized patients: which lead residents to more correct diagnoses? Acad Med. 2011;86(3):384–8.

33. Amichai-Hamberger Y, Wainapel G, Fox S. "On the internet no one know i'm an introvert': extroversion, neuroticism, and internet interaction. CyberPsychol Behav. 2002;5(2):125–8.

34. Alklind Taylor A-S, Backlund P, Niklasson L. The coaching cycle: a coaching-by-gaming approach in serious games. Simul Gaming. 2012;43(5):648–72.

35. Ferlitsch A, Schoefl R, Puespoek A, Miehsler W, Schoeniger-Hekele M, Hofer H, Gangl A, Homoncik M. Effect of virtual endoscopy simulator training on performance of upper gastrointestinal endoscopy in patients: a randomized controlled trial. Endoscopy. 2010;42(12):1049–56.

36. Blum M, Powers TW, Sundaresan S. Bronchoscopy simulator effectively prepares junior residents to competently perform basic clinical bronchoscopy. Ann Thorac Surg. 2004;78(1):287–91.

37. Koch AD HJ, Schoon EJ, de Man RA, Kuipers EJ. A second-generation virtual reality simulator for colonoscopy: validation and initial experience. Endoscopy. 2008;40(9):735–8.

38. Davoudi M, Osann K, Colt HG. Validation of two instruments to assess technical bronchoscopic skill using virtual reality simulation. Respiration. 2008;76:92–101.

39. Andreatta P, Woodrum DT, Birkmeyer JD, Yellamanchilli RK, Doherty GM, Gauger PG, Minter RM et al. Laparoscopic skills are improved with LapMentor training: results of a randomized, double-blinded study. Ann Surg. 2006;243(6):854–60.

40. Tanoue K IS, Konishi K, Yasunaga T, Okazaki K, Yamaguchi S, Yoshida D, Kakeji Y, Hashizume M. Effectiveness of endoscopic surgery training for medical students using a virtual reality simulator versus a box trainer: a randomized controlled trial. Surg Endosc. 2008;22(4):985–90.

41. Hodge T, Deakin JM. Deliberate practice and expertise in the martial arts: the role of context in motor recall. 1998;20(3):260–79.

42. Lehmann A, Ericsson KA. Research on expert performance and deliberate practice: implications for the education of amateur musicians and music students. Psychomusicology. 1997;16(1–2):40–58.

43. Kessler D, Auerbach M, Pusic M, Tunik MG, Foltin JC. A randomized trial of simulation-based deliberate practice for infant lumbar puncture skills. Simul Healthc. 2011;6(4):197–203.

44. Wayne D, Barsuk JH, O'Leary KJ, Fudala MJ, McGaghie WC. Mastery learning of thoracentesis skills by internal medicine residents using simulation technology and deliberate practice. J Hosp Med. 2008;3(1):48–54.

45. Ericsson K. Deliberate practice and acquisition of expert performance: a general overview. Acad Emerg Med. 2008;15(11):988–94.

46. Ericsson K. Deliberate practice and the acquisition and maintenance of expert performance in medicine and related domains. Acad Med. 2004;79(Suppl 10):S70–81.

47. Garris R, Ahlers R, Driskell JE. Games, motivation, and learning: a research and practice model. Simul Gaming. 2002;43(1):118–32.

48. Cohen J, Cohen SA, Vora KC, Xue X, Burdick JS, Bank S, et al. Multicenter, randomized, controlled trial of virtual-reality simulator training in acquisition of competency in colonoscopy. Gastrointest Endosc. 2006;64(3):361–8. Epub 2006/08/23.

49. Luciano C, Banerjee PP, Sorenson JM, FOley KT, Ansari SA, Rizzi S, Germanwala AV, Kranzler L, Chittiboina P, Roitberg BZ. Percutaneous spinal fixation simulation with virtual reality and haptics. Neurosurgery. 2013;72(Suppl 1):89–96.

50. Posel N, Fleiszer D, Shore BM. 12 tips: guidelines for authoring virtual patient cases. Med Teach. 2009;31:701–8.

51. McGee J. Designing, developing and implementing branched-narrative virtual patients for medical education, training and assessment: a guide for authors of virtual patients. http://vpsim.pitt.edu/shell/documents/Virtual_Patient_Authoring_Best_Practices.pdf. Accessed 1 Sept 2014 [16p].

52. Triola M, Campion N, McGee JB, Albright S, Greene P, Smothers V, Ellaway R. An XML standard for virtual patients: exchanging case-based simulations in medical education. AMIA Annu Symp Proc. 2007;2007:741–5.

53. Medbiquitous Consortium Virtual Patient Implementors. (World Wide Web) 2013. http://www.medbiq.org/virtual_patient/implementers. Accessed 30 Aug 2014.

54. Dabbagh N. Pedagogical models for E-Learning: a theory-based design framework. Int J Technol Teach Learn. 2005;1(1):25–44.

55. Moreno-Ger P, Torrente J, Hsieh YG, Lester WT. Usability testing for serious games: making informed design decisions with user data. Adv Hum-Computer Interact. 2012;2012:13.

Mannequin-Based Simulators and Task Trainers

Arielle Levy, Dominic Allain, Afrothite Kotsakis and
Terry Varshney

Simulation Pearls

1. Level of fidelity should target the educational needs guided by the training objectives of the program. Ask yourself three questions: (1) What are your educational needs? (2) How does the fidelity relate to the needs? (3) What is the optimal combination of simulation tools and technologies to meet these needs?
2. Part task trainers can be used to teach novices basic psychomotor skills and can allow experts to maintain more advanced skills.
3. Having a case facilitator and/or having visual cues prepared to prompt the learners can help overcome limitations inherent to all mannequins.
4. Although extremely effective, hybrid models are time- and cost-consuming, thus should only be used if they will enhance the learners' educational objectives.

A. Levy (✉)
Department of Pediatric Emergency, Department of Pediatrics,
University of Montreal, Sainte-Justine Hospital University Centre,
Montreal, Quebec, Canada
e-mail: arielle.levy007@gmail.com

D. Allain
Department of Emergency Medicine, Dalhousie University, Halifax,
NS, Canada
e-mail: Dominic.Allain@iwk.nshealth.ca

A. Kotsakis
Department of Pediatrics, Department of Critical Care Medicine,
University of Toronto, The Hospital for Sick Children, Toronto, ON,
Canada
e-mail: afrothite.kotsakis@sickkids.ca

T. Varshney
Department of Pediatric Emergency, Children Hospital of Eastern
Ontario, University of Ottawa, Ottawa, ON, Canada
e-mail: Terryv1984@gmail.com

Introduction

Mannequin-based simulators were first developed in the 1960s [1]. Over the past few decades, their design has undergone tremendous change and the models available today, including pediatric models, offer specialized functions with compact control systems and increasingly smaller physical footprints with greater flexibility. Compared to desktop or screen-based simulations, these computerized, mannequin-based simulators offer the advantage of recreating a realistic patient for use within a realistic simulated environment. Also referred to as high-fidelity simulators, they are capable of recreating a wide variety of human functions. These include physical examination findings such as heart and lung sounds, as well as physiological parameters, such as changes in respiratory rate or heart rate. Mannequin-based simulators offer both instructors and participants real-time display of electronically monitored physiological parameters. Operators have the capacity to pre-program simulation scenarios and modify a range of parameters in response to changes in the patient's clinical condition as well as participant interventions. By programming effectively and adjusting the inputs to the mannequin and to the environment, the operator is able to maximize the realism of the interaction, and contribute positively to the learner experience, as well as optimize the simulator's use as a research and assessment tool. Invasive procedures, such as inserting a catheter for intravenous access, performing endotracheal intubation, or defibrillating a patient in cardiac arrest, can all be practiced, depending on the type of mannequin. Mannequin-based simulators can be used in a dedicated simulation facility or transported to a specific clinical setting, such as a clinic, a ward, or an emergency department room, based on the resource availability and learner needs and numbers.

Key differences exist between pediatric and adult mannequin, reflecting the real-life distinctions seen between pediatric and adult patients. Some of these differences are anatomical, some are physiological and based on underlying medical conditions, while others are based on responses to treatments. This chapter will explore, compare and contrast (where possible) the various task trainers and whole body mannequins available in the market today. Finally, the chapter will explore the programming of whole body mannequins and highlight how the understanding of both the features and limitations of the current generation of simulation mannequins is essential to create and deliver clinically authentic and realistic scenarios that will help with simulation education delivery.

Fidelity/Realism

In simulation-based education, fidelity can be classified into three types: *semantical* (or conceptual), *emotional* (or phenomenal), and *physical* [2]. Semantical or conceptual fidelity concerns concepts such as information presented via text, pictures, sounds, or progression in clinical events. For example, a scenario can be conceptually realistic if the information given is interpretable regardless if it is lacking physical realism and if the clinical progression is consistent with what would be experienced with a real patient (e.g., in a patient with hypovolemic shock, the heart rate improves after a fluid bolus is given). Emotional or phenomenal fidelity includes emotions or beliefs that learners directly experience when emerged in a situation. This is an important issue in simulation because it describes the different elements of the experience such as complex real-time situation and an educational experience resembling a real situation [2].

Physical fidelity classically refers to the degree to which a simulator looks, feels, and acts like a human patient. The definition of physical fidelity has a tendency to emphasize technical and physical advances over pedagogical principles and objectives. Although some studies report that training with realistic mannequins improves clinical performance [3, 4], several studies have demonstrated that the degree of physical fidelity is independent of educational effectiveness [5, 6]. Nevertheless, trainees do report increased satisfaction with more realistic high physical fidelity mannequins [7]. However, fidelity should not just refer to the physical resemblance of the simulator but should consider the functional aspect of fidelity, that is, the degree to which learners are required to use the same performance strategies and competencies in the simulation and in the real clinical environment [8]. As such, simulation should not be simply considered high or low fidelity.

It is not uncommon for practitioners to simplify fidelity into a one-dimensional construct that results in categorization on a continuum from low to high. However, a one-dimensional conceptualization of fidelity can be misleading when trying to select appropriate simulators for a given training need. A simulation that has the look and feel of the real world is often considered high fidelity, when in fact only one dimension of overall fidelity (i.e., physical fidelity) is high. A simulation can replicate the outward appearance of the operational environment (e.g., an operating room, OR) quite effectively yet still be ineffective at helping learners meet the training goals. Ultimately, the focus should be to match the various types of simulation fidelity to best meet educational targets (Fig. 10.1). For example, team training involves high emotional, high conceptual, and high physical fidelity. Patient assessment will target high conceptual and physical fidelity. In communication training, the focus will be on high conceptual and emotional fidelity. Keeping in mind the following questions is mandatory when considering fidelity options for a simulation: What are the educational *needs* of the learner group, and what are the educational *objectives* of the session? What level of *fidelity* is required to best meet those needs? What is the best *combination* of simulation tools and technologies available to achieve that level of fidelity and meet the aforementioned needs [9]? Figures 10.2 and 10.3 illustrate an example of the choice of simulation modalities according to educational objectives.

The term Human Factors (HF) represents a set of physical and psychological characteristics that are needed to successfully match humans to equipment and systems. It integrates technology, policies, processes and environment, training, skills, and experiences of the personnel involved in the simulation. HF tools originating in aviation and other safety critical industries have been proven effective [11]. The latter are currently being applied effectively in health care because they may support fidelity decisions and design. Incorporating HF techniques into simulation-based education may lead to better decisions on appropriate use of fidelity. Many frameworks have been suggested to classify and understand elements of fidelity. A simple and common framework of HF called the PTE (Patient-Task-Environment; Fig. 10.4) is one example where after determining the learning objectives, educators can choose simulation elements within the PTE dimension for each stage of the scenario and match the appropriate level of fidelity to target specific objectives within each stage. Systematically reviewing the training objective relevant to the simulation element and matching the element fidelity against the training objective will further guide educators to select the most appropriate level of fidelity to target educational needs.

A recent review examining key concepts and assumptions surrounding the topic of fidelity in simulation suggests that concepts such as transfer of learning, learner engagement, and suspension of disbelief are not only useful in explaining educational effectiveness but also directly influence properties of the learning experience. The authors suggest

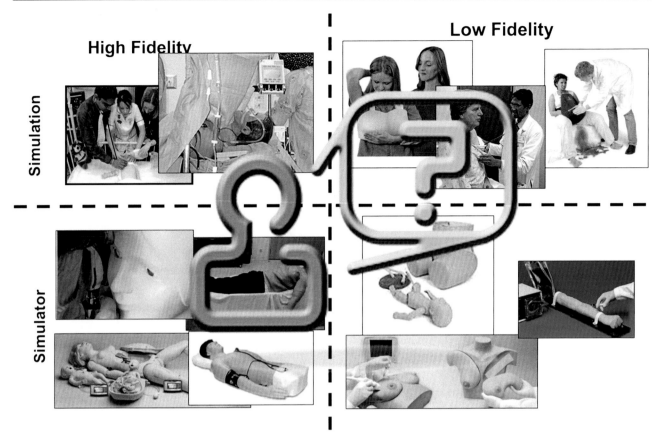

Fig. 10.1 Matching simulation fidelity to educational needs. (Photo courtesy of CAE Healthcare [10])

Fig. 10.2 Choosing a 3D training program best used to train knowledge of endotracheal intubation. (Photo courtesy of CAE Healthcare [10])

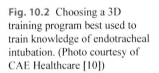

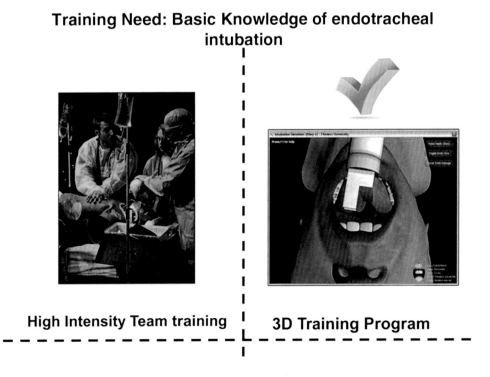

Fig. 10.3 High-intensity team training best used to train for team skills during trauma intubation. (Photo courtesy of CAE Healthcare [10])

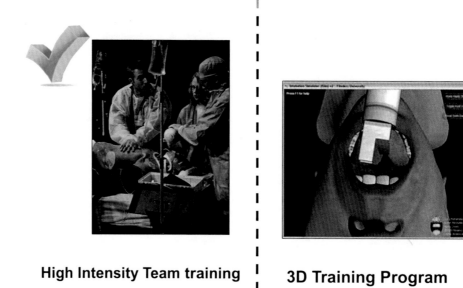

Training Need: Team Skills for Trauma Intubation

High Intensity Team training | **3D Training Program**

Fig. 10.4 PTE framework to choose simulation elements. *PTE* patient-task-environment. (Photo courtesy of CAE Healthcare [10])

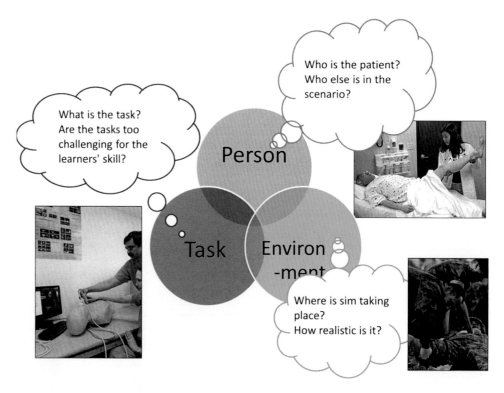

What is the task? Are the tasks too challenging for the learners' skill?

Who is the patient? Who else is in the scenario?

Person

Task

Environ -ment

Where is sim taking place? How realistic is it?

abandoning the term fidelity in simulation-based education and replacing it with terms reflecting the underlying physical resemblance and functional task alignment. They also suggest shifting away from the current emphasis on physical resemblance to a focus on functional link between the simulator and the desired educational context. Finally, they recommend that educators focus on methods to enhance educational effectiveness such as principles of transfer of learning, learner engagement, and suspension of disbelief [12].

Pediatric Partial Task Trainers

When teaching a particular procedural skill, it may only be necessary to reproduce specific portions of the patient or task. Partialtask physical trainers replicate only a portion of a complete process or system [13], provide key elements of the procedure being learned, and allow learners to acquire the basic skills needed to accomplish the same task on real

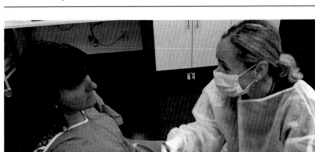

Fig. 10.5 Partial task trainers for suturing lacerations.(From https://web.mail.comcast.net/service/home/~/?id=176615&part=2.2&auth=co&disp=i)

patients (see Chap. 11). Some examples of homemade task trainers include using oranges to learn injection techniques or chicken bones to learn intraosseous line placement [14], among others. Commercially produced pediatric partial task trainers (PTTs), usually composed of plastic and rubber allow the same procedural practice, albeit in a safe (and cleaner) environment. In contrast to whole body mannequins, they incorporate only the anatomical section required for a particular procedural skill. Hybrid simulations involve combining a PTT with a live standardized patient (SP) actor to help enhance the physical fidelity of the overall educational experience. Examples include partial task trainers for suturing lacerations consisting of a pad with a wound cut on the surface. Such a pad can be strapped onto the arm of an SP and then draped appropriately. The learner not only has to perform the elements of suturing the wound but also has to do so while speaking to the patient, thus emulating a real-life situation (Fig. 10.5).

PTTs are a commonly utilized modality due to cost and size. They can be effectively used to teach novices the basics of psychomotor skills [15] and can allow experts to maintain and practice more advanced skills. Currently, a significant amount of PTTs are available or are in development. The following section will focus on various PTTs that are currently available on the market, divided into five categories:

1. Airway trainers
2. Vascular and intraosseous (IO) access trainers
3. Invasive torso-based task trainers (including lumbar puncture (LP) trainers, chest tube, and pericardiocentesis trainers)
4. Surgical task trainers
5. Miscellaneous trainers

Airway Trainers

Airway Management

Airway management skills demand a significant amount of practice in order to achieve competency standards [16–20]. Infant and child PTTs that realistically reproduce different parts of an anatomic airway allow for practicing basic and advanced airway management skills. They permit skill development in bag-valve mask ventilation, placement of nasopharyngeal and oropharyngeal airways, and placement of endotracheal tubes (Fig. 10.6). Many studies have shown that trainees can develop responses to and skill in management of emergency airway situations when practicing with airway trainers [16]. Furthermore, studies have also demonstrated that recent tracheal intubation training is associated with immediate refresher training effectiveness and trainer outcome [17–20].

Airway trainers may have certain mechanical and visual limitations. For example, not all trainers allow for a good seal to practice effective bagging during ventilation. In other models, the tongue and the epiglottis may be semirigid in structure and are distinctly separated from the posterior pharynx. The epiglottis is suspended anteriorly and superiorly away from the laryngeal inlet. Identifying laryngeal structures and controlling the tongue and epiglottis on an airway trainer may not represent a realistic clinical challenge. Along with the mechanical and visual limitations of airway trainers, most institutions provide trainees with practice on only one type of intubation trainer. This fosters a very limited understanding of anatomy and mechanical variation encountered in actual patients. Studies support the use of several types of airway trainers to enhance learning. [21, 22]

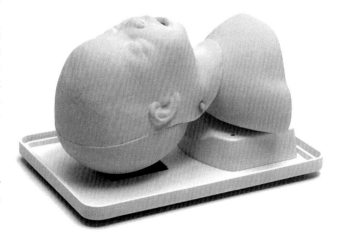

Fig. 10.6 Infant Airway Management Trainer. (Image used courtesy of Laerdal Medical [23])

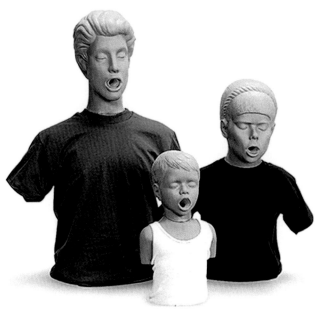

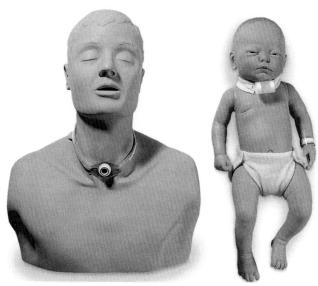

Fig. 10.8 Infant tracheostomy trainer. (Photo courtesy of North American Strategy for Competitiveness (NASCO) [25])

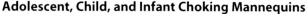

Fig. 10.7 Adolescent, Child, and Infant Choking Mannequins. (Photo courtesy of Simulaids [24] Corporation)

Adolescent, Child, and Infant Choking Mannequins

Some airway PTTs also offer opportunities to practice foreign body removal (Fig. 10.7). Some adolescent, child, and infant choking mannequins include a rib cage, xiphoid process, and jugular notch to provide anatomical reference points for the demonstration of proper hand placement for the technique inherent to the clearing of impacted airway foreign bodies. Each life-size head and upper torso allows practice of abdominal thrusts, chests thrusts, and back blows for clearing foreign body obstruction. When correct clearing procedures are performed, the mannequin will expel the object causing the blockage. The choking objects provided make excellent practice of obstructions.

Cricothyrotomy and Tracheotomy Insertion and Care

PTTs have been developed for training in rescue airway skills such as cricothyrotomy and tracheotomy. Infant tracheostomy trainers also provide an opportunity to teach basic tracheostomy care skills to patients and caregivers (Fig. 10.8). Procedures such as dressing changes, stoma cleansing, changing of tracheostomy tube, and tracheostomy ties as well as cuff inflation can be performed on this infant trainer. These trainers have the advantage of filling lungs and stomach with fluid for realistic practice of tracheostomy care and tracheal suctioning. They also allow for practice of various steps for tracheostomy insertion and care. However, they are limited in their ability to mimic human anatomy and tissues, but may be used to gain familiarity with the different equipment available for percutaneous tracheostomy.

Cricothyrotomy trainers are designed for learning and practicing the technique of emergency cricothyrotomy. Palpable landmarks include both the cricoid and thyroid cartilage. All landmarks are accurately placed and allow for a rapid procedure. As the airway passes completely through from top to bottom, the trachea in this simulator is replaceable. This allows checking the stylet and obturator placement once the stab has been made. Complete with a full-size neck, ties can be used to hold the obturator in a secure position (Fig. 10.9). Advantages include the opportunities for trainees to practice various steps of a high-stakes procedure such as this one, as well as preparing necessary equipment mandatory to ensure a successful procedure. However, disadvantages include variable realism and fixed anatomy specific to the model. Models cannot bleed and certain tissues may not feel realistic. In addition, because most emergent airways are done in patients who have altered anatomy (e.g., a patient with an expanding hematoma after undergoing branchial cyst resection, a teenager with massive trauma to the face or neck, a syndromic child with a short, fat, thick neck, etc.), these *fixed* models may not be the ideal method for training [26].

Vascular Access and Intraosseous Trainers

Venipuncture and Intravenous Catheter Insertion

Venipuncture PTTs are commonly used for training healthcare providers. Intravenous access arms come in different colors, sizes, and depths of veins (Fig. 10.10). Not only do they allow for the procedures of venipuncture and

Fig. 10.9 Life/form® Cricothy-rotomy Simulator Kit. (Photo courtesy of NASCO [25])

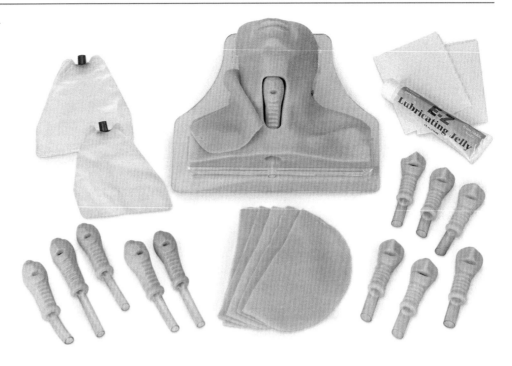

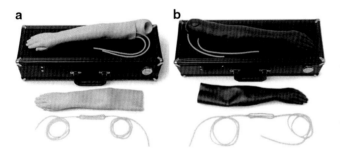

Fig. 10.10 Pediatric Multi-Venous IV Training Arm Kits (**a, b**). (Images courtesy of Laerdal Medical [23])

models that are currently available include subclavian, internal jugular, and femoral veins (Fig. 10.11). Anatomic landmarks can be palpated and identified. There is good evidence to support the positive impact of practicing these skills before experiencing similar procedures in clinical settings [28]. Studies have shown higher confidence levels and knowledge gain, and improved clinical performances of trainees after

intravenous catheter insertion, they also permit learners to practice the ancillary procedures of preparation, wearing gloves, and respecting sterility. Proper needle placement can be confirmed on these models by a flashback of simulated blood, as well as the possibility of infusing fluids and withdrawing blood. These trainers allow for review of principles, skills and tools necessary for insertion, assessment, dressing care, securement and maintenance of vascular access devices in children. Disadvantages include minimal adhesion when placing dressings on certain models due to the nonstaining properties of the tissuelike material. Studies have shown improvements in peripheral intravenous vein placement and higher scores on knowledge examinations of pediatric house staff after simulated procedural skill training [27].

Central Venous Catheter Insertion

Central line PTTs are widely available, with some of the newer models allowing for the use of ultrasound in ultrasound-guided central venous catheter insertion. Pediatric

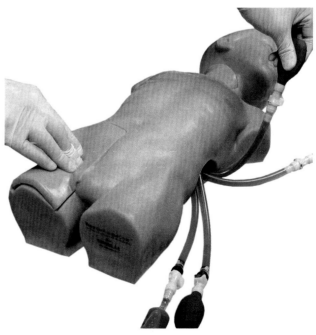

Fig. 10.11 VascularAccessChild. (Photo courtesy of Simulab Corporation [32])

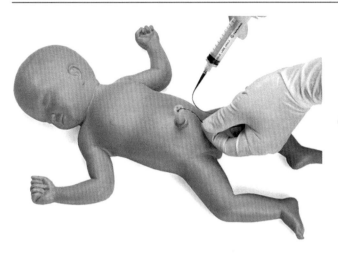

Fig. 10.12 Baby Umbi. (Photo courtesy of Laerdal Medical [23])

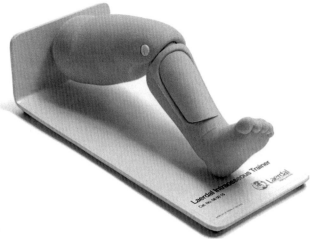

Fig. 10.13 Laerdal Intraosseous Trainer. (Image used courtesy of Laerdal Medical [23])

simulated training with these task trainers [29, 30]. A recent study demonstrated how dissemination of a simulation-based mastery learning intervention reduced central-line-associated bloodstream infections [31].

Umbilical Venous Catheter Insertion

Neonatal trainers are available for the practice of umbilical venous and arterial line catherization (Fig. 10.12). These trainers offer an opportunity to practice blood withdrawal and fluid infusion. The lifelike umbilicus allows the repeated accessing of the umbilical vein, with proper placement verified by blood return. Advantages include flashback of simulated blood, and certain models can mimic the curves of the umbilical vein after it enters the body, making placement more realistic. However, in some models, the cord is secured poorly and thus does not adequately mimic placement in a newborn. Other models are limited in their ability to mimic the curves of the umbilical vein after it enters the body, representing a more unrealistic placement.

Intraosseous Access Trainers

IO trainers are designed for teaching infant intraosseous infusion techniques and permit both intraosseous needle insertion and aspiration of simulated bone marrow (Fig. 10.13). IO access trainers can be used to train to competency as assessed by validated assessment instruments [33]. Advantages include the ability to use either manual IO introducers or powered IO insertion devices such as guns or drills. However, some models offer only one size and do not provide flashback. In addition, current models do not allow external rotation of the hip to permit proper positioning. Most models do not allow practicing insertion in other sites other than the proximal tibia, such as proximal humerus, distal femur, and malleola.

Invasive Torso-Based Task Trainers

Chest Tube Placement (Tube Thoracostomy) and Pericardiocentesis

Many high-fidelity full-body mannequins offer the possibility of performing needle thoracostomy, chest tube placement, paracentesis, and even pericardiocentesis. However, there is the potential for increased wear and tear on the mannequins and likely an earlier need to replace the mannequin. Because of the high costs associated with high-fidelity full-body mannequins, specific PTTs are available to acquire necessary skill and experience in performing the same procedures, as well as the ancillary concepts of setting up and maintaining closed water-seal drainage systems. Many programs use torso-based surgical PTTs as part of pediatric emergency medicine, critical care, and surgery procedural skills training programs for needle and tube thoracostomy as well as pericardiocentesis (Fig. 10.14). A recent study developed and validated an assessment tool for chest tube insertion competency (Tool for Assessing Chest Tube Insertion Competency; TACTIC) in children and identified areas where training is required for pediatric emergency physicians. They demonstrated significant improvement in scores after targeted training, providing a way to document acquisition of skill, guide individualized teaching, and assist with the assessment of the adequacy of clinician training [34].

Limitations in using torso-based surgical PTTs for chest tube insertion (CTI) include gaps in the procedural fidelity of current training models and their insufficiency to support training of procedural mastery potentially leading to iatrogenic complications associated with these procedures. A recent study developed, piloted, and implemented a novel CTI bench model for usability by volunteer pediatric residents

Fig. 10.14 TraumaChild® (**a, b**). (Photos courtesy of Simulab Corporation [32])

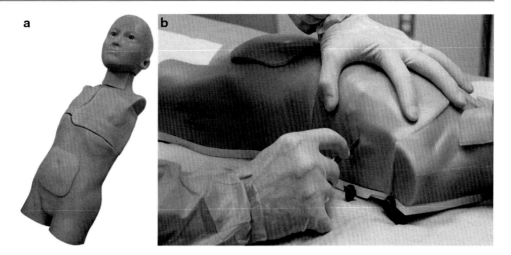

and pediatric emergency fellows during training courses. Their study highlights the feasibility of creating homemade task trainer models to teach CTI skills [35].

Lumbar Puncture Trainers

Several infant and pediatric LP PTTs are available for practice of the LP technique (Figs. 10.15 and 10.16). Neonatal models can be positioned in lateral decubitus or upright position. They possess a realistic interchangeable spine with spinal cord that may be palpated for location of correct puncture site. Simulated cerebrospinal fluid (CSF) may also be removed as part of the procedure. Pediatric models have soft and flexible body tissue resistance, which adds to the realism of the procedure. Puncture blocks can be quick and easy to replace. Successful LP is confirmed by the flow of simulated CSF. CSF pressure can also be measured with a manometer. The neonatal model also replicates the iliac crests and spinous process for appropriate landmarking during the procedure. There is evidence that the majority of pediatric interns at the start of residency have little experience, poor knowledge, low confidence, and are not prepared to perform infant

LPs [36]. A recent study demonstrated that a task-trainer-based course improved the confidence and knowledge about infant LP procedure and that this confidence and knowledge can translate to actual clinical practice [37]. The LP technique in particular has been a target for medical education simulation research concerning knowledge transfer from a simulated setting to the real clinical setting [15]. A recent assessment tool for LP procedure, objective structured assessment of technical skills for neonatal LP (OSATS-LP), has recently been developed and has shown evidence of validity for the instrument. In addition, this tool may provide real-time formative and summative feedback to improve resident skills and patient care [38].

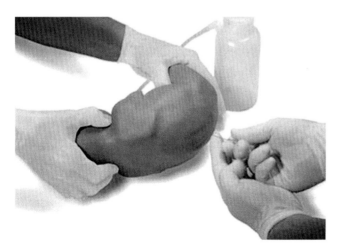

Fig. 10.15 Lumbar Puncture (LP) Simulator, Neonatal—Baby Stap. (Image used courtesy of Laerdal Medical [23])

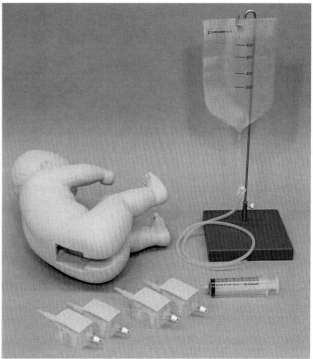

Fig. 10.16 Lumbar Puncture (LP) Simulator, Pediatric. (Photo courtesy of Limbs and Things LTD [39])

Fig. 10.17 Deluxe Basic Open Surgical Skills Simulator. (Photo courtesy of SIMULAB Corporation [18])

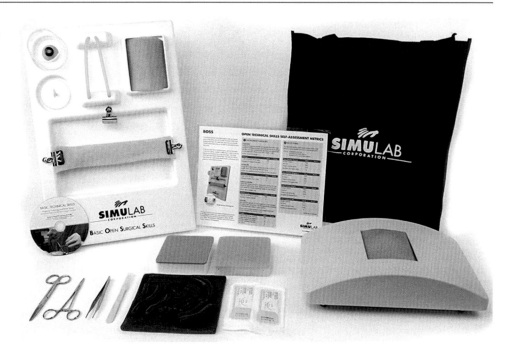

Surgical Trainers

Many challenges are encountered during medical school training and in surgical residency, including limited operative exposure and a lack of autonomy (see Chap. 22). These issues may limit trainees' opportunities to learn or apply technical skills intraoperatively or in the course of their surgical rotations [40]. Hence, even students graduating from the same medical school may enter residency with differing levels of proficiency in knot tying, suturing, and handling of laparoscopic instruments [41, 42]. Simulation and structured preparatory skills sessions have emerged as interventions to standardize developing proficiency in basic surgical skills and serve as an adjunct to potentially limited intraoperative application [43, 44]. Because new surgical technologies increase the number of skills, trainees are expected to acquire during residency, targeting early skill development by using simulation for surgical skills training and evaluation may aid in achieving the proficiency levels necessary to optimize patient care, operative experience, and skill refinement.

Suturing Trainers

The Deluxe Basic Open Surgical Skills Simulator shown in Fig. 10.17 is an example of suturing and knot tying trainer that consists of a specialized board and surgical skills development platform offering trainees the opportunity to practice these procedures. Suture practice arms as well as trainers with vinyl skin over foam can be stitched and used to train laceration repair and incision. Other models replicate layers of the abdominal wall to teach layered opening and closing during laparotomy.

Laparoscopic Skills Box Trainers and Virtual Reality Laparoscopic Trainers

Training to proficiency with a laparoscopic simulator has resulted in improving performance in the OR and has shown transferability of basic laparoscopic skills gained on a physical simulator to the OR, emphasizing the value of laparoscopic simulators for training purposes [45]. A recent systematic review strengthened the evidence that simulation-based training, as part of a structured program and incorporating predetermined proficiency levels, results in skills transfer to the operative setting [46]. In addition, laparoscopic box model training appears to improve technical skills compared with no training in trainees with no previous laparoscopic experience [47]. Both video-box model physical simulator and mirrored-box model physical simulators are available options. Figure 10.18 shows the Fundamentals of Laparoscopic Surgery (FLS) Trainer Box Simulator. The Laparoscopic Trainer Box facilitates the development of psychomotor skills and dexterity required during the performance of basic laparoscopic surgery. Advantages include transferring, precision cutting, placement and securing of ligation loop, and simple suturing with intracorporeal- and extracorporeal knot. Targeted skills include eye–hand coordination and the ability to perform three-dimensional actions of organs being operated on using a two-dimensional screen as a guide. Eye–hand coordination is improved by both visual feedback, by way of a screen, as well as tactile feedback that simulates the manipulation of organs and tissue. Various surgical tools or gloves are connected to motion sensors and haptic or tactile feedback mechanisms where the user can physically feel

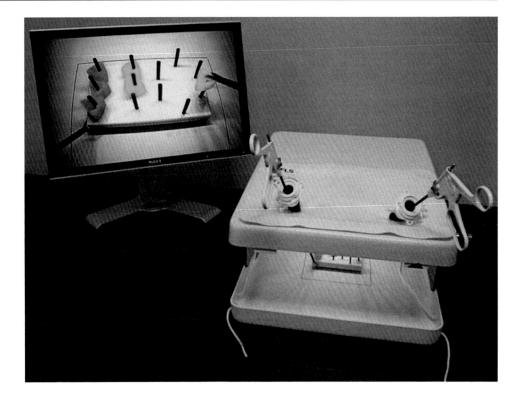

Fig. 10.18 FLS trainer box simulator. (Fundamentals of Laparoscopic Surgery® (FLS) Program is owned by Society of American Gastrointestinal and Endoscopic Surgeons and American College of Surgeons. Used with permission)

the difference in simulated tissue and organs. Virtual reality training appears to decrease the operating time and improve the operative performance of surgical trainees with limited laparoscopic experience when compared with no training or with box-trainer training [48].

Miscellaneous Trainers

Circumcision Trainer

Circumcision trainers have been developed for realistic training of this special procedure (Fig. 10.19). Trainees can improve their skills on the surgical removal of the foreskin

Fig. 10.19 Infant circumcision trainer. (Photo courtesy of NASCO [25])

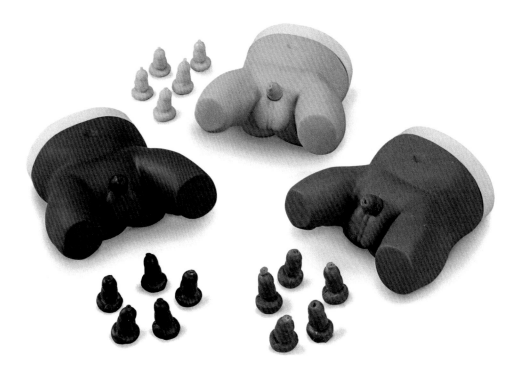

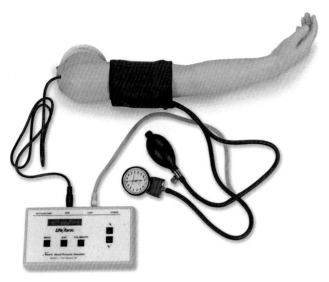

Fig. 10.20 Blood pressure trainer. (Photo courtesy of NASCO [25])

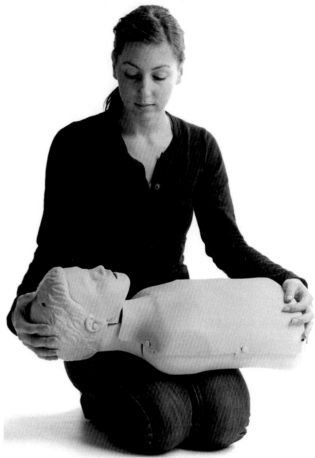

on the glans penis and can be used to demonstrate aftercare skills to parents and family members. Most trainers have the advantages of being designed for various circumcision methods such as Mogen clamp method, the Guillotine clamp method, the Gomco clamp method, the Plastibell method, the dorsal slit method, the forceps-guided method, and the sleeve circumcision. However, certain disadvantages include the fact that the glans is not fused to the foreskin as it is in reality, and so there is no sensation of ripping the foreskin from the glands. The trainer does not bleed and because it is not attached to a body, trainees will need to be reminded the importance of properly constraining the infant and provide necessary sedation.

Fig. 10.21 Little Junior CPR. CPR cardiopulmonary resuscitation (Image courtesy of Laerdal Medical [23])

Blood Pressure Trainers

Pediatric blood pressure (BP) arms are available for teaching the skill of BP acquisition. The model reproduces the arm of an 8-year-old child that can attach to the right shoulder of the mannequin away from the body for easy accessibility (Fig. 10.20). These trainers allow for practice listening to and distinguishing the different BP sounds. Korotkoff sounds may be synchronized with pulses, and systolic and diastolic pressure may be individually set and pulse strength depending on BP. However, BP will still respond appropriately even if the student selects the wrong size cuff.

Cardiopulmonary Resuscitation Trainers

Many cardiopulmonary resuscitation (CPR) trainers have been developed to practice the skills of effective CPR by providing immediate feedback in various ways. These PTTs are widely used in both basic life support (BLS) and advanced life support (ALS) courses around the world (Figs. 10.21, 10.22, and 10.23). Some trainers have built in real-time and

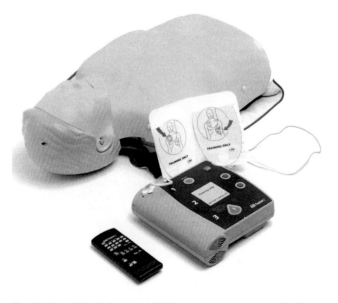

Fig. 10.22 AED Little Anne. AED Automated external defibrillator (Image courtesy of Laerdal Medical [23])

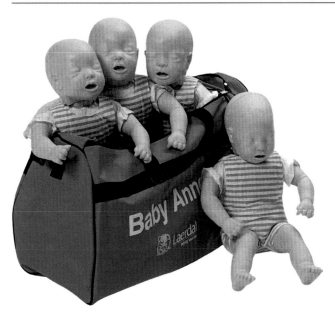

Fig. 10.23 Baby Anne CPR. CPR cardiopulmonary resuscitation (Image courtesy of Laerdal Medical [23])

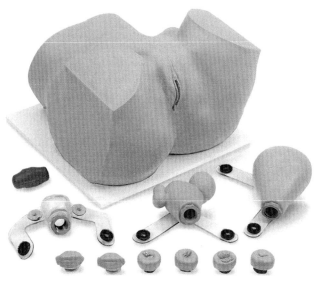

Fig. 10.24 Sim Gynnie. (Photo courtesy of NASCO [25])

summative feedback on the quality of CPR (depth and rate), which has been shown to improve acquisition and retention of CPR skills. When purchasing CPR trainers, educators should verify that trainers are manufactured to allow compressions to be provided to guideline-specific standards (i.e., does the trainer allow for compression of the chest to >5 cm for a child). Training on a mannequin that is not designed with guidelines in mind may have deleterious effects on skill acquisition. In addition, using CPR training in the form of rolling refreshers, a portable mannequin/defibrillator system with chest compression sensor providing automated corrective feedback to optimize CPR skills, demonstrated benefit for improving skill acquisition and performance of CPR in simulated (and real) cardiac arrests. Indeed, more frequent refreshers resulted in significantly shorter times to achieve proficient CPR skills [49].

Adolescent Gynecology Task Trainers

Lifelike female pelvis task trainers are available for developing diagnostic skills in gynecological procedures and anatomical instruction (Fig. 10.24). These trainers permit learners to practice abdominal palpation, bimanual and rectovaginal examination, and speculum insertion and removal. Certain models also provide practice for intrauterine device (IUD) insertion and removal, including uterine sounding. Elements of realism include viewing cervical normality and abnormality as well as normal and abnormal uteri. Fundus Skills and Assessment Task Trainer features the normal anatomy of the status-post or postpartum female abdomen designed for training fundus assessment and fundus skills. These trainers include female pelvis w/upper thighs, a firm

and boggy fundus, as well as simulated blood. Physical realism is highlighted by upper thighs articulating for positioning and realistic landmarks of the symphysis pubis as well as interchangeable uteri, either firm and well contracted or boggy.

Ear and Eye Exam Models

Innovative eye PTTs have been designed for fundoscopic examination using an ophthalmoscope. Various scenarios can be set up for trainees using combinations of pathology slides, as well as difference in both the retinal depth and pupil diameter. Soft and supple material allows hands-on simulation of real examination procedures, such as raising the eyelid to achieve better visualization of the eye (Fig. 10.25). PTTs are also available for direct examination of the tympanic membrane with an otoscope. The ear trainers also allow practice of the technique of foreign body removal (Fig. 10.26).

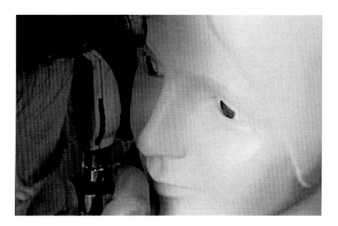

Fig. 10.25 Ophthalmologic Exam Trainer. (Photo courtesy of Kyoto Kagaku Co. Ltd. [50])

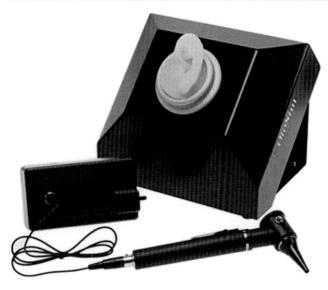

Fig. 10.26 OtoSim Otoscopy Trainer—OtoSim™. (Photo courtesy of Otosim [51])

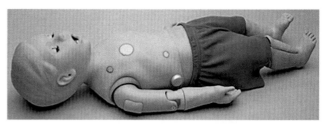

Fig. 10.28 Toddler Gaumard mannequin. (Photo courtesy of Gaumard Scientific [2])

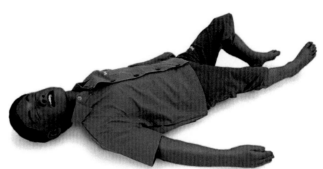

Fig. 10.29 SimJunior mannequin. (Image courtesy of Laerdal Medical [1])

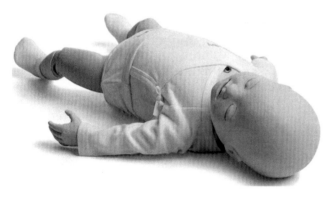

Fig. 10.27 Infant Laerdal mannequin. (Image courtesy of Laerdal Medical [1])

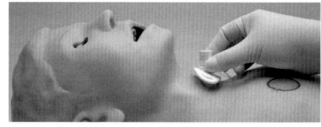

Fig. 10.30 Pediatric Gaumard mannequin. (Photo courtesy of Gaumard Scientific [2])

Whole Body Simulators

A variety of whole body pediatric simulator models are currently present in health care. This section will be devoted to discussing the frequently used models and their various features and capabilities. See figures for examples of the Infant Laerdal (Fig. 10.27), Toddler Gaumard (Fig. 10.28), Laerdal SimJunior (Fig. 10.29), Pediatric Gaumard (Fig. 10.30), and Pediatric CAE (Fig. 10.31) mannequins.

Features

In the following tables, the features of each commercially available pediatric simulator are divided into various categories: airway (Table 10.1), breathing (Table 10.2), circulation (Table 10.3), central nervous system (Table 10.4), gastrointestinal (Table 10.5), procedures (Table 10.6), and miscellaneous/equipment sizing (Table 10.7). The tables were generated from data extrapolated from product catalogues from

Fig. 10.31 Pediatric CAE mannequin. (Photo courtesy of CAE Healthcare)

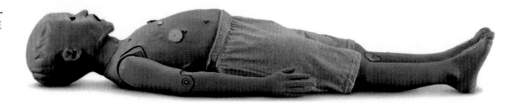

Table 10.1 Airway

Sim model	Gaumard	Gaumard	Gaumard	Gaumard	Gaumard	Laerdal	Laerdal	Laerdal	Laerdal	CAE/Meti
	Adult HAL®3201	Child Pediatric HAL® S3005	Toddler Pediatric HAL® S3004	Newborn	Premie	SimBaby	SimNewB	SimJunior	SimMan	Ped
Age	Adult	5 year	1 year	Newborn	Prem			6 year		6 year
Speech	Prerecord manual	Prerecord manual	Prerecord manual	Crying	Crying sync with breathing	Cry cough hiccup			Prerecord manual	Prerecord manual
Upper airway sounds	✓	✓	✓	✓	✓					
Trismus									✓	
Airway obstruction	✓ (pharyngeal swelling)	✓	✓			✓	✓		✓	✓
Laryngospasm	✓					✓			✓	✓
Airway resistance						✓				
Airway insertion				✓	✓	✓	✓	✓	✓	
Oral intubation	✓	✓	✓	✓	✓	✓	✓	✓	✓	✓
Nasal intubation	✓	✓	✓	✓	✓	✓	✓	✓	✓	✓
Intubation depth detection	✓	✓	✓	✓						
Tongue edema	✓	✓	✓			✓		✓	✓	✓
Head tilt/chin lift			✓	✓		✓			✓	
Jaw thrust				✓					✓	
Sellick maneuver			✓	✓		✓	✓	✓	✓	

Table 10.2 Breathing

Sim model	Gaumard Adult HAL®3201	Gaumard Child Pediatric HAL® S3005	Gaumard Toddler Pediatric HAL® S3004	Gaumard Newborn	Gaumard Premie	Laerdal SimBaby	Laerdal SimNewB	Laerdal SimJunior	Laerdal SimMan	CAE/Meti Ped
Spontaneous breathing	✓		✓	✓		✓				✓
Chest rise	✓	✓	✓	✓	✓		✓	✓		
Cyanosis central	✓	✓	✓	✓	✓	✓	✓		✓	
Cyanosis peripheral										
O₂ sat probe	✓								Hand	✓
CO₂ exhalation	✓					✓	✓		✓	✓
Unilateral breath sounds	✓	✓	✓	✓	✓	✓	✓	✓		✓
Unilateral chest rise		✓	✓	✓		✓				✓
R mainstem intubation	✓	✓	✓				✓		✓	✓
Different breath sounds	✓	✓	✓	✓	✓	✓	✓	✓	✓	✓
Bronchial obstruction										✓
Lung compliance	✓	Only get chest rise with 20 cm H₂O	Only get chest rise with 20 cm H₂O			✓			✓	✓
Thorax compliance										
Chest rise with appropriate ventilation		✓	✓							
Insp/exp ratio			✓	✓						✓
Seesaw resp						✓				✓
Retractions						✓				
Bag mask ventilation	✓	✓	✓	✓	✓					✓
Ventilation through LMA	✓	✓	✓	✓						
Ventilation through ETT	✓	✓	✓	✓	✓					✓
Attach to real ventilator	✓								✓	
Trans tracheal jet ventilation									✓	
Limitation		Abnormal breath sounds disappear at high RR / Need to bring RR = 0 to allow assisted ventilation								

R mainstem intubation right mainstem intubation, *Insp/exp ratio* inspiration/expiration ratio, *Seesaw resp* seesaw respiration, *LMA* laryngeal mask airway, *ETT* endotracheal tube, *RR* respiratory rate

Table 10.3 Circulation

Sim model	Gaumard	Gaumard	Gaumard	Gaumard	Gaumard	Laerdal	Laerdal	Laerdal	Laerdal	CAE/Meti
	Adult HAL®3201	Child Pediatric HAL® S3005	Toddler Pediatric HAL® S3004	Newborn	Premie	SimBaby	SimNewB	SimJunior	SimMan	Ped
Carotid pulse (mmHg where absent)		Bilat	Bilat					✓	✓	✓ (60)
Brachial pulse		Bilat	Bilat	Bilat	Bilat	L	R	✓	L	✓ (70)
Absent pulse one side			✓	✓						
Radial pulse		Bilat	Bilat			L			L	✓ (90)
Femoral pulse			Bilat		Bilat	Bilat			Bilat	✓ (80)
Pedal									✓	✓ (80)
Popliteal										✓
Fontanel pulse				✓	✓					
Umbilical artery pulse				✓	✓		✓			
Arterial blood temp										✓
CVP										✓
Pulses sync to ECG			✓	✓	✓	✓				✓
Heart sound variety	✓	✓	✓	✓	✓	✓	✓	✓	✓	✓
Heart sounds sync to ECG		✓	✓	✓	✓	✓	✓	✓	✓	✓
ECG generated to real time			✓	✓						
BP measurements (palp/ausc)	✓ left arm	✓	✓			✓	✓	✓	✓	✓
Korotkoff sounds	✓	✓	✓	✓		✓	✓	✓	✓	
Chest wall recoil with CPR	✓		✓							
CPR generates palpable pulses						✓				✓
CPR generate palpable BP wave form and ECG artifacts	✓		✓	✓						✓
Defibrillation	✓	✓	✓			✓		✓	✓	✓
Auto conversion ECG with defibrillation								✓	✓	✓
Pacing		✓	Anterior			✓		✓	✓	✓
Arterial waveform change										✓
Limitation		Not enough depth for adequate CPR	No fluctuation for the art line							

CVP *central venous pressure*, ECG *electrocardiogram*, BP *blood pressure*, CPR *cardiopulmonary resuscitation*

Table 10.4 Central nervous system

Sim model	Gaumard Adult HAL®3201	Gaumard Child Pediatric HAL® S3005	Gaumard Toddler Pediatric HAL® S3004	Gaumard Newborn	Gaumard Premie	Laerdal SimBaby	Laerdal SimNewB	Laerdal SimJunior	Laerdal SimMan	CAE/Meti Ped
Fontanel										
Eyes open/close	✓	✓	✓			✓			✓	Close if $O_2 < 75$ Spontaneous min vent < 1500 ml
Blink rate	✓	✓	✓						✓	✓
Pupil response	✓	✓	✓			Interchange			✓	Manual
Seizure	✓	✓	✓	✓		✓	✓	✓	✓	
Muscle tone—active, reduce, limp				Unifocal Arms only		Spasm				
Cardio response to symp/parasymp										
Limitation		For seizure, need to stay supine								
Limitation		Stop breathing when having seizure								

Table 10.5 Gastrointestinal

Sim model	Gaumard Adult HAL®3201	Gaumard Child Pediatric HAL® S3005	Gaumard Toddler Pediatric HAL® S3004	Gaumard Newborn	Gaumard Premie	Laerdal SimBaby	Laerdal SimNewB	Laerdal SimJunior	Laerdal SimMan	CAE/Meti Ped
Bowel sounds	✓	✓		✓				✓	✓	✓
Stomach ausc								✓	✓	
Esophageal intubation								✓	✓	✓
Stomach decompression						✓		✓	✓	
Gastric distension	✓	✓	✓			✓				✓
Enema		✓								
Abdominal thrust									✓	

ausc *ausculation*

Table 10.6 Procedures

Sim model	Gaumard Adult HAL®3201	Gaumard Child Pediatric HAL® S3005	Gaumard Toddler Pediatric HAL® S3004	Gaumard Newborn	Gaumard Premie	Laerdal SimBaby	Laerdal SimNewB	Laerdal SimJunior	Laerdal SimMan	CAE/Meti Ped
IV insertion	Arms	Arms	Arms	Arms	Dorsum hands / Left foot	Ante fossa / Dorsum hand / Long saph		Ante fossa / Dorsum hand / Median, basilic and cephalic vein	✓	Right jug / Right arm
Umbilical catheterization				✓	✓					
IM	Deltoid/quads	Deltoid/quads	Deltoid/quads	✓					✓	
Subcutaneous			✓	✓						
IO	Tibia	Tibia	Tibia	Tibia	Tibia	Tibia		Medial and lateral malleolus	Tibia / Sternum	Right tibia
Pulmonary artery cath										
NG		✓	✓	✓		✓	✓	✓	✓	✓
G-tube						✓				
Suction			✓			✓	✓	✓		
Foley	✓	10F	8F	✓	✓				✓	
Temperature				✓	✓				✓	✓
Tracheotomy	✓	✓	Too much space	✓		✓			✓	✓
Crichothyrotomy	✓	✓							✓	✓
Needle decompression	✓					✓	✓		✓	Bilat
Chest tube insertion						L mid-axillary			L mid-axillary	Bilat
MEC aspiration							✓			

IO *intraosseous*, NG *nasogastric*, IM *intramuscular*, G-tube *gastrostomy tube*, MEC aspiration *meconium aspiration*

Table 10.7 Miscellaneous/equipment sizing

Sim model	Gaumard Adult HAL®3201	Gaumard Child PediatricHAL® S3005	Gaumard Toddler PediatricHAL® S3004	Gaumard Newborn	Gaumard Premie	Laerdal SimBaby	Laerdal SimNewB	Laerdal SimJunior	Laerdal SimMan	CAE/Meti Ped
Secretions										✓
Bleeding									✓	
EQUIPMENT	Adult	Child	Toddler	Newborn	Premie	SimBaby	SimNewB	SimJunior	SimMan	Ped
Laryngoscope	Miller 4, mac 3.5	Miller 2, mac 3	Miller 1	Miller 0	Miller 0	Miller 1				
ETT size	7–7.5	5.5.5	3.5	3	2.5	3.5			7.5–8	
NTT size	8			3		3			7–7.5	
Foley size				6F		n.a			16F	10F
Nasal trumpet size										
OPA				0.5		2				
LMA	4	2–2.5	1.5–2	1–1.5	1	1			4	
NG		10F	10F	8F	8F	8F				
MOBILITY (wireless)	✓	✓	✓	✓	✓				✓	✓
Battery life (h)	4	3	3	4	2					
Wireless range (m)	300	300	300	300	300					
Extra AC adaptor			✓	✓	✓					

ETT endotracheal tube, *NTT* nasotracheal tube, *OPA* oropharyngeal airway, *LMA* laryngeal mask airway, *NG* nasogastric the various manufacturer [14, 22, 23]. These tables should aid in both acquisition of the appropriate mannequin(s) for a simulation program, as well as aid individual educators at choosing the optimal simulator to fit the scenario being developed.

Limitations

It is equally important to understand the limitations of the various simulators being used. Some limitations are currently present in all whole body mannequins, such as a marker of capillary refill time and changes to the color or temperature of the skin of the mannequin, both which are considered essential in the rapid assessment of an acutely ill pediatric patient. Based on these limitations, the most significant overall limitation to whole body mannequin use is the inability of the mannequins to provide an accurate instantaneous assessment of whether a child is *sick* or *not sick* (vital sign changes alone are often a late manifestation of abnormal physiology). Facilitators must do their best to provide a mixture of mannequin and verbal or other visual clues (pictures and videos) in order to overcome this very real limitation, until the fidelity of the current generation of mannequins is improved to better simulate these clinical features.

Furthermore, in order to optimize the learners' preparedness for the simulation experience, it is also imperative to prebrief the mannequins' limitations, and how these will be overcome, prior to running the scenario.

Programming Principles

The foundation for simulation programming are the objectives of the simulation itself: research, teaching, or assessment, the intended learning outcomes, and the learners' level of training. Simulation scenarios developed for research or summative assessment must be programmed to progress and respond to actions taken by participants in a tightly standardized fashion every time they are used [52]. These simulations must therefore be pre-programmed so that vitals and triggers/findings are presented in the same time sequence and the same time intervals. Programmers must also try to anticipate all possible actions that can be taken by participants and the appropriate simulator responses to these actions when pre-programming. These simulation scenarios should be pilot-tested to ensure the proper fidelity has been chosen, the feasibility of the scenario is appropriate, and the standardized scenario is consistent before use [53].

Simulation scenarios developed for teaching or formative evaluation can allow for some variability in how they progress depending on the performance and responses of the learners. This flexibility allows for the facilitator/teacher to allow participants to follow an unintended path, if this presents a teaching opportunity. Similarly, flexibility in programming allows the facilitator to manipulate complexity depending on the skill set of the learners [54]. When programming simulation scenarios, the primary goal is to aim for clinical authenticity. Scenario progress and changes to vital signs in response to actions taken by participants should all follow a time course that is realistic [54].

Autonomous simulators and manual simulators are both currently available and have their own unique advantages and disadvantages. Autonomous simulators use an adult physiology platform that require pre-programming and may be more difficult to run on the fly [54]. The programming inherent in the simulators themselves are a predefined physiologic algorithm where each change or trend in a vital sign or action leads to a cascading change in all vital signs and the mannequin itself [10]. For example, the programmer does not necessarily need to program the time over which heart rate, respiratory rate, and BP change following a fluid bolus, unless they want to slow down the change in vitals to augment learning for novice participants. Another concrete example would be the use of neuromuscular blockade. If this one action is chosen, the mannequin platform understands that this one action means the simulator must stop breathing, display a respiratory rate of zero, start lowering oxygen saturation levels, close the mannequin's eyes and have the mannequin stop chest rise/fall and breathing sounds, all of which are done automatically with the choice of neuromuscular blockade. Although the benefits of this may be more realistic, it may also take the simulation irreversibly off-course. Additionally, the current autonomous platforms do not allow for common pediatric physiology to be represented, including hypoxemia, cyanosis, and tachycardia without entering a so-called *death-spiral*, whereby the mannequin irreversibly deteriorates to the point of cardiac arrest or at minimum requiring the programmer to incorporate complicated work modifications to save the scenario.

Manual simulators, on the other hand, follow programming absolutely. Once the programmer makes a change to the mannequin platform, the change is absolute. As such, the programmer must understand how patients behave in the real world in order to incorporate transition times for vital signs and clinical findings. For example, the hemodynamic response to a fluid bolus should occur over the five or so minutes it would take to administer that bolus, and therefore in order to maintain realism the heart rate, BP, and respiratory rate would not change instantaneously and would follow different time courses. This does not happen automatically on a manual simulator and needs to be played out in real time [23]. In the example of neuromuscular blockade given above, each of the individual features of neuromuscular blockade would have to be chosen individually on the fly or pre-programmed to be packaged into one option that a programmer could use while the scenario is taking place. In general, most simulation facilitators prefer manual simulators because the basic platforms are straightforward and easier to run on the fly, although facilitators with clinical backgrounds must be present to ensure clinical authenticity [1].

Understanding the specific features of the simulator being used is important for three reasons: (1) It allows the facilitator to provide missing cues to participants if the simulator is leading them down the wrong diagnostic path, (2) adds to the authenticity of the experience by filling in the missing gaps that the simulator cannot simulate, and (3) anticipates how the lack of authenticity can be overcome/minimized (including a review of simulator capabilities when pre-briefing the participants to the mannequin and the environment). Other features that can be incorporated to improve the realism of the simulation and trigger learners to respond include vocalizations (high-pitched cry, microphone through which patient can talk), pupillary size, blink control, seizures, and anterior fontanel, differential in upper versus lower limb pulses, among many others (refer to Tables 13.1–13.7; [54]). A concrete example of the interplay of all these features is the irritable child, where irritability is an important sign for possible neurologic as well as cardiac pathology. The fontanel is examined on all neonates to determine volume status as well as possible intracranial pathology. Incorporating vocalization (high-pitched cry) can also provide cues to the learner. An irritable child in supraventricular tachycardia (SVT) who suddenly stops crying may be a cue that stable SVT has suddenly become unstable SVT. Similarly, a blinking child who stops blinking and closes its eyes is a cue to a change in the level of consciousness or a potential change to the cardiac output. Some simulators can be programmed for seizure activity. However, simulators that do not have seizures as a feature can also mimic the other physiologic features of seizures, such as enlarged pupils and associated vital sign changes. So, understanding the diverse features of each simulator, as well as their limitations and how to overcome them, are essential to anyone programming or facilitating a simulation session.

Conclusions

Mannequin-based simulators have evolved significantly since their first conception in the 1960s. Today, a wide variety of specialized pediatric and adult models exist, in the form of full-body autonomous and manual simulators, as well as partial task trainers. Educators now have the capacity to optimize their learners' experiences by creating and programming realistic clinical scenarios by modifying the inputs to both the mannequins and task trainers, as well as the immersive physical environment. Mannequin-based simulators have become a very important tool for the education,

training, and evaluation of healthcare professionals, providing unique opportunities in a wide variety of settings. They have also become integral to research involving simulation-based education. As computer hardware and software technology continues to progress, along with advances in mannequin design, future simulators are likely to offer even more lifelike characteristics and realistic patient responses, which will enhance the simulated experiences for educators and researchers, as well as for participants of all levels.

References

1. Epps C, White ML, Tofil N. Manikin based simulators. In: Levine AI, DeMaria S Jr, Schwartz AD, Sim AJ, editors. The comprehensive textbook of healthcare simulation. 1st ed. New York: Springer; 2013. p. 721.
2. Dieckmann P, Gaba D, Rall M. Deepening the theoretical foundations of patient simulation as social practice. Simul Healthc. 2007;2(3):183–93.
3. Donoghue AJ, Durbin DR, Nadel FM, Stryjewski GR, Kost SI, Nadkarni VM. Effect of high-fidelity simulation on pediatric advanced life support training in pediatric house staff: a randomized trial. Pediatr Emerg Care. 2009;25(3):139–44.
4. Fraser K, Wright B, Girard L, Tworek J, Paget M, Welikovich L, et al. Simulation training improves diagnostic performance on a real patient with similar clinical findings. Chest. 2011;139(2):376–81.
5. Knudson MM, Khaw L, Bullard MK, Dicker R, Cohen MJ, Staudenmayer K, et al. Trauma training in simulation: translating skills from SIM time to real time. J Trauma. 2008;64(2):255–63. (discussion 63–4).
6. Hoadley TA. Learning advanced cardiac life support: a comparison study of the effects of low- and high-fidelity simulation. Nurs Educ Perspect. 2009;30(2):91–5.
7. Campbell DM, Barozzino T, Farrugia M, Sgro M. High-fidelity simulation in neonatal resuscitation. Paediatr Child Health. 2009;14(1):19–23.
8. Rehmann A, Mitman R, Reynolds M. A handbook of flight simulation fidelity requirements for human factors research. In: Crew System Ergonomics Information Analysis Center (CSERIAC) 2255 H Street B, Wright-Patterson AFB O-, editors.: Crew System Ergonomics Information Analysis Center (CSERIAC). Wright-Patterson; 1995. p. 46.
9. Gaba DM. The future vision of simulation in healthcare. Simul Healthc. 2007;2(2):126–35.
10. Healthcare H. CAE healthcare. 2013. http://www.caehealthcare.com. Accessed 3 Nov 2014.
11. DeLucia P. Definitions of human factors and ergonomics. 2014. http://www.hfes.org/web/educationalresources/hfedefinitions-main.html. Accessed 26 Oct 2014.
12. Hamstra SJ, Brydges R, Hatala R, Zendejas B, Cook DA. Reconsidering fidelity in simulation-based training. Acad Med. 2014;89(3):387–92.
13. Cooper JB, Taqueti VR. A brief history of the development of mannequin simulators for clinical education and training. Postgrad Med J. 2008;84(997):563–70.
14. Ota FS, Yee LL, Garcia FJ, Grisham JE, Yamamoto LG, Which IO. model best simulates the real thing? Pediatr Emerg Care. 2003;19(6):393–6.
15. Kessler DO, Auerbach M, Pusic M, Tunik MG, Foltin JC. A randomized trial of simulation-based deliberate practice for infant lumbar puncture skills. Simul Healthc. 2011;6(4):197–203.

16. Ellis C, Hughes G. Use of human patient simulation to teach emergency medicine trainees advanced airway skills. J Accid Emerg Med. 1999;16(6):395–9.

17. Owen H, Plummer JL. Improving learning of a clinical skill: the first year's experience of teaching endotracheal intubation in a clinical simulation facility. Med Educ. 2002;36(7):635–42.

18. Nishisaki A, Scrattish L, Boulet J, Kalsi M, Maltese M, Castner T, et al. Advances in patient safety effect of recent refresher training on in situ simulated pediatric tracheal intubation psychomotor skill performance. In: Henriksen K, Battles JB, Keyes MA, Grady ML, editors. Advances in patient safety: new directions and alternative approaches (Vol 3: performance and tools). Rockville: Agency for Healthcare Research and Quality (US); 2008.

19. Advances in Patient Safety. New directions and alternative approaches (Vol. 4: Technology and Medication Safety). Rockville (MD). 2008. http://www.ncbi.nlm.nih.gov/books/NBK43770/.

20. Nishisaki A, Nadkarni V, Berg R. Intensive care medicine annual update 2009. In: Vincent J, editor. Pediatric advanced airway management training for non-anesthesia residents. New York: Springer; 2009. p. 322–31.

21. Plummer JL, Owen H. Learning endotracheal intubation in a clinical skills learning center: a quantitative study. Anesth Analg. 2001;93(3):656–62.

22. Parry K, Owen H. Small simulators for teaching procedural skills in a difficult airway algorithm. Anaesth Intensive Care. 2004;32(3):401–9.

23. ® LM. Laerdal internet. 2014. http://www.laerdal.com/ca. Accessed 23 Sept 2014.

24. ® Simulaids. 2014. http://www.simulaids.com. [updated 2014]

25. Nasco. Nasco [Internet]. Internet. 2014. http://www.enasco.com. [updated 2014; cited 2014]

26. Bowyer MW, Manahl M, Acosta E, Stutzmen J, Liu A. Far forward feasibility: testing a cricothyroidotmy simulator in Iraq. Stud Health Technol Inform. 2008;132:37–41.

27. Gaies MG, Morris SA, Hafler JP, Graham DA, Capraro AJ, Zhou J, et al. Reforming procedural skills training for pediatric residents: a randomized, interventional trial. Pediatrics. 2009;124(2):610–9.

28. Britt RC, Novosel TJ, Britt LD, Sullivan M. The impact of central line simulation before the ICU experience. Am J Surg. 2009;197(4):533–6.

29. Macnab AJ, Macnab M. Teaching pediatric procedures: the Vancouver model for instructing Seldinger's technique of central venous access via the femoral vein. Pediatrics. 1999;103(1):E8.

30. Velmahos GC, Toutouzas KG, Sillin LF, Chan L, Clark RE, Theodorou D, et al. Cognitive task analysis for teaching technical skills in an inanimate surgical skills laboratory. Am J Surg. 2004;187(1):114–9.

31. Barsuk JH, Cohen ER, Potts S, Demo H, Gupta S, Feinglass J, et al. Dissemination of a simulation-based mastery learning intervention reduces central line-associated bloodstream infections. BMJ Qual Saf. 2014;23(9):749–56.

32. Simulab. Simulab corporation Internet. 2014. http://www.simulab.com. [cited 2014]

33. Oriot D, Darrieux E, Boureau-Voultoury A, Ragot S, Scepi M. Validation of a performance assessment scale for simulated intraosseous access. Simul Healthc. 2012;7(3):171–5.

34. Shefrin AE, Khazei A, Hung GR, Odendal LT, Cheng A. The TACTIC: development and validation of the tool for assessing chest tube insertion competency. CJEM. 2014;16(0):32–9.

35. Al-Qadhi SA, Pirie JR, Constas N, Corrin MS, Ali M. An innovative pediatric chest tube insertion task trainer simulation: a technical report and pilot study. Simul Healthc. 2014;9(5):319–24.

36. Auerbach M, Chang TP, Reid J, Quinones C, Krantz A, Pratt A, et al. Are pediatric interns prepared to perform infant lumbar punctures? A multi-institutional descriptive study. Pediatr Emerg Care. 2013;29(4):453–7.

37. White ML, Jones R, Zinkan L, Tofil NM. Transfer of simulated lumbar puncture training to the clinical setting. Pediatr Emerg Care. 2012;28(10):1009–12.

38. Iyer MS, Santen SA, Nypaver M, Warrier K, Bradin S, Chapman R, et al. Assessing the validity evidence of an objective structured assessment tool of technical skills for neonatal lumbar punctures. Acad Emerg Med. 2013;20(3):321–4.

39. Things LA. Limbs and things Canada Internet. 2014. http://www.limbsandthings.com/ca/home. [cited 2014 Sept 24]

40. Bridges M, Diamond DL. The financial impact of teaching surgical residents in the operating room. Am J Surg. 1999;177(1):28–32.

41. Naylor RA, Hollett LA, Castellvi A, Valentine RJ, Scott DJ. Preparing medical students to enter surgery residencies. Am J Surg. 2010;199(1):105–9.

42. Parent RJ, Plerhoples TA, Long EE, Zimmer DM, Teshome M, Mohr CJ, et al. Early, intermediate, and late effects of a surgical skills "boot camp" on an objective structured assessment of technical skills: a randomized controlled study. J Am Coll Surg. 2010;210(6):984–9.

43. Gershuni V, Woodhouse J, Brunt LM. Retention of suturing and knot-tying skills in senior medical students after proficiency-based training: results of a prospective, randomized trial. Surgery. 2013;154(4):823–9. (discussion 9–30).

44. Fernandez GL, Page DW, Coe NP, Lee PC, Patterson LA, Skylizard L, et al. Boot cAMP: educational outcomes after 4 successive years of preparatory simulation-based training at onset of internship. J Surg Educ. 2012;69(2):242–8.

45. Sturm LP, Windsor JA, Cosman PH, Cregan P, Hewett PJ, Maddern GJ. A systematic review of skills transfer after surgical simulation training. Ann Surg. 2008;248(2):166–79.

46. Dawe SR, Pena GN, Windsor JA, Broeders JA, Cregan PC, Hewett PJ, et al. Systematic review of skills transfer after surgical simulation-based training. Br J Surg. 2014;101(9):1063–76.

47. Nagendran M, Toon CD, Davidson BR, Gurusamy KS. Laparoscopic surgical box model training for surgical trainees with no prior laparoscopic experience. Cochrane Database Syst Rev. 2014;1:Cd010479.

48. Nagendran M, Gurusamy KS, Aggarwal R, Loizidou M, Davidson BR. Virtual reality training for surgical trainees in laparoscopic surgery. Cochrane Database Syst Rev. 2013;8:Cd006575.

49. Niles D, Sutton RM, Donoghue A, Kalsi MS, Roberts K, Boyle L, et al. "Rolling Refreshers": a novel approach to maintain CPR psychomotor skill competence. Resuscitation. 2009;80(8):909–12.

50. Kagaku K. Kyoto Kagaku Co, Ltd. 2014. http://www.kyotokagaku.com. [updated 2012].

51. OtoSim. OtoSim better ear and eye training internet. 2014. http://www.otosim.com. [updated 2014; cited 2014].

52. Downing S, Yudkowsky R. Assessment in health professions education. New York: Routledge; 2009. (Downing S, Yudkowsky R. editors)

53. Issenberg SB, Scalese RJ. Simulation in health care education. Perspect Biol Med. 2008;51(1):31–46.

54. Forrest K, McKimm J, Edgar S. Essential simulation in clinical education. West Sussex: Wiley-Blackwell; 2013.

Task and Procedural Skills Training

Marjorie Lee White, Anne Ades, Allan Evan Shefrin and Susanne Kost

Simulation Pearls

1. Task trainers are available commercially for most major pediatric procedures
2. Multiple recipes for homemade task trainers are available
3. Curricular development is an important component for pediatric procedural skills training
4. Simulation enables the learner to practice potentially life-saving but rarely performed emergency procedures

Introduction

Procedures are a fundamental part of healthcare delivery. Learning procedures on task trainers has been a practice for centuries. Task trainers are devices that replicate a portion of a complete process or system [1]. They may take many forms, ranging from foods (e.g., using oranges to practice injection techniques or pig's feet to practice suturing) to more developed plastic molds, which allow for repetitive

M. L. White (✉)
Department of Pediatrics, Office of Interprofessional Simulation, Pediatric Simulation Center, University of Alabama at Birmingham, Children's of Alabama, Birmingham, AL, USA
e-mail: mlwhite@peds.uab.edu

A. Ades
Department of Pediatrics, Perelman School of Medicine, University of Pennsylvania, Philadelphia, PA, USA
e-mail: ades@email.chop.edu

Department of Pediatrics, Neonatology Division, The Children's Hospital of Philadelphia, Philadelphia, PA, USA

A. E. Shefrin
Department of Pediatrics, Division of Pediatric Emergency Medicine, University of Ottawa, Children's Hospital of Eastern Ontario, Ottawa, ON, Canada
e-mail: ashefrin@cheo.on.ca

S. Kost
Department of Pediatrics, Sidney Kimmel Medical College, Thomas Jefferson University, Philadelphia, PA, USA
e-mail: skost@nemours.org

use. In addition, virtual reality trainers are now being developed and used with increasing frequency and effectiveness. In pediatrics, there are added challenges for development of procedural competency, which include the limited opportunities in clinical practice and the technical complexity inherent in the variability of patient size and physiology. As such, learning procedures on a partial task trainer, particularly those that are uncommon and high risk, is a preferred learning modality.

The use of simulation for psychomotor skills acquisition has received significant attention in the literature [2, 3]. Its use is advocated by major medical accrediting bodies including the Accreditation Council for Graduate Medical Education (ACGME) and the Royal College of Physicians and Surgeons of Canada [4, 5]. Table 11.1 lists the specific procedures required of pediatric medical trainees. Several meta-analyses have shown that simulation-based procedural skills training results in improved skill acquisition [6–10].

Review of Procedural Task Trainers

Airway

Successful completion of a procedural task is a function of knowledge, skill, and judgment. The learner requires knowledge and judgment as to when an airway maneuver is necessary and skills practice to perform the action competently and with consistency. Airway task trainers were among the first devices to become available for simulated medical skills training [11]. A variety of devices are currently marketed to assist the learner in understanding the anatomy of the pediatric airway and to facilitate learning and practice of physical airway-related skills. Airway task trainers may comprise partial- or whole-task training and may include both virtual and/or physical components. Live animals (e.g., cats, ferrets) have traditionally served as pediatric airway task trainers, but cost and ethical considerations limit the practicality of

© Springer International Publishing Switzerland 2016
V. J. Grant, A. Cheng (eds.), *Comprehensive Healthcare Simulation: Pediatrics*,
Comprehensive Healthcare Simulation, DOI 10.1007/978-3-319-24187-6_11

Table 11.1 Procedures required by selected accrediting organizations for Pediatric certification

Procedure	ACGME (2012)[a]	Royal College (2008)[b]	Royal College of Pediatrics and Child Health (2014)[c]
Intravenous access/peripheral venous cannulation	Y	Y	Y
Venipuncture	Y		Y
Umbilical venous cannulation	Y	Y	Y
Umbilical arterial cannulation		Y	
Arterial puncture		Y	
Suture of a one layer laceration, simple wound closure	Y	Y	
Cardiopulmonary resuscitation (neonatal and pediatric)	Y	Y	
Chest tube placement and thoracentesis		Y (patient or model)	
Intraosseous insertion	Y (simulated)	Y (patient or model)	
Gastric tube placement (oro or nasogastric)		Y	
Bladder catheterization and/or suprapubic aspiration	Y	Y	
Lumbar puncture		Y	Y
Bag-mask ventilation	Y	Y	Y
Tracheal intubation	Y (neonate)	Y (neonatal and pediatric)	Y (term and preterm 28–34 weeks)
Gastric tube placement		Y	
Giving immunizations	Y		
Incision and drainage of abscesses	Y		
Reduction of a simple dislocation	Y		
Removal of foreign body	Y		
Temporary splinting of a fracture	Y		

[a] ACGME 2013. https://www.acgme.org/acgmeweb/Portals/0/PFAssets/2013-PR-FAQ-PIF/320_pediatrics_07012013.pdf. Accessed 21 Oct 2014
[b] The Royal College of Physicians and Surgeons of Canada
[c] Royal College of Pediatrics and Child Health, Directly Observed Procedures *(DOPS)*. Compulsory procedures listed. http://www.rcpch.ac.uk/system/files/protected/page/DOPS%20Guidance%20June%202014.pdf. Accessed 21 Oct 2014

this approach. The remainder of this section will focus on inert physical airway task trainers.

Airway-related tasks in pediatric medical training generally consist of techniques that enable maintenance of a patent airway and ventilation when anesthesia, illness, or trauma hinder the patient's ability to do so independently. Insertion of airway adjuncts, such as nasopharyngeal and oral pharyngeal airways, and artificial airways, such as laryngeal mask airways and endotracheal tubes, are techniques well suited for skills training on physical task trainers. Some airway task trainers also have simulated lungs that allow the learner to practice ventilation skills, either via a bag-mask device placed directly on the simulated face or via an artificial airway.

The most basic physical airway task trainer consists of a simulated head with a realistic face, nose, and mouth. The simplest models have an externally anatomically correct nose and mouth with a simple opening in the mouth connected to rudimentary simulated lungs that will inflate with appropriate positive-pressure ventilation. The lungs may be as simple as a pair or balloons attached to a simulated trachea, or may be embedded within a whole torso or whole-body mannequin, where ventilation is assessed by chest rise. When provided in a variety of sizes (neonate, infant, child, adolescent), even the most basic airway task trainers allow practice in the selection of an appropriately sized

facial mask, proper technique for holding the mask, and an approximation of ventilation volume required for patients of various sizes.

The next level of airway task trainer increases human physical resemblance with the addition of a patent nasopharynx and an anatomically realistic oropharynx and upper airway, including tongue, epiglottis, larynx with vocal cords, and upper esophagus. Again, a variety of ages and sizes enable instruction in the anatomic differences among these age groups. For example, the neonatal and infant task trainers allow emphasis on the anterior placement of the infant larynx and the smaller caliber of the airway, and the child and adult task trainers include teeth.

In addition to the normal anatomically correct airway models, task trainers have also been designed to allow practice with a more difficult airway. Even in the absence of electronics, some models include features such as a controllable degree of mouth opening, changeable limit of neck flexibility, and an inflatable tongue.

With the addition of high-fidelity electronic components, airway task trainers can mimic functional as well as anatomic features of the airway, and these features may be activated remotely in real time, changing the difficulty of the task. For example, the tongue can be inflated to mimic airway swelling and the vocal cords can be clamped to mimic laryngospasm. Some simulators can produce sounds that mimic stertor or

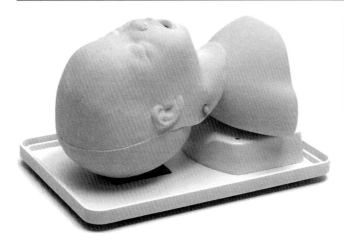

Fig. 11.1 Pediatric airway task trainer. (Image courtesy: Laerdal Medical)

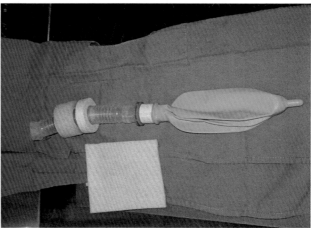

Fig. 11.2 Cricothyrotomy model showing equipment needed. (Photo courtesy: Canadian Medical Education Journal [98])

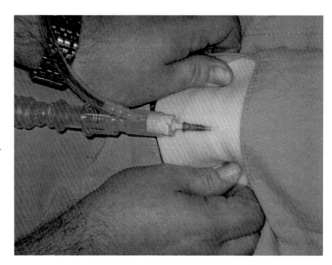

Fig. 11.3 Cricothyrotomy model with cannula. (Photo courtesy: Canadian Medical Education Journal [98])

stridor, suggestive of airway obstruction. High-tech models can also be used for assessment purposes, with sensors that enable the facilitator to assess technique and success of the desired task from a remote location via computer monitor. High-fidelity airway simulators can detect airway repositioning, tracheal versus esophageal placement of an endotracheal tube, adequacy of ventilation, and even pressure on teeth during laryngoscopy.

Advantages of airway task trainers include the ability of learners to practice a skill in a variety of patient sizes and as many times as necessary, all without potentially causing trauma to an actual patient. Depending on the fidelity of the device, airway trainers may also provide valuable feedback to the instructor, without having to look directly over the shoulder of the learner. Direct and indirect (video) laryngoscopy and endotracheal tube placement are difficult skills to master, and studies of groups of new learners have shown that these skills can be mastered well with the aid of airway task trainers (see Fig. 11.1) [11, 12].

However, some of the features of a human airway do not lend themselves well to practice with a rigid, plastic airway task trainer. Mandibular positioning and flexibility with a jaw thrust is not replicated well with most plastic head models or mannequins. Many of the trainers and mannequins have a stiff feel compared to actual tissue. Control of secretions is also an important skill in the management of a pediatric airway, yet simulator technology has not yet reached the point where task trainers or mannequins can produce drool, mucus, or emesis. Clever post-marketing modifications have been described, including gluing a nasal cannula inside out inside the nose of a mannequin head skin, enabling fake mucus to be pumped from an infant nose [13], and recipes for simulated mucus, blood, and emesis are also available [14, 15].

In addition to *standard* techniques for insertion of artificial airways, task trainers can also facilitate surgical airway practice. The simplest of these models involves the creation of a permanent stoma (drilling a hole) into a doll or mannequin with a hollow neck to enable practice of tracheostomy tube replacement. Animal models, commercial head and neck task trainers, and high-fidelity mannequins are available for practicing cricothyrotomy, all enabling study of the speed and efficacy of various devices and techniques as well as retention of skills [16, 17]. In addition, artificial models can be created using easily accessible medical equipment, as well as real models such as pig tracheas can also be used (See Figs. 11.2 and 11.3). Unfortunately, the majority of research on the topic of surgical airways focuses on the adult trauma victim, and the majority of the task trainers therefore also reflect adult anatomy. Porcine tracheas provide a close physical approximation of adult human airway anatomy. Some work is being done with other animal models including rabbits, which more closely approximate the pediatric airway in size. One published study evaluated the efficacy

Fig. 11.4 Virtual intravenous access trainer. (Photo courtesy: Sue Kost)

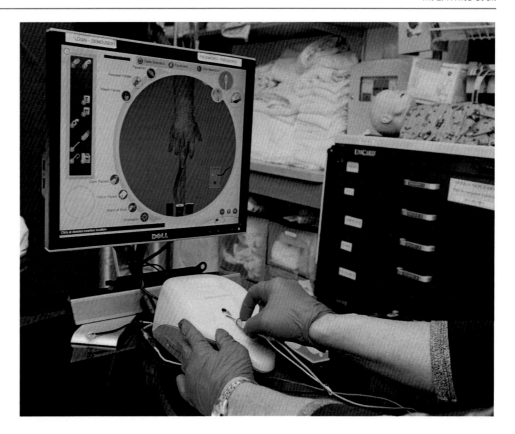

of a commercial device for rapid percutaneous cricothyrotomy in pediatric patients using adult rabbit cadavers [18]. All learners were successful in inserting the device and in providing adequate ventilation, with two of the ten tracheas suffering minor trauma.

Vascular Access

Vascular access is a critically important yet technically difficult skill to master in the pediatric patient. The insertion of a catheter into a blood vessel is again a procedure that lends itself well to practice with a task trainer before engaging in this technique on a real patient. A variety of devices have been developed and implemented to facilitate this practice. These trainers can be divided into three basic categories: computerized models with haptic feedback, animal models with artificial blood vessels embedded within, and simulated plastic limbs with embedded blood vessels. Some of these trainers are geared specifically for practicing peripheral venous access while others for central venous access, with or without the aid of ultrasound guidance. Trainers also exist for practicing more invasive vascular access procedures such as intraosseous access, which typically consists of either animal tissue (e.g., chicken leg) or plastic bone models, with or without overlying simulated soft tissue [19].

The virtual intravenous (IV) access trainer consists of computer software that provides didactic education as well as a stepwise approach to the entire task, from preparation through completion (see Fig. 11.4). Both adult and infant versions are marketed. The software provides feedback to the learner when steps are missed during the practice session. The computer monitor also provides visual feedback, with the ability to vary features such as skin tone, body size, and habitus. The computer is attached to a haptic device with a simulated IV catheter, which allows some level of sensory feedback as to features such as skin compliance, arterial pulse, and vessel depth. Incorrect insertion is met with visual feedback, such as bleeding or bruising visible on the monitor. The virtual trainer has some useful features, including the ability to provide didactic education and skills assessment in the absence of an instructor. The device is expensive, but can be used by many learners without the need to supply tissue or actual IV catheters, and the risk of needle sticks during training is eliminated. However, a realistic sensation of a needle entering tissue and the *pop* of puncturing the vessel are lacking in this device.

Animal tissue models typically consist of the muscle mass and overlying skin, with plastic tubing of various thickness and diameter inserted within the tissue to simulate vessels. The artificial vessels may be cannulated via traditional palpation-based localization or via ultrasound-guided techniques. A chicken tissue model was shown to improve comfort levels in physician trainees learning ultrasound-guided central line placement [20]. The tubing can be filled with simulated blood under pressure to enable a flash in the hub of

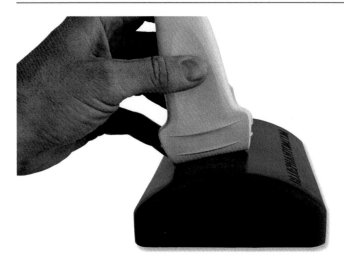

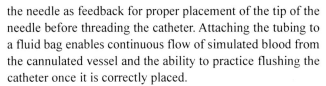

Fig. 11.5 Ultrasound for venous access. (Photo courtesy: CAE Healthcare)

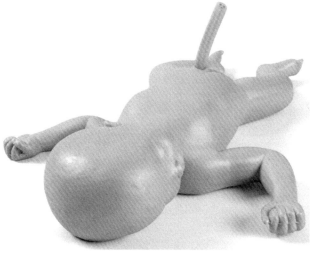

Fig. 11.6 Female newborn infant reproduction designed for the practice of umbilical catheterization. (Image courtesy: Laerdal Medical)

the needle as feedback for proper placement of the tip of the needle before threading the catheter. Attaching the tubing to a fluid bag enables continuous flow of simulated blood from the cannulated vessel and the ability to practice flushing the catheter once it is correctly placed.

Plastic limbs with embedded blood vessels work in a manner similar to the animal tissue models described earlier, without the potential risk of infectious disease transmission and need for cold storage. Drawbacks to the plastic models include the lack of true tissue feel and the retention of permanent holes in the plastic (needle *tracks*) when the same site is punctured repeatedly. Some models have replaceable simulated skin and tubing that alleviates this problem.

Commercial central venous access task trainers include torso models for subclavian, internal jugular, and femoral venous access. Simulation for central venous access training has been shown to be an effective teaching tool in numerous studies over the past decade. Training programs that have embraced vigorous, simulation-based medical education have seen patient and unit-based improvements in clinical care. Outcomes documented include improved success rates in performing procedures by novice learners in the clinical setting and decreased central line infections. The incorporation of ultrasound guidance further improves the success rate of simulated central venous access, with this skill having been shown to translate to improved success in real patients [21–24]. Specific task trainers for teaching ultrasound-guided access *(phantoms)* are readily available (See Fig. 11.5), both commercially and with homemade versions [25].

One final vascular access technique unique to the pediatric setting is that of umbilical vessel catheterization in neonates. Task trainers utilized for practicing this procedure include using actual tissue (e.g., discarded umbilical cords) as well as plastic models. The plastic models are available on their own and as part of whole-body infant mannequins (See

Fig. 11.6). In addition, post-market modifications to commercially available models have been described [26].

Surgical Procedures

Task training in pediatric surgery has focused on laparoscopic surgery skills, trauma procedures, and suturing. Surgical simulators may be in the form of cadaveric or animal models, commercially produced models, or virtual reality computer simulators [27, 28]. The specific skill that is being taught will determine which trainer should be used and the environment best suited for training. Trainers have been developed for circumcision, gastroschisis repair, pyloromyotomy, and thoracoscopic repair of tracheoesophageal fistulas [29–33]. Other procedures for which models exist include models to assist with extracorporeal membrane oxygenation training, endoscopy, and cardiac surgery planning [34–36]. The Society of American Gastrointestinal and Endoscopic Surgeons has developed and validated an adult-sized "fundamentals of laparoscopic surgery" simulator [37]. A pediatric version of this simulator has been developed using smaller components [27]. These simulators teach object transfer, pattern cutting, ligating loops, and suturing using laparoscopic equipment, and have become a mandatory part of surgical training across North America. For further details, please refer to Chap. 22.

Ear, Nose, and Throat Procedures

Children undergo a proportionately higher percentage of procedures on the head and neck than adults, and task trainers have been developed for a variety of these ear, nose, and throat (ENT) procedures. Both commercially available and homemade devices have been described for practicing tasks ranging from simple ENT procedures (e.g., removal of cerumen from the external auditory canal) to the more complex (e.g., cleft palate repair). A comprehensive review of the use of simulators in the field of otolaryngology concluded that dozens of task trainers are available or under development in this field. Nearly 100 peer-reviewed publications were reviewed, demonstrating the burgeoning potential of simulation for teaching and evaluating ENT skills [38]. This section will focus on ENT procedures in children that are typically performed outside of the operating room.

A common ENT problem in the pediatric population is that of insertion of foreign material into an orifice, and the large proportion of foreign bodies ends up being inserted into the ears, nose, and respiratory tract. Foreign body removal is a procedure that is easily practiced with a task trainer. Commercial ear simulators are marketed (with replaceable ears) that enable practice of otoscopy and cerumen removal as well as removal of foreign bodies of various shapes and sizes. Bone wax or beeswax serve as reasonable substitutes for cerumen, and beads and small toys can serve as real examples of foreign bodies. One model provides both auditory and visual feedback when too much pressure is applied to the ear canal or tympanic membrane [39].

Treatment of epistaxis is another common problem amenable to practicing in a simulated environment. Mannequin heads and task trainers can both be modified to mimic epistaxis [40–41]. Commercial devices are available in adult sizes, including one that enables control of the amount and speed of nasal bleeding. These devices enable the learner to practice various packing techniques for the control of hemorrhage [42].

Procedures in the oral cavity can also be simulated; however, there are currently no commercially available pediatric models. Dental procedures can be taught with a virtual reality device that combines graphics on-screen with a haptic device for practicing drilling and implant techniques [43]. A recent publication describes the creation of an inexpensive model of peritonsillar abscess with latex moulage of an oral cavity to enable practice of drainage procedures (see Fig. 11.7) [44]. Existing mannequins and airway task trainers can be modified to allow practice of removal of foreign material from the upper airway.

Cardiovascular and Pulmonary Procedures

Given that the illnesses and conditions requiring cardiovascular and pulmonary procedures in pediatrics are rare, practitioners have limited real-life experience performing these potentially lifesaving procedures, including chest tube insertion and pericardiocentesis [45–47]. A wide variety of task trainers have been developed and used to fill these gaps.

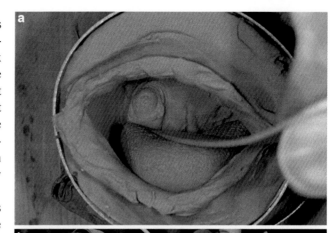
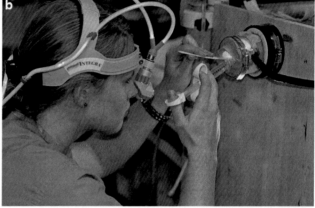

Fig. 11.7 Task trainer for drainage of a peritonsillar abscess. (Reproduced with permission of SAGE publications [44])

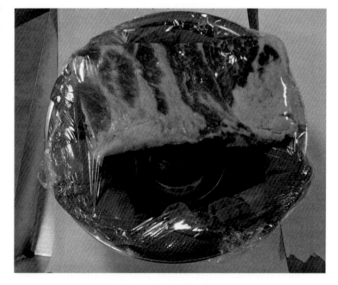

Fig. 11.8 Pork rib model. (Photo courtesy: Allan Shefrin)

Homemade task trainers are generally of lower cost and are simple to construct. A pediatric chest can be simulated using a rack of pork or lamb ribs (see Figs. 11.8 and 11.9) [48]. Animal models best approximate human tissue as the

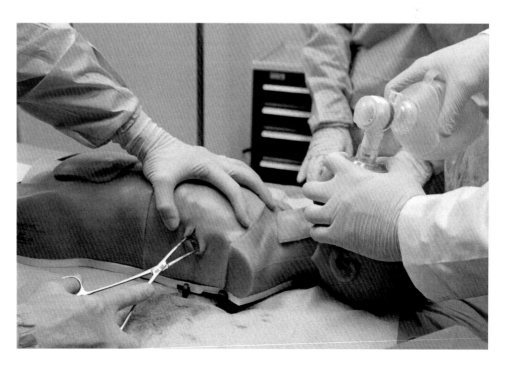

Fig. 11.9 Pork rib model with skin and chest tube. (Photo courtesy: Allan Shefrin)

learner can feel what intercostal muscle feels like in relation to the bony ribs and parietal pleura. The use of animal tissue again involves potential ethical implications as well as requires proper storage, handling, and hygiene. Homemade task trainers are also becoming more widely used in the neonatal setting [49–50].

Commercially available thoracic task trainers come in a variety of configurations. Some offer only a thorax while others are part of an entire upper-body or whole-body mannequin. Some trainers allow connection to drainage tubing so that this part of the procedure may be practiced. These models are considerably more expensive than homemade task trainers, and while progress has been made in making models look and feel more human-like, a gap still remains.

An important consideration is the requirement for replacement parts as there are a limited amount of practice attempts that can be performed on a given model. Most commercially available trainers are adult-sized, although pediatric models are increasingly becoming available. Commercially available trauma simulators are available (see Fig. 11.10). These allow the learner to perform multiple trauma-oriented procedures such as chest tube insertion, pericardiocentesis, and cricothyroidotomy. Some models allow for diagnostic peritoneal lavage, while others can be set up to practice focused assessment with sonography for trauma (FAST).

Finally, commercially available pericardiocentesis models allow the learner to drain red fluid from an anatomic location in the thorax, although no model currently simulates a beating heart or the possible adverse effects of the procedure (e.g., ventricular puncture). Some practitioners prefer to perform pericardiocentesis under ultrasound visualization. Gelatin can be used to create an ultrasoundable model with placement of red dye in a balloon to simulate ultrasound-guided pericardial sac aspiration (see Figs. 11.11 and 11.12) [51]. A similar model can be made out of gel wax with an embedded balloon [52–53].

Neurologic Procedures

Many high-fidelity mannequins incorporate features that enable the learner to practice diagnostic procedures related to neurologic conditions. These features include the ability to reproduce a bulging anterior fontanel in an infant, to alter pupillary size and reactivity, and to mimic seizure activity.

Fig. 11.10 Pediatric surgical simulator "Traumachild". (Photo courtesy: SimuLab Corporation)

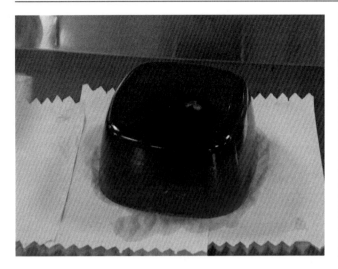

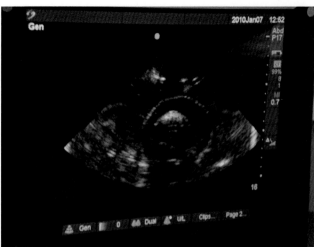

Fig. 11.11 Pericardiocentesis model using low-fidelity mold. (Photo courtesy: Canadian Medical Education Journal [98])

Fig. 11.12 Pericardiocentesis model ultrasound image (Photo courtesy: Canadian Medical Education Journal [98])

Although focal neurologic findings are difficult to replicate with high-fidelity mannequins, simulators have been combined with video clips to aid in the recognition and treatment of stroke, and this approach could likely be applied to other diagnostic challenges in neurology [54].

In terms of invasive neurologic procedures, the most common pediatric procedure performed is that of the lumbar puncture (LP). LP task trainers are available in a variety of sizes, everything from neonate to adult. These devices provide a realistic approximation of the lumbar anatomy for an LP performed in either the lateral recumbent or (in some models) sitting positions. These models typically include internal tubing containing clear fluid simulating cerebral spinal fluid that allows instant feedback in the event of a successful procedure. One model provides negative feedback as well, with an ancillary set of tubing containing simulated blood acting as the epidural venous plexus around the spinal canal resulting in a *bloody tap* if the procedure is performed incorrectly. These models also suffer from repetitive use, as repeated procedures leave multiple puncture marks, which can potentially lead to leaks in the tubing. This is remedied in most models by the replacement of the simulated skin tissue just over the puncture sites as well as the internal tubing (where possible).

Orthopedic Procedures

Task trainers are available to teach normal musculoskeletal anatomy and function. One of the oldest models, the skeleton, is ubiquitous in the training of health professionals. There are a number of commercially available spine and joint task trainers for practicing arthrocentesis; however, there are currently no pediatric models specifically. With the increasing availability of 3D printing, this may be an area where much growth is expected.

Other Procedures

Skin suturing has been traditionally taught by using either animal (e.g., pig skin) or commercially available silicone or rubber models. Soft tissue infections and foreign bodies may be simulated as well. Animal parts with embedded objects may be used. Educators may purchase trainers or make their own out of gelatin [55–56]. As pediatric care providers increase their use of ultrasound in clinical practice, educators have begun to use gelatin to create ultrasound models for various procedures. Table 11.2 provides a set of suggestions for making a gelatin model [57]. Simulation has also been used for teaching nerve blocks [58, 59].

Table 11.2 Recipe for creating homemade gelatin models

1. Gelatin blocks made at a lower temperatures result in a more desirable consistency. Caution should be used with hot water as it can burn gelatin
2. Use a 10 % solution of gelatin (e.g., 100 g of gelatin per 1 L of water)
3. Heat until gelatin is liquid, cool to solidify
4. Use food coloring as gelatin is clear. Consider adding chlorhexidine or EDTA for bacteriostatic properties
5. Layered production process is advised for any kind of inclusions such as cysts, foreign bodies, or vessels
a. Cysts can be simulated using water filled balloons, liquid pills
b. Masses can be simulated with vegetable pieces, pasta, deli meats, or hot dogs
c. Penrose drains can be used to simulate blood vessels
6. Refrigerate the models when not in use to extend their durability, but do not freeze them to avoid cracking
7. Clear adhesive plastic, a strip of gelatin-impregnated gauze, reusable latex coating, or hydrocolloid skin dressings can be used to protect the model, making it more durable
8. Models should be stored in airtight containers when not in use
9. Gelatin blocks can be melted down and recycled

There are many other models available for teaching procedures associated with routine medical care including: care of the tracheostomy and gastrostomy tube, pelvic exams, and bladder catheterization [60–62]. In terms of bladder catheterization, no specific pediatric models are currently available.

Instructional Design for Procedural Skills Training

While having task trainers that can provide a realistic look and feel is one significant factor to augment the transfer of skill acquisition to a real patient, the most significant factor is how the procedure is taught and how it fits within the curriculum it is embedded in. It is critical that the procedural skills curriculum does not simply impart the physical mechanics of a procedure (e.g., how to hold an endotracheal tube, how to advance the catheter, where to put your hand to stabilize the patient, etc.), but equally how to properly select the equipment, how to position and prepare the patient, as well as knowing and anticipating complications from the procedure, among others. Developing a well-designed curriculum is key to ensure educational goals are met and efficiency is maintained. Evidence-based conceptual models should be used to help guide the curriculum design [63].

Simulation Session

Maximizing the time spent in the simulation setting is one of the most important aspects of a procedural training session. Several key considerations to maximize the learning in the simulation lab include (1) use of prework, (2) use of expert modeling (3) use of deliberate practice and mastery learning, (4) skills assessment, and (5) feedback.

Use of Prework

In terms of procedural skill training, it can be very useful to have learners arrive already prepared with the background knowledge required before they come to the hands-on session. This prework may include watching videos of an *expert* performing the procedure. The New England Journal of Medicine (http://www.nejm.org/multimedia/medical-videos) has developed a number of procedural videos, and work is being done to develop pediatric-specific procedural training [64]. Other examples of prework could include reviewing the relevant steps and associated considerations in detail (e.g., indications, anatomic considerations, complications, pearls) as well as the checklist that will be used to evaluate the learner. Assessment of knowledge with a pretest has also been recommended. Additional consideration should be given as to whether a passing grade on a pretest is required before participating in the actual hands-on session. This will

ensure that your learners have completed and understood the background material and should improve the efficiency of your time in the simulation setting [65]. The ultimate goal of this prework is for learners to acquire the requisite cognitive knowledge [66].

Setting the Stage and Use of Expert Modeling

As with any simulation-based medical education session, important first steps are setting the expectation and structure of the session, familiarizing learners with the equipment and the task trainer, and answering any questions the learners have from any associated prework. Expert modeling is a technique by which an expert demonstrates the procedure in its entirety and then may break down the procedure into its component parts. Expert modeling or watching an expert video may also be considered prior to having the learners start their practice [67–71].

Expert modeling is a tool that can ensure learners know the expectations for their performance. In addition, expert modeling may decrease ineffective cognitive load associated with unnecessary problem-solving, and allow the learner to concentrate on building muscle and working memory during their practice. One study showed that expert modeling improved performance with simulated bronchoscopy training and builds on the evidence that shows the effectiveness of expert modeling in different realms [72]. If expert modeling is being included, the facilitator should talk through the steps (including what they are thinking of and anticipating) as they perform each one. Once the learners have seen the expert performance and are given a chance to play around with the equipment, the real practice begins.

Use of Deliberate Practice and Mastery Learning

One useful framework that provides a foundation to guide curriculum development for procedural skills training is the mastery learning model [73], which includes the following steps:

a. Baseline or diagnostic testing
b. Clear learning objectives, sequenced as units in increasing difficulty
c. Engagement in educational activities focused on reaching the objectives
d. A set minimum passing standard for each educational unit
e. Formative testing to gauge unit completion at a preset minimum passing standard for mastery
f. Advancement to the next educational unit, given measured achievement at or above the mastery standard
g. Continued practice or study on an educational unit until the mastery standard is reached

Mastery learning has been shown to lead to improved learner and patient outcomes [74]. It can therefore be used as the foundation to build a simulation-based procedural skills curriculum. See Table 11.3 for an example of how this might be applied.

Table 11.3 Procedural skills training process

Steps	Description	Curricular components
Baseline or diagnostic testing	Baseline testing: ensures prerequisite knowledge obtained Diagnostic testing: identifies gaps	Prework
Clear learning objectives sequenced	Organizes learning activities, ensures learners have basics before proceeding	Setting the stage, expert modeling
Engagement	Directs learning to the key steps needed to achieve the objectives	Deliberate practice; feedback/debriefing
Minimum passing standard	To ensure learners are able to proceed to next educational unit	Checklists
Formative testing	Allows for continued practice if not ready to advance	Deliberate practice
Advancement	Summative evaluation	Assessment: global rating
Continued practice	Ensures learners achieve goals	

Deliberate practice is a key component of mastery learning and includes repetitive performance of the desired skill, rigorous skills assessment, and specific formative feedback. Deliberate practice involves coaching learners through each procedural skill step. Each time the steps are repeated allows for refinement of the skill towards the desired performance level. The initial training towards skill acquisition using deliberate practice does not end until the learners can successfully perform the procedure to a *mastery* standard without any prompting or coaching. Thus, learners who have completed procedural skills training using deliberate practice, as part of a mastery learning model, by definition have mastered that skill and are ready to advance to the next educational unit (performance with supervision on a live patient or progression to practice with more advanced scenarios). Deliberate practice has been successfully applied to procedural training, central venous line placement, and laparoscopic skills, and has shown significant benefit translating to improved learner and patient outcomes [73].

Assessment

Two of the most common types of assessment used for procedural skills testing are global rating scales and specific procedure-based checklists (see Chap. 7). There is growing evidence that suggests global rating scales may be as good, if not better than procedure-specific checklists [75]. Some task trainers and training devices incorporate scoring into their use, by meeting predefined criteria or achieving a passing score.

Having well-developed checklists is important for rigorous skills assessment in procedural skills training (see Chap. 7). Many checklists available have been developed describing key steps for various procedures. These checklists can be a very useful adjunct for teaching the procedures. Significant resources are required to develop a checklist which has a strong validity argument [76]. Checklists have been published with evidence of validity in the simulated setting for pediatric LP, intraosseous lines, and chest tubes. In addition, there is an active effort on the part of the International Network for Simulation-based Pediatric Innovation, Research and Education (INSPIRE) research network to develop checklists for the major pediatric procedures expected of pediatric trainees [77–81].

Feedback

One key feature of mastery learning with deliberate practice is the provision of formative feedback to learners. Feedback may be from the instructor, a peer, or generated from the simulator. In addition, feedback may be delivered concurrently, while the trainee is actively performing the skill or may be delivered terminally, at the end of the skill practice. One example of real-time feedback is that provided by Q-CPR devices, which provide real-time feedback on cardiac compression depth, rate, and leaning force. Real-time feedback during training improves learning and retention of cardiopulmonary resuscitation (CPR) skills, and, most importantly, improves performance during actual resuscitations [82]. Evidence suggests CPR performance in actual resuscitations by in-hospital and prehospital providers, alike, improves when using real-time feedback as guidance [83, 84]. Scenario-based training with real-time feedback and use of real-time feedback during actual resuscitations was correlated with dramatic increases in CPR quality and survival [85]. In addition, some laparoscopic trainers report specific metrics in addition to time and error rates [86–88].

Feedback has been shown to improve skill outcomes with no difference noted whether the feedback was concurrent or terminal. There was also no significant effect found for instructor-given feedback compared to feedback from the simulator [7]. Another key consideration is ensuring that facilitators are skilled at delivering the formative feedback to improve the learner's abilities. As debriefing (see Chap. 3) can be considered feedback that involves interaction, bidirectional communication between the instructor and trainee, and reflection, trained simulation facilitators should be skilled at this step [6].

Just-in-Time Training

Another important consideration for running a procedural skills session is how it will be run temporally and geographically. For the initial exposure to a skill, it is reasonable to learn that skill removed from the actual clinical environment. This may occur in a skills lab or simulation center.

Once a skill is learned and applied to clinical practice, subsequent training would be more valuable when incorporated into the clinical environment, specifically if the skill is not encountered frequently. Maintaining skills can be done effectively using a *just-in-time* and/or *just-in-place* technique. The just-in-place technique describes training that occurs in the clinical environment where the skill will be used (i.e., at the bedside). The addition of just-in-time training creates *a training session conducted directly prior to a potential intervention and at/near the site of the potential intervention.* One example of the just-in-time and just-in-place technique is *rolling refresher,* where a cart with a mannequin and a CPR feedback device allowed staff to practice CPR skills with automated and instructor feedback in close proximity to their patient. Specific staff were chosen to practice these CPR skills, namely those caring for patients deemed most likely to need CPR that day. This type of approach has been described in the literature as a successful, timely, and efficient way to ensure skills are appropriate prior to being performed in an actual clinical situation [89–91].

Challenges and Limitations

One of the biggest challenges with procedural skills training lies in the realism and fidelity of most task trainers, as well as their inability to incorporate the additional stress of performing the procedure in the clinical environment with parents watching, colleagues assisting, monitors ringing, and possible patient instability. This could be partly overcome by ensuring the learner can still adequately perform the procedure to the predefined standards as part of full-scale simulations with these stressors added in. A developmental framework has been described whereby novices first learn, see, practice, and prove. This framework allows for a layered approach in which a skill is first learned in isolation and then placed in simple context. Additional layers of complexity, be they cognitive or behavioral, can then be added on with the development of expertise [92].

Another significant challenge is the inability to predict procedural competence in a real patient. This appears to be somewhat procedure dependent. Simulation-based training for central line placement and cardiac compressions have been shown to improve performance in the clinical realm [20, 76, 79]; however, simulation-based training for others procedures, such as neonatal and pediatric endotracheal intubation, have not [93]. Further research needs to be performed in order to understand better what techniques will enhance procedural training and lead to better translation in the clinical realm. The eventual goal must be to achieve population-based (T3) outcomes that improve patient/public health outcomes [94].

The final challenges that need to be overcome in terms of planning procedural training, as described in this chapter, are the requirements of human, space, and equipment resources and availability. Deliberate practice, in particular, requires a low learner-to-facilitator ratio in order to allow for immediate formative feedback. Intensive training of facilitators may be required to ensure their effectiveness and ability to provide appropriate feedback and use the appropriate rating scales for assessment. As learners may require variable amounts of time to master the material, scheduling becomes increasingly difficult as it is hard to predict how much time each learner will need to attain competence, if that is the goal. Just-in-time and just-in-place training have the additional challenges of finding the time for the clinical healthcare providers to leave their clinical assignments and perform the training as well as the organization and upkeep of the equipment [95–97].

Conclusions

This chapter has demonstrated that a wide spectrum of task trainers exist for pediatric procedural training as well as established models for the creation of curriculum associated with procedural training. While some significant limitations exist, it is clear that simulation-based procedural training will continue to be an integral part of pediatric simulation in the future. Future work needs to be focused on improving the realism and fidelity of the models, the development of valid and reliable tools for the evaluation of various procedural skills, and evaluation of what techniques will enhance procedural training and lead to better translation in the clinical realm and actual patient outcomes.

References

1. Cooper JB, Taqueti VR. A brief history of the development of mannequin simulators for clinical education and training. Qual Saf Health Care. 2004;13(Suppl 1):i11–8.
2. Ross J. Simulation and psychomotor skill acquisition: a review of the literature. Clin Simul Nurs. 2012;8(9):e429–e35.
3. Lenchus JD. End of the "see one, do one, teach one" era: the next generation of invasive bedside procedural instruction. J Am Osteopath Assoc. 2010;110(6):340–6.
4. Philbert I, editor. Accreditation Council for Graduate Medical Education (ACGME) Bulletin. Published December 2005. Accessed Oct 2014.
5. Al-Eissa M, Chu S, Lynch T, Warren D, Seabrook JA, Rieder MJ, et al. Self-reported experience and competence in core procedures among Canadian pediatric emergency medicine fellowship trainees. CJEM. 2008;10(6):533–8.
6. Cheng A, Lang TR, Starr SR, Pusic M, Cook DA. Technology-enhanced simulation and pediatric education: a meta-analysis. Pediatrics. 2014;133(5):e1313–23. Epub 2014 April 14.
7. Hatala R, Cook DA, Zendejas B, Hamstra SJ, Brydges R. Feedback for simulation-based procedural skills training: a meta-anal-

ysis and critical narrative synthesis. Adv Health Sci Educ Theory Pract. 2014;19(2):251–72.

8. Gurusamy K, Aggarwal R, Palanivelu L, Davidson BR. Systematic review of randomized controlled trials on the effectiveness of virtual reality training for laparoscopic surgery. Br J Surg. 2008;95(9):1008–97.

9. Ma IWY, Brindle ME, Ronksley PE, Lorenzetti DL, Sauve RS, Ghali WA. Use of simulation-based education to improve outcomes of central venous catherization: a systematic review and meta-analysis. Acad Med. 2011;86(9):1137–47.

10. Sutherland LM, Middleton PF, Anthony A, Hamdorf J, Cregan P, Scott D, et al. Surgical simulation: a systematic review. Ann Surg. 2006;243(3):291–300.

11. Howells TH, Emery FM, Twentyman JE. Endotracheal intubation training using a simulator. An evaluation of the Laerdal adult intubation model in the teaching of endotracheal intubation. Br J Anaesth. 1973;45:400–2.

12. Kennedy CC, Cannon EK, Warner DO, Cook DA. Advanced airway management simulation training in medical education: a systematic review and meta-analysis. Crit Care Med. 2014;42:169–78.

13. Rowland J. http://www.jumpsimulation.org/blog/building-nasal-secretions-simulator/. Accessed 31 Oct 2014.

14. Chez Moulage. www.laerdal.com/usa/SUN/ppt/Chez_Moulage.pdf. Accessed 28 Jan 2015.

15. Merica BJ. Medical moulage: How to make your simulations come alive. Philadelphia: F. A. Davis Company; 2012. (Chap. 3 Blood, p. 32–43; Chap. 7 Drainage and Secretions, p. 74–81; Chap. 27 Vomit, p. 32–43).

16. Deransy R, Dupont H, Duwat A, Hubert V, Mahjoub Y, et al. Effect of simulation training on compliance with difficult airway management algorithms, technical ability, and skills retention for emergency cricothyrotomy. Anesthesiology. 2014;120(4):999–1008.

17. Boet S, Borges BC, Bould MD, Chandra D, Joo HS, Naik VN, Riem N, Siu LW, et al. Complex procedural skills are retained for a minimum of 1 year after a single high-fidelity simulation training session. Br J Anaesth. 2011;107(4):533–9.

18. Frommer M, Graf BM, Kwok P, Metterlein T, Sinner B, et al. Emergency cricothyrotomy in infants—evaluation of a novel device in an animal model. Paediatr Anaesth. 2011;21(2):104–9.

19. Ault B, Ault MJ, Rosen BT, et al. The use of tissue models for vascular access training: phase I of the procedural patient safety initiative. J Gen Intern Med. 2006;21(5):514–7.

20. Barsuk JH, Cohen ER, Feinglass J, McGaghie WC, Wayne DB. Use of simulation-based education to reduce catheter-related bloodstream infections. Arch Intern Med 2009;169:1420–3.

21. Barsuk JH, McGaghie WC, Cohen ER, Blachandran JS, Wayne DB. Use of simulation-based mastery learning to improve the quality of central venous catheter placement in a medical intensive care unit. J Hosp Med. 2009;4(7):397–403.

22. Cherry RA, West CE, Hamilton MC, Rafferty CM, Hollenbeak CS, Caputo GM. Reduction of central venous catheter associated blood stream infections following implementation of a resident oversight and credentialing policy. Patient Saf Surg. 2011;5:15.

23. Zingg W, Cartier V, Inan C, Touveneau S, Clergue F, Pittet D, Walder B. Sustained reduction of catheter-associated bloodstream infections by simulator-training and self-assessment. BMC Proc. 2011;5(Suppl 6):O13.

24. Cohen ER, Feinglass J, Barsuk JH, Barnard C, O'Donnell A, McGaghie WC, Wayne DB. Cost savings from reduced catheter-related bloodstream infection after simulation-based education for residents in a medical intensive care unit. Simul Healthc. 2010;5:98–102.

25. Kendall JL, Faragher JP. Ultrasound-guided central venous access: a homemade phantom for simulation. CJEM. 2007;9(5):371–3.

26. Berg B, Chan DS, Hara K, Thompson MW, Sawyer T, et al. Modification of the Laerdal SimBaby to include an integrated umbilical cannulation task trainer. Simul Healthc. 2009;4(3):174–8.

27. Azzie G, Farcas M, Gerstle JT, Green J, Henao O, Lasko D, Okrainec A, et al. Development and validation of a pediatric laparoscopic surgery simulator. J Pediatr Surg. 2011;46(5):897–903.

28. Evgeniou E, Loizou P, et al. Simulation-based surgical education. ANZ J Surg. 2012;83(9):619–23.

29. Korets R, Liu DB, Maizel M, Smith A, Stiener M, Sutherland RW, et al. A novel method of teaching surgical techniques to residents—computerized enhanced visual learning (CEVL) with simulation to certify mastery of training: a model using newborn clamp circumcision. J Pediatr Urol. 2013;9(6 Pt B):1210–3.

30. Alvarado C, Farooq S, Hill-Engstler EA, Stausmire JM, et al. Effectiveness of a simulated training model for procedural skill demonstration in neonatal circumcision. Simul Healthc. 2012;7(6):362–73.

31. Bacarese-Hamilton J, Pena V, Haddad M, Clarke S, et al. Simulation in the early management of gastroschisis. Simul Healthc. 2013;8(6):376–81.

32. Davenport D, French J, Hoskins J, Iocono JA, Plymale M, Ruzic A, Skinner SC, Yuhas M, et al. A middle fidelity model is effective in teaching and retaining skill set needed to perform a laparoscopic pyloromyotomy. J Laparoendosc Adv Surg Tech A. 2010;20(6):569–73.

33. Chin AC, Davis LM, Rooney DM, et al. Validation of measures from a thoracoscopic esophageal atresia/tracheoesophageal fistula repair simulator. J Pediatr Surg. 2014;49(1):29–32.

34. Biffar D, Grisham LM, Hamilton AJ, Jarred J, Mogan C, Prescher H, Thompson JL, et al. Construction of a reusable, high-fidelity model to enhance extracorporeal membrane oxygenation training through simulation. Adv Neonatal Care. 2014;14(2):103–9.

35. Jabbour N, Reihsen T, Sidman JD, Sweet RM, et al. Psychomotor skills training in pediatric airway endoscopy simulation. Otolaryngol Head Neck Surg. 2011;145(1):43–50.

36. Costello JP, Jonas RA, Krieger A, Marshall MB, Nath DS, Thabit O, Yoo SJ, et al. Utilizing three-dimensional printing technology to assess the feasibility of high-fidelity synthetic ventricular septal defect models for simulation in medical education. World J Pediatr Congenit Heart Surg. 2014;5(3):421–26.

37. Derossis AM, Fried GM, Abrahamowicz M, et al. Development of a model for training and evaluation of laparoscopic skills. Am J Surg. 1998;175:482–7.

38. Javia L, Deutsch E, Javia L, et al. A systematic review of simulators in otolaryngology. Otolaryngol Head Neck Surg. 2012;147(6):999–1011.

39. See http://limbsandthings.com/global/products/ear-examination-simulator-ii. Accessed 31 Oct 2014.

40. Atchison P, Kharasch M, Pettineo CM, Vozenilek JA, Wang E, et al. Epistaxis simulator: an innovative design. Simul Healthc. 2008;3(4):239–41.

41. Lammers RL, et al. Learning and retention rates after training in posterior epistaxis management. Acad Emerg Med. 2008;15(11):1181–9.

42. See http://en.honglian8.com/p/429/gdlv17-advanced-nasal-hemorrhage-simulator. Accessed 31 Oct 2014.

43. Louloudiadis K, Papadopoulos L, Pentzou AE, Tsiatsos TK, et al. Design and evaluation of a simulation for pediatric dentistry in virtual worlds. J Med Internet Res. 2013;15(11):e240.

44. Taylor SR, Chang CW. Novel peritonsillar abscess task simulator. Otolaryngol Head Neck Surg. 2014;151(1):10–3.

45. Al-Eissa M, Chu S, Lim R, Lynch T, Rieder MJ, Seabrook JA, Warren D, et al. Self-reported experience and competence in core procedures among Canadian pediatric emergency medicine fellowship trainees. CJEM. 2008;10(6):533–8.

46. Gaies MG, Hafler JP, Landrigan CP, Sandora TJ, et al. Assessing procedural skills training in pediatric residency programs. Pediatrics. 2008;120(4):715–22.

47. King L, Paul RI, et al. Technical skills experiences in pediatric emergency medicine fellowship programs. Pediatr Emerg Care. 1996;12(1):10–2.

48. Pirie J. Pork rib model in hospital for sick children simulation centre manual. (Personal communication by AS, August 2014).

49. Gupta AO, Ramasethu J, et al. An innovative nonanimal simulation trainer for chest tube insertion in neonates. Pediatrics. 2014;134(3):798–805.

50. Barsness KA, Davis LM, Rooney DM, et al. Collaboration in simulation: the development and initial validation of a novel thoracoscopic neonatal simulator. J Pediatr Surg. 2013;48(6):1232–8.

51. Girzadas DV Jr, Harwood R, Tommaso L, Zerth H, et al. An inexpensive, easily constructed, reusable task trainer for simulating ultrasound-guided pericardiocentesis. J Emerg Med. 2012;43(6):1066–69.

52. Al-Qadhi SA, Ali M, Constas N, Corrin MS, Pirie JR, et al. An innovative pediatric chest tube insertion task trainer simulation: a technical report and pilot study. Simul Healthc. 2014;9(5):319–24.

53. Breitkreutz R, Campo dell'Orto M, Hannemann U, Hempel D, Seibel A, Starzetz A, Walcher F. Assessment of a low-cost ultrasound pericardiocentesis model. Emerg Med Int. 2013;2013:376415.

54. Garside MJ, Rudd MP, Price CL, et al. Stroke and TIA assessment training: a new simulation-based approach to teaching acute stroke assessment. Simul Healthc. 2012;7(2):117–22.

55. Heiner JD, et al. A new simulation model for skin abscess identification and management. Simul Healthc. 2010;5(4):238–41.

56. Ackley SH, Lo MD, Solari P, et al. Homemade ultrasound phantom for teaching identification of superficial soft tissue abscess. Emerg Med J. 2012;29(9):738–41.

57. Hampton K, et al. Homemade tastes better. http://sonokids.wordpress.com/2014/05/19/homemade-tastes-better/. Accessed 9 Nov 2014.

58. Bretholz A, Cheng A, Doan Q, Lauder G, et al. A presurvey and postsurvey of a web- and simulation-based course of ultrasound-guided nerve blocks for pediatric emergency medicine. Pediatr Emerg Care. 2012;28(6):506–9.

59. Ding L, Moore DL, Sadhasivam S, et al. Novel real-time feedback and integrated simulation model for teaching and evaluating ultrasound-guided regional anesthesia skills in pediatric anesthesia trainees. Pediatr Anesth. 2012;22(9):847–53.

60. Black A, Dumont T, Fleming N, Hakim J, et al. Enhancing postgraduate training in pediatric and adolescent gynecology: evaluation of an advanced pelvic simulation session. J Pediatr Adolesc Gynecol. 2014 Sept (available online).

61. Finkenzeller D, Ibrahim S, Lovelss MB, Satin AJ, et al. A simulation program for teaching obstetrics and gynecology residents the pediatric gynecology examination and procedures. J Pediatr Adolesc Gynecol. 2011;24(3):127–36.

62. Lendvay TS, et al. Surgical simulation in pediatric urologic education. Curr Urol Rep. 2011;12(2):137–43.

63. Hsu DC, Macias CG, et al. Rubric evaluation of pediatric emergency medicine fellows. J Grad Med Educ. 2010;2(4):523–9.

64. Auerbach M, Chang TP, Gerard JM, Kessler DO, Krantz A, Pratt A, Quinones C, Reid J, et al. Are pediatric interns prepared to perform infant lumbar punctures? A multi-institutional descriptive study. Pediatr Emerg Care. 2013;29(4):453–7.

65. McGaghie WC, Issenberg SB, Cohen ER, Barsuk JH, Wayne DB. Does simulation-based medical education with deliberate practice yield better results than traditional clinical education? A meta-analytic comparative review of the evidence. Acad Med. 2011;86(6):706–11.

66. Kovacs G. Procedural skills in medicine: linking theory with practice. J Emerg Med. 1997;15(3):387–91.

67. Srivastava G, Roddy M, Langsam D, Agrawal. An educational video improves technique in performance of pediatric lumbar punctures. Pediatr Emerg Care. 2012;28(1):12–6.

68. Ventres W SJ. Introducing a procedure using videotape instruction: the case of the lateral birth position. Fam Med. 1994;26(7):434–6.

69. Dubrowski A, Xeroulis G. Computer-based video instructions for acquisition of technical skills. J Vis Commun Med. 2005;28(4):150–5.

70. Jowett N, Leblanc V, Xeroulis G, et al. Surgical skill acquisition with self-directed practice using computer-based video training. Am J Surg. 2007;193(2):237–42.

71. Porte MC, Xeroulis G, Reznick RK, Dubrowski A. Verbal feedback from an expert is more effective than self-accessed feedback about motion efficiency in learning new surgical skills. Am J Surg. 2007;193(1):105–10.

72. Bjerrum AS, Hilberg O, van Gog T, Charles P, Eika B. Effects of modeling examples in complex procedural skills training: a randomized study. Med Educ. 2013;47:888.

73. Ericsson K. Deliberate practice and the acquisition and maintenance of expert performance in medicine and related domains. Acad Med. 2004;79:S70–81.

74. Cook DA, Brydges R, Zendejas B, Hamstra SJ, Hatala R. Mastery learning for health professionals using technology-enhanced simulation: a systematic review and meta-analysis. Acad Med. 2013;88(8):1178–86.

75. Adler MD, Vozenilek JA, Trainor JL, Eppich WJ, Wang EE, Beaumont JL, Aitchison PR, Pribaz PJ, Erickson T, Edison M, McGaghie WC. Comparison of checklist and anchored global rating instruments for performance rating of simulated pediatric emergencies. Simul Healthc. 2011;6(1):18–24.

76. Gawande A. The checklist manifesto: how to get things right. New York: Metropolitan Books; 2009. http://www.projectcheck.org/checklist-for-checklists.html. Accessed 31 Jan 2015.

77. Boureau-Voultoury A, Darrieux E, Oriot D, Ragot S, Scèpi M, et al. Validation of a performance assessment scale for simulated intraosseous access. Simul Healthc. 2012;7(3):171–5.

78. Auerbach M, Foltin JC, Kessler D, Pusic M, Tunik MG, et al. A randomized trial of simulation-based deliberate practice for infant lumbar puncture skills. Simul Healthc. 2011;6(4):197–203.

79. Bradin S, Chapman R, House JB, Iyer MS, McAllister J, Nypaver M, Santen SA, Warrier K, Accreditation Council for Graduate Medical Education Committee, Emergency Medicine and Pediatrics Residency Review Committee, et al. Assessing the validity evidence of an objective structured assessment tool of technical skills for neonatal lumbar punctures. Acad Emerg Med. 2013;20(3):321–4.

80. Auerbach M, Braun C, Gerard JM, Kessler DO, Mehta R, Scalzo AJ, et al. Validation of global rating scale and checklist instruments for the infant lumbar puncture procedure. Simul Healthc. 2013;8(3):148–54.

81. Shefrin AE, Khazei A, Hung GR, Odendal LT, Cheng A. The TACTIC: development and validation of the Tool for Assessing Chest Tube Insertion Competency. CJEM. 2015;17(2):140–7. doi:10.2310/8000.2014.141406.

82. Yeung J, Meeks R, Edelson D, Gao F, Soar J, Perkins GD. The use of CPR feedback/prompt devices during training and CPR performance: a systematic review. Resuscitation. 2009;80(7):743–51.

83. Abella BS, Edelson DP, Kim S, Retzer E, Myklebust H, Barry AM, O'Hearn N, Hoek T, Becker LB. CPR quality improvement during in-hospital cardiac arrest using a real-time audiovisual feedback system. Resuscitation. 2007;73(1):54–61.

84. Kramer-Johansen J, Mykelbust H, Wik L, Fellows B, Svensson L, Sorebo H, Steen PA. Quality of out-of-hospital cardiopulmonary resuscitation with real time automated feedback: a prospective interventional study. Resuscitation. 2006;71(3):283–92.

85. Bobrow BJ, Vadeboncoeur TF, Stolz U, Silver AE, Tobin JM, Crawford SA, Mason TK, Schirmer J, Smith GA, Spaite DW. The influence of scenario-based training and real-time audiovisual feedback on out-of-hospital cardiopulmonary resuscitation quality and survival from out-of-hospital cardiac arrest. Ann Emerg Med. 2013. 62(1):47–56.

86. Larsen DP, Butler AC, Roediger HL. Repeated testing improves long-term retention relative to repeated study: a randomised controlled trial. Med Educ. 2009;43(12):117–34.

87. Cosman PH, Cregan PC, Martin CJ, Cartmill JA. Virtual reality simulators: current status in acquisition and assessment of surgical skills. ANZ J Surg. 2002;72(1):30–4.

88. Choy I, Okrainec A. Simulation in surgery: perfecting the practice. Surg Clin North Am. 2010;90(3):457–73.

89. Niles D, Sutton RM, Donoghue A, Kalsi MS, Roberts K, Boyle L, et al. "Rolling refreshers": a novel approach to maintain CPR psychomotor skill competence. Resuscitation. 2009;80(8):909–12.

90. Brown CA, Colborn S, Donoghue AJ, Helfaer MA, Meyer A, Nadkarni VM, Nishisaki A, Walls RM, Watson C, et al. Effect of just-in-time simulation training on tracheal intubation procedure safety in the pediatric intensive care unit. Anesthesiology. 2012;113(1):214–23.

91. Kalynych CJ, Kaminski A, Konzelmann J, Matar-Joseph M, McIntosh MS, Schneider H, Smith J, Wears RL, Wylie T Stabilization and treatment of dental avulsions and fractures by emergency physicians using just-in-time training. Ann Emerg Med. 2009;54(4).585–92.

92. Sawyer T, White M, Zaveri P, Chang T, Ades A, French H et al. Learn, see, practice, prove, do, maintain: an evidence-based pedagogical framework for procedural skill training in medicine. Acad Med. In press.

93. Finan E, Bismilla Z, Campbell C, LeBlanc V, Jefferies A, Whyte HE. Improved procedural performance following a simulation training session may not be transferable to the clinical environment. J Perinatol. 2012;32:539–44.

94. Monographs from the First Research Consensus Summit for the society for simulation in healthcare. Simulation in Healthcare. August 2011. supplement.

95. Conlon T, Nadkarni V, Nishisaki A Simulation-based procedural training for pediatric residents: one small step for a program … one giant leap for mankind! Pediatr Crit Care Med. 2013;14(9):908–9.

96. Denmark KT, Eppich WJ, Joseph MM, Kim I, Mahajan P, Nypaver MM, et al. The role of high-fidelity simulation in training pediatric emergency medicine fellows in the United States and Canada. Pediatr Emerg Care. 2013;29(1):1–7.

97. Calaman S, McGregor RS, Spector ND How can we assure procedural competence in pediatric residents in an era of diminishing opportunities? The answer is simulation-based training. J Pediatr. 2010;156(6):865–6.

98. Shefrin A, Khazei A, Cheng A. Realism of procedural task trainers in pediatric emergency medicine procedures course. Can Med Educ J. 2015;6(1):e68–73.

In Situ Simulation

Tensing Maa, Ellen Heimberg and Jennifer R. Reid

Simulation Pearls

1. In addition to predetermined learning objectives, in situ simulation can concurrently identify latent safety threats and opportunities for process and systems improvement.
2. In situ training may be better suited for intermediate and experienced practitioners. The novice learner, who is still developing basic knowledge, skills, and attitudes, may benefit from the controlled environment of a center: without time limits, distractions, risk of unintended observers, and lesscomplex physical and functional fidelity.
3. Unique challenges include scheduling interprofessional teams, frequent distractions, lastminute room and staff cancellations, and missing or malfunctioning equipment. Facilitators need to be resilient to this lack of consistency and work to adjust learning objectives to the changing learning environment.
4. Mobile simulation, taking simulation to hospitals or clinics in the community, can make in situ simulation methodologies accessible across institutions, geographical regions, and international boundaries. It can inspire interest in simulation, patient safety, and cultural change in these institutions.

T. Maa (✉)
Department of Pediatrics, Department of Critical Care Medicine, Ohio State University College of Medicine, Nationwide Children's Hospital, Columbus, OH, USA
e-mail: Tensing.Maa@nationwidechildrens.org

E. Heimberg
Department of Pediatric Cardiology, Pulmology, Intensive Care Medicine, University Children's Hospital, Tuebingen, Germany
e-mail: e.heimberg@paedsim.de

J. R. Reid
Department of Pediatrics, Division of Emergency Medicine, University of Washington School of Medicine, Seattle Children's Hospital, Seattle, WA, USA
e-mail: Jennifer.reid@seattlechildrens.org

Introduction

In situ simulation describes training that occurs in real patient care environments, rather than in a simulation center or off-site training area. By utilizing actual patient care spaces, simulation training can be performed in specialized settings such as a trauma bay, operating room (OR), hospital lobby, or prehospital site. Mobile simulation, taking simulation to hospitals or clinics in the community or to rural environments, can make in situ simulation methodologies accessible across institutions, broad geographical regions, and international boundaries.

This chapter reviews opportunities and challenges specific to in situ simulation, including applications where it has been shown to be particularly effective as compared to center-based training. We outline guidelines on setting up a successful in situ session, common challenges that may be encountered, as well as possible solutions. Strategies for planning and executing effective multi-institutional mobile in situ simulations are included.

Advantages

One of the main advantages of in situ simulation is that of increased fidelity, both from physical and functional perspectives. Physical fidelity refers to the realism of the physical environment. Performing simulation exercises in actual patient care locations and using real equipment minimizes environmental and physical differences between simulation training versus real patient care. This may make it easier for the learner to suspend disbelief and identify the relevance of the simulation. Functional fidelity refers to the realism of the content and process. Training that occurs in a native work setting can provide functional fidelity of content (what to do) and context (how to do it) combined in one educational session. Choosing clinical scenarios that approximate real patient experiences can support generalization of acquired competencies. By integrating physical and functional fidelity, in situ simulation can maximize transfer of knowledge, skills, and behaviors learned during training to actual practice [1, 2].

In situ simulation offers improved efficiency when it comes to space and cost. Highly specialized environments such as a cardiac catheterization lab or an operating room are difficult and expensive to fully replicate. In 2009, the estimated cost to start up an in situ program, including a high-fidelity human simulator, was US$41,000 versus US$472,000 for a simulation center [3]. Rather than a dedicated simulation space, in situ sessions borrow from clinical space, needing only a smaller secured storage area. Figure 12.1 shows two examples of an in situ cart for storing and transporting a high-fidelity simulator and equipment. Figure 12.2 shows a hospital stretcher modified for carrying a mannequin, simulation equipment, and supplies, which can be wheeled through the hospital for in situ simulation. Additional savings come from being able to use real but expensive equipment, such as a defibrillator or bronchoscope, rather than purchasing those separately for training or using decommissioned units that have been collected for training use and are out of date. Furthermore, the authenticity of the environment provides such high fidelity that learning objectives may still be successfully accomplished using less costly, lower fidelity mannequins.

The core staff needed to run an in situ session (e.g., operator and facilitator) is similar to that at a center [3]. However, more time is required for transport of equipment, setup, and tear-down for sessions, and this must be taken into account when considering human resource costs [4]. Some institutions utilize creative solutions for deferring staffing costs such as redirecting mandatory academic educational time of faculty members who act as facilitators and content experts for simulation sessions [5]. The affordability of starting an in situ program has allowed institutions with fewer resources to benefit from simulation-based education.

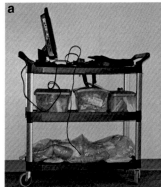
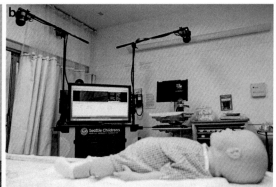

Fig. 12.1 Examples of in situ simulation carts. **a** Minimal equipment needed: mannequin, basic supplies, and monitor versus **b** comprehensive console that contains mannequin, supply storage, technician console, cameras for video, and debriefing capabilities and connections to power sources. (Photo courtesy of Seattle Children's Hospital)

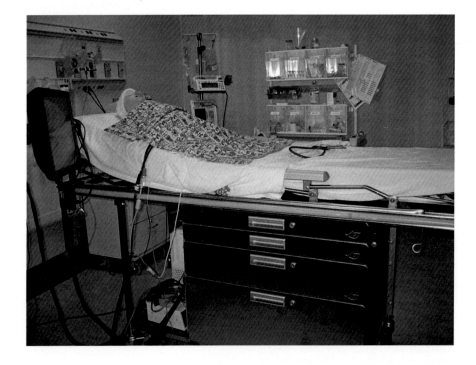

Fig. 12.2 Example of an in situ stretcher modified for carrying a mannequin, simulation equipment and supplies, which can be wheeled through the hospital for in situ simulation. (Photo courtesy of KidSIM Pediatric Simulation Program, Calgary, Canada)

Additional potential cost savings benefits can come from educating healthcare personnel while they are on duty rather than having to set aside separate time and money for off-site education. By bringing training to the learners, in situ sessions can be incorporated throughout all clinical shifts, promoting increased access to learning experiences for a larger number of staff.

Challenges

There are unique challenges with in situ simulation. Educational time may be limited as simulations may happen while staff are working and thus cannot leave their clinical responsibilities for long. There are increased distractors such as frequent interruptions from pagers, phone calls and patient care duties. Last-minute cancellations can occur when staff or patient rooms become unavailable due to high patient census or acuity. Debriefings, arguably the most important part of the simulation experience, may not be optimal; physical space may be confining and interfere with confidential debriefing or make video feedback challenging. Alternatively, in situ space may not physically accommodate all participants and observers that would like to attend.

The physical and cognitive demands on the simulation educator team are different for in situ simulation than for simulations performed within a center. For each simulation session, there is more time and effort needed for transportation of equipment, set-up, and tear-down, particularly for elaborate simulations (e.g., extracorporeal membrane oxygenation (ECMO)) [4, 6]. Inadequate cleanup after an in situ session has the potential to harm patients if real medical equipment or medications become contaminated with those used for simulation, and thus not for patient use. If the clinical area is not appropriately restocked, this may result in inadvertent threats to safety during a real-patient emergency if key supplies are missing or damaged [3, 7]. Rehearsal of the simulation may not be possible until just prior to training, if at all, due to limited availability of clinical simulation space. This may place additional cognitive burden on the educator team when equipment is forgotten or unexpectedly malfunctioning, and there are no resources immediately available for replacement.

Finally, there are psychological safety concerns for participants and unintended observers. A goal of simulation is to provide a safe learning environment but confidentiality may be difficult to preserve while in the hospital setting. During team training, an individual's clinical weaknesses and knowledge gaps may be revealed to teammates who then later need to trust each other and work together. Other healthcare personnel who are not part of the educational session may potentially observe and cast judgment on faults and mistakes that are made. In addition, families, patients, and visitors may experience anxiety after seeing chest compressions or procedures performed, not understanding that it was a simulation [3, 7].

Effectiveness of In Situ Simulation

In situ simulation makes it easier to gather and train intact, interprofessional teams if the sessions occur while they are already on duty together. Training is more effective when healthcare teams rehearse communication and nontechnical skills in their normal clinical setting, using real medical equipment, and learners function in their actual professional roles (e.g. nurse, respiratory, physician, pharmacy) [3, 8–10]. Hearing the perspectives of other healthcare professionals or clinical disciplines can further enrich the debriefing process. Immersive simulation training in teamwork and communication has been shown to improve recognition and management of deteriorating pediatric inpatients [11], survival outcomes after pediatric cardiac arrest, and time to task completion and team communication in the trauma bay [12–14].

In situ simulation also has the unique ability to examine the clinical environment, specific care processes, and healthcare systems in action for previously unidentified patient and staff safety concerns (see Chap. 5). Latent safety threats can be defects in design, organization, training, or maintenance and can include equipment failure, personnel/system resource failures, and procedural failures. They can occur at the microsystem level (e.g., patient unit), or they might be rooted in organizational processes, at a macrosystem level (see Chap. 6). The simulation group of Cincinnati Children's Hospital Medical Center performed a series of unannounced, recurring multidisciplinary in situ training sessions in an emergency department (ED) and on inpatient units and discovered a higher rate of latent safety threats with in situ compared to lab-based trainings [10, 15, 16]. Multiple examples in the literature have used in situ to test existing and newly designed clinical space and have shown discovery of missing or malfunctioning equipment, unsuitable room layout, medication errors, and knowledge and clinical skill deficits [10, 15, 17–20].

Setting Up a Successful In Situ Simulation

Depending on the specific needs and target learners, in situ simulations have unique considerations to ensure that objectives are met. In this section, we will discuss the *why, who, what, where, when,* and *how* of in situ simulation: the practical considerations of conducting successful in situ simulation.

Why?

Determining the specific learning objectives is one of the most critical steps in planning. Learning objectives should be *observable, measurable,* and *meaningful.* Objectives can focus on (1) *instruction* to develop and facilitate application of cognitive, technical, or teamwork competencies, (2) *assessment* of performance or a healthcare delivery process, or (3) *diagnostics* of potential risks or system defects [21]. Most learning objectives depend on target learners. Target learners may be at the level of an individual (e.g., physician, nurse, or therapist), a healthcare team (e.g., code response team), a unit (e.g., representatives of all professions within an emergency department), or an organization (e.g., representatives of various departments, enterprise-wide systems, and leadership or culture influencers) [22].

Let us examine three examples to illustrate how target objectives and learners drive practical decisions (who, what, where, when, and how).

Example One: Intubation Process in the Emergency Department

1. Target objective—instruction of technical and teamwork competencies.
2. Target learners—healthcare team.

The focus is training in the emergency department, with specific objectives including selection and preparation of equipment and medications, securement of the airway, and arrangement for safe patient transport.

Example Two: A New Chemotherapy Verification Process

1. Target objective—assessment of healthcare delivery process.
2. Target learners—inpatient cancer unit.

The focus is assessment of a new process requiring a physician review of chemotherapy orders and medications with two nurses, immediately prior to administration.

Example Three: Evaluation of a New Critical Care Unit

1. Target objective—identification of patient safety and environmental threats.
2. Target learners—organization.

The goal is to identify and mitigate patient safety risks prior to opening a new critical care unit.

Who?

In situ training may be better suited for intermediate and experienced practitioners because the sessions and debriefings are often time-limited, leaving less time for teaching new concepts. The novice learner, who is still developing basic knowledge, skills, and attitudes, may benefit more from instruction in the controlled environment of a center: without time limits, distractions, and risk of unintended observers.

Target objectives and learners define the participants, content experts, and observers required. Participants may be part of active patient care teams, pulled from clinical duties, or be on standby, ready to simulate. Using on-duty teams provides an opportunity to assess competing clinical demands and the full impact of a process. Some programs use *just-in-time* training to simulate the likely deterioration of a current patient. This type of training acts as a *dress rehearsal* if that situation occurs. At risk is lack of engagement if participants remain focused on actual patient care, and the potential creation of real-patient safety risks while removed from their clinical duties. Choosing observers or facilitators with knowledge of the specific unit's protocols and practices can maximize the richness of the debrief.

Let us examine our examples to help ensure you include WHO; you will need to participate in your simulation-based event to reach your target learners.

Example One: Intubation Process in the Emergency Department

The participant team would include the physician who makes medication selections for intubation and physically performs the procedure, the respiratory therapist who sets up and assists with all the equipment, the nurse who administers the medications and prepares all supplies for patient transfer, and the technician who assists with transport. Observers may include educators responsible for training other team members or departmental quality improvement leaders who determine policies and procedures. As the target objective involves technical and teamwork competencies, the facilitator should be capable of providing feedback on the medical knowledge and clinical skill specific to the procedure (endotracheal intubation) as well as communication among team members.

Example Two: A New Chemotherapy Verification Process

Participants should include individuals physically and mentally involved in each step of the process. In this example, a unit clerk notifies providers that medications have arrived, and then a physician and two nurses review chemotherapy orders and the medication in the patient room independently. Use of staff actively involved in patient care to participate in the simulation would provide the richest insight into identifying barriers and tracking delays. Using auxiliary staff, designated only for the simulation, may fail to identify disruptions in workflow or patient safety risks created as real-team members attempt to implement the new process. In this example, target learners include stakeholders who developed this process and educators who will implement and support the change. Stakeholders are good candidates to monitor for safety risks, process breakdown, and opportunities for improvement.

Example Three: Evaluation of a New Critical Care Unit

Participants could include a representative care team: attending and resident physicians, nurses, technicians, respiratory therapists, unit clerks, environmental services, security, pharmacy, and family representatives. Observers could include leadership for each of these groups plus engineering, supply delivery, construction, patient safety, human factors, marketing, etc. The more complete the participant and observer team, the broader the range of experience available to identify safety risks, and the more invested and prepared the organization will be to respond.

What?

The target objectives determine the content of the session, including necessary equipment and issues to discuss in the debrief. Best practice is to utilize only existing equipment in the clinical environment. If training materials are substituted, placing them in the exact locations of actual equipment will facilitate the learners going through as many of the real mental and physical steps in the process as possible. With higher levels of physical fidelity, participants may be able to suspend their disbelief with lower fidelity mannequins or task trainers.

Example One: Intubation Process in the Emergency Department

The objective of instruction includes the acquisition of all medications and equipment, the physical placement, confirmation and securement of the endotracheal tube, and the application of all safety monitors and devices for transport, in addition to teamwork competencies. A low-fidelity simulator could meet the technical and teamwork objectives. However, if recognition of respiratory failure is also a learning objective, a high-fidelity patient simulator may be needed to provide the appropriate physical cues.

Example Two: A New Chemotherapy Verification Process

Content of this simulation and debrief should focus on the new process from arrival of the chemotherapy, to physician and nurse notification, to completion of medication verification. Equipment should include all communication systems (e.g., paging systems or phones) utilized in real time. Skipping the real-time use of communication systems may fail to identify barriers or delays. Since the target objective does not involve administration of the medication or a patient, this scenario may not include a patient simulator.

Example Three: Evaluation of a New Critical Care Unit

The scope of this simulation could include a *day in the life* series of simultaneous simulations that mimic an actual day on that unit: for example, admissions, transfers, procedures, medication administration, complete care teams rounding on patients, and unexpected patient decompensation. Alternatively, it may focus on a limited number of high risk, low frequency patient scenarios such as cardiopulmonary arrest. Both approaches could meet the objective of testing the new environment and identification of latent safety hazards. A broader scope will uncover a more exhaustive list of risks but require more resources.

Discussions with key stakeholders should weigh benefits of risk identification against resource limitations such as availability of staff, equipment, and simulators, in deciding the scope of testing. Ideally, any new technology (e.g., new defibrillator or bedside monitor) to be rolled out with the new unit should be incorporated into the scenarios. Equipment should be stocked in the expected locations where it will be once the unit is functional. Simulators may include multiple low- and high-fidelity mannequins and standardized patients being utilized in tandem, or in a resource-limited setting, one mannequin progressing through a series of simulations.

Where?

Clinical space availability may be volatile, affecting the duration or scope of planned simulations and can be challenging to standardize, particularly for high-stakes assessment or research [21, 22]. If the space is needed for real patient care and participants/observers have been scheduled, it helps to have an alternate plan. This could be an unconventional space, such as a treatment room, bathroom, stairwell, or hallway, if it still addresses target objectives and learners. If not, rescheduling the session may be the best way to achieve targets. In either case, the more the simulation educator can anticipate and prepare participants and observers for contingency plans, the more likely the session and future sessions are to be successful.

Progressive simulations follow a patient as they move from one clinical area to the next and can involve different clinical teams. Patient flow processes, transport skills, environmental challenges, handovers, and communication issues or systems can be examined with a simulation that physically transitions from one space (e.g., ED to elevator to OR) and team (e.g., ED team to OR team) to the next.

Finding private space for participants to debrief can be challenging. Instructors can facilitate this process by moving participants away from the site of care, even if it is to the side of the room. Reconfiguring the group, or drawing a curtain, to visually separate them from the patient care area can be helpful. If there are no alternatives other than to debrief at the bedside, minimizing distractors, such as turning off auditory stimuli and discouraging cleaning up of the simulation/clinical equipment, is a must. Additional efforts should be made to ensure that other providers, family members, and unintended observers not involved in the simulation cannot overhear the debrief.

When?

When is the best time to have your in situ simulation? Conduct the simulation to maximize your chance of guaranteeing both your space and learner availability while still addressing your objectives. Let us revisit our examples.

Example One: Intubation Process in the Emergency Department

As the target objective is instruction of technical and teamwork skills, this simulation can be scheduled. There are advantages and disadvantages to choosing different times of day. At low-census times, the emergency department intubation room and staff participants are more likely to be available. Planning this session in coordination with other department meetings or trainings may make it easier to enlist team members. However, if the target objective is to assess the system under stress and identify latent safety threats, the simulation should be conducted during the busiest hours of the day.

Example Two: A New Chemotherapy Verification Process

Perform your simulation in *real time* to best examine how the process is expected to integrate into daily work flows. If the chemotherapy verification process is expected to occur at a time that potentially interrupts morning rounds, you should conduct the simulation at that time only. If this is not possible, include a discussion of how modifications made for the simulation might impact your discoveries during the debriefing. It is useful to conduct the simulation after most of the new process has been developed but prior to initiation of staff education. This ensures that safety concerns discovered during the in situ testing can be remediated, alterations to the process made, and staff trained to a refined process.

Example Three: Evaluation of a New Critical Care Unit

For the richest experience, the new unit should be patient ready before the in situ session. New technologies, such as communication systems, emergency alarms, computers, staff tracking devices, patient locator boards, and patient monitors, should be in place. All equipment should be stocked in their new location. In addition, allow an adequate period of time following the simulation to mitigate risks, prior to opening of the unit for patient care.

HOW?

A common challenge with in situ is time limitations due to participants having concurrent clinical responsibilities. One solution is to use brief, individually targeted *just-in-time* in situ training to improve psychomotor skills. For example, a *rolling refresher* approach to maintain high-quality chest compression skills among pediatric intensive care staff has been shown to be effective [23]. This training is limited to less than 10 min at the start of the clinicians' shifts. Another effective and efficient training and debriefing technique, particularly applicable to in situ simulation, is "Rapid Cycle Deliberate Practice" [24]. Directed feedback is given to the participant team as they repeatedly drill through a scenario, allowing multiple opportunities for deliberate practice of resuscitation skills and teamwork competencies in one session.

Another common challenge is providing training for staff from all shifts, including nights and weekends. Mitigation strategies include scheduling in situ sessions just before or after shift changes or including in situ sessions as part of mandatory training and meetings.

Scheduled Versus Impromptu Simulations

Scheduled simulations allow participants to mentally and emotionally prepare. It allows time for them to review knowledge or skill gaps, equipment, and processes. It also prepares them to set aside time to learn. For participants unaccustomed to simulation, scheduled sessions allow facilitators to provide a *prebriefing* for setting expectations and potentially alleviating performance anxiety. This can help prime participants and optimize the learning experience.

Impromptu simulations promote the opportunity to examine the environment and processes in *real time*. If an impromptu simulation pulls clinical staff away from actual patient care, the team can examine safety risks and unintended consequences. But, without preparation beforehand or time to debrief, the learning potential may be diminished. By reviewing goals, creating a safe learning environment, and maintaining a clear agenda, a facilitator can mitigate feelings of resentment due to the disruption to the work day. This can prevent development of poor attitudes towards in situ simulation.

Target objectives and learners inform the mechanism by which performance will be measured and how feedback is provided. If the target learner is the participating healthcare team, a verbal and/or written summary may be sufficient to reinforce learning objectives. There are multiple teamwork assessment tools available in the literature that may be useful. If the target learners are enterprise-wide leadership, a formal written summary of findings and a reporting system may be required for dissemination. Regardless of the system, identified deficiencies and mitigation strategies should be provided to stakeholders in a timely fashion.

The In Situ Simulation Educator

"The key factor to success lies less so in the site or technology delivered, but in the faculty that deliver it" [25]. In situ simulation educators will encounter challenges with scheduling interprofessional teams, frequent distractions, last-minute room and staff cancellations, and missing or malfunctioning equipment. These can provide unexpected learning opportunities that can complement or compete with target goals. Facilitators need to be resilient to this lack of consistency and innovative in adjusting learning objectives to the changing learning environment [4]. Educators need to be able to debrief an interprofessional and multidisciplinary team with learners of various subspecialty training and experience levels while concurrently identifying latent safety threats and opportunities for system-level improvement. Balancing these in situ challenges may require a different skill set than at a simulation center, and it has been suggested that faculty development specific to in situ simulation may be helpful [22].

Multi-institutional Mobile Simulation

Community hospitals in some regions and countries have limited access to simulation-based education and team training. Mobile simulation has the potential to inspire interest in simulation, patient safety issues, and cultural change in these institutions. It offers the opportunity to bring simulation and team training to a wide range of healthcare providers in their own clinical environment. This can promote direct translation of lessons learned during simulation to the local environment, including individual knowledge and skill, teamwork and human resources, patient care systems and supports, and physical space and equipment.

Multi-institutional mobile simulation is both resource and labor-intensive. Outreach education may need to occur over the course of one to several days in order to accomplish desired objectives. Multi-institutional mobile simulation educators are challenged with conducting training in an unfamiliar environment and with participants who may be entirely unacquainted with simulation-based education. The facilitator team needs to be flexible, adapting scenarios and learning objectives to the in situ environment promptly, particularly if the medical setting and team composition is different than

anticipated or unforeseeable safety issues appear. Table 12.1 lists some common complications and recommended solutions for mobile simulation.

Clear communication and extensive advance planning with the host institution to determine their specific needs and set expectations is essential to create a safe environment for conducting a successful experience. Helpful information to exchange includes: (1) learning objectives and opportunities of in situ training including identification of latent safety threats; (2) the size of the simulation team and equipment storage needs; (3) the time frame including setup and dismantling of equipment, (4) course schedule; (5) multidisciplinary team composition and number of participants; (6) requirements for clinical space and use of real medical equipment.

It is essential to engage stakeholders for input. Consider creating a common curriculum that meets the needs of multiple institutions, which can promote consistency between and predictability for educators and stakeholders. This organization can help create additional benefits such as attaining continuing education credits for various professional organizations.

In addition, carefully consider the participants and their native teams. The format of the simulations may need to change from institution to institution, to reflect their healthcare teams. One institution may have a team of ten people; another may be limited to only two or three. Creativity regarding the format of the simulations (e.g., one simulation with observers vs. multiple smaller rotating simulations) will have dramatic effects on both the participants' experience as well as the number of educators and patient care spaces, which are required.

Figure 12.3 shows the extent of equipment required for transport to an institution for a successful mobile simulation. Figures 12.4 and 12.5 show a mobile simulation unit that has been modified to accept the in situ stretcher from Fig. 12.2, as well as the team that will perform the training. There should always be an opportunity for the institution to address questions and concerns with the simulation team. The more information the simulation team has obtained in advance, the fewer unexpected distractions will occur during the training.

Conclusions

In situ and mobile simulations allow participants to experience and examine their native work environment. Target learners can include the individual and team, as is common in center-based simulation, or extend to the hospital unit or an organization as a whole. In situ offers the unique ability to explore complex systems and interrelationships, at all levels of the healthcare delivery process.

Table 12.1 Multi-institutional mobile simulation: lessons learned

Potential obstacle	Recommendations
People	
Difficulty coordinating staff at outside institution	Identify both nursing and physician contacts and provide detailed communication to them
	Obtain participants' e-mail or contact information and directly provide schedules and prebrief to them
Participants unfamiliar with simulation training	E-mail prebrief, which includes explanation and expectations for the day
	Do not use unannounced simulation session for initial exposure
Participant performance anxiety	Provide a verbal prebrief before starting simulations to explain the safe learning environment and purpose of the training
	Ensure local press or leadership does not unexpectedly come to observe without notice
	Keep initial debriefing focused at the team and system level before addressing an individual's performance
Trainees are unmotivated to participate in simulation and debriefing	Identify a local champion to advertise your visit and role model enthusiastic behavior during the sessions
	Consider using the "Rapid Cycle Deliberate Practice" approach to encourage participation in groups that need *warming up* to simulation
Underestimated size of simulation team needed	Ideally requires at least two facilitators or facilitator and technician. To minimize participant down time, bring enough staff to set up/clean up for next simulation while participants are being debriefed
	Can enlist additional help from hosting facility
Equipment/devices	
Audiovisual (AV) system is not wireless but video debriefing is desired	Verify with host institution the maximum distance between simulation and debriefing rooms
	Arrange for AV staff at host facility to be available to help if needed
Storage of simulation equipment if training is > 1 day	Secure storage area of sufficient size needs to be pre-arranged
	A local responsible person should be named
Host institution did not account for set-up and tear down time	Prewarn that mobile simulation team may need up to 3 h on site before the training starts and 1–2 h after training for tear down
	Clinical simulation space needs to be reserved
Equipment unexpectedly malfunctions or is missing	Bring replacements or repair tools for critical items
	Create checklist of critical items and quantity needed
	Prepare a back-up simulation plan
Institution refuses to use real medical equipment	Ask institution to create a similar crash cart using simulation training equipment or bring a simulated crash cart (or at least contents)
	Double-check similarity before training
Host site promised to provide equipment but it does not show up and no one is aware of the request	Verify equipment needed with on-site contact the day prior to training
	Bring replacements/substitutes for critical items

Table 12.1 (continued)

Potential obstacle	Recommendations
A real patient emergency occurs during the training session	If you are using host site's real medical equipment, alternative crash carts and clinical equipment need to be determined beforehand
	Ensure the entire healthcare team is aware of the plan
Real medical equipment and simulation equipment could be merged after training	A local responsible person should be named to check the medical equipment
Specific adapters required to use local defibrillator with the mannequin	Pre-check the type of defibrillator with the institution
The *simulated* patient care room has no compressed air supply	Pre-check with the institution if a compressor is needed
Facility/space	
Physical space for simulation session is unknown to your team	If possible, perform a site inspection prior to the simulation date or allow time to orient to the local environment and medical equipment before simulation. A standardized approach using a checklist may be useful. LSTs may be uncovered in advance
	Ask host site to send pictures or video of the simulation space
	Provide host site with a schematic of your room needs (simulation and debrief space, lecture room, storage)
	Perform a rehearsal after setting up simulation equipment but before educational session
Did not consider logistics of parking and equipment unloading/loading	Arrange all logistics beforehand (equipment transport vehicle, hotel rooms, meals, infection control in operating rooms, etc.)
In situ simulation space is limited or unexpectedly occupied for patient care	Be creative in finding in situ simulation space: bathroom, treatment rooms, nursing station, etc. And debriefing rooms: parent consultation rooms, balconies, staff room, etc.
	A back-up room plan should be prearranged
System/cultural	
Parents might be intimidated by noise and action	Prebrief parents and display an information sheet at the unit
Significant LSTs were discovered but not remediated	Contact host institution's key stake holders, particularly from quality improvement or patient safety departments, and request their involvement during the simulation day
	Take pictures of faulty equipment or physical layout to include in the follow-up report

LSTs latent safety threats

Fig. 12.3 Equipment needed to provide a comprehensive multi-institutional mobile simulation. **a** Packed and ready for transport. **b** During unpacking and setting up. (Photo courtesy of PAEDSIM e.V., Germany)

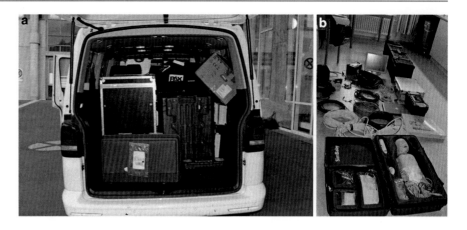

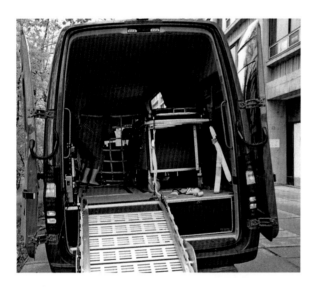

Fig. 12.4 Example of a *mobile simulation unit* modified to accommodate the in situ stretcher from Fig. 12.2. (Photo courtesy of eSIM Provincial Simulation Program, Albert Health Services)

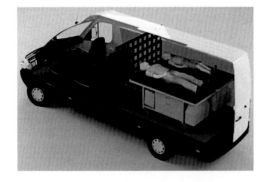

Fig. 12.5 Schematic of the *mobile simulation unit* shown in Fig. 12.4 is designed to accommodate stretchers, simulation equipment, clinical equipment, and the education team that will perform the training. (Photo courtesy of eSIM Provincial Simulation Program, Albert Health Services)

References

1. Hays RT, Singer MJ. Simulation fidelity in training system design: bridging the gap between reality and training. New York: Springer-Verlag; 1988.
2. Allan CK, Thiagarajan RR, Beke D, Imprescia A, Kappus LJ, Garden A, et al. Simulation-based training delivered directly to the pediatric cardiac intensive care unit engenders preparedness, comfort and decreased anxiety among multidisciplinary resuscitation teams. J Thorac Cardiovasc Surg. 2010;140(3):646–52.
3. Weinstock PH, Kappus LJ, Garden A, Burns JP. Simulation at the point of care: reduced-cost, in situ training via a mobile cart. Pediatr Crit Care Med. 2009;10:176–81.
4. Clapper TC. In situ and mobile simulation: lessons learned… authentic and resource intensive. Clin Simul Nurs. 2013;9(11):e551–7.
5. Calhoun AW, Boone MC, Peterson EB, Boland KA, Montgomery VL. Integrated in-situ simulation using redirected faculty educational time to minimize costs: a feasibility study. Simul Healthc. 2011;6:337–44.
6. Patterson MD, Blike GT, Nadkarni VM. In situ simulation: challenges and results. In: Henriksen K, Battles JB, Keyes MA, et al., editors. Advances in patient safety: new directions and alternative approaches (Vol. 3: Performance and tools). Rockville: Agency for healthcare research and quality (US); 2008. http://www.ncbi.nlm.nih.gov/books/NBK43682/.
7. Raemer DB. Ignaz Semmelweis Redux? Simul Healthc. 2014;9:153–5.
8. Kobayashi L, Patterson MD, Overly FL, Shapiro MJ, Williams KA, Jay GD. Educational and research implications of portable human patient simulation in acute care medicine. Acad Emerg Med. 2008;15:1166–74.
9. Miller KK, Riley W, Davis S, Hansen HE. In situ simulation: a method of experiential learning to promote safety and team behavior. J Perinat Neonatal Nurs. 2008;22(2):105–13.
10. Wheeler DS, Geis G, Mack EH, LeMaster T, Patterson MD. High-reliability emergency response teams in the hospital: improving quality and safety using in situ simulation training. BMJ Qual Saf. 2013;22:507–14.
11. Theilen U, Leonard P, Jones P, Ardill R, Weitz J, Agrawal D, Simpson D. Regular in situ simulation training of paediatric medical emergency team improves hospital response to deteriorating patients. Resuscitation. 2013;84(2):218–22.
12. Andreatta P, Saxton E, Thompson M, Annich G. Simulation-based mock codes significantly correlate with improved pediatric patient cardiopulmonary arrest survival rates. Pediatr Crit Care Med. 2011;12(1):33–7.

13. Steinemann S, Berg B, Skinner A, DiTulio A, Anzelon K, Terada K, et al. In situ, multidisciplinary, simulation-based teamwork training improves early trauma care. J Surg Educ. 2011;68(6):472–7.

14. Miller D, Crandall C, Washington C, McLaughlin S. Improving teamwork and communication in trauma care through in situ simulations. Acad Emerg Med. 2012;19(5):608–12.

15. Patterson MD, Geis GL, Falcone RA, LeMaster T, Wears RL. In situ simulation: detection of safety threats and teamwork training in a high risk emergency department. BMJ Qual Saf. 2013;22:468–77.

16. Wetzel EA, Lang TR, Pendegrass TL, Taylor RG, Geis GL. Identification of latent safety threats using high-fidelity simulation-based training with multidisciplinary neonatology teams. Jt Comm J Qual Patient Saf. 2013;39(6):268–73.

17. Kobayashi L, Shapiro MJ, Sucov A, Woolard R, Boss RM 3rd, Dunbar J, et al. Portable advanced medical simulation for new emergency department testing and orientation. Acad Emerg Med. 2006;13(6):691–5.

18. Geis GL, Pio B, Pendergrass TL, Moyer MR, Patterson MD. Simulation to assess the safety of new healthcare teams and new facilities. Simul Healthc. 2011;6(3):125–33.

19. Guise JM, Mladenovic J. In situ simulation: identification of systems issues. Semin Perinatol. 2013;37(3):161–5.

20. O'Leary F, McGarvey K, Christoff A, Major J, Lockie F, Chayen G, et al. Identifying incidents of suboptimal care during pediatric emergencies—an observational study utilizing in situ and simulation center scenarios. Resuscitation. 2014;85:431–6.

21. Groom JA. Creating new solutions to the simulation puzzle. Simul Healthc. 2009;4(3):131–4.

22. Rosen MA, Hunt EA, Pronovost PJ, Federowicz MA, Weaver SJ. In situ simulation in continuing education for the health care professions: a systematic review. J Contin Educ Health Prof. 2012;32(4):243–54.

23. Niles D, Sutton RM, Donoghue A, Kalsi MS, Roberts K, Boyle L, et al. "Rolling Refreshers": a novel approach to maintain CPR psychomotor skill competence. Resuscitation. 2009;80:909–12.

24. Hunt EA, Duval-Arnould JM, Nelson-McMillan KL, Bradshaw JH, Diener-West M, Perretta JS, et al. Pediatric resident resuscitation skills improve after "rapid cycle deliberate practice" training. Resuscitation. 2014;85:945–51.

25. Weinstock P. Weathering the perfect storm: a deeper look at simulation applied to pediatric critical care. Pediatr Crit Care Med. 2012;13(2):226–7.

Simulation Along the Pediatric Healthcare Education Continuum

Aaron William Calhoun, Elaine Sigalet, Rebekah Burns and Marc Auerbach

Simulation Pearls

1. The healthcare education process spans a wide continuum, with each phase possessing unique characteristics and challenges.
2. Simulation has been demonstrated to be an effective tool for addressing the challenges at each level of the healthcare education continuum, including the teaching of basic knowledge, teamwork, procedural skills, attitudes, and team performance constructs such as communication skills.
3. Simulation is an ideal venue for introducing stakeholders to the concept of interprofessional (IP) education. It provides an opportunity for them to learn from, with, and about each other as they learn to work effectively together to manage pediatric illness.
4. Future developments in simulation across the healthcare education continuum should focus on improving learner transitions between educational phases.

A. W. Calhoun (✉)
Department of Pediatrics, Division of Critical Care, University of Louisville School of Medicine, Kosair Children's Hospital, Louisville, KY, USA
e-mail: Aaron.calhoun@louisville.edu

E. Sigalet
Department of Education, Sidra Research and Medical Center, Doha, Qatar
e-mail: esigalet@sidra.org

R. Burns
Department of Pediatrics, Division of Emergency Medicine, University of Washington School of Medicine, Seattle, WA, USA
e-mail: Rebekah.burns@seattlechildrens.org

M. Auerbach
Department of Pediatrics, Section of Emergency Medicine, Yale University School of Medicine, New Haven, CT, USA
e-mail: marc.auerbach@yale.edu

Introduction

Educational needs change considerably as learners progress from undergraduate to graduate educational environments and then from graduate to the ongoing professional education that occurs during clinical practice. Despite advances in curricula design and instructional methods, medical, nursing, and other students in healthcare programs perform a significant fraction of their education in preclinical settings using didactic sessions, small group discussions, and problem-based learning to acquire and master new knowledge and skills. As they graduate, however, this environment changes. At this phase, emphasis is on delivery of care in an IP context, but given the pace at which new knowledge is generated, ongoing educational processes are still needed to assure that practitioners can maintain a current knowledge base and skill set. While clinicians often rely on conferences and other continuing professional development (CPD) activities for this education, studies indicate that these methods often have little impact [1].

Medical students are required to go through an additional transitional phase of residency (and possibly fellowship education) that exists between these two environments. Increased supervision and decreased autonomy, however, may lead to residents feeling unprepared for the transition to independent practice [2]. Furthermore, in the graduate medical environment, they experience more stringent time constraints due to both the demands of clinical practice and government mandate while still being expected to maintain their role as learners [3]. Scheduling issues may become even more a barrier as graduates transition into the independent practitioner role. Salient differences between these environments are graphically depicted in Fig. 13.1.

Given these challenges, technology-enhanced educational modalities, such as e-learning and simulation, are being increasingly relied upon to assist learners in transitioning between these environments [4]. In particular, simulation-based educational methodologies have been utilized across the spectrum of medical education [3, 5]. In this chapter,

© Springer International Publishing Switzerland 2016
V. J. Grant, A. Cheng (eds.), *Comprehensive Healthcare Simulation: Pediatrics*,
Comprehensive Healthcare Simulation, DOI 10.1007/978-3-319-24187-6_13

Fig. 13.1 The spectrum of educational environments in health care. This figure depicts the relationships between educational and clinical time within the undergraduate, graduate, and continuing professional development environments. As learners progress from preclinical education to graduate education and finally to practice, the relative balance between educational and clinical time shifts substantially. Common educational methodologies used in each phase have been included.

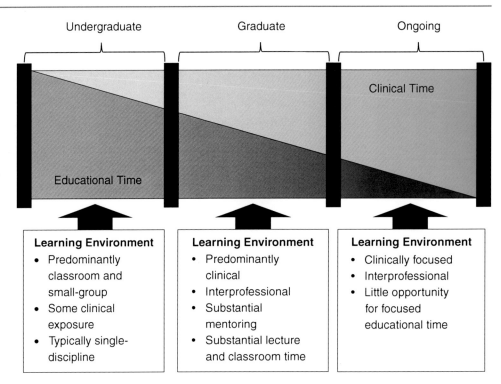

we describe the use of simulation to address the educational needs of diverse groups of learners and the science behind the implementation of various strategies in the hopes of allowing educators to more effectively engage with their learners.

The structure of the chapter includes a discussion of:

- Pediatric simulation in undergraduate education
- Pediatric simulation in graduate medical education
- Pediatric simulation in CPD
- Pediatric IP simulation across the education continuum
- A consideration of the research needs and future pedagogical directions of simulation-based education (SBE) across the healthcare education continuum

Initial discussion in each area will focus on both the *science of simulation* as it has been applied to the specific problems inherent to each level of education. We will then discuss *program implementation,* both within and across these domains. It is our hope that this chapter will inform readers as to what is known and enhance their ability to address educational issues that transcend the domains presented.

Undergraduate Education

The paradigm shift in undergraduate health professional education from a traditional apprenticeship model to a competency-based model has led to many programs integrating the basic sciences with clinical sciences early in training [6]. As a result, students must be prepared to interact in the clinical environment at an earlier phase in their training. Programs are accountable for this change and need to ensure that new curricula are designed to address these goals. Educators must

understand the theory of skill acquisition so they can develop learning objectives appropriate to novices. In particular, students require earlier experience with deliberate practice. Deliberate practice, or mastery-based learning theory, refers to an instructional method where learners continue to rehearse the application of knowledge or a specific task in a mentored setting until mastery is achieved [7]. Simulation potentiates this technique by providing a standardized educational environment where the skill in question can be practiced as many times as the learner's assigned educational time and need allows. Deliberate practice-based simulations require students to be attentive, reflect on performance, and repeat actions until they feel confident and demonstrate a specified level of competence [8]. This design gives students the opportunity to increase their confidence and level of competency before being asked to interact with real patients.

SBE also facilitates planned experiences to support curriculum delivery via timely exposure, in a controlled educational environment, and with enhanced mechanisms for student feedback [9]. This approach gives learners an opportunity to experiment with clinical practice, facilitating conceptualization of principles supporting best practice in healthcare delivery [10]. The element of facilitator control is an important facet of SBE. Educators make decisions about what type of experiences will support the learning objectives and the required level of complexity to facilitate learning for a specific group or individual [9]. This approach can move the learner along the continuum of competency from entry to graduation in a more efficient manner by creating a bridge between classroom learning and the clinical environment without creating risk to real patients and families [11].

State of the Science

The past four decades have seen an explosion of publications in SBE, from two publications in 1972 to almost 1200 publications today [12, 13]. Most of the literature focuses on undergraduate medical and nursing education, though a limited number of articles exist providing scientific support for the effective use of simulation in the education of allied health professions such as physiotherapy and pharmacy [14, 15]. This suggests that institutions, faculty, and stakeholders are committing resources to simulation in undergraduate health professional education. The majority of these studies focus on curriculum development, assessment, and strategies for addressing technical skill acquisition. In a recent systematic review, 19 studies noteworthy for the rigor of their research designs were identified [16]. The majority of these studies focused on technical skills, with three also addressing nontechnical skills [17–19]. In all but one study, assessment of the curricula supported an increase in student knowledge [16]. Only one of these studies, however, focused on the technical skill needed to effectively manage pediatric illnesses [19]. Unfortunately, little research has examined skill transfer to actual patient care in medical education. However, in undergraduate nursing education there is good evidence to support the efficacy of curricula that transfers to clinical practice. Noteworthy is a recently published study that examined the impact of replacing a percentage of clinical practice with SBE. Results show that SBE can replace up to 50 % of clinical practice in North America in undergraduate nursing programs with no significant impact on student performance as measured by the national nursing exam scores (national council licensure examination, NCLEX). Importantly, there was no adverse effect on the transition to real practice settings measured at 6 months after graduation [20]. This is the first known study to achieve this level of outcome in undergraduate SBE. In addition to knowledge and procedural skills, critical thinking may be improved with SBE. Although there are few studies that evaluate the effectiveness of this approach, what can be found is encouraging. One study of 237 nursing students noted a significant improvement in critical thinking after engagement with simulation-based coursework [21].

Simulation may also overcome barriers to engagement that can be experienced when educational programs are overly reliant on didactic teaching and assessment of knowledge. A study examining perceptions of traditional medical education curricula uncovered that many students feel checked out or intellectually disengaged in classroom sessions and believe that their time was better spent memorizing knowledge for an upcoming test [22]. This suggests that some programs are still reliant on knowledge-based assessments and may need a greater focus on the application of knowledge to adequately prepare undergraduate students for the demands of the clinical environment. A number of studies in the field of undergraduate nursing education also support this. A recent meta-analysis in undergraduate nursing education demonstrated the effectiveness of SBE in improving attitudes, knowledge, and skills, as well as the application of these to actual practice [23]. The study did reveal, however, that there is a paucity of pediatric focused simulation-based curricula.

Overall, the existing literature supports the use of carefully constructed simulation-based educational opportunities in the preparation of students for the demands of real practice, and that these interventions can result in good knowledge transfer to the real environment. Given that required clinical rotations often reach capacity, particularly for nursing students, simulation appears to offer a viable alternative for undergraduate learners [24].

Program Implementation

As is evident from the breadth of the literature discussed above, simulation-based programs have already found widespread acceptance in the undergraduate nursing and medicine contexts. In 2011, the Association of American Medical Colleges conducted a survey on the prevalence of simulation at the medical school level [25]. According to this study, 92 % of participating medical schools used simulation in some way, and 86 % of associated teaching hospitals also used simulation. This finding is also supported by a national survey of pediatric clerkship directors completed in 2012 [26]. In this study, 89 % of 72 responding clerkship directors reported using simulation in some form. These surveys indicate that SBE has already achieved an overwhelming prevalence at the undergraduate level, and mastering this means of delivering educational curricula will likely continue to pay dividends well into the future.

When incorporating simulation into undergraduate education, it is important to follow established steps in curricula design [9]. The first step is problem identification. Who are the learners (profession, phase in training program, and current level of experience) and what do the learners need to know and do? Step two is a needs analysis. Are there specific needs of the learners that you need to understand before developing learning objectives? In step three, learning objectives are developed based on information from the needs analysis or educational program leaders. Objectives should challenge the learner's cognitive entry behaviors but not overwhelm the learner. Engaging simulation as a learning modality is appropriate when the learner achievement of the learning objectives would benefit from deliberate practice or the theory of experiential learning. Scenario development is the curriculum content, the first step of the educational strategy detailed in step four. For less experienced learners, a simpler scenario intended to teach basic paradigms of care in a distraction-free environment may be best. Although high environmental fidelity is often held out as the ideal, this must be balanced with the increased cognitive load produced by such environments. Excessive cognitive load has been associated with diminished retention of knowledge (Chap. 1) [27]. For more experienced learners, however, higher environmental fidelity may be desired, as this will allow for a more realistic experience that may translate more readily to the clinical environment. Additionally, in this phase it is necessary to be sure that adequate personnel, equipment, and space exists to efficiently move the large groups of learners through their required coursework. Step five is implementation. A related consideration is how far the case should progress toward a negative outcome, as a number of recent articles have been published focusing on emotionally difficult scenarios that suggest mitigating the impact of these cases to undergraduate learners may be best [28–31]. The last step is feedback and evaluation. Faculty need to make a judgment about the efficacy of the curriculum. Did the learners achieve the learning objectives and if not, why not? This information should be used to revise the curriculum before delivering it to another cohort of learners. Stand-alone simulation centers, unless directly associated with the academic training center, provide capacity for engaging simulation; however, there are usually financial implications for the program that must be planned for in the early phases of curricula design.

Postgraduate Education

The application of simulation-based educational methodologies to pediatric postgraduate training has been widespread, and, correspondingly, has produced a robust literature [32]. One telling study sought to quantify the number of pediatric emergency medicine programs that incorporated high-fidelity simulation into their routine training activities. A total of 66 programs throughout the USA and Canada were surveyed. Of the 51 programs that responded, 63 % were using high-fidelity simulation to teach a broad array of skills including management of medical emergencies, procedural skills, and medical decision-making [33]. The past decades have also seen the development of simulation *boot camps* designed to train incoming interns and fellows in an attempt to avoid the July effect, seen as novice trainees begin to fill new patient care roles [34]. Programs of this nature have been described for internal medicine and pediatric critical care medicine [34, 35]. They have been shown to be logically feasible and to result in improved clinical performance and trainee confidence [34].

State of the Science

A number of publications focus on the application of high-fidelity simulation to resuscitation training. This is not surprising, given the roots in airline crew resource management and the correlation between the skills needed in that environment with those required during a medical crisis (Chap. 4) [36]. Studies have demonstrated the positive effect of simulation training on team performance, timeliness of essential procedures, resuscitation team self-perception and confidence, and hospital survival rates for pediatric arrests [37–39]. Several studies have also addressed the addition of a deliberate practice educational methodology to team training [38, 40]. This technique has been used to good effect in simulated environments and should be strongly considered when developing curricula. [35, 40–42].

Another area in which simulation has found particular applicability to postgraduate pediatric education is in the domain of procedural skills (see Chap. 11) and sedation. Given current work-hour restrictions, it is becoming increasingly difficult for pediatric residents to obtain adequate practice with crucial procedures [43–45]. Simulation is becoming a growing modality used to fill this gap [46]. One common procedure that has been extensively studied is lumbar puncture (LP), with data suggesting that performance skills can be significantly improved using simulation-based training methodologies, though it is less clear how many sessions are needed to effect this change [47–49]. LP skills have also been shown to transfer between the simulated and real environments [49]. Another procedure that has been extensively investigated is endotracheal intubation, a procedure that is both critical and high risk. Simulation-based training has been demonstrated to significantly improve airway team interpersonal interactions, intubation success rates, and to decrease time to successful intubation among trainees [50–52]. Unlike LP, however, the literature on skill transfer is mixed [52, 53].

Finally, a number of publications have addressed the area of communication skills training in pediatrics (see Chap. 23). Skills that have been taught in the postgraduate environment using simulation include the delivery of difficult news, communication surrounding medical error, and conflict resolution both within the medical team and between the team and patient family members [54–61]. While some of these studies are descriptive in nature, many have shown positive improvements in learner confidence, perceived skill, and qualitative measures of emerging conversational themes that could be traced to the intervention [54, 58, 60]. IP team communication in graduate medical education has also been addressed using simulation. In particular, crisis team communication and communication regarding errors have been addressed [28, 38, 62]. Some factors, such as the effect of hierarchy and authority gradients on medical errors during crises, can be difficult to address without recourse to medical simulation [28, 62].

Program Implementation

It is clear that a great deal of research has been performed with regard to graduate level simulation in pediatrics, with value demonstrated in a myriad of ways. Still, the practical issues of how such a program can be implemented remain. Many graduate level simulation programs opt to use a freestanding simulation center affiliated with their institution, and, if such is available, this can be an excellent approach. If, however, such a program is not available, or is available but requires a prohibitive transit time, then other options exist. One technique is the creation of an in-hospital simulation suite [63, 64]. Such an approach has been successfully adopted by a number of institutions, and requires the conversion of one or more clinical beds into part-time or full-time simulation spaces. While still potentially costly, this approach effectively removes the distance issue from the equation. Having a simulation program on-site can significantly enhance the ease at which IP activities can be conducted, as it is often much more difficult to free nursing staff from clinical duties than it is to generate resident educational time [63, 64]. One exemplar program that has adopted this strategy reported an initial construction cost of $290,000, and ongoing costs of approximately $67,875 per year [63].

As space is at a premium in many hospitals such a strategy may not work at many institutions. For those in this situation, adopting an *in situ* approach may be the most cost and space effective. In situ simulation refers to the use of simulation equipment in functional clinical space to achieve an impromptu educational environment (see Chap. 12) [65]. While sometimes used in an unannounced fashion to perform systems testing, it is also possible to use in situ methodology to develop graduate level simulation programs that require no permanent educational space. Using this approach, simulators are placed on mobile carts that allow for easy transport to different clinical domains, and sessions are scheduled based on predicted space availability [64, 66]. Such programs are often more cost-effective as there is no need for large-scale infrastructure. One program reported an initial startup cost of $128,921, and ongoing yearly costs of $11,695 for the first 2 years of operation [64]. Current operational data shows that this program presently conducts approximately 360–370 simulation sessions per year with 440–420 education hours provided. In situ programs do have their limitation, such as the possibility of session cancellation due to capacity issues necessitating the need to identify backup spaces in which to conduct simulations. Still, this approach offers a means by which graduate medical programs with little space and financial support can conduct SBE. Table 13.1 depicts the strengths and weaknesses of each approach.

At present, curricula are frequently developed locally, which can lead to significant divergence and a concurrent need for standardization. Here, reference to national guidelines such as the Accreditation Council for Graduate Medical Education Milestones Project (in the USA), can be of use, as these provide a global framework to which curricula can adhere [67]. Despite this anchor, however, the temptation will always be present to develop material without reference

Table 13.1 A comparison of different approaches to graduate medical simulation

	Off-site simulation center	On-site simulation center	In situ program
Benefits	Resource-rich	Lack of transit time makes learner attendance easier	Lower startup and ongoing costs
	Often easy to schedule sessions	Easy scheduling	Lack of transit time makes learner attendance easier
	Low cancellation rate	Easy to organize interprofessional sessions	Easy to organize interprofessional sessions
	Ease of audiovisual recording	Low cancellation rate	High environmental fidelity
		Possible ease of audiovisual recording (site-specific)	
Drawbacks	Location and resulting transit time can make attendance difficult	Costly to build and maintain	Higher cancellation rate due to lack of required space
	Can be difficult to organize interprofessional sessions	Requires adequate clinical space	Higher cancellation rates due to competing clinical demands
	Costly to build and maintain		Dependence of audiovisual recording on portable devices
	Lower environmental fidelity		

This table lists the strengths and benefits of different simulation program operational structures as they pertain to graduate level simulation. Off-site and on-site simulation centers as well as in situ approaches are included to the strategies other institutions have used to approach the same issues. Overcoming this will require deliberate collaboration among educators during all phases of curriculum design as well as thorough searches of the literature to uncover existing curricula that could be built upon. To that end, we have cited here a number of published curricula for this purpose [4, 35, 68–70].

An additional consideration for standardization is that of outcome assessment, as different curricula often focus on different primary educational outcomes. While this is often unavoidable, defining similar outcomes in a more cohesive manner would improve inter-curricular crosstalk and allow for a more transferable understanding of a given learner's or team's skillset. With this in mind, a group of educators have embarked on the development of simulation data registry with standardization of case outcomes as a primary goal [71]. Though this is a pilot effort at present, we are enthusiastic that this could represent a move toward a more cohesive inter-programmatic approach.

Continuing Professional Development

CPD programs, such as continuing medical education, traditionally utilize didactic conferences or self-guided reading with multiple-choice questions. Participation in CPD is a component of lifelong learning and is often required for maintenance of certification and/or licensure in one's profession, such as pediatric medicine, nursing, or other related subspecialties. While most simulation-based educational techniques and technology have historically been used to target undergraduate and graduate learners, their use in CPD is increasing. Simulation interventions also offer the ability to explicitly utilize IP approaches that engage participants across specialties and along the continuum of training. Additionally, computer-based simulation and e-learning has grown exponentially in the past decade through the adoption of online learning management systems at academic medical centers as part of the accreditation process [72]. These programs are leveraging web-based and experiential learning theory to provide ongoing education to their members.

Continuing education can involve the application of simulation for both formative and summative assessment. In professional situations such as this, the consequences of assessment are greater (perhaps even involving maintenance of licensure and credentialing) and thus require a significantly higher level of evidence for validity than at the undergraduate or graduate level. For further discussion on the process needed to obtain this level of validity, please refer to the chapter on assessment (Chap. 7). A number of pediatric certifying bodies are utilizing simulation-based techniques including the American Heart Association (AHA) through its Basic Life Support and Pediatric Advanced Life Sup-

port programs, the American Academy of Pediatrics, and the American College of Surgeons [73–75]. While, at present, the American Board of Pediatrics has not tied maintenance of certification to simulation-based training, pediatrics is likely to follow fields such as anesthesia, surgery, and family medicine in offering simulation-based options for this process [75–81].

State of the Science

Few studies have compared the use of simulation for CPD to traditional didactic or reading programs. A recent systematic review examined the effectiveness of SBE on independently practicing acutecare physicians. This comprehensive review reported on 30 studies that utilized simulation as an educational intervention and found that a majority reported increases in self-confidence and/or knowledge or skill performance afterwards. Most studies where quasi-experimental and used single group designs with pre–post repeated measures, and very few randomized clinical trials were reported [82]. In a meta-analysis of research pertaining to pediatric simulation, only 11 articles reported on physician CPD programs (along with an additional, unspecified number of studies pertaining to nursing CPD), and many also included data on undergraduate and graduate medical education [83]. The outcomes reported were largely knowledge, resuscitation, and procedural skills based. The summary data for pediatric simulation-based educational research involving physicians in practice included seven studies with a total of 490 participants and demonstrated a standardized mean difference effect size of 0.75, much lower than those seen for undergraduate and graduate level studies.

Individual studies have sought to evaluate the effect of SBE on communication and procedural skills. Neonatology research has reported improvements in practicing physicians' teamwork, communication, and psychomotor skills after participation in simulation [84–87]. Similar results were seen in studies involving practicing pediatric intensivists [88–90]. Simulation has been applied to teach and assess physicians in the novel technique of ultrasound-guided nerve blocks in pediatric emergency medicine [91]. It has also been successfully used to teach trauma team management and pain management within the emergency department [92–94]. While many of these studies included graduate-level learners, the data obtained from them should be easily translatable into pure CPD education environments. Two studies exclusively assessing CPD showed positive results [95, 96]. One found that physicians and clinic staff felt more confident in performing resuscitation skills after simulation training, while the other demonstrated improved laparoscopic skills in surgeons with limited preceding experience. Another study demonstrated that the use of *just-in-time* training before cardiopulmonary resuscitation performance improved provider's performance, supporting the contention that more intermittent, shorter duration programs can have a positive effect [97]. Such programs may be easier and more time-efficient to provide in many professional environments. Under the wider umbrella of CPD, the Helping Babies Breathe program has been successful in using simulation to improve practicing healthcare provider resuscitation skills and patient outcomes in Africa and India [98, 99]. Despite the relative lack of CPD-specific studies, this field has the potential to generate higher level outcomes data than undergraduate and graduate level of studies due to the longitudinal nature of such programs and the availability of more data regarding unsupervised practitioner performance and actual patient outcomes.

Program Implementation

In situ simulation is currently being integrated into a number of CPD programs as a key component. There are several institutions at which a minimum number of simulations are required to maintain privileges or are used to incentivize malpractice programs [100, 101]. The use of in situ simulation as a safety intervention is discussed in detail in Chap. 5. Programs such as these, however, can also have an educational impact at the provider level [102]. In situ simulation also has the benefit of providing IP CPD in the workplace to frontline providers. The location of the intervention may have a significant impact on faculty participation as these practitioners have a higher cost associated with their time and may find it logistically difficult to be pulled away from clinical duties. The strategy of workplace-based training has also been effectively implemented in a number of Children's Hospitals as part of ongoing in situ simulations (Chap. 12).

Interprofessional Simulation Across the Healthcare Education Continuum

While simulation has been used to effectively address the educational needs within each phase of training in a myriad of ways, it has less often addressed the transition between these domains. The transition between medical school and residency, or between nursing school and clinical practice, comes with many abrupt changes. IP SBE is strongly endorsed in all professions, yet there remains a paucity of evidence to support its integration into the various phases of the health professional education continuum (Chap. 15) [25].

In order to successfully develop and integrate IP simulation-based curricula, there needs to be some shared understanding of team performance concepts, an understanding of the dose-dependency between exposure to a curriculum and

learner outcomes, and defined levels of competency required for the learner to progress. IP SBE is grounded by contact theory, the need for a purposeful and controlled learning experience, and the constructs of effective teamwork to optimize patient safety [103–106]. Intergroup contact theory identifies the importance of leveling hierarchies, articulating common goals, and creating opportunities for intergroup cooperation as powerful moderators of effective group function [105]. Translated to health professional education, it reinforces the importance of creating opportunities for healthcare professionals to learn about each other, from each other, and with each other as they acquire the knowledge and skill necessary to work effectively in a team context [107]. The value of simulation for providing a realistic clinical context whilst integrating a purposeful and controlled curriculum has already been discussed. Evidence to support the relationship between patient safety and effective team performance continues to expose communication as a contributing element [103]. Additionally, there is evidence to support a correlation between a higher level of group culture and higher levels of patient safety, again contributing to the science behind IP SBE [108].

In the undergraduate environment, contact with other allied healthcare professionals is at a minimum. Then, almost overnight, the new graduate must learn to navigate the complex IP environment of a modern hospital. This leads to the question of how we can use simulation to better integrate medical and nursing student educational activities in order to optimize this transition.

State of the Science

Undergraduate learners benefit from engaging in a clinical environment early in their training [109]. The use of IP SBE creates another venue to support IP deliberate practice when clinical placements may be challenging to acquire. Additionally, it provides an element of control in the learning experience. A number of studies have been performed to assess the value of IP education, the majority of which involved nursing and medical students in their final year. These studies reported increased learner satisfaction, improved perception of confidence in the team role, and increased awareness of the scope of practice of other professions [110–115]. Several studies have also examined measurements of teamwork after IP SBE with promising results, including one study specifically examining pediatric simulation that found an increase in self-perceived knowledge and skills, communication and teamwork, professional identity and role awareness, and attitudes about shared learning in both participating medical and nursing students [19, 110, 116, 117]. Two preliminary studies examining curriculum design for IP education reported that mixed sessions including didactic components

Fig. 13.2 Breaking down barriers on the educational continuum. This diagram depicts ways in which new developments in simulation-based education can bridge existing educational divisions. Such approaches could provide a more seamless experience as learners advance from novice to practicing professional.

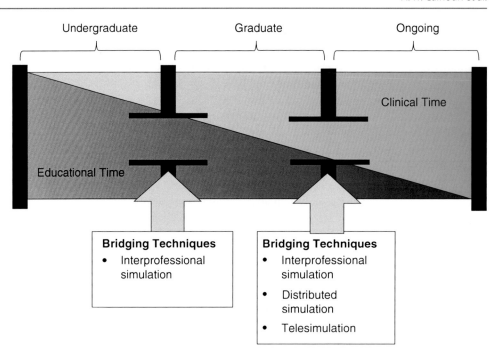

intended to enhance learner knowledge regarding concepts of team performance, expert modeling, and response to hierarchy were associated with higher team performance [115, 118, 119]. Interestingly, a dose-dependency effect was reported in one of the studies in which teams failed to exceed a threshold with complex team performance concepts such as cross-monitoring, situation summaries, and resource utilization. This suggests that educators should initially focus curriculum on simple team performance concepts like role clarity, leadership, and communication [118].

In postgraduate contexts, IP SBE has focused on improving skills inclusive of the ability to improve communication, the enhanced ability to speak up to a physician or other clinician, and the increased ability to assess and manage acute pain [120–122]. The majority of studies focus on effective management of the deteriorating patient in acute care areas such as emergency departments, pediatric cardiac intensive care units, neonatal intensive care units, obstetrical delivery rooms, and the operating room [38, 123–130]. Although reported outcomes are predominantly related to a change in knowledge, skill, and/or behavior, one study was able to demonstrate relevance to real patientclinical outcomes; a decrease in brachial palsy post -shoulder dystocia in neonates after training teams using SBE [131].

Program Implementation

Given that most studies currently address undergraduate and graduate learners, our discussion thus far has focused on these levels only [132]. This approach, however, is being extended to the level of CPD. One organization notable for promoting IP education hosts curricula including student-,

graduate-, and professional-level learners [133]. Another potential benefit of this approach is the ability of IP curricula to offer courses with learners that span stages of training. By creating an environment that promotes discussion and collaboration between student-level and professional-level learners, mentoring relationships could be promoted that could assist learners of all levels in bridging the natural gaps created by the training process. Figure 13.2 illustrates the potential effect of this approach on the continuum of education.

Future Directions

Enhanced Outcome Measures

While much research has been performed on simulation across the educational spectrum, the level of evidence provided by these studies must be addressed. The Kirkpatrick hierarchy is a useful tool to categorize study outcomes [134]. In this system, as applied to medical education, level one evidence corresponds with learner reactions to the educational environment; level two evidence corresponds with measured improvement in knowledge, attitudes, or skills in the educational environment; level three evidence corresponds with an alteration in learner behavior or skill in the actual clinical environment; and level four evidence represents the effect on patient outcomes. See Table 13.2 for further details regarding the adapted Kirkpatrick hierarchy [135].

When assessing simulation-based research using this rubric, it is clear that there is much work yet to be done. In the meta-analysis of pediatric simulation studies cited above, 76 articles were classified by outcome category and the results indicated a historical focus on lower levels of evidence. Over

Table 13.2 Adapted Kirkpatrick hierarchy for evaluating educational outcomes

Evidence level	Target	Outcomes assessed
1	Reaction	Learner's opinions on the educational intervention, its organization, presentation, content, methods, materials, and quality of instruction
2a	Learning: Change in attitudes/perceptions	Change in attitudes/perception deriving from the educational experience
2b	Learning: Change in knowledge or skills	Acquisition of knowledge and/or problem-solving, psychomotor or communication skills
3	Behavior	Transfer of learning to the workplace or willingness to apply new knowledge and skills
4a	Results: Changes in professional practice	Change in organizational practices, delivery of care
4b	Results: Benefit to patients	Improvement in patient health and outcomes

This table delineates levels of evidence within research pertaining to medical education and simulation as classified by the adapted Kirkpatrick hierarchy [135]

95 % of the articles uncovered report only levels one or two evidence. While studies addressing outcomes related to participant opinion of the curriculum and changes in knowledge, attitudes and skills are often useful in a preliminary fashion, more rigorous approaches are needed if we are to clarify the effect of simulation-based educational interventions on provider skills and behaviors with actual patients and the effect of that practice alteration on actual patient outcomes.

Mobile and Distributed Simulation

As the value of simulation throughout the educational spectrum is increasingly recognized, providers and educators may see the need to develop novel approaches to gaining access to technologies and curriculum. One promising development is the use of portable, low-cost simulated environments to bring training to sites currently without simulation capability, an approach often called *distributed simulation*. At present, little literature exists on these modalities, and what is present consists mostly of studies of this approach's feasibility [136–138]. Despite this, distributed simulation has the potential to lower barriers between the academic environments in which most simulation-based training occurs, and the community practice domains in which it is needed [1].

Another innovative means of bridging this gap is telesimulation [139–142]. While distributed simulation takes simulation training materials to community settings, telesimulation utilizes the internet to connect simulators virtually, allowing for the educators at centralized locations to easily share their expertise with more remote sites. Many of the initial studies in this area have focused on resource-restricted countries, but there is no reason why this technique could not be used in a more widespread fashion to unite the graduate medical and the community practice environments.

At present the undergraduate, graduate, and CPD environments function in a largely independent manner. By leveraging new developments in IP SBE, distributed simulation, and telesimulation, this independence can be challenged, allowing for a more seamless integration of the educational experience (Fig. 13.2). Future research in these areas should focus on increasing the level of evidence available in the literature and on exploring new means of applying these techniques to all areas along the education spectrum.

References

1. Davis DA, Thomson MA, Oxman AD, Haynes RB. Changing physician performance. A systematic review of the effect of continuing medical education strategies. JAMA. 1995;274(9):700–5.
2. Rosenberg AA, Kamin C, Glicken AD, Jones MD Jr. Training gaps for pediatric residents planning a career in primary care: a qualitative and quantitative study. J Grad Med Educ. 2011;3(3):309–14.
3. Harden RM. Trends and the future of postgraduate medical education. Emerg Med J. 2006;23(10):798–802.
4. Cheng A, Goldman RD, Aish MA, Kissoon N. A simulation-based acute care curriculum for pediatric emergency medicine fellowship training programs. Pediatr Emerg Care. 2010;26(7):475–80.
5. Ruiz JG, Mintzer MJ, Leipzig RM. The impact of E-learning in medical education. Acad Med. 2006;81(3):207–12.
6. Hodges BD, Albert M, Arweiler D, Akseer S, Bandiera G, Byrne N, et al. The future of medical education: a Canadian environmental scan. Med Educ. 2011;45(1):95–106.
7. Hastings RH, Rickard TC. Deliberate practice for achieving and maintaining expertise in anesthesiology. Anesth Analg. 2015;120(2):449–59.
8. Dreyfus S, Dreyfus R. A five stage model of the mental activities inovlved in directed skill acquistion. Berkley: University of California Berkley; 1980.
9. Kern D, Thomas P, Howard D, Bass E. Curriculum development for medical education. 2 ed. Maryland: John Hopkins University Press; 1998.
10. Dewey J. Experience and education. Toronto: Collier-MacMillan; 1938.
11. Hodges HF. Preparing new nurses with complexity science and problem-based learning. J Nurs Educ. 2011;50(1):7–13.
12. De Dombal FT, Smith RB, Modgill VK, Leaper DJ. Simulation of the diagnostic process: a further comparison. Br J Med Educ. 1972;6(3):238–45.
13. Meadow R, Hewitt C. Teaching communication skills with the help of actresses and video-tape simulation. Br J Med Educ. 1972;6(4):317–22.

14. Blackstock FC, Watson KM, Morris NR, Jones A, Wright A, Mc-Meeken JM, et al. Simulation can contribute a part of cardiorespiratory physiotherapy clinical education: two randomized trials. Simul Healthc. 2013;8(1):32–42.

15. Tofil NM, Benner KW, Worthington MA, Zinkan L, White ML. Use of simulation to enhance learning in a pediatric elective. Am J Pharm Educ. 2010;74(2):21.

16. Michael M, Abboudi H, Ker J, Shamim Khan M, Dasgupta P, Ahmed K. Performance of technology-driven simulators for medical students–a systematic review. J Surg Res. 2014;192(2):531–43.

17. Deering SH, Hodor JG, Wylen M, Poggi S, Nielsen PE, Satin AJ. Additional training with an obstetric simulator improves medical student comfort with basic procedures. Simul Healthc. 2006;1(1):32–4.

18. Hallikainen J, Vaisanen O, Randell T, Tarkkila P, Rosenberg PH, Niemi-Murola L. Teaching anaesthesia induction to medical students: comparison between full-scale simulation and supervised teaching in the operating theatre. Eur J Anaesthesiol. 2009;26(2):101–4.

19. Stewart M, Kennedy N, Cuene-Grandidier H. Undergraduate interprofessional education using high-fidelity paediatric simulation. Clin Teach. 2010;7(2):90–6.

20. Hayden JK, Smiley RA, Alexander M, Kardong-Edgren S, Jeffries PR. Supplement: the NCSBN National Simulation Study: a longitudinal, randomized, controlled study replacing clinical hours with simulation in prelicensure nursing education. J Nurs Regul. 2014;5(2):C1–64.

21. Shin H, Ma H, Park J, Ji ES, Kim DH. The effect of simulation courseware on critical thinking in undergraduate nursing students: multi-site pre-post study. Nurse Educ Today. 2015;35(4):537–542.

22. White C, Bradley E, Martindale J, Roy P, Patel K, Yoon M, et al. Active learning, the accreditation process and 20-something students. Med Educ. 2014;48(7):733.

23. Shin S, Park JH, Kim JH. Effectiveness of patient simulation in nursing education: meta-analysis. Nurse Educ Today. 2015;35(1):176–82.

24. Reierson IA, Hvidsten A, Wighus M, Brungot S, Bjork IT. Key issues and challenges in developing a pedagogical intervention in the simulation skills center–an action research study. Nurse Educ Pract. 2013;13(4):294–300.

25. Passiment M, Sacks H, Huang G. Medical simulation in medical education: results of an AAMC Survey: Association of American Medical Colleges; 2011 [cited 2014 September 26]. https://www.aamc.org/download/259760/data/medicalsimulationinmedicaleducationanaamcsurvey.pdf.

26. Vukin E, Greenberg R, Auerbach M, Chang L, Scotten M, Tenney-Soeiro R, et al. Use of simulation-based education: a national survey of pediatric clerkship directors. Acad Pediatr. 2014;14(4):369–74.

27. Haji F, Cheung J, deRibaupierre S, Dubrowski A, Regehr G, Woods N. Performance and cognitive load among novices training on simple vs. complex simulation scenarios during procedural skills training: a prospective randomized study. International Meeting on Simulation in Healthcare; New Orleans, LA: Simulation in Healthcare; 2014. p. 414–5.

28. Calhoun AW, Boone MC, Miller KH, Pian-Smith MC. Case and commentary: using simulation to address hierarchy issues during medical crises. Simul Healthc. 2013;8(1):13–9.

29. Gaba DM. Simulations that are challenging to the psyche of participants: how much should we worry and about what? Simul Healthc. 2013;8(1):4–7.

30. Truog RD, Meyer EC. Deception and death in medical simulation. Simul Healthc. 2013;8(1):1–3.

31. Corvetto MA, Taekman JM. To die or not to die? A review of simulated death. Simul Healthc. 2013;8(1):8–12.

32. McLaughlin S, Fitch MT, Goyal DG, Hayden E, Kauh CY, Laack TA, et al. Simulation in graduate medical education 2008: a review for emergency medicine. Acad Emerg Med. 2008;15(11):1117–29.

33. Eppich WJ, Nypaver MM, Mahajan P, Denmark KT, Kennedy C, Joseph MM, et al. The role of high-fidelity simulation in training pediatric emergency medicine fellows in the United States and Canada. Pediatr Emerg Care. 2013;29(1):1–7.

34. Cohen ER, Barsuk JH, Moazed F, Caprio T, Didwania A, McGaghie WC, et al. Making July safer: simulation-based mastery learning during intern boot cAMP. Acad Med. 2013;88(2):233–9.

35. Nishisaki A, Hales R, Biagas K, Cheifetz I, Corriveau C, Garber N, et al. A multi-institutional high-fidelity simulation "boot camp" orientation and training program for first year pediatric critical care fellows. Pediatr Crit Care Med. 2009;10(2):157–62.

36. Rosen KR. The history of medical simulation. J Crit Care. 2008;23(2):157–66.

37. Andreatta P, Saxton E, Thompson M, Annich G. Simulation-based mock codes significantly correlate with improved pediatric patient cardiopulmonary arrest survival rates. Pediatr Crit Care Med. 2011;12(1):33–8.

38. Cordero L, Hart BJ, Hardin R, Mahan JD, Nankervis CA. Deliberate practice improves pediatric residents' skills and team behaviors during simulated neonatal resuscitation. Clin Pediatr (Phila). 2013;52(8):747–52.

39. van Schaik SM, Von Kohorn I, O'Sullivan P. Pediatric resident confidence in resuscitation skills relates to mock code experience. Clin Pediatr (Phila). 2008;47(8):777–83.

40. Hunt EA, Duval-Arnould JM, Nelson-McMillan KL, Bradshaw JH, Diener-West M, Perretta JS, et al. Pediatric resident resuscitation skills improve after "rapid cycle deliberate practice" training. Resuscitation. 2014;85(7):945–51.

41. Pukenas EW, Dodson G, Deal ER, Gratz I, Allen E, Burden AR. Simulation-based education with deliberate practice may improve intraoperative handoff skills: a pilot study. J Clin Anesth. 2014;26(7):530–8.

42. Udani AD, Macario A, Nandagopal K, Tanaka MA, Tanaka PP. Simulation-based mastery learning with deliberate practice improves clinical performance in spinal anesthesia. Anesthesiol Res Pract. 2014;2014:659160.

43. Falck AJ, Escobedo MB, Baillargeon JG, Villard LG, Gunkel JH. Proficiency of pediatric residents in performing neonatal endotracheal intubation. Pediatrics. 2003;112(6 Pt 1):1242–7.

44. Bismilla Z, Finan E, McNamara PJ, LeBlanc V, Jefferies A, Whyte H. Failure of pediatric and neonatal trainees to meet Canadian Neonatal Resuscitation Program standards for neonatal intubation. J Perinatol. 2010;30(3):182–7.

45. Sectish TC, Zalneraitis EL, Carraccio C, Behrman RE. The state of pediatrics residency training: a period of transformation of graduate medical education. Pediatrics. 2004;114(3):832–41.

46. Schinasi DA, Nadel FM, Hales R, Boswinkel JP, Donoghue AJ. Assessing pediatric residents' clinical performance in procedural sedation: a simulation-based needs assessment. Pediatr Emerg Care. 2013;29(4):447–52.

47. Kessler DO, Auerbach M, Pusic M, Tunik MG, Foltin JC. A randomized trial of simulation-based deliberate practice for infant lumbar puncture skills. Simul Healthc. 2011;6(4):197–203.

48. Kessler DO, Arteaga G, Ching K, Haubner L, Kamdar G, Krantz A, et al. Interns' success with clinical procedures in infants after simulation training. Pediatrics. 2013;131(3):e811–20.

49. White ML, Jones R, Zinkan L, Tofil NM. Transfer of simulated lumbar puncture training to the clinical setting. Pediatr Emerg Care. 2012;28(10):1009–12.

50. Ernst KD, Cline WL, Dannaway DC, Davis EM, Anderson MP, Atchley CB, et al. Weekly and consecutive day neonatal intubation training: comparable on a pediatrics clerkship. Acad Med. 2014;89(3):505–10.

51. Sudikoff SN, Overly FL, Shapiro MJ. High-fidelity medical simulation as a technique to improve pediatric residents' emergency airway management and teamwork: a pilot study. Pediatr Emerg Care. 2009;25(10):651–6.

52. Gerard JM, Thomas SM, Germino KW, Street MH, Burch W, Scalzo AJ. The effect of simulation training on PALS skills among family medicine residents. Fam Med. 2011;43(6):392–9.

53. Finan E, Bismilla Z, Campbell C, Leblanc V, Jefferies A, Whyte HE. Improved procedural performance following a simulation training session may not be transferable to the clinical environment. J Perinatol. 2012;32(7):539–44.

54. Peterson EB, Porter MB, Calhoun AW. A simulation-based curriculum to address relational crises in medicine. J Grad Med Educ. 2012;4(3):351–6.

55. Bell SK, Pascucci R, Fancy K, Coleman K, Zurakowski D, Meyer EC. The educational value of improvisational actors to teach communication and relational skills: perspectives of interprofessional learners, faculty, and actors. Patient Educ Couns. 2014;96(3):381–8.

56. Browning DM, Meyer EC, Truog RD, Solomon MZ. Difficult conversations in health care: cultivating relational learning to address the hidden curriculum. Acad Med. 2007;82(9):905–13.

57. Meyer EC, Brodsky D, Hansen AR, Lamiani G, Sellers DE, Browning DM. An interdisciplinary, family-focused approach to relational learning in neonatal intensive care. J Perinatol. 2011;31(3):212–9.

58. Meyer EC, Sellers DE, Browning DM, McGuffie K, Solomon MZ, Truog RD. Difficult conversations: improving communication skills and relational abilities in health care. Pediatr Crit Care Med. 2009;10(3):352–9.

59. Waisel DB, Lamiani G, Sandrock NJ, Pascucci R, Truog RD, Meyer EC. Anesthesiology trainees face ethical, practical, and relational challenges in obtaining informed consent. Anesthesiology. 2009;110(3):480–6.

60. Gough JK, Frydenberg AR, Donath SK, Marks MM. Simulated parents: developing paediatric trainees' skills in giving bad news. J Paediatr Child Health. 2009;45(3):133–8.

61. Tobler K, Grant E, Marczinski C. Evaluation of the impact of a simulation-enhanced breaking bad news workshop in pediatrics. Simul Healthc. 2014;9(4):213–9.

62. Calhoun AW, Boone MC, Porter MB, Miller KH. Using simulation to address hierarchy-related errors in medical practice. Perm J. 2014;18(2):14–20.

63. Weinstock PH, Kappus LJ, Kleinman ME, Grenier B, Hickey P, Burns JP. Toward a new paradigm in hospital-based pediatric education: the development of an onsite simulator program. Pediatr Crit Care Med. 2005;6(6):635–41.

64. Calhoun AW, Boone MC, Peterson EB, Boland KA, Montgomery VL. Integrated in-situ simulation using redirected faculty educational time to minimize costs: a feasibility study. Simul Healthc. 2011;6(6):337–44.

65. Patterson M, Blike G, Nadkarni V In-situ simulation, challenges and results. 2008. http://ahrq.hhs.gov/downloads/pub/advances2/vol3/Advances-Patterson_48.pdf.

66. Weinstock PH, Kappus LJ, Garden A, Burns JP. Simulation at the point of care: reduced-cost, in situ training via a mobile cart. Pediatr Crit Care Med. 2009;10(2):176–81.

67. Holmboe ES, Edgar L, Hamstra S. Accreditation Council for Graduate Medical Education: milestones project: Accreditation Council for Graduate Medical Education. 2015 [cited 2015 February 5]. http://www.acgme.org/acgmeweb/tabid/430/ProgramandInstitutionalAccreditation/NextAccreditationSystem/Milestones.aspx.

68. Sam J, Pierse M, Al-Qahtani A, Cheng A. Implementation and evaluation of a simulation curriculum for paediatric residency programs including just-in-time in situ mock codes. Paediatr Child Health. 2012;17(2):e16–20.

69. Bank I, Snell L, Bhanji F. Pediatric crisis resource management training improves emergency medicine trainees' perceived ability to manage emergencies and ability to identify teamwork errors. Pediatr Emerg Care. 2014;30(12):879–83.

70. Bank I, Cheng A, McLeod P, Bhanji F, Group. ftPEMSC. A National Simulation Curriculum for pediatric emergency medicine training. Can J Emerg Med. in press.

71. Kurrek M, Calhoun AW. Simulation registry pilot project. 2014. [cited 2014 April 15]. simulationregistry.academicanesthesia.com.

72. Healthstream. HealthStream. 2015 [cited 2015 January 30]. www.healthstream.com.

73. Association AH. American Heart Association: life is why 2015 [cited 2015 January 30]. http://www.heart.org/HEARTORG/.

74. Pediatrics AAo. American Academy of Pediatrics: dedicated to the health of all children. 2015 [cited 2015 January 30]. http://www.aap.org/en-us/Pages/Default.aspx.

75. Surgeons ACo. American College of Surgeons: inspiring quality: highest standards, better outcomes. 2015. [cited 2015 January 30]. https://www.facs.org/.

76. Anesthesiologists ASo. American Society of Anesthesiologists Education Center. 2015. [cited 2015 January 30]. http://education.asahq.org/simulation-education.

77. Johnson KA, Sachdeva AK, Pellegrini CA. The critical role of accreditation in establishing the ACS Education Institutes to advance patient safety through simulation. J Gastrointest Surg. 2008;12(2):207–9.

78. Hagen MD, Ivins DJ, Puffer JC, Rinaldo J, Roussel GH, Sumner W, et al. Maintenance of certification for family physicians (MC-FP) self assessment modules (SAMs): the first year. J Am Board Fam Med. 2006;19(4):398–403.

79. Wayne DB, Butter J, Siddall VJ, Fudala MJ, Wade LD, Feinglass J, et al. Mastery learning of advanced cardiac life support skills by internal medicine residents using simulation technology and deliberate practice. J Gen Intern Med. 2006;21(3):251–6.

80. Vassiliou MC, Dunkin BJ, Marks JM, Fried GM. FLS and FES: comprehensive models of training and assessment. Surg Clin North Am. 2010;90(3):535–58.

81. Medicine ABoF. American Board of Family Medicine. Maintenance of certification: part II-self-assessment and lifelong learning. 2011. [cited 2013 November 1]. http://www.theabfm.org/moc/part2.aspx.

82. Khanduja PK, Bould MD, Naik VN, Hladkowicz E, Boet S. The role of simulation in continuing medical education for acute care physicians: a systematic review*. Crit Care Med. 2015;43(1):186–93.

83. Cheng A, Lang TR, Starr SR, Pusic M, Cook DA. Technology-enhanced simulation and pediatric education: a meta-analysis. Pediatrics. 2014;133(5):e1313–23.

84. Sawyer T, Laubach VA, Hudak J, Yamamura K, Pocrnich A, Improvements in teamwork during neonatal resuscitation after interprofessional TeamSTEPPS training. Neonatal Netw. 2013;32(1):26–33.

85. Dadiz R, Weinschreider J, Schriefer J, Arnold C, Greves CD, Crosby EC, et al. Interdisciplinary simulation-based training to improve delivery room communication. Simul Healthc. 2013;8(5):279–91.

86. Mosley CM, Shaw BN. A longitudinal cohort study to investigate the retention of knowledge and skills following attendance on the newborn life support course. Arch Dis Child. 2013;98(8):582–6.

87. Schilleman K, Witlox RS, Lopriore E, Morley CJ, Walther FJ, te Pas AB. Leak and obstruction with mask ventilation during simulated neonatal resuscitation. Arch Dis Child Fetal Neonatal Ed. 2010;95(6):F398–402.

88. Stocker M, Allen M, Pool N, De Costa K, Combes J, West N, et al. Impact of an embedded simulation team training programme in a paediatric intensive care unit: a prospective, single-centre, longitudinal study. Intensive Care Med. 2012;38(1):99–104.

89. Macnab AJ, Macnab M. Teaching pediatric procedures: the Vancouver model for instructing Seldinger's technique of central venous access via the femoral vein. Pediatrics. 1999;103(1):E8.

90. Lopez-Herce J, Ferrero L, Mencia S, Anton M, Rodriguez-Nunez A, Rey C, et al. Teaching and training acute renal replacement therapy in children. Nephrol Dial Transplant (Official Publication of the European Dialysis and Transplant Association—European Renal Association). 2012;27(5):1807–11.

91. Bretholz A, Doan Q, Cheng A, Lauder G. A presurvey and postsurvey of a web- and simulation-based course of ultrasound-guided nerve blocks for pediatric emergency medicine. Pediatr Emerg Care. 2012;28(6):506–9.

92. Augarten A, Zaslansky R, Matok Pharm I, Minuskin T, Lerner-Geva L, Hirsh-Yechezkel G, et al. The impact of educational intervention programs on pain management in a pediatric emergency department. Biomed Pharmacother. 2006;60(7):299–302.

93. Falcone RA Jr, Daugherty M, Schweer L, Patterson M, Brown RL, Garcia VF. Multidisciplinary pediatric trauma team training using high-fidelity trauma simulation. J Pediatr Surg. 2008;43(6):1065–71.

94. Hunt EA, Heine M, Hohenhaus SM, Luo X, Frush KS. Simulated pediatric trauma team management: assessment of an educational intervention. Pediatr Emerg Care. 2007;23(11):796–804.

95. Toback SL, Fiedor M, Kilpela B, Reis EC. Impact of a pediatric primary care office-based mock code program on physician and staff confidence to perform life-saving skills. Pediatr Emerg Care. 2006;22(6):415–22.

96. Nakajima K, Wasa M, Takiguchi S, Taniguchi E, Soh H, Ohashi S, et al. A modular laparoscopic training program for pediatric surgeons. JSLS. 2003;7(1):33–7.

97. Cheng A, Brown LL, Duff JP, Davidson J, Overly F, Tofil NM, et al. Improving cardiopulmonary resuscitation with a CPR feedback device and refresher simulations (CPR CARES Study): a randomized clinical trial. JAMA Pediatr. 2015;169(2):137–44.

98. Singhal N, Lockyer J, Fidler H, Keenan W, Little G, Bucher S, et al. Helping babies breathe: global neonatal resuscitation program development and formative educational evaluation. Resuscitation. 2012;83(1):90–6.

99. Musafili A, Essen B, Baribwira C, Rukundo A, Persson LA. Evaluating helping babies breathe: training for healthcare workers at hospitals in Rwanda. Acta Paediatr. 2013;102(1):e34–8.

100. Gardner R. Malpractice insurance incentives for teamwork training via simulation. 2014. [cited 2015 January 30]. http://halldale.com/files/halldale/attachments/Gardner_0.pdf.

101. Hospital SFG. Privileges for San Francisco General Hospital. 2015. [cited 2015 January 30]. https://www.sfdph.org/dph/files/hc/JCC/SFGH/Agendas/2015/Jan%2027/09c%20CREDS_05%20FCM%20MDDO%20Privilege%20Form_Sept2014%20AV%20edits-1.pdf.

102. Rubio-Gurung S, Putet G, Touzet S, Gauthier-Moulinier H, Jordan I, Beissel A, et al. In situ simulation training for neonatal resuscitation: an RCT. Pediatrics. 2014;134(3):e790–7.

103. Heideveld-Chevalking AJ, Calsbeek H, Damen J, Gooszen H, Wolff AP. The impact of a standardized incident reporting system in the perioperative setting: a single center experience on 2,563 'near-misses' and adverse events. Patient Saf Surg. 2014;8(1):46.

104. Kohn LT, Corrigan JM, Donaldson MS. To err is human: building a safer health system. (Medicine Io. editor). Washington, DC: National Academy Press; 1999.

105. Pettigrew TF, Tropp LR. A meta-analytic test of intergroup contact theory. J Pers Soc Psychol. 2006;90(5):751–83.

106. Baker GR, Norton P. Addressing the effects of adverse events: study provides insights into patient safety at Canadian hospitals. Healthc Q (Toronto, Ont). 2004;7(4):20–1.

107. Barr H, Low H. Centre for the advancement of interprofessional education: the definition and principles of interprofessional education. 2011. http://caipe.org.uk/about-us/the-definition-and-principles-of-interprofessional-education/.

108. Singer SJ, Falwell A, Gaba DM, Meterko M, Rosen A, Hartmann CW, et al. Identifying organizational cultures that promote patient safety. Health Care Manage Rev. 2009;34(4):300–11.

109. Liljedahl M, Boman LE, Falt CP, Bolander Laksov K. What students really learn: contrasting medical and nursing students' experiences of the clinical learning environment. Adv Health Sci Educ Theory Pract. 2014.

110. Alinier G, Harwood C, Harwood P, Montague S, Huish E, Ruparelia K, et al. Immersive clinical simulation in undergraduate health care interprofessional education: knowledge and perceptions. Clin Simul Nurs. 2014;10(4):e205–e16.

111. Atack L, Parker K, Rocchi M, Maher J, Dryden T. The impact of an online interprofessional course in disaster management competency and attitude towards interprofessional learning. J Interprof Care. 2009;23(6):586–98.

112. Ker J, Mole L, Bradley P. Early introduction to interprofessional learning: a simulated ward environment. Med Educ. 2003;37(3):248–55.

113. Sigalet E, Donnon T, Grant V. Undergraduate students' perceptions of and attitudes toward a simulation-based interprofessional curriculum: the KidSIM ATTITUDES questionnaire. Simul Healthc. 2012;7(6):353–8.

114. Wakefield A, Cooke S, Boggis C. Learning together: use of simulated patients with nursing and medical students for breaking bad news. Int J Palliat Nurs. 2003;9(1):32–8.

115. Sigalet E, Donnon T, Cheng A, Cooke S, Robinson T, Bissett W, et al. Development of a team performance scale to assess undergraduate health professionals. Acad Med. 2013;88(7):989–96.

116. Luctar-Flude M, Baker C, Pulling C, McGraw R, Dagnone D, Medves J, et al. Evaluating an undergraduate interprofessional simulation-based educational module: communication, teamwork, and confidence performing cardiac resuscitation skills. Adv Med Educ Pract. 2010;1:59–66.

117. Bandali K, Parker K, Mummery M, Preece M. Skills integration in a simulated and interprofessional environment: an innovative undergraduate applied health curriculum. J Interprof Care. 2008;22(2):179–89.

118. Sigalet EL, Donnon TL, Grant V. Insight into team competence in medical, nursing and respiratory therapy students. J Interprof Care. 2015;29(1):62–7.

119. Osman A. Undergraduate interprofessional paediatric simulation in a district general hospital. Med Educ. 2014;48(5):527–8.

120. Salam T, Saylor JL, Cowperthwait AL. Attitudes of nurse and physician trainees towards an interprofessional simulated education experience on pain assessment and management. J Interprof Care. 2015;29(3):276–278.

121. Nicksa GA, Anderson C, Fidler R, Stewart L. Innovative approach using interprofessional simulation to educate surgical residents in technical and nontechnical skills in high-risk clinical scenarios. JAMA Surg. 2015;150(3):201–7.

122. Pian-Smith MC, Simon R, Minehart RD, Podraza M, Rudolph J, Walzer T, et al. Teaching residents the two-challenge rule: a simulation-based approach to improve education and patient safety. Simul Healthc. 2009;4(2):84–91.

123. Nishisaki A, Nguyen J, Colborn S, Watson C, Niles D, Hales R, et al. Evaluation of multidisciplinary simulation training on clinical performance and team behavior during tracheal intubation procedures in a pediatric intensive care unit. Pediatr Crit Care Med. 2011;12(4):406–14.

124. Manser T, Harrison TK, Gaba DM, Howard SK. Coordination patterns related to high clinical performance in a simulated anesthetic crisis. Anesth Analg. 2009;108(5):1606–15.

125. Auerbach M, Roney L, Aysseh A, Gawel M, Koziel J, Barre K, et al. In situ pediatric trauma simulation: assessing the impact and feasibility of an interdisciplinary pediatric in situ trauma care quality improvement simulation program. Pediatr Emerg Care. 2014;30(12):884–91.

126. Siassakos D, Fox R, Draycott T. Training to reduce adverse obstetric events with risk of cerebral palsy. Am J Obstet Gynecol. 2011;204(5):e15–6.

127. Atamanyuk I, Ghez O, Saeed I, Lane M, Hall J, Jackson T, et al. Impact of an open-chest extracorporeal membrane oxygenation model for in situ simulated team training: a pilot study. Interact Cardiovasc Thorac Surg. 2014;18(1):17–20. discussion.

128. Crofts JF, Fox R, Draycott TJ, Winter C, Hunt LP, Akande VA. Retention of factual knowledge after practical training for intrapartum emergencies. Int J Gynaecol Obstet. 2013;123(1):81–5.

129. Reynolds A, Ayres-de-Campos D, Lobo M. Self-perceived impact of simulation-based training on the management of real-life obstetrical emergencies. Eur J Obstet Gynecol Reprod Biol. 2011;159(1):72–6.

130. Daniels K, Arafeh J, Clark A, Waller S, Druzin M, Chueh J. Prospective randomized trial of simulation versus didactic teaching for obstetrical emergencies Simul Healthc. 2010;5(1):40–5.

131. Draycott TJ, Crofts JF, Ash JP, Wilson LV, Yard E, Sibanda T, et al. Improving neonatal outcome through practical shoulder dystocia training. Obstet Gynecol. 2008;112(1):14–20.

132. Abu-Rish E, Kim S, Choe L, Varpio L, Malik E, White AA, et al. Current trends in interprofessional education of health sciences students: a literature review. J Interprof Care. 2012;26(6):444–51.

133. Studies IfSaI. ISIS Institute for Simulation and Interprofessional Studies. About the center. 2015. [cited 2015 February 5]. http://isis.washington.edu/about/learners.

134. Kirkpatrick DI. Evaluating training programs: the four levels. 2nd ed. San Francisco: Berrett-Koehler; 1998.

135. Issenberg SB, McGaghie WC, Petrusa ER, Lee Gordon D, Scalese RJ. Features and uses of high-fidelity medical simulations that lead to effective learning: a BEME systematic review. Med Teach. 2005;27(1):10–28.

136. Harris A, Kassab E, Tun JK, Kneebone R. Distributed Simulation in surgical training: an off-site feasibility study. Med Teach. 2013;35(4):e1078–81.

137. Kassab E, Tun JK, Arora S, King D, Ahmed K, Miskovic D, et al. "Blowing up the barriers" in surgical training: exploring and validating the concept of distributed simulation. Ann Surg. 2011;254(6):1059–65.

138. Kneebone R, Arora S, King D, Bello F, Sevdalis N, Kassab E, et al. Distributed simulation–accessible immersive training. Med Teach. 2010;32(1):65–70.

139. Mikrogianakis A, Kam A, Silver S, Bakanisi B, Henao O, Okrainec A, et al. Telesimulation: an innovative and effective tool for teaching novel intraosseous insertion techniques in developing countries. Acad Emerg Med. 2011;18(4):420–7.

140. Henao O, Escallon J, Green J, Farcas M, Sierra JM, Sanchez W, et al. Fundamentals of laparoscopic surgery in Colombia using telesimulation: an effective educational tool for distance learning. Biomedica. 2013;33(1):107–14.

141. Okrainec A, Henao O, Azzie G. Telesimulation: an effective method for teaching the fundamentals of laparoscopic surgery in resource-restricted countries. Surg Endosc. 2010;24(2):417–22.

142. Treloar D, Hawayek J, Montgomery JR, Russell W, Medical Readiness Trainer T. On-site and distance education of emergency medicine personnel with a human patient simulator. Mil Med. 2001;166(11):1003–6.

Simulation Curriculum Development, Competency-Based Education, and Continuing Professional Development

14

Jonathan Pirie, Liana Kappus, Stephanie N. Sudikoff
and Farhan Bhanji

Simulation Pearls

- There are increasing calls for healthcare professionals to fulfill their social contract with society and ensure competence of all professionals in order to maintain the privilege of self-regulation. Competency-based education (CBE) offers promise, as an outcome-based model of education, to help address the gap between actual and desired performance.
- Simulation-based education (SBE) curricula should be based on needs analysis. Prior to designing, clear goals should be defined to measure the success of the training program.
- Specific learning objectives, instructional strategy, simulation technology, training environment, and debriefing models should be carefully selected based on the level of learner.

- Challenges to CBE include defining learning objectives that are not excessively comprehensive, trainees focusing on milestones rather than achieving excellence, administrative logistics, instructor expertise and availability, and cost.
- Optimal education will require a change in our current approach to assessment. Assessment needs to be programmatic and conceptualized as part of instructional design with a shift away from assessment of learning to assessment for learning.
- SBE is increasingly used for high-stakes, summative purposes such as local program-based examinations, achieving certification, and demonstrating ongoing competence to maintain certification.

Introduction

In 1999 the Institute of Medicine's landmark report "To Err is Human: Building a Safer Health System" highlighted that as many as 98,000 deaths are due to medical error [1]. In response, accrediting bodies, healthcare organizations, and medical educators across all disciplines have embraced SBE as one solution to improving what many believe was a root cause, namely poor communication and team functioning [2]. A burgeoning literature in SBE has demonstrated that simulation can improve knowledge, skills, and behaviors as well as result in some improvement in patient outcomes [3–7]. Despite the success and large uptake of SBE many programs are ad hoc with variable and inconsistent instruction, curricula, and evaluation of competency. In response, educators have turned their focus to developing comprehensive curricula for continuing professional development (CPD) and the use of mastery learning/CBE. This chapter will describe a model for curriculum development and the promotion of professional development through CBE. We conclude by reviewing barriers and challenges to CPD and CBE and explore future directions.

J. Pirie (✉)
Department of Medicine, Department of Paediatrics, University of Toronto, The Hospital for Sick Children, Toronto, ON, Canada
e-mail: Jonathan.pirie@sickkids.ca

L. Kappus · S. N. Sudikoff
SYN:APSE Center for Learning, Transformation and Innovation, Yale New Haven Health System, New Haven, CT, USA
e-mail: Liana.kappus@ynhh.org

S. N. Sudikoff
e-mail: Stephanie.Sudikoff@ynhh.org

S. N. Sudikoff
Pediatric Critical Care, Yale School of Medicine, New Haven, CT, USA
e-mail: Stephanie.Sudikoff@ynhh.org

F. Bhanji
Department of Pediatrics, Centre for Medical Education, McGill University, Royal College of Physicians and Surgeons of Canada, Montreal, QC, Canada
e-mail: Farhan.bhanji@mcgill.ca

© Springer International Publishing Switzerland 2016
V. J. Grant, A. Cheng (eds.), *Comprehensive Healthcare Simulation: Pediatrics*,
Comprehensive Healthcare Simulation, DOI 10.1007/978-3-319-24187-6_14

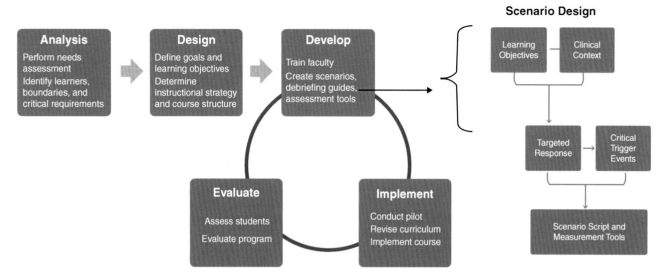

Fig. 14.1 Curriculum development process/scenario design based on the analysis, design, development, implementation, and evaluation (ADDIE) Model of Instructional Design and the Simulation Module for Assessment of Resident-Targeted Event Responses (SMARTER) approach to creating measurement tools for simulation-based education [8, 10]. The first two steps of the process, (1) analysis and (2) design, occur sequentially. (3) Development, (4) implementation, and (5) evaluation may be cyclical. Revisions may continue after piloting as evaluation informs further development

Curriculum Development in Competency-Based Education

Some key challenges to developing simulation curricula for CBE across the healthcare education continuum include the heterogeneity of learners, the variable experiences they bring, the feasibility of teaching, and the validity and reliability of assessing competencies through simulation within the professional environment. This section outlines a curriculum development process for CBE for all disciplines that follows the analysis, design, development, implementation, and evaluation (ADDIE) model of instructional design and incorporates concepts from Kern's six-step approach to curriculum development for medical education and the Simulation Module for Assessment of Resident-Targeted Event Responses (SMARTER) approach of developing measurement tools for simulation-based training [8–10]. The process can be applied for curriculum development for any level of learner and unfolds in five phases including ADDIE (Fig. 14.1). We will describe these five phases and discuss the key considerations in each phase specific to CBE.

Analysis

The process begins with a needs assessment which includes identifying the target audience and level(s) of expertise, defining boundaries to conducting training, and crystallizing the critical requirements to include in the educational initiative. The subject matter expert must understand the gap in knowledge, skills, and attitudes (KSA) to be addressed

with simulation-based training as well as anticipated outcomes. For students or trainees, focus may be placed on learning outcomes including cognitive outcomes, skill-based outcomes, and changes in attitudes. Additionally, cost of training must be justified with specific outcomes included, such as patient safety outcomes and/or financial components [11].

Needs assessments can be accomplished through literature review, review of institutional data surrounding patient safety events or quality improvement activities, direct observation in the actual clinical or simulated environment, written surveys, in-person or telephone interviews, and/or focus group discussions. The latter three strategies can be completed with learners, their colleagues, their educators or managers, and patients. The rationale for including many perspectives in the needs assessment is that competence in the professional healthcare environment encompasses not only an individual's knowledge or ability to perform a skill but rather one's ability to apply this knowledge or skill among interprofessional teams. Perspectives from colleagues and patients will further inform the identification of training needs. For example:

A needs analysis for students suggests that in order to adhere to curriculum standards, learners need to describe the indications for central venous line (CVL) placement. Within the hospital, a needs analysis suggests that physicians in training must demonstrate competence in placing CVLs in order to comply with accrediting body regulations. Furthermore, institutional data may also suggest that there is a high blood stream infection rate in a particular intensive care unit where staff does not feel empowered to speak up, based upon results of a safety attitude survey.

Based on the results of the needs analysis, the target audience, and level(s) of expertise, the critical requirements to include in the educational initiative should be identified. The target audience must be defined in consideration of whether the group is uniprofessional or interprofessional, the varying expertise levels inherent in the group, and the approximate size of the target audience. Because we work in teams in health care, we are interdependent. In this way, increased consideration and effort should be made to determine feasibility and applicability of interprofessional education.

In the next step, the expertise level or range of expertise within the target audience must be determined (see Table 14.1 for a description of each learner type). The level of expertise is not presumed by the learner's level of training but rather should be assessed in each learner to determine their individual starting point. The characteristics of each learner type will inform the entire instructional design and development process. For example, a novice learner may have few past experiences upon which to base judgment. As a result, they are more reliant on established rules, standards, and protocols. In this way, the novice must gain knowledge prior to applying the material in a simulation. Moreover, the simula-tion should remain focused on a specific task or process and may include some direct coaching (scaffold building) during the simulation. Alternatively, a competent learner is less dependent on rules, algorithms, and analytic decision-making but rather relies on pattern recognition, previous experiences, and gut-feeling to make decisions. A competent learner therefore requires more autonomy in the learning process. This group of learners will benefit from more complex simulations that require decision-making without coaching during the simulation so that the learner can observe the results of their decisions. In professional environments, there may be a mix of expertise present for any learning situation. As the curriculum development process progresses, the design team must develop objectives and a range of expected learner actions for each level of expertise [12–15].

The size of the target audience has implications for both feasibility and scheduling. For small uniprofessional groups, a few training sessions to capture all learners may suffice. When the target audience spans an entire department or institution, the design team must determine the appropriate group size for each training class, the appropriate complement of caregivers that should be present for interprofessional train-

Table 14.1 Levels of expertise [12–15]

Level of expertise	Characteristics	Simulation-based education design considerations
Novice	Has virtually no experience in an actual situation upon which to base judgment	Consider prework to enhance knowledge base
	Solves problems using rules and analytic reasoning	High instruction and low facilitation
		Simplify scenarios. Ensure opportunities for success and validation by offering multiple scenarios
		Use reflection-in-action with clinical pauses
Advanced beginner	Has enough experience in actual situations to begin seeing patterns	Consider including several scenarios with slight variation to compare and contrast
	Solves problems using analytic reasoning and pattern recognition	Begin with common and move to more complex
	Often not able to prioritize	High instruction and low facilitation
		Reflection-in-action with clinical pauses or reflection-on-action
Competent	Has broader experience in actual situations	Consider challenging with low-frequency clinical situations in order to continue to build experience
	Beginning to see big picture	Balance instruction and facilitation
	Solves problems more often through pattern recognition	Encourage autonomy and self-reflection in debriefing
	Approaches uncommon or complex problems with analytical reasoning	
	Feels personal responsibility	
Proficient	Has a bank of past experiences. Approaches all situations with a lens or perspective based on past experiences	Continue adding more complexity to scenarios such as communication with family members, teamwork, delegation, and assertion
	Can look at the whole picture rather than "aspects"	Low instruction and high facilitation
		Draw from experience in the room to crystallize learning points
Expert	Has intuitive grasp of the whole situation	Continue to keep the expert challenged to use technical and nontechnical skills
	Uses intuition to recognize problems, respond and manage situations	Encourage the expert to discuss, coach, or mentor during simulations and debriefings
		Train the expert to facilitate and debrief

ing, the frequency at which the training should be offered to capture all individuals in a reasonable amount of time, and the number of faculty it will take to complete the training. Drawing upon social learning theory, all individuals may not need to participate in the simulation in order to learn. There may be a benefit to observing the simulation event. Special consideration should be made to engage observers more directly in the learning process by assigning specific areas of focus to direct their observations [16].

Boundaries to training must also be considered before designing a program. For students, educators may be constrained by the timing of the academic year, faculty who can implement simulations, and finding and training raters to assess competency. In professional environments, the design team must consider *institutional policies for education of learners* (is the education part of 'mandatory' education or do learners need to be paid for their time?), *scheduling* (are there particular days or times of day to avoid?), *timing* (does the training need to be completed by a certain date for regulatory purposes?), and *location* (based on the goals of the program, does the training need to occur in situ or in a simulation laboratory?). In response to these boundaries or constraints, the design team must brainstorm solutions to overcome these challenges to determine feasibility, appropriate length of the training, and an achievable timeline and plan for training and assessment.

Finally, the critical requirements or competencies should be defined. It should be determined if there are core competencies already described by a recognized accrediting body (e.g., the National League of Nursing, the Accreditation Council for Graduate Medical Education (ACGME) in the USA, or the Royal College of Physicians and Surgeons of Canada, CanMEDS) or by the home institution. The aforementioned accrediting bodies have outlined comprehensive competency frameworks and defined key competencies in terms of KSA, by level of learner, required to be a competent clinician. This information should be reviewed to determine which competencies can be included and observed in simulation-based training. If formal requirements are not predefined, the design team must list the competencies that will be included in the training. Once a comprehensive needs analysis is complete, the design team can begin designing the specific educational initiative.

Design

The first step in the design phase is to write a goal statement against which the success of the training initiative will be measured. Goal statements should be specific, measurable, achievable, result-focused, and time-bound [17]. Building on the example provided earlier, a goal statement for novice learners might be to provide simulation-based training for fourth-year medical students during the first 6 months of the academic year on placing CVLs using the Seldinger technique in order to increase their self-efficacy by x%. For an interprofessional group of learners that spans the expertise gradient (novice through expert), a goal might be to decrease blood stream infection rates in the intensive care unit (ICU) by 20% in the following year by providing interprofessional simulation-based training on central line placement, teamwork, and communication.

Next, the specific learning objectives should be defined. Learning objectives describe the specific changes that the training course is meant to produce in the KSA of the learner: What can you reasonably expect the learner *to know* and *be able to do* at the end of the program and what *change in attitudes* are you aiming to achieve? For each objective, a performance statement, a set of conditions, and a set of standards should be incorporated. Knowledge and attitude objectives are less likely to be observable than skill. Learning objectives should be written using strong action verbs (see Table 14.2 for a reference on developing learning objectives) [18].

Following the setting of goals and objectives, the next step is to select an instructional strategy based on several learning theories including self-determination theory, experiential learning theory, and cognitive load theory. *Self-determination theory,* which describes a learner's willingness to learn, posits that learners must feel related to the group, feel a sense of competence, and feel a sense of autonomy. A safe environment for learning must be established at the start of all simulation-based training by establishing rules of engagement and maintaining confidentiality [19, 20]. *Experiential learning theory* suggests that adult learners learn through experiences and must engage in a continuous cycle which includes a concrete experience (a simulation), time to observe and reflect, the formation of abstract concepts

Table 14.2 Learning objectives [18]

Dimension		Example verbs
Knowledge	Cognitive: What should the learner be able to know?	Identify, list, recall, summarize, classify, describe, explain, calculate, differentiate, conclude, compose
Skills	Psychomotor: What should the learner be able to do?	Arrange, build, construct, design, deliver, display, fix, operate, sketch, use, perform
Attitude	Affective: What should the learner value?	Commit to, challenge, discuss, dispute, follow, justify, integrate, judge, question, resolve, synthesize

(facilitated debriefing), and testing or experimenting in new situations (a second simulation or real-life experience) [21]. While simulation and debriefing map quite nicely on the cycle, the design team should also consider any prework and didactic information specifically for the novice learner who has no previous experience to draw from but relies on rules, algorithms, policies, etc. *Cognitive load theory* describes that in order to achieve effective learning, the cognitive load of learners should be kept at a minimum during the learning process as short term memory can only contain limited elements. It follows that prework, as well as the complexity of the simulations, should match the level of the learner so as not to impede learning by incorporating information and protocols that overcomplicate rather than simplify [19]. Moreover, providing learners with the tools to gain knowledge prior to coming to the experiential simulation lab will allow learners to process the information independently and then apply this knowledge in the simulation setting thereby avoiding a common pitfall of lecturing by the simulated bedside.

A second piece of designing the instructional strategy involves selecting the appropriate type of simulation or simulation technology and environment to achieve the objectives to match the level of the learner. Simulation technology can include screen-based simulation, task trainers, human patient simulators, live actors, or hybrid simulation which combines live actors and task trainers. In the example above, the appropriate technology for novice students learning the procedural steps of placing a CVL would be a task trainer designed for this purpose. This training could be accomplished in a simulation laboratory as opposed to the actual clinical environment because the goals of training are narrowly focused to the procedural skill. Novices benefit from time and space to learn, practice, and apply the step-by-step procedure, void of additional complexities and distractions that might be present in the actual clinical environment. On the other hand, if an interprofessional team is learning how to work together to maintain a sterile environment while placing a central line, the design team may utilize a task trainer and conduct the training in situ. In this way, the learners can practice maintaining sterility while placing a CVL surrounded by the physical barriers that are present in their native clinical environment.

Facilitation strategies for implementing the simulations and debriefing must be considered, again, based upon the level of the learner. For example, novice learners require more instruction and less facilitation. A strategy to consider for novices is *scaffolding*. This strategy allows the facilitator to provide support where cognitive structures are not sufficiently developed [22]. One way to incorporate scaffolds is to provide expert modeling and then coaching during skills training. Another is to build clinical pauses into simulations with human patient simulators at critical decision-making points to allow the facilitator to prompt *reflection-in-action*

[23]. During this pause, the facilitator can expose the learners' mental model, frame of mind, or thought process. The facilitator can then provide a scaffold by modeling their own thought process to create new mental models on the part of the learner. The facilitator can then coach or guide the learner to continue in the simulation. These scaffolds can be reorganized or eliminated as learners' understanding increases. Competent, proficient, and expert groups require less instruction and more facilitation. The design of the course may include simulations without any pause followed by debriefing, allowing learners to *reflect-on-action* and form new concepts [24]. Furthermore, the course may include opportunities to practice or experiment with new knowledge. This can be accomplished either by allowing learners multiple opportunities to practice with procedural skills or by allowing learners to run through a clinical scenario a second time to apply new theories discovered during a debriefing. There are several models of debriefing described elsewhere in this book (see Chap. 3). An appropriate approach should be determined based on the level of the learner(s).

Development

Once the course is designed, the faculty, the simulation exercises (see Chap. 2), debriefing guides (see Chap. 3), and assessment tools (see Chap. 7) must be developed. The content experts, who may also serve as faculty for the training, should be taught the art and science of simulation design, implementation, and debriefing. It is important for faculty to have a general understanding of adult learning principles in order to create psychological safety for learners. Additionally, faculty should understand how to design simulation exercises, whether it is procedural skills on trainers or clinical scenarios, and implement them to achieve learning objectives. Finally, because deep learning may not happen with experience alone, faculty need to be trained on facilitating debriefing exercises and matching their instruction during debriefing to the level of learner. For example, debriefing novice learners may include more directed teaching methods, whereas debriefing competent, proficient, and even expert learners may require more guided reflection and discovery of mental models of the learner(s) or rationale for their specific behavior. Once a mental model is discovered, the faculty member can facilitate discussion among the group to explore multiple perspectives on that mental model and facilitate learning. Faculty development is described elsewhere in this book (see Chap. 15).

Once the faculty members are adequately trained, they can better engage in the development of simulation exercises to achieve learning objectives. In the design phase of the curriculum development process, learning objectives for the course are defined while in the development phase, specific objectives and clinical context for each simulation exercise are defined. Selecting the appropriate context is important as it establishes meaningful linkages with experiences and promotes connections among, knowledge, skill and experiences [19, 22]. Context can and should even be defined in procedural skills training so that learners can understand when and how the skill is utilized. One group describes a process of "identifying competencies within the context of a particular profession such that the assessment of competence is tied to learner's performance of essential clinical activities that define the profession." This cluster of competencies has been referred to as *entrustable professional activities* (EPAs). An EPA requires a learner to not only possess knowledge, skill, and attitude but to apply these through specific activities in the clinical environment to achieve optimal results [25, 26]. In this way, the design team should consider identifying EPAs upon which to base scenarios. This allows learners to acquire not only knowledge but also a sense of when and how to use that knowledge in the actual clinical setting. As an example, the context for novice student learners in the CVL example might be devoid of context and simply focus on the steps of line placement while the context for the interprofessional team might be placing the line while ensuring maximal sterility in a septic patient in the ICU, as well as performing the time-out, sterile field preparation, and necessary documentation.

The design team must next define the expected actions using the event-based approach to training (EBAT). This list of expected actions for any competency may look different for each level of expertise. In order to create an opportunity for these actions, the design team should also embed *triggers* within the scenario script (see Chap. 2). Triggers are prompts for the facilitator to provide necessary events to meet the learning objectives. Please see Table 14.3 for an example of how to embed triggers into scenario script.

This list of expected actions and triggers allow the educator to establish a controlled and standardized learning experience. Moreover, this list can be easily combined with observational measurement tools to aid in debriefing and evaluation. For successful EBAT training, the design team should match learning objectives to triggers, define acceptable observable behaviors or expected actions, and script the scenario to ensure triggers are executed according to plan.

Finally, the design team should develop debriefing guides that outline the phases of debriefing, sample narrative text, and sample questions to include during each phase. Debriefing guides or scripts can assist the novice debriefer in following a structure to guide the learning process and ensure that key learning points are addressed in a standardized way (see Chap. 3) [27]. Furthermore, the guide can be structured to serve dual purposes: an instructor guide and an assessment tool to evaluate faculty on debriefing competencies such that it sets the stage for an engaging learning experience,

Table 14.3 Embedding triggers into scenario scripts

Learning objective	Expected action	Trigger
Novice After participating in this activity, the learner will be able to demonstrate the steps of placing a central venous line sterilely	*Novice* 1. Don gown and gloves 2. Prepare the sterile field 3. Clean the insertion area 4. Identify appropriate landmarks 5. Place a central venous line using Seldinger technique	None
Competent After participating in this activity, the learner will be able to do the following: 1. Demonstrate the steps of placing a central venous line sterilely 2. Utilize assertion to alert team of breach in sterility	*Competent* 1. Don gown and gloves 2. Prepare the sterile field 3. Perform a pre-procedural time-out. 4. Clean the insertion area 5. Identify appropriate landmarks 6. Place a central venous line using Seldinger technique 7. Recognize breach in sterility and alert the team	Facilitator should be able to do the following: 1. Encourage learner to quickly begin procedure 2. Contaminate the field by positioning IV tubing across the sterile field

facilitates the debriefing in an organized way, or provides feedback to participants on their performance [28].

Implementation

The course should be piloted and refined as needed. The goals of the pilot are to provide an opportunity for faculty to practice implementation of the course and to test the simulations. Faculty should practice creating a safe environment, trial any task trainers, practice directing any clinical scenarios using the scenario template to execute triggers, and practice debriefing using the debriefing guide. The pilot may include other faculty or a subset of the target audience willing to participate and offer feedback to further shape the course. During the pilot, the design team should determine if the simulation activity allows faculty to properly observe and assess the predefined competences and if the debriefing guide adequately promotes discussion of these competencies. Following the pilot, the prework, simulation exercises, and facilitation guides should be revised and potentially piloted again.

Evaluation

The final phase in the curriculum development process is evaluation. Evaluation should include the assessment of the performance of the learners, as will be described in the next section of the chapter, and the evaluation of the effectiveness of the educational program. The evaluation plan should be developed alongside the curriculum development process. Ideally data should be collected, analyzed, and reviewed prior to the implementation of the program, and throughout the program to guide continuous improvement for learners, faculty, and the design team [9].

There are several evaluation types, including formative and summative assessments for both the individual and the program. Formative assessments matched with predefined competencies should be performed at each course offering, with the goal of identifying areas for improvement for the learner and the program, respectively. Alternatively, summative assessments of the learner focus on judging individual competence at a particular skill, or achievement of a milestone. Summative assessment of a program may determine if it has had an impact and if resources will continue to be allocated for future implementation [9].

Kirkpatrick describes four levels of evaluation of training programs: Level 1—Reaction, Level 2—Learning, Level 3—Behavior, and Level 4—Results (Table 14.4 [29]. Level 1 measures how learners reacted to the training and helps identify any topics that might be missing from the curriculum. This can be accomplished through a post-event questionnaire or focus group discussion. Level 2 measures what the learner has actually learned as a result of the training. In order to measure learning, KSAs should be measured prior to and after the training. This can be accomplished by observing expected actions during a simulation or on a written test. Pre-/post-evaluations may also be valuable. Level 3 describes how behavior has changed as a result of training and if the learners can apply what they have learned. Measuring behavior requires observation over time, either in the actual clinical environment or in the simulation laboratory. Observation tools can be generated during the scenario design process and should include the expected critical actions for each learning objective. Finally, Level 4 measures the impact of the training, using the problem and goal statements as described above (see Chap. 7).

Program evaluation is critical to the educational process but challenging to measure. Due to time and resource constraints and ongoing learning in the actual clinical environment, it is challenging and often not feasible to determine how an educational intervention has impacted clinical outcomes, patient safety outcomes, or financial outcomes. Competency-based medical education (CBME) educators can more realistically focus on the impact their program has had on learning and transfer of that learning to application in a simulated environment and then the actual clinical environment.

Simulation for Competency-Based Education

CBE has gained considerable momentum over the past few years and may prove to be a catalyst that transforms health professional education worldwide. CBE can be conceptualized as "the education for the medical professional that is targeted at a fixed level of ability in one or more medical competencies" [30]. This description relies on a trajectory of development from the preclinical phase of professional school to the healthcare provider in practice. Ultimately, the goal of CBE is to produce graduates who provide high quality patient care from the moment they enter clinical medicine in school to the time of retirement. Traditional training models have fallen considerably short of this goal with substantial rates of preventable error that occur across different healthcare systems [31–33]. While that error cannot be attributed entirely to individual practitioners (a large portion may relate to the teams and system they work within), there is also substantial variability in patient outcomes depending on where clinical training occurred [34], suggesting an opportunity to improve patient care through a competency-based approach to education. CBE focuses on accountability and curricular outcomes organized around competencies, promoting greater learner-centeredness and de-emphasizing time-based curricular design [35]. Achievement of competence is demonstrated through a progression of milestones or

Table 14.4 Kirkpatrick's adapted hierarchy of evaluating educational outcomes [29]. (Reproduced with permission)

Level 1	Reaction	Covers learners' views on the learning experience, its organization, presentation, content, teaching methods, and aspects of the instructional organization, materials, quality of instruction
Level 2a	Learning: change in attitudes/perception	Modification of attitudes/perceptions—outcomes here relate to changes in the reciprocal attitudes or perceptions between participant groups towards intervention/simulation
Level 2b	Learning: modification of knowledge or skills	Modification of knowledge/skills—for knowledge, this relates to the acquisition of concepts, procedures, and principles; for skills, this relates to the acquisition of thinking/problem-solving, psychomotor, and social skills
Level 3	Behavior	Documents the transfer of learning to the workplace or willingness of learners to apply new knowledge and skills
Level 4a	Results: change in the professional practice	Change in organizational practice—wider changes in the organizational delivery of care, attributable to an education program
Level 4b	Benefits to patients	Any improvement in the health and well-being of patients/clients as a direct result of an educational program

EPAs [25, 26]. As an example, the field of medicine holds a social contract with society where physicians receive status and respect, are granted the privilege to self-regulate their profession and receive substantial remuneration in exchange for the promise to provide competent, altruistic, and moral care that addresses the needs of individuals and society [36]. Multiple high-profile cases have outlined how medicine can improve its performance in this implicit agreement [37, 38].

Inherent to the use of CBE is the use of a competency framework such as CanMEDS [39], ACGME competencies [40], and the Scottish Doctor [41]. While the frameworks differ and are chosen to reflect the needs of the local environment, they all extend beyond medical knowledge/expertise and include domains such as communication and collaboration which align well with SBE—particularly as it is applied to crises resource management or team training (see Chap. 4). Additionally, SBE holds the promise to support skill development and demonstrate baseline competence before trainees perform complex procedures on patients, reducing complications and healthcare costs [42, 43]. This foundational simulation training may function to accelerate the development of expertise in the clinical environment, allowing for system optimization (e.g., expensive operating room (OR) time) [44]. Collateral effects of simulation-based instruction may influence the learning environment and improve skill acquisition of learners that do not actually participate in the simulation [45].

Current models of health professional education retain the silos of undergraduate education, postgraduate education (in the case of medicine), and CPD which may focus learners on the current tasks of the training (particularly during formal training programs) and impede the development of reflection and lifelong learning skills that are critical to improve future practice in an ongoing manner. Medical science is rapidly evolving and there needs to be greater investment to support practicing healthcare providers to incorporate new knowledge into their practice in real time [46]. Evidence from the CPD literature suggests that physician performance and health outcomes improve when the CPD activities are more interactive, use multiple methods, involve multiple exposures, are longer in duration, and are focused on activities that the physician believes to be important [47]. Well-designed SBE has the potential to meet many of these criteria and can form an important piece of CPD. Novel methods of instruction, such as debriefing without a formal debriefer present in the room, may help build capacity to integrate more simulation into CPD course offerings [48].

Two international CBE collaborative summits have been held over the past 5 years (2009 and 2013), with both scholarly and practical outputs [49]. Implementation of CBE has occurred in multiple specialties in multiple jurisdictions with several others planning to move to a CBE model in the coming years [49]. SBE can align very well with CBE as it allows for feedback from experts, repetitive practice across a range of difficulties that are required in skill development, and curricular integration [3].

Shifting the Assessment Paradigm for Competency-Based Education

CBE will require substantial change in our current approach to assessment. Assessment should be conceptualized as part of instructional design with a shift away from assessment *of* learning to assessment *for* learning [50]. This will require an emphasis on a robust, programmatic approach to assessment that ideally focuses on workplace-based formative assessment, rather than isolated high-stakes point in time-summative examinations. This is not to imply that there is not a role for high-stakes examination, as it can be useful to predict future patient outcomes [24], but rather that the opportunity for lower-stakes, more frequent assessment may be invaluable for learning on an ongoing basis [51]. Moving up to Miller's top level of "Does" (Fig. 14.2) can only be achieved in the clinical environment, but simulation reaches the level of "Shows" and can be helpful as a piece of the assessment program to inform judgments on the overall competence of practitioners [52].

Simulation educators have historically focused on promoting high-fidelity training in order to improve the quality of education and assessment. Yet, the term fidelity has been problematic to define and qualify in the simulation community—we may therefore benefit by considering functional task alignment (the alignment between the simulator's functional properties and the functional requirements of the task) to reflect how well the simulation-based assessment (SBA) truly allows the learner to "Show" how they might perform [53]. Ultimately, judgment of competence needs to be conducted by a collective, using the wisdom of the crowd (e.g.,

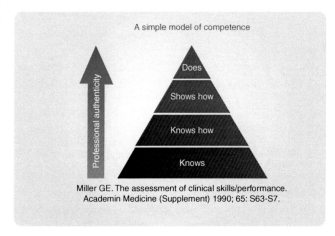

Fig. 14.2 Miller's framework for assessment. (Reproduced with permission of [52])

competence committee) to incorporate multiple assessments from multiple assessors using multiple tools across multiple situations to help determine competence and make progression decisions on the trainee. Subjective assessments and narrative descriptions may also form an important part of that assessment program [54]. The negative connotations of biased and unfair with subjective assessment do not hold true (though they can occur—as they also might with an objective measure). Much like the clinical environment, there may be opportunities to reduce information to a numerical score when appropriate (e.g., Glasgow Coma Scale score of 3 is identified universally as having the same clinical meaning to every healthcare provider), while there may be other instances where a more complete description would be helpful to make judgments (e.g., one would not hand over a pediatric ICU patient simply with a validated risk of mortality score (such as the Pediatric Index of Mortality 2, PIM2), but one would want more detailed, narrative descriptions of the patient on which to make important judgments and decisions).

Assessment programs should continue to be evaluated by their reliability, validity, acceptability, and cost (both financial and resource related) but should also be judged by their educational impact and catalytic effect where results and feedback are used in a manner that creates, enhances, and supports education [55]. Assessment will certainly need to be more continuous and frequent. It needs to be criterion-based and support learners to achieve developmental milestones [56]. Viewed with this lens, SBE may be important to CBE allowing the achievement of milestones that are associated with rare presentations in the clinical environment, as well as those that would pose significant risk to patients if they were not first assessed outside of clinical care. The educational as well as catalytic effect of SBE could be very positive, but further work needs to be conducted on how best to maintain a safe learning environment where trainees and faculty can feel comfortable making mistakes (and learning from them).

Robust assessment instruments/tools with evidence of validity and reliability will continue to be required, and faculty development around their use may be even more critical (see Chap. 7). Tools are only as good as the individual using them—it may be time for the healthcare professions to mandate teaching faculty to learn a core set of competencies in assessment, with accredited training programs providing ongoing professional development in assessment [57]. As any simulation-based researcher will report, it takes a substantial amount of time to calibrate assessors even with a tightly regulated script for the scenario.[48]. Assessment in the workplace complicates the ability to standardize scoring with tremendous variability in case presentation and will require clinical supervisors to understand some of these complexities and basic psychometrics of assessment. Reliability will only be achieved with rater training and adequate sampling of performance (i.e., content specificity should not

Table 14.5 Assessment in competency-based education

Key points
Assessment needs to be programmatic with multiple observations, performed by multiple observers, using multiple tools at multiple times
The focus of assessment needs to move to the level of "Does" in Miller's framework. Simulation can be helpful to assess the level of "Shows" to demonstrate competence for rare clinical events or to ensure baseline competence before learners are allowed to perform tasks on actual patients
There needs to be a greater emphasis on assessment *for* learning rather than exclusive focus on assessment *of* learning
Faculty development on assessment and faculty support to implement assessment strategies will be critical to the implementation of CBE
Collective decision-making will be needed to determine overall competence as learners progress from one stage to another of training
Assessment strategies need to support reflection on the part of learners, allowing them to *own* the responsibility for learning for their ongoing development as clinicians
Narrative descriptions of learners, rather than absolute reliance on numerical scores, may be particularly helpful to support learning. Additionally, the reflective use of *subjective* assessment may be valuable in allowing *experts* to judge performance

CBE competency-based education

allow overreliance on a single case). Additionally, there are likely to be content domains in which faculty need to develop their own knowledge and skills before they are able to accurately assess their junior colleagues (e.g., patient safety is a very important part of medical education in this decade, yet many of the practitioners trained previously would have limited formal knowledge in how to teach or assess it). See Table 14.5.

Challenges of Continuing Professional Development and Competency-Based Simulation Education

Challenges in Continuing Professional Development

Many concerns still exist about the feasibility and efficacy of SBE to solve the problem of improving quality of care. The many challenges of SBE used for CPD have been highlighted [58]. Although there is mounting evidence that lectures and bolus CPD courses are not effective for long-term knowledge and skills retention, it is often the preferred method for educational delivery. Simulation activities, despite attempts to create a safe learning environment are by their nature anxiety producing. Exposing deficiencies especially for more senior healthcare practitioners is a common concern and dissuades engagement by those participants. Reluctance to engage in interprofessional learning has been rooted in the traditional teaching models where meeting different learners'

Table 14.6 Barriers and solutions to continuing professional development (CPD)

Barriers	Potential solutions
Lectures and courses	Evidence-based, outcome-focused educational models to persuade the use of SBE
Simulation anxiety	Privacy of learners Educators skilled in nonthreatening debriefing styles
Interprofessional learning	Train teams using simulation Support teamwork with protocols and procedures Develop an organizational culture—need for *senior champions*
Lack of simulation education experts	Promotion of faculty development Promotion of simulation fellowships

SBE Simulation-based education

objectives has been challenging. SBE offers the ability to engage in learning that mirrors the real working environment, yet uptake for CPD activities is still slow despite its inherent advantages. Finally, SBE requires educators with expertise in case preparation, facilitation, and in debriefing. Limited faculty with these skills and the considerable time required to prepare for these sessions are both barriers to implementing CPD programs, especially in smaller centers. Table 14.6 outlines these barriers and offers potential solutions to the implementation of SBE into our continuing education programs.

Challenges in Competency-Based Simulation Education

Ultimately SBE is a tool that offers many advantages over traditional education delivery such as lectures, courses, and workshops [2]. However, it cannot work in isolation and must be integrated into curricula to achieve the competencies or learning objectives set out by governing bodies across the various disciplines.

At the same time that SBE has flourished, CBE has become the new paradigm in professional medical education. Many specialties have embraced its theoretical advantages: focus on outcomes, emphasis on abilities derived from societal needs over knowledge, de-emphasis of time-based training, and promotion of learner-centered training to achieve milestones [35]. Despite these advantages, many concerns exist. Defining learning objectives that are both comprehensive yet not exhaustive is a challenge to medical educators. There is a fear that endless lists of competencies will overwhelm learners and reduce competencies into a series of tasks rather than what truly makes a healthcare provider. Another concern is that learners will focus on achieving milestones, "jumping over the hurdle" and achieving bare competence rather than striving for excellence. Scheduling of trainees

at different stages has the potential to create administrative logistical challenges while trying to balance clinical needs. Although most trainees will complete training in a similar time frame as traditional curricula, some trainees will take considerably longer and will add to increased resources [35]. Simulation training embedded into these programs is expensive and requires educational expertise that is already in high demand. Finally, as highlighted previously, assessment tools and processes will need to be developed that are "more continuous and frequent, criterion-based, developmental, work-based where possible, …and involve the wisdom of group process in making judgments about trainee progress" [56].

Conclusions

High-Stakes Testing

SBE is being increasingly used for summative purposes [59]. These high-stakes decisions include passing a program, gaining certification or licensure, and maintenance of competence. SBE is ideally suited to measure competencies beyond traditional knowledge-based exams. Organizing bodies such as the ACGME and Royal College of Physicians and Surgeons of Canada (RCPSC) require that examinations are tailored towards skills that mimic the actual practice behaviors [4]. Assessment of most of the six core competencies of the ACGME/American Board of Medical Specialties (ABMS) and the seven CANMEDs roles of the RCPSC, for example, can readily be achieved using simulation-based environments. Use of simulation for high-stakes testing is emerging in many specialties. One example is the use of procedural simulation for carotid stenting where training and passing examinations are required for certification [60]. Use of simulation in high-stakes examination has also been reported in anesthesia, surgery, and internal medicine [61].

Another use of SBA is in the maintenance of certification. Many specialties require either recertification examinations (ABMS) or aggregation of hours in learning activities (RCPSC) in order to maintain certification. Pressure to ensure that these activities reflect patient care competencies rather than knowledge acquisition has led educators to incorporate simulation into these programs [62]. The use of simulation in maintenance of certification in anesthesia and surgery has been described [63]. In Canada, as part of its maintenance of certification program, the RCPSC recognizes and gives credits for learning activities. For example, attending a conference receives 1 credit per hour and reading a journal article 1 credit per article. In contrast, learners receive 3 credits for each hour of approved assessment-driven simulation activity [64].

Although there has been tremendous uptake of SBA, challenges still exist. Frequently, curricula do not always match the assessment. The concept that "assessment drives education" should serve as impetus to curricular development in SBE that is comprehensive and standardized. SBA-scoring strategies must be robust and achieve high degrees of reliability and validity. Experts in the clinical field (content experts), simulation, and measurement are all essential for high-stakes examinations. Further, SBA raters need to be qualified and properly trained with appropriate review of scoring rubrics and emphasis on rater consistency [59]. Finally, SBA is an expensive methodology and must be supported by professional and regulatory boards with the view that patient safety is worth the investment.

Role of National/Shared Curricula

Until recently, simulation programs have been built haphazardly. Sessions were developed locally and dependent on educators with simulation experience, on labs and equipment of variable quality, and on participant availability. Typically, programs were considered an add-on to other components of the education curriculum. As a result, there has been a push to develop standardized trainee-focused curricula that cover the core competencies of accredited training programs. Examples exist in the undergraduate medical education literature of attempts to incorporate a disaster management [65] and simulation-based pediatric clinical skills [66] into the curriculum. In postgraduate medical education, many centers have reported the development and evaluation of standardized simulation curricula. Examples include the specialties of pediatrics, surgery, emergency medicine, and pediatric emergency medicine [67]. Despite these recent attempts to develop simulation-based educational curricula, there is the absence of acceptance of standardized curricula at a national or international level. However, this is likely to change. Currently, in Canada, a group of pediatric emergency medicine physicians have just developed a national standardized simulation curriculum [68]. Additionally, a national pediatric residency program simulation curriculum is being developed while the anesthesiology specialty program is moving towards CBE and incorporating simulation into their curricula and evaluation process. It is only a matter of time before many programs follow suit, and SBE becomes an integral component of training and CPD programs.

References

1. Kohn LT, Corrigan JM, Donaldson MS (Institute of Medicine). To err is human: building a safer health system. Washington, DC: National Academy Press; 1999.
2. Dow AW, Salas E, Mazmanian PE. Improving quality in systems of care: solving complicated challenges with simulation-based continuing professional development. J Contin Educ Health Prof. 2012;32(4):230–5.
3. Issenberg SB, McGaghie WC, Petrusa ER, Lee Gordon D, Scalese RJ. Features and uses of high-fidelity medical simulations that lead to effective learning: a BEME systematic review. Med Teach. 2005;27(1):10–28.
4. McGaghie WC, Issenberg SB, Petrusa ER, Scalese RJ. A critical review of simulation-based medical education research: 2003–2009. Med Educ. 2010;44(1):50–63.
5. Cook DA, Hatala R, Brydges R, Zendejas B, Szostek JH, Wang AT, et al. Technology-enhanced simulation for health professions education: a systematic review and meta-analysis. JAMA. 2011;306(9):978–88.
6. Cheng A, Lang TR, Starr SR, Pusic M, Cook DA. Technology-enhanced simulation and pediatric education: a meta-analysis. Pediatrics. 2014;133(5):e1313–e23.
7. Knight LJ, Gabhart JM, Earnest KS, Leong KM, Anglemyer A, Franzon D. Improving code team performance and survival outcomes: implementation of pediatric resuscitation team training. Crit Care Med. 2014;42(2):243–51.
8. Grafinger DJ. Basics of instructional systems development. INFO-LINE Issue 8803. Alexandria: American Society for Training and Development; 1988.
9. Kern DE. Curriculum development for medical education: a six-step approach. Baltimore: Johns Hopkins University Press; 1998.
10. Rosen MA, Salas E, Silvestri S, Wu TS, Lazzara EH. A measurement tool for simulation-based training in emergency medicine: the simulation module for assessment of resident targeted event responses (SMARTER) approach. Simulation in healthcare: journal of the Society for. Simul Healthc. 2008;3(3):170–9.
11. Kraiger K, Ford JK, Salas E. Application of cognitive, skill-based, and affective theories of learning outcomes to new methods of training evaluation. J Appl Psychol. 1993;78(2):311–28.
12. Benner P. From novice to expert. Am J Nurs. 1982;82(3):402–7.
13. Benner P. Using the dreyfus model of skill acquisition to describe and interpret skill acquisition and clinical judgment in nursing practice and education. Bull Sci Technol Soc. 2004;24(3):188–99.
14. Carraccio CL, Benson BJ, Nixon LJ, Derstine PL. From the educational bench to the clinical bedside: translating the Dreyfus developmental model to the learning of clinical skills. Acad Med. 2008;83(8):761–7.
15. Daley BJ. Novice to expert: an exploration of how professionals learn. Adult Educ Q. 1999;49(4):133–47.
16. Bandura A. Social learning theory. New York: General Learning Press; 1977.
17. Bogue R. Use S.M.A.R.T goals to launch management by objectives plan; 2014 [cited 2014 September 20]; http://www.techrepublic.com/article/use-smart-goals-to-launch-management-by-objectives-plan/.
18. Anderson LW, Krathwohl DR, Bloom BS. A taxonomy for learning, teaching. and assessing: a revision of Bloom's taxonomy of educational objectives. Harlow: Longman; 2001.
19. Schumacher DJ, Englander R, Carraccio C. Developing the master learner: applying learning theory to the learner, the teacher, and the learning environment. Acad Med. 2013;88(11):1635–45.
20. Knowles MS. Self-directed learning: a guide for learners and teachers. New York: Cambridge, the Adult Education Co.; 1975.
21. Kolb DA. Experiential learning: experience as the source of learning and development. Englewood Cliffs: Prentice-Hall; 1984.
22. Choi J-I, Hannafin M. Situated cognition and learning environments: roles, structures, and implications for design. ETR&D. 1995;43(2):53–69.
23. Schon DA. Educating the reflective practitioner: toward a new design for teaching and learning in the professions. New Jersey: Wiley; 1987.
24. Sharp LK, Bashook PG, Lipsky MS, Horowitz SD, Miller SH. Specialty board certification and clinical outcomes: the missing link. Acad Med. 2002;77(6):534–42.

25. Ten Cate O, Snell L, Carraccio C. Medical competence: the interplay between individual ability and the health care environment. Med Teach. 2010;32(8):669–75.

26. Carraccio CL, Englander R. From Flexner to competencies: reflections on a decade and the journey ahead. Acad Med. 2013;88(8):1067–73.

27. Cheng A, Hunt EA, Donoghue A, Nelson-McMillan K, Nishisaki A, Leflore J, et al. Examining pediatric resuscitation education using simulation and scripted debriefing: a multicenter randomized trial. JAMA Pediatr. 2013;167(6):528–36.

28. Brett-Fleegler M, Rudolph J, Eppich W, Monuteaux M, Fleegler E, Cheng A, et al. Debriefing assessment for simulation in healthcare: development and psychometric properties. Simul Healthc. 2012;7(5):288–94.

29. Khanduja PK, Bould MD, Naik VN, Hladkowicz E, Boet S. The role of simulation in continuing medical education for acute care physicians: a systematic review. Crit Care Med. 2015;43(1):186–93.

30. Ten Cate O. Medical Education Competency-based. The Wiley Blackwell encyclopedia of health, illness, behavior, and society. New Jersey: Wiley; 2014.

31. Kohn LT, Corrigan JM, Donaldson MS (Institute of Medicine). To err is human: building a safer health system. Washington, DC: National Academy Press; 2000.

32. Baker GR, Norton PG, Flintoft V, Blais R, Brown A, Cox J, et al. The Canadian adverse events study: the incidence of adverse events among hospital patients in Canada. CMAJ. 2004;170(11):1678–86.

33. Shaw R, Drever F, Hughes H, Osborn S, Williams S. Adverse events and near miss reporting in the NHS. Qual Saf Health Care. 2005;14(4):279–83.

34. Asch DA, Nicholson S, Srinivas S, Herrin J, Epstein AJ. Evaluating obstetrical residency programs using patient outcomes. JAMA. 2009;302(12):1277–83.

35. Frank JR, Snell LS, Cate OT, Holmboe ES, Carraccio C, Swing SR, et al. Competency-based medical education: theory to practice. Med Teach. 2010;32(8):638–45.

36. Cruess SR. Professionalism and medicine's social contract with society. Clin Orthop Relat Res. 2006;449:170–6.

37. Quebec mammogram review finds 109 errors. 2012; http://www.cbc.ca/news/canada/montreal/quebec-mammogram-review-finds-109-errors-1.1221134.

38. Medical Scan Mistakes. What's behind the problems? 2012; http://www.cbc.ca/news/canada/medical-scan-mistakes-what-s-behind-the-problems-1.1161747.

39. Frank JR, Danoff D. The CanMEDS initiative: implementing an outcomes-based framework of physician competencies. Med Teach. 2007;29(7):642–7.

40. Batalden P, Leach D, Swing S, Dreyfus H, Dreyfus S. General competencies and accreditation in graduate medical education. Health Aff (Millwood). 2002;21(5):103–11.

41. Simpson JG, Furnace J, Crosby J, Cumming AD, Evans PA, Friedman Ben David M, et al. The Scottish doctor–learning outcomes for the medical undergraduate in Scotland: a foundation for competent and reflective practitioners. Med Teach. 2002;24(2):136–43.

42. Cohen ER, Feinglass J, Barsuk JH, Barnard C, O'Donnell A, McGaghie WC, et al. Cost savings from reduced catheter-related bloodstream infection after simulation-based education for residents in a medical intensive care unit. Simul Healthc. 2010;5(2):98–102.

43. Barsuk JH, Cohen ER, Feinglass J, Kozmic SE, McGaghie WC, Ganger D, et al. Cost savings of performing paracentesis procedures at the bedside after simulation-based education. Simul Healthc. 2014;9(5):312–8.

44. Sroka G, Feldman LS, Vassiliou MC, Kaneva PA, Fayez R, Fried GM. Fundamentals of laparoscopic surgery simulator training to proficiency improves laparoscopic performance in the operating room-a randomized controlled trial. Am J Surg. 2010;199(1):115–20.

45. Barsuk JH, Cohen ER, Feinglass J, McGaghie WC, Wayne DB. Unexpected collateral effects of simulation-based medical education. Acad Med. 2011;86(12):1513–7.

46. Bastian H, Glasziou P, Chalmers I. Seventy-five trials and eleven systematic reviews a day: how will we ever keep up? PLoS Med. 2010;7(9):e1000326.

47. Cervero RM, Gaines JK. Effectiveness of continuing medical education: updated synthesis of systematic reviews. Chicago: Accreditation Council for Continuing Medical Education; 2014.

48. Boet S, Bould MD, Bruppacher HR, Desjardins F, Chandra DB, Naik VN. Looking in the mirror: self-debriefing versus instructor debriefing for simulated crises. Crit Care Med. 2011;39(6):1377–81.

49. Carraccio C, et al. Competency-based medical education: a charter for clinician-educators. Personal Correspondence; 2014.

50. Schuwirth LW, Van der Vleuten CP. Programmatic assessment: from assessment of learning to assessment for learning. Med Teach. 2011;33(6):478–85.

51. Norcini JJ, Boulet JR, Opalek A, Dauphinee WD. The relationship between licensing examination performance and the outcomes of care by international medical school graduates. Acad Med. 2014;89(8):1157–62.

52. Miller GE. The assessment of clinical skills/competence/performance. Acad Med. 1990;65(9 Suppl):S63–7.

53. Hamstra SJ, Brydges R, Hatala R, Zendejas B, Cook DA. Reconsidering fidelity in simulation-based training. Acad Med. 2014;89(3):387–92.

54. Hodges B. Assessment in the post-psychometric era: learning to love the subjective and collective. Med Teach. 2013;35(7):564–8.

55. Norcini J, Anderson B, Bollela V, Burch V, Costa MJ, Duvivier R, et al. Criteria for good assessment: consensus statement and recommendations from the Ottawa 2010 Conference. Med Teach. 2011;33(3):206–14.

56. Holmboe ES, Sherbino J, Long DM, Swing SR, Frank JR. The role of assessment in competency-based medical education. Med Teach. 2010;32(8):676–82.

57. Holmboe ES, Ward DS, Reznick RK, Katsufrakis PJ, Leslie KM, Patel VL, et al. Faculty development in assessment: the missing link in competency-based medical education. Acad Med. 2011;86(4):460–7.

58. McGaghie WC, Siddall VJ, Mazmanian PE, Myers J. Lessons for continuing medical education from simulation research in undergraduate and graduate medical education: effectiveness of continuing medical education: American College of Chest Physicians Evidence-Based Educational Guidelines. Chest. 2009;135(3 Suppl):62S–8S.

59. Feldman M, Lazzara EH, Vanderbilt AA, DiazGranados D. Rater training to support high-stakes simulation-based assessments. J Contin Educ Health Prof. 2012;32(4):279–86.

60. Gallagher AG, Cates CU. Approval of virtual reality training for carotid stenting: what this means for procedural-based medicine. JAMA. 2004;292(24):3024–6.

61. Hatala R, Kassen BO, Nishikawa J, Cole G, Issenberg SB. Incorporating simulation technology in a Canadian internal medicine specialty examination: a descriptive report. Acad Med. 2005;80(6):554–6.

62. Levine AI, Schwartz AD, Bryson EO, Demaria S Jr. Role of simulation in U.S. physician licensure and certification. Mt Sinai J Med. 2012;79(1):140–53.

63. Gallagher CJ, Tan JM. The current status of simulation in the maintenance of certification in anesthesia. Int Anesthesiol Clin. 2010;48(3):83–99.

64. Royal College of Physicians and Surgeons of Canada. The Royal College's MOC Program: Short Users Manual. [cited 2014 December 12]; http://www.royalcollege.ca/portal/page/portal/rc/members/moc.

65. Ingrassia PL, Ragazzoni L, Tengattini M, Carenzo L, Della Corte F. Nationwide program of education for undergraduates in the field of disaster medicine: development of a core curriculum centered on blended learning and simulation tools. Prehosp Disaster Med. 2014;29(5):508–15.

66. Dudas RA, Colbert-Getz JM, Balighian E, Cooke D, Golden WC, Khan S, et al. Evaluation of a simulation-based pediatric clinical skills curriculum for medical students. Simul Healthc. 2014;9(1):21–32.

67. Cheng A, Goldman RD, Aish MA, Kissoon N. A simulation-based acute care curriculum for pediatric emergency medicine fellowship training programs. Pediatr Emerg Care. 2010;26(7):475–80.

68. Bank I, Cheng A, McLeod C, Bhanji F. Determining content for a simulation-based curriculum in pediatric emergency medicine: results from a National Delphi Process. CJEM. 2015:1–8.

Interprofessional Education

Janice C. Palaganas, Ella Scott, Mary E. Mancini
and Glenn Stryjewski

Simulation Pearls

1. Interprofessional education (IPE) occurs when two or more members of different professions come together in the same space for an educational event. IPE involves learning with, from, and about each other to improve collaboration and/or the delivery of patient care.
2. Healthcare simulation with debriefing can be used to deliberately create an experience for an interprofessional team to not only allow practitioners from different professions to learn alongside each other but to also learn from and about each other.
3. Using healthcare simulation for effective IPE requires much forethought and planning. There are ways to overcome challenges in the implementation, debriefing, and evaluation of simulation-based IPE (SimBIE).
4. Debriefing is where the skills most relevant to interprofessional practice are gained.

5. While pediatric SimBIE requires preplanning, professional development occurs in the doing. Therefore, planning paralysis during the professional development process is to be avoided.

Introduction

A review of the historical progression of health care reveals an organic fragmentation of healthcare disciplines into specializations. Specialization has allowed advances in knowledge and technology while increasing the complexity of today's patient care. Moreover, the resulting specialization and fragmentation have created some gaps in patient care that over time have widened, negatively affecting specific patient outcomes. Adverse outcomes as a result of fragmented care continue to highlight the need for unification of information, communication skills, and hence collaborative care [1].

Clinicians, patient safety officers, and educators continue to search for effective methods that can assist in achieving the goal of collaborative care. This effort comes with many challenges that have created a renewed focus on IPE, a perceived bridge toward more effective and efficient care, and ultimately greater patient safety. IPE is defined as learning with, from, and about each other for the purpose of improving interprofessional collaboration and improving patient outcomes [2]. IPE can:

- Develop the ability to share knowledge and skills collaboratively
- Enable students to become competent in teamwork
- Decompartmentalize curricula
- Integrate new skills and areas of knowledge
- Ease interprofessional communication
- Generate new roles
- Promote interprofessional research
- Improve understanding and cooperation between educational and research institutions
- Permit collective consideration of resource allocation according to need

J. C. Palaganas (✉)
Department of Anesthesia, Critical Care & Pain Medicine, Harvard University, Massachusetts General Hospital, Boston, MA, USA
e-mail: jpalaganas.cms@gmail.com

E. Scott
Department of Simulation, Sidra Medical & Research Center, Doha, Qatar
e-mail: ellaannscott@yahoo.com.au

M. E. Mancini
College of Nursing and Health Innovation, The University of Texas at Arlington, Arlington, TX, USA
e-mail: Mancini@uta.edu

G. Stryjewski
Department of Pediatrics, Jefferson Medical College, Philadelphia, PA, USA

Division of Pediatric Critical Care, Nemours/Alfred I. duPont Hospital for Children, Wilmington, DE, USA
e-mail: gstryjew@nemours.org

© Springer International Publishing Switzerland 2016
V. J. Grant, A. Cheng (eds.), *Comprehensive Healthcare Simulation: Pediatrics*,
Comprehensive Healthcare Simulation, DOI 10.1007/978-3-319-24187-6_15

- Ensure consistency in curriculum design [2]
- Assist with systems processes, interprofessional clinical guidelines, and procedures

Healthcare simulation has been growing simultaneously with patient quality and safety improvement strategies and is increasingly used as the platform for team training, including skills training for communication and teamwork (see Chap. 5). Recent advances in using healthcare simulation for team training have stemmed from findings in the fields of aviation, crisis resource management (CRM) training, nuclear energy teams, organizational behavior, business management, and patient safety (see Chap. 4). As in these other fields, team training in health care has revealed many valuable areas for interprofessional improvement. Given the value of learning within a relative context or environment, simulation-based education (SBE) is increasingly becoming a preferred platform for IPE [1]. While healthcare simulation as a platform for IPE continues to be defined and refined, this chapter seeks to provide pediatric-focused simulation educators with knowledge around using healthcare simulation for IPE, specifically how to overcome its many challenges.

Gaps in Simulation and IPE Literature

Analytical reviews (i.e., critical synthesis and meta-analysis) of simulation and the IPE literature have found similar gaps that make it difficult to determine the factors that lead to positive or negative interprofessional learning [3–18]. These common gaps include:

- Lack of common language
- Lack of conceptual models/frameworks
- Lack of a theoretical foundation to guide program development
- Lack of rigor in teaching and research methodology with too many unaccounted variables
- Lack of validated or reliable measures of evaluation

The identified gaps underscore challenges for educators looking to create simulation-enhanced IPE. Given these gaps, this chapter provides common language, a conceptual model, theories that educators can use, variables to consider when implementing activities (specifically, how to develop, implement, debrief, and evaluate interprofessional simulations, IPsim), reporting frameworks, and areas for future research as a guide for simulation educators.

Creating a Common Language

Human communication depends on given names. In order to create and maintain common understanding, names are used. Healthcare simulation and IPE has the inherent potential for wide creativity. Programs and organizations around the world continue to pioneer innovative methods, creating their own terminology [19]. This leads to a disjointed community with difficulty in understanding each other's work and findings and often making individual interpretations of others' terminology.

A common language is essential in developing knowledge and for facilitating discussions that will build knowledge. In an attempt to decrease varying terminology across geography, professions, and institutions, some key terms and definitions are suggested for the field in Table 15.1. These terms and definitions stem from sentinel articles in the fields and have been confirmed with current and leading group work in lexicography for both fields: the Taxonomy and Terminology Committee for the Society for Simulation in Healthcare and the interprofessional work published by the Institute of Medicine, World Health Organization, and Centre for the Advancement of Interprofessional Education [20–24].

A Conceptual Model for Simulation-Enhanced IPE

Conceptual models often provide clarity in understanding and can serve as a guide for development of programs. We offer here a model to clarify understanding of the field (Fig. 15.1) [25]. A model for developing valid, reliable, and measurable SimBIE is provided later in the chapter, as well as an implementation model for SimBIE (Fig. 15.2).

Simulation-Enhanced IPE

SBE is only one type of methodology used in IPE but is increasingly becoming the preferred methodology in the healthcare field. IPE is one type of purpose used in SBE. As depicted in Fig. 15.1, simulation-enhanced IPE is the mergence of both sciences into one field.

The elements of simulation that make it an attractive method for IPE are as follows: (a) It provides a safe environment by keeping real patients safe; (b) there is, otherwise, a lack of opportunities in clinical settings for skill development; (c) it provides a realistic experience; (d) students are more engaged in experiential and active learning; (e) it is deliberate practice; and (f) it provides a standardized experience. Simulation was seen to be more effective than other IPE activities at achieving interprofessional objectives due to the following attributes: realism, practice, debriefing and reflection, increased student engagement, relevance of the experience, fostered interaction, safe environment, opportunity for feedback, immediacy of feedback, immersive experience, framework for learning communication, and the emotional experience [48].

Table 15.1 Simulation-enhanced interprofessional education terms of reference

Crisis resource management (CRM) is an approach to managing critical situations in a healthcare setting. CRM training emphasizes communication skills. Originally developed in aviation and, as a result, also called crew resource management, CRM emphasizes the role of *human factors*—the effects of fatigue and perceptual errors, as well as the effects of different management styles and organizational cultures in high-stress, high-risk environments [20, 21]

Interdisciplinary learning (IDL) "involves integrating the perspective of professionals from two or more professions, by organizing the education around a specific discipline, where each discipline examines the basis of their knowledge" [22]

Interprofessional education/training (IPE) "describes those occasions when two or more professions learn with, from and about each other to improve collaboration and the quality of care" [23]. "It is an initiative to secure interprofessional learning and promote gains through interprofessional collaboration in professional practice" [24]. *"Formal interprofessional education* aims to promote collaboration and enhance the quality of care; therefore it is an educational or practice development initiative that brings people from different professions together to engage in activities that promote interprofessional learning. The intention for formal interprofessional education is for curricula to achieve this aim" [24]. *"Informal (or serendipitous) interprofessional education* is unplanned learning between professional practitioners or between students on uniprofessional or multi-professional programs, which improves interprofessional practice. At its inception, it lacks the intention of interprofessional education. At any point in time after that it may be acknowledged that learning with, from and about each other is happening between participants. However, in many such initiatives, this remains unacknowledged or is only recognized on reflection in and on the learning practice" [24]

Interprofessional learning (IPL) is "learning arising from interaction between members (or students) of two or more professions. This may be a product of interprofessional education or happen spontaneously in the workplace or in education settings (e.g., from serendipitous interprofessional education)" [24]

Interprofessionalism is "the effective integration of professionals through mutual respect, trust, and support, from various professions who share a common purpose to mold their separate skills and knowledge into collective responsibility and awareness that can be achieved through learned processes for communication, problem solving, conflict resolution, and conducting evaluation" [48]

Intraprofessional involves activity between or among individuals within the same profession with similar or different specialties or levels of practice (e.g., surgeons and emergency physicians; clinical nurses and nurse practitioners; and residents and physicians)

Multidisciplinary (MD) involves bringing professionals with different perspectives together to provide a wider understanding of a particular problem [22]

Multiprofessional education (MPE) is "when members (or students) of two or more professions learn alongside one another: in other words, parallel rather than interactive learning. Also referred to as common or shared learning" [24]

Simulation-enhanced IPE is the use of healthcare simulation modalities for IPE. *Simulation-based interprofessional education (SimBIE)* describes simulations that are created using interprofessional learning objectives, and students from two or more professions learn with, from, and about each other during the simulation; whereas *interprofessional simulations (IPsim)* describe simulations that are created using clinical, diagnosis-centered, or task-focused learning objectives, and students from two or more professions participate in the simulation, learning in parallel and not necessarily from and about each other during the simulation [48]

Transdisciplinary is a strategy that crosses many disciplinary boundaries to create a holistic approach to development and attempts to overcome the confines of individual disciplines to form a team that crosses and recrosses disciplinary boundaries and thereby maximizes communication, interaction, and cooperation among team members [24]

Uniprofessional education is when members (or students) of a single profession learn together [22, 24]

Relevant Theories as Frameworks for Development

While ongoing research and publications strengthen the foundation of this field, there are a number of educational theories that serve as a tool for development of simulation-enhanced IPE programs. An understanding of the common theories used to support the development of simulation activities and those used to support the development of IPE provides educators with a deeper understanding of the purposes and benefits of both fields. This understanding will guide educators when choosing methods to create effective and high-quality simulation-enhanced IPE. Theories are derived from years and years of collective experience and reflective thought of experts. The use of theories to guide practice creates an informed and intelligent approach to the educational activity [34]. Relevant theoretical frameworks for healthcare simulation are presented in Table 15.2 (for more background, see Morrison and Deckers [35]). Relevant theoretical frameworks for IPE are presented in Table 15.3 (for more information on these frameworks, see the *Journal of Interprofessional Care*, Theoretical Special Issue 27 [36]).

Variables to Consider in SimBIE: Development, Implementation, Debriefing Considerations, and Evaluation

While educators across the globe nod their heads in agreement on the need for IPE using healthcare simulation (HCS), the difficulty is in the doing. Many educators feel insecure about their knowledge in either IPE or SBE; however, given the relatively young phase of this science [3], this is expected. Simulation and IPE educators are currently pioneers developing this educational science.

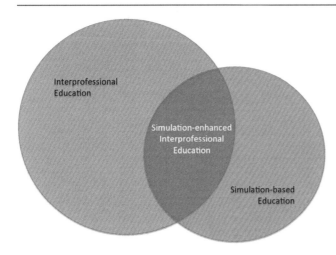

Fig. 15.1 The field of simulation-enhanced interprofessional education (IPE). (Reproduced with permission [25])

Many programs have successfully provided team training and published findings for years; however, each program has different unaccounted variables for success and failure (e.g., characteristics of the educator, students, simulation program) [3]. The collective recommendations toward successful programs suggested in this chapter come from the experience of the authors and are offered to help faculty develop their own simulation-enhanced IPE programs. While a reader of this chapter may gain insight into developing a simulation-enhanced IPE program, skills and knowledge of developing simulation-enhanced IPE are gained in the process of creating, implementing, and evaluating an activity. By these experiences, one may understand the unique programmatic variables that support or oppose IPE efforts in their own particular organizational culture.

Recall from Table 15.1 the difference between IPsim and SimBIE. IPsim may be created by recreating an actual clinical event that involved different professions performing their profession-specific goals simultaneously. Many simulation programs developing interprofessional activities create IPsim where the objectives are a mix of profession-specific clinical objectives. While this may create interprofessional learning in the process, it is not guaranteed. Different from IPsim, SimBIE simulations are based on interprofessional objectives (competencies required for effective interprofessional collaboration and practice) and have interprofessional opportunities (e.g., communication or communication challenges) embedded into and facilitated throughout the simulated case (e.g., via an embedded simulated provider (ESP)/confederate). These simulations require an interprofessional focus during the development of the case. As a method that is more secure in achieving IPE objectives and in alignment with the scope of this chapter, we will be focusing on pediatric SimBIE when describing how to develop, implement, and evaluate cases. To distinguish the terminology used in this chapter, simulation-enhanced IPE is the umbrella term for any simulation used for IPE, whereas SimBIE are simulations that have interprofessional objectives embedded into the experiential activities.

Fig. 15.2 Implementation model for simulation-enhanced interprofessional education (IPE). *PA* physician assistant. (Reproduced with permission [3])

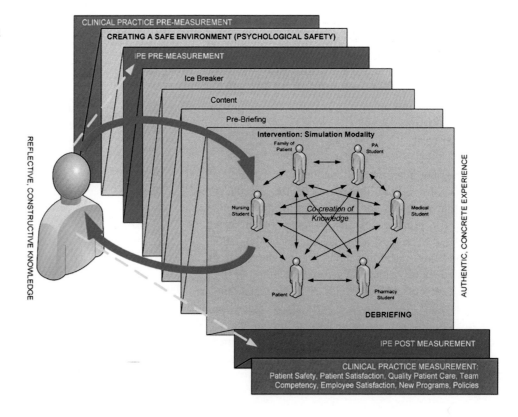

Table 15.2 Relevant theoretical frameworks for healthcare simulation

Theory	Description
Adult learning [26]	Andragogy is the study of adult learning. Malcolm Knowles states six assumptions that motivate adults to learn. These assumptions include that (1) adults need to know the reason why they are learning what they are learning, (2) adults need to be involved in their plan and decisions around education (be self-directing), (3) adults bring vast experiences to the discussion, (4) adults are most interested in material that is relevant to their lives, (5) adults learn best when the activity is problem-centered, and (6) adults are internally driven [26]
Experiential learning [27, 28]	David Kolb and Roger Fry developed a model of learning that conceptualizes learning as a process through the transformation of experience from the work of Dewey, Lewin, and Piaget [27]. The model posits four cycles: experience (e.g., work, real-world experience, simulations), reflection (e.g., reflecting on a specific action), conceptualization (e.g., analyzing and understanding what drove the action and effect), and experimentation (e.g., planning and executing a course of action) [28]. This highlights the crucial role of debriefing in SBE
Situated learning [29]	Lave and Wenger describe a social process where knowledge is cocreated within the context of how that skill or knowledge is applied [29]. Situated learning theory also embraces a concrete experience (i.e., simulation) and reflective observation on the experience (i.e., debriefing). Learning is constructed in a way where knowledge is contextualized. This deep understanding of the context becomes the means for understanding that situation and the meaning made by the learner. This dynamic perspective adds a larger context to debriefing and suggests that learning is supported and altered through the exchange and interaction of individuals
Reflective practice [30, 31]	Donald Schön's work describes how we create new meaning through the analysis and understanding of actions and values. There are two types of reflection: reflection-in-action (i.e., during the simulation) and reflection-on-action (i.e., after the simulation) during debriefing [30]. Debriefing should also allow for a third type of reflective practice identified by Thompson and Pascal [31]: reflection-for-action (i.e., how to apply new meaning for new action in practice or for the next simulation)
Deliberate practice [32, 33]	K. Anders Ericsson outlines essential components of deliberate practice that optimize learning and performance including internal motivation to engage in a task to improve; building upon previous experience, skill, and knowledge; immediate feedback on the performance; and repetition of the task [32]. Ericsson underscores the point that healthcare students need representations that can support planning and practice of the actual performance to allow for adjustments toward mastery, and there is a need where feedback can be immediate [33]. With careful planning and skilled facilitation, simulation with debriefing helps to fill this need

SBE simulation-based education

Developing SimBIE

Performing a Needs Assessment

When developing simulation-enhanced IPE, a needs assessment should be performed. Education created to address identified needs are likely to be more successful in achieving support (i.e., institutional and funding), as well as generating a more significant impact. Findings from a needs assessment can serve as goals or objectives for simulation-enhanced IPE. Needs may be identified at the macro-, meso-, and microlevels (see Fig. 15.3).

At the macrolevel, professional societies identify needs for the community and for the profession. More and more professional societies are recognizing and promoting the need for and developing specific competencies around interprofessional collaboration. External funding is often available for organizations that look to meet this need. Team competencies have been developed by international and national, professional, and interprofessional committees [49–51]. These competencies can be used as objectives that structure the simulation experience.

Programmatic competencies, areas for improvement as identified by accreditation organizations, and actual patient safety or risk management cases can identify needs at the mesolevel. Internal funding and human resources for programs structured around needs at the mesolevel are often easier to obtain. Programs developed around mesolevel needs often foster interdepartmental and interprofessional collaboration within the institutional system.

A needs assessment performed at the microlevel may seek to answer questions identified by the patient and family, individual learner or learner group, educators, or supervisors. These can be done via survey, focus groups, town halls, or from meeting reports. Questions that can assist in identifying needs include:

Patient and Family
- Describe situations where you experienced what you considered to be great teamwork and poor teamwork for you or your child?
- What did you see or would have liked to have experienced?

Individual Learner
- What intimidates you about working in a team of healthcare providers?
- What does good interprofessionalism look like to you? What are the gaps in your clinical experience?

Table 15.3 Relevant theoretical frameworks for interprofessional education

Theory	Description
Psychodynamic theory [37]	Bion brings to light psychodynamic perspectives where learning depends on cultivating critical awareness of behavior in, as, and between groups [37]
Contact hypothesis/theory [38]	Allport posits that contact modifies prejudice and stereotypes between professions and, therefore, modifies relationships between professional groups [38]
Identity theories [39–41]	In *social identity theory*, Tajfel and Turner describe how our identity comes from our membership of social groups in which we perceive our group more positively than others [39]. Turner explores *self-categorization theory* as an expansion of social identity theory in the context of one's organization [40]. Brown et al. focuses on group objectives in *realistic conflict theory* where the objectives in each group surface through attitude and behavior [41]
Practice theory (Bourdieu, 1977)	Bourdieu describes how professional identity is acquired through one's culture and how each profession has its own *cultural capital*. Under this theory, IPE should be a common, long, and consistent experience [42].
Situated learning [29]	See description in Table 15.2. Lave and Wenger complement situated learning with the concept of a *community of practice*. The learning in IPE should include the same members with their perspectives and contribution of the event explored [29]
Sociology perspectives	The field of sociology has many social theories that could explain how professions are socialized into the values and mental models of each and the behaviors that ensue
General systems theory [43]	Von Bertalanffy views the whole individual–community–environment as beyond professional and political bounds typically of focus, taking into account each profession's complexity. Cause and effect are interdependent, and this theory seeks to unify how each profession relates their work to the needs of all involved components [43]
Organizational theory [44]	Senge describes conditions that nurture learning, creating *a culture of enquiry*. An environment capable of a respectful, proactive, innovative, continuous, and iterative process of change and reframing allows this culture of inquiry [44]
Activity theory [45]	Engestrom focuses on understanding and intervening in interactions to effect change in relations at the microlevel (individual) and macrolevel (community rules). This requires a joint activity [45]
Complexity theory [46]	Fraser and Greenhalgh account for the unpredictable, complex, adaptive systems in organizations, professions, and learners. Learning takes place between familiar and unfamiliar tasks and environments. To address each complexity, multiple remedies are more effective [46]
Transformative learning theory [47]	Transformational learning is a branch of adult learning (see Table 15.2). Mezirow describes a 10-step process for transformative learning to offer a guideline in developing the skills needed for optimal team performance in a complex environment [47]

IPE interprofessional education

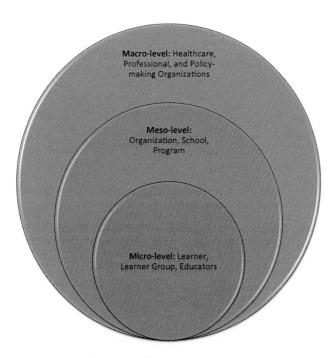

Learner Group
- What surprises or scares you about working in a healthcare team?
- What are your stereotypes of other professions, and how does that impact clinical behavior?

Educators
- What are the things about working in teams that you wish your clinical students would know prior to beginning a clinical rotation?
- What learning gaps exist between professions?
- What team-related gaps have you observed in simulations?

Supervisors
- What are your fears around patient safety that are relevant to team collaboration or communication?
- What practice gaps exist between professions?

Fig. 15.3 Assessing interprofessional education (IPE) needs at the macro-, meso-, and microlevels

Authoring a SimBIE Case

Once the needs have been determined, interprofessional objectives may be written. When writing objectives for SimBIE, depending on time allotted for the simulation and for debriefing, it is important to choose achievable and observable interprofessional objectives. Faculty from each target learner group should come to consensus on objectives. Once objectives are determined, the simulation case can be chosen or written.

A common occurrence when authoring IPE scenarios is the use of existing scenarios developed for one profession. If this is done, each scenario needs to be revised to meet the needs of each professional group involved in the learning to ensure equal opportunity for learning.

If/Thens Each scenario should have progression plans with if/thens outlined for scenario facilitators. If/thens are written plans for "If X occurs, then the facilitators will do Y." Faculty from each learner group should be involved in developing a robust list of if/thens for the scenario. Faculty should become familiar with these progression plans and be prepared to facilitate in these situations.

Simulation, in the context of an educational tool, should be validated prior to implementation. Validity is not only established by making sure that faculty proponents from each target learner group have reviewed and revised the scenario to make it realistic and achievable for their group but also through dry runs (e.g., implementation of the simulation with a pilot group). A dry run with practicing providers from each learner group can confirm or disconfirm the realism of the case. A dry run with a sample of the intended target learner groups helps confirm or disconfirm that opportunities to demonstrate objectives are adequately embedded in the scenario, are realistic, achievable, and observable (Table 15.4).

Implementing SimBIE

An Implementation Model for Simulation-Enhanced IPE

The model provided in Fig. 15.2 outlines nine steps that have been identified to create strong simulation-enhanced IPE and suggests points of measurement to assist in evaluating the education, as well as its practice impact:
1. Clinical practice premeasurement
2. Creating a safe physical and psychological environment
3. IPE premeasurement
4. Ice breaker
5. IPE content
6. Pre-briefing
7. Simulation + debriefing
8. IPE post-measurement
9. Clinical practice post-measurement

Clinical Practice Pre- and Post-measurement

Gaps in the literature call for programs to measure and think about IPE impact at the clinical practice or healthcare systems level [8, 11, 16, 18]. We present this as a beginning and end goal of IPE and recognize that this presents as a current challenge to many educators and IPE activities. In the case that these pre- and post-clinical practice measurement steps are difficult to achieve, it is good practice to consider how the simulation-enhanced IPE translates from and to the clinical practice setting, informing future IPE activities and bridging the education-to-practice gap [52, 53].

Table 15.4 Simulation-based interprofessional education development: challenges and tips

Developing simulation-based IPE	
Challenge	*Tips*
Scheduling faculty to assist in development	There are often faculty in each profession who are simulation or IPE enthusiasts. Ask your simulation program staff and each school. These proponent faculty are often eager to participate and flexible in their scheduling
Deciding on a scenario	It is often easy for a group of interprofessional faculty to come to consensus on objectives. Deciding on a scenario usually presents more challenges based on each faculty's preference/specialty. Explore each faculty's ideas and see if you could come to consensus on which scenario best meets the agreed upon objectives
The dry run with target learners did not meet the objectives	Simplify. Choose 1–2 objectives and rerun. Run a focus group following the dry run to determine how they think you could have achieved the objectives. Make sure you are choosing the right modality—is a mannequin better for this scenario or a standardized patient? Is simulation the best method for these objectives?

IPE interprofessional education

Creating a Safe Physical and Psychological Environment

Given social barriers of unfamiliarity, hierarchy, stereotypes, and individual and group identity, the importance of establishing psychological safety is heightened when bringing together learners from different professions. Four important practices have been suggested with the goal of establishing a psychologically safe environment: declaring and enacting a commitment to respecting learners and concern for their psychological safety; attending to logistic details; clarifying expectations and establishing a *fiction contract* (i.e., informing participants that educators and staff have done their best to make the simulation as real as possible, acknowledging that it is not real, while asking participants to act as though it is real for the purpose of individual and group learning) with participants [54]. While the steps of creating a safe environment are beyond the limits of this chapter, it is noted that team engagement and reflection depends on the safe container created by the faculty where one feels safe to take risks with the potential to make mistakes, speak up, share his/her thoughts, and provide peer-to-peer feedback despite the social challenges faced in IPE [55].

IPE Pre- and Post-measurement

The literature identifies the challenges of understanding which variables in simulation-enhanced IPE actually influence the learning [3, 56–58]. This is because the methods are often not directly studied or reported. Pre- and post-IPE measurement is necessary in order to replicate successful IPE. One example of a pre-post measurement tool for IPE was created and used to assess student perspectives on SimBIE [59]. The methodology should be examined in a way where, if it were to be adopted by another program or be implemented again, the same (or higher) level of interprofessional learning will be achieved. While rigorous measurement (e.g., controlled, randomized, longitudinal, mixed methodology) is ideal for these steps, it is beyond the scope of this chapter (see Chap. 7).

Ice Breaker

A brief introductory and interactive activity allows the learners and faculty to learn about each other in a less formal way, establishing a team environment, flattening hierarchy, creating group unity, and contributing to the future engagement of the learners [60].

IPE Content

In a recent report of team training and patient outcomes, the use of simulation was found to enhance learning outcomes, and the use of combined training strategies with simulated practice, information, and demonstration is more effective than simulation alone for learning, behavioral transfer, and organizational outcomes [16]. Additionally, a supplemental team training curriculum, in addition to SimBIE, was found to have a significant effect on team performance and behavior [61]. This suggests that explicit information around the objectives should be provided to the learners in addition to simulation.

Pre-briefing

Depending on the objectives of the session, faculty who developed the case should determine what information is needed and appropriate for the learners to know prior to the simulation, particularly the learners' roles. Many simulation programs believe that simulation is most powerful for the learner when they are exactly who they are rather than another role, for example, a physician should be a physician in the simulation rather than pretending to be a nurse. This school of thought believes that it subtracts from necessary learning for that individual, tends to make the simulation environment more confusing for participants, and may reinforce stereotypes that IPE seeks to breakdown—stereotypes that have been shown to negatively impact patient care. These programs will give a general assignment to the participants that allows freedom for them to be who they are clinically in their profession (e.g., "you are the rapid response team"). Some simulation programs predetermine the roles of the learners to provide variety and realistic composition of involved teams in the simulation case and under the belief that playing a role other than one's clinical role may provide insight into this other role [62]. Based on our interprofessional experience, the authors recommend against the predetermination of individual roles unless role exposure is one of the main objectives—and if that is the case, the simulation debriefing should be carefully facilitated to address role issues.

The Simulation

Environment

As highlighted in the section on theoretical frameworks influencing SBE and IPE, an authentic concrete experience where teams of professions can demonstrate team behaviors can create rich and relevant experiences for reflection and debriefing. Whether the program developed is for an undergraduate or a postgraduate group of learners, it is essential to determine the time, date, and venue well in advance. Resource and logistical implications of developing and running IPsim is often concerned with undergraduate programs where large cohorts from multiple sites are common [63]. The size of the group may encourage restructuring of the simulation, change in methodology, or change in venue [13].

Clinical practice scenarios using high-technology pediatric simulation may be conducted in the clinical area. This is called in situ simulation. In situ simulation provides a naturalistic environment with actual and familiar clinical equipment, enhancing the fidelity or realism of the case (see Chap. 12 for details). There are advantages to conducting the IPE in a simulation center, including decreased distraction affecting a clinical workload, providing a private and safe environment, removing the learners from social barriers that are associated with the actual environment, and unifying the learners by holding the simulation in a less familiar environment.

The Pediatric Patient

Mannequins are typically used as the pediatric patient. The voice and verbal mannerisms of the mannequin (if applicable) should be realistic for the patient size, age, and condition (see Chap. 10 for details). Voice altering software or realistic sound files may be used to enhance fidelity.

Standardized pediatric patients are rare. While some programs find ways to employ actual children as pediatric patients, most programs do not and are uncomfortable seeking this methodology. The idea or effect of using children to play roles as a pediatric patient needs further exploration and is listed as an area of future study (see Chap. 8 for details).

Embedded Simulated Family/Caregivers

Because pediatric care involves care of the family or caregiver, pediatric simulations should have embedded simulated family and caregivers. The roles should have clear if/ thens and should be dry run for the purpose of training for realistic acting. The inclusion of family and caregivers allows opportunity for other healthcare professions (e.g., social work, marriage and family therapy, etc.). Such roles can be performed by embedded simulated family or caregivers who will be familiar with the case and the script, and facilitate the learning by providing realistic cues (e.g., providing additional information if an objective was missed by the group for a period of time).

Embedded Simulated Providers

Depending on the objectives of the education, ESPs, also known as "confederates" or "actors," may be used. It is imperative that these roles be structured and dry run cautiously. To prevent the reinforcement of stereotypes or offense to the profession, the portrayal of the role must be realistic and the ESP screened for the ability to play a realistic role.

Debriefing Simulation-Enhanced IPE

Debriefing is necessary in the most critical phase in simulation-enhanced IPE. It allows for reflection on team processes and feedback (see Chap. 3 for details). In debriefing, the team is able to cocreate new knowledge based on their behaviors in the simulation merged with thoughts and beliefs from past experiences. A general rule for debriefing is that it is twice the amount of time allotted to the simulation scenario. If the objectives chosen for the educational experience were carefully built into the simulation, they often naturally make their way to the debriefing conversation. While the simulation provides a common experience as material for discussion, the debriefing is the discussion and that is where team excellence and barriers could be explored to deepen each learner's understanding of interprofessional practice in ways that are relevant to them and applicable to their practice.

Debriefers

Faculty often wonder who should debrief interprofessional groups. Interprofessional groups can be debriefed by a member or members of any of the healthcare professions. It is best that the individual has formal training in the debriefing process. There are a number of training programs for interprofessional debriefing [64]. The debriefer should not only be competent in facilitating discussions and facilitating challenging discussions but should also be aware of their own stereotypes and beliefs around different professions and interprofessional practice. These beliefs often leak out in the conversation with risk of reinforcing existing stereotypes or creating negative interprofessional learning.

Co-debriefing

Because of learner diversity, a model of co-debriefing might be chosen. Co-debriefers should meet beforehand to become familiar with each other including areas of expertise and debriefing comfort. Proactive planning and planning for reactive strategies (e.g., plan to do X if Y occurs during the debriefing) assist in well-facilitated co-debriefings.

Subject Matter Experts

Many programs feel as though subject matter experts from each profession should be part of the debriefing. If subject matter experts are used, guidelines should be provided regarding the debriefing to prevent multiple facilitations of the debriefing. Generally, it works well for the subject matter expert to be called on by the debriefer when consultation on clinical or practice content is needed. Other programs will have separate short uniprofessional debriefings with subject matter experts following the interprofessional debriefing or vice versa. Further research is needed with regard to how subject matter experts are best integrated.

Video

The debriefing discussion may be facilitated through the use of video. The video clips played should allow opportunities for each learner's profession to visualize its impact on the team and case. Previewing the discussion topic prior to playing the video helps learners view the video from the perspective of an objective.

Tools for Evaluating SimBIE

Evaluation of the event can measure and analyze areas for improvement in the program (content, simulation, and debriefing), in student learning, and in the impact that this IPE activity has on actual patient care. Unfortunately, many programs use homegrown tools that have not been tested for validity or reliability. A tool is considered valid if it has been tested in a rigorous way and shown that it measures what it intends to measure. A tool is considered reliable when it has been shown to provide consistent and stable results (see Chap. 7 for details). It often takes years to develop a valid and reliable tool. Novice educators should seek assistance from experts in assessment or psychometrics when choosing and implementing an evaluation tool and analyzing data. The National Center for Interprofessional Practice and Education has information and tools that may fit the purpose of a study (https://nexusipe.org/measurement-instruments).

A Framework for Reporting

Findings from simulation-enhanced IPE should be disseminated. This allows the field to synthesize existing work in a way that promotes scientific excellence and determines which variables (e.g., methodology, equipment, techniques) in simulation-enhanced IPE contribute to effective learning. Table 15.5 suggests variables that should be reported when publishing simulation-enhanced IPE work. Current reporting mechanisms may limit the details necessary for replication (e.g., word limits, journal requirements for methods used). Finding additional venues (e.g., MedEdPortal, Web addendums to journals) to report details is necessary to addressing gaps in this science. Recognizing the limitations in reporting, when a published model is chosen, more thorough details should be sought via direct inquiry with the authors or researchers.

Table 15.5 Suggested variables to report in simulation-enhanced IPE. (Reproduced with permission [3])

Suggested reporting items for future simulation-enhanced IPE
Objectives
Aims and purpose of study (manuscript)
Objectives of educational activity
Objectives of simulation activity
Background
Terminology and definitions used by author
Current existing literature
Learners
Sample sizes (total and per professional group)
Profession or program
Grade level
Team composition in simulation
Educators/researchers
Backgrounds/credentials
Composition for development of study and educational activity
Composition for implementation of study and educational activity
Method
Design
Theoretical framework
Interventions
Simulation modality
Type, model, and version
Details of scenario (consider video supplement and scenario appendix)
Structure of debriefing if incorporated (consider video supplement and appendix if structured or semi-structured)
Measures
Why chosen
Validity
Reliability
Results
Discussion
Simulation factors that may have led to positive outcomes
Simulation factors that may have led to negative outcomes
Challenges encountered
Strengths of study design
Limitations of study design
Areas for future study

IPE interprofessional education

Examples of Simulation-Enhanced IPE

Example 1

This study aimed to develop, implement, and evaluate an interprofessional undergraduate program using technology-enhanced pediatric simulation to learn clinical competencies and communication and teamwork skills [65]. The authors developed and delivered workshops to an undergraduate interprofessional group of medical and nursing students. Learning outcomes for this group included the clinical management of sick children, learned competencies, communication and teamwork. Six clinical scenarios were developed (bronchiolitis, croup, asthma, meningococcal septicemia, acute gastroenteritis, and heart failure). Students undertaking this program were in a simulation suite comprising two rooms within a clinical skills center. The setting is described as a typical pediatric accident and emergency treatment room. Questionnaires received from 95 students resulted in positive feedback in that the groups felt that the experience allowed them to learn essential skills for the management of acutely ill children in a risk-free environment with the opportunity to practice and reflect on performance.

Example 2

This program was developed for preregistration interns, third-year nursing students, physiotherapy students, and pharmacy interns focused on team communication, professionalism, shared problem-solving and clinical decision-making within an interprofessional team in the simulated environment [66]. The authors describe the approach as scheduling three 2-h sessions encompassing a series of short didactic lectures, followed by appropriate discipline skills workshops and two concurrent simulated *pause and discuss* clinical scenarios. All students were involved at the same time, and no video replay was used for these sessions. Topics based on a needs analysis included the deteriorating child, pain management, and the child with asthma. Each session addressed discipline-specific objectives in addition to shared competencies. In a post-session 5-point Likert questionnaire with comments, all four disciplines stated that it was constructive to explore the interaction and roles within allied health and medical and nursing staff working together. However, the internal medicine group were unable to participate in the plastering skills session due to time constraints. They expressed their interest and disappointment in not attending. This session was only scheduled for participation from the physiotherapy group. Faculty feedback from this study highlighted the difficulty in scheduling for learners from multiple university facilities while on a clinical placement. Interprofessional faculty are required to facilitate such a program, and this may also cause scheduling challenges in balance with a clinical workload.

Example 3

This program was developed in the undergraduate setting with five different professional groups [67]. This study describes the development of half-day pilot sessions involving prequalifying students from the disciplines of medicine, nursing, physiotherapy, radiography, and operating department practice. Faculty from three universities worked collaboratively to develop the adult scenarios and learning out-

comes that included a patient (standardized) with chest pain, another with chronic obstructive pulmonary disease (COPD) and a mannequin-based cardiac arrest sequence. The scenarios were conducted with those students not involved observing their peers through live video feed. The pre- and post-session student questionnaires reported related both to attitudes to interprofessional learning and perceptions of elements imperative to good patient care. From the data collected, most students reported an increase in confidence levels in interacting with other professional groups. The usefulness of video feedback differed between the professional groups with a post hoc Dunn's test demonstrating that medical students were less positive about this than nursing students.

Example 4

This program was created with the intent to help guide educators on the design, delivery, and assessment of simulation-enhanced IPE. The authors developed a measurement instrument to evaluate team-based performance during simulated pediatric acute care scenarios. The KidSIM Team Performance Scale checklist was developed and tested with 196 undergraduate medical, nursing, and respiratory therapy students using a quasi-experimental research design. The student teams underwent two 20-min acute illness management scenarios followed by 40 min of facilitated debriefing. Teams comprised one medical student, one to two respiratory therapy students, and two to four nursing students. Teams underwent scenarios of sepsis, seizures, asthma, and anaphylaxis. The objectives focused on the CRM concepts of leadership, roles and responsibilities, communication, situation awareness, and resource utilization. Students in the intervention group received a 30-min team training presentation, discussion, and a short video module prior to the simulation. In the establishment to the reliability and validity of this instrument, the investigators discovered three dimensions of team performance that align with team performance literature and show that team performance relies on these dimensions: (1) roles and responsibilities, (2) communication, and (3) patient-centered care. The study also found that a supplementary team training curriculum further enhances team performance [61].

Conclusion

This chapter provides a brief overview of terms, theoretical frameworks, conceptual models, considerations for development, implementation, evaluation, and reporting of simulation-enhanced IPE. While information, suggestions, and guidelines are provided in this chapter, learning how to do simulation-enhanced IPE occurs in the doing. There

Table 15.6 Areas for pediatric simulation-enhanced IPE future research

Foundational areas
What areas of pediatric simulation-enhanced IPE differ from adult simulation-enhanced IPE?
What effect do individual students have on IPL? How can simulation-enhanced IPE be measured taking into account unique individuals involved in an IPE activity?
Are multisite studies in simulation-enhanced IPE feasible given the variability of simulation programs?
What is more effective at achieving IPL: SimBIE or IPsim?
Lab design
What effect does IPE have on IPL in required courses versus elected courses?
What is the most effective number of members and disciplines composing a team for simulation-enhanced IPE?
Is it more effective for students to engage in simulation-enhanced IPE in their current role as students or in their post-licensure role?
Evaluation
What valid and reliable tools effectively measure teamwork and collaboration in simulation?
Faculty
To what degree is faculty a confounding variable in simulation-enhanced IPE?
What faculty characteristics can best predict highest IPL?
How are subject matter experts best used? In debriefing?
Students
How much does previous clinical experience affect IPL?
What creates better IPL outcomes? Existing teams or ad hoc teams?
Hybrid methods
Comparison of hybrid approaches in simulation-enhanced IPE
Simulation methods
What are the effects on the child actor when using pediatric standardized patients?
What characteristics exist in pediatric standardized patients and mannequin-based simulations?

IPE interprofessional education, *IPL* interprofessional learning, *SimBIE* simulation-based interprofessional education, *IPsim* interprofessional simulations

are many areas in need of further study, which are listed in Table 15.6. Thought, planning, and consideration of simulation-related and IPE-related variables lead to effective simulation-enhanced IPE programs.

References

1. Palaganas JC, Epps C, Raemer D. A history of simulation-enhanced interprofessional education. J Interprof Care. 2014;28(2):110–5.
2. World Health Organization. Framework for action on interprofessional education and collaborative practice. Geneva: WHO; 2010.
3. Palaganas JC. Exploring healthcare simulation as a platform for interprofessional education [Dissertation]. Loma Linda: Loma Linda University; 2011.
4. Zhang C, Thompson S, Miller C. A review of simulation-based interprofessional education. Clin Sim Nurs. 2011;7:e117–26.
5. Issenberg SB, McGaghie WC, Petrusa ER, Gordon DL, Scalese RJ. Features and uses of high-fidelity medical simulations that lead to effective learning: a BEME systematic review. Med Teach. 2005;27:10–28.
6. McGaghie W, Issenberg SB, Petrusa E, Scalese R. A critical review of simulation-based medical education research: 2003–2009. Med Edu. 2010;44:50–63.
7. Reeves S, Goldman J, Gilbert J, Tepper J, Silver I, Suter E, Zwarenstein M. A scoping review to improve conceptual clarity of interprofessional interventions. J Interprof Care. 2011;25(3):167–74.
8. Reeves S, Perrier L, Goldman J, Freeth D, Zwarenstein M. Interprofessional education: effects on professional practice and healthcare outcomes (update). Cochrane Database Syst Rev. 2013; 3:CD002213.
9. Thistlethwaite J. Interprofessional education: a review of context, learning and the research agenda. Med Educ. 2012;46(1):58–70.
10. Abu-Rish E. Current trends in interprofessional education of health sciences students: a literature review. J Interprof Care. 2012; 26:444–51.
11. Zwarenstein M, Reeves S, Barr H, Hammick M, Koppel I, Atkins J. Interprofessional education: effects on professional practice and health care outcomes. Cochrane Database Syst Rev, 2001.
12. Barr H, Koppel I, Reeves S, Hammick M, Freeth D. Effective interprofessional education: argument, assumption and evidence. Oxford: Blackwell; 2005.
13. Hammick M, Freeth D, Reeves S, Koppel I, Barr H. A best evidence systematic review of interprofessional education. Med Teach. 2007;29(9):735–51.
14. Barr H, Helme M, D'Avray L. A review of interprofessional education in the UK, 1997–2013. London: CAIPE; 2014.
15. Frenk J, Chen L, Bhutta Z, Cohen J, Crisp N, Evans E, et al. Health professionals for a new century: transforming education to strengthen health systems in an interdependent world. Lancet. 2010;376(9756):1923–58.
16. Sonesh S, Salas E. Team training and patient outcomes. Proceedings of the Institute of Medicine Measuring the Impact of Interprofessional Education on collaborative practice and patient outcomes consensus study; 2014 Oct 7; Washington, DC (USA).

17. Pauze E, Reeves S. Examining the effects of interprofessional education on mental health providers: findings from an updated systematic review. J Ment Health. 2010;19(3):258–71.

18. Brashers V. Review: measuring the impact of interprofessional education on collaborative practice and patient outcomes. Proceedings of the Institute of Medicine Measuring the Impact of Interprofessional Education on collaborative practice and patient outcomes consensus study; 2014 Oct 7; Washington, DC (USA).

19. Huang YM, Rice J, Spain AE, Palaganas J. Terms of reference. In: Palaganas J, Maxworthy J, Epps C, Mancini ME, editors. Defining excellence in healthcare simulation. Philadelphia: Wolters Kluwer/Lippincott Williams & Wilkins; 2014.

20. Helreich R, Merritt A, Willhelm J. The evolution of crew resource management training in commercial aviation. Int J Aviat Psychol. 1999;9(1):19–32.

21. Gaba D, Howard S, Fish K, Smith B, Sowb Y. Simulation-based training in anesthesia crisis resource management (ACRM): a decade of experience. Simul Gaming. 2001;32(2):175–93.

22. Howkins E, Bray J. Preparing for interprofessional teaching. Oxon: Radcliffe Publishing Ltd; 2008.

23. Centre for the Advancement of Interprofessional Education (CAIPE). Interprofessional education—a definition. London: CAIPE; 2005.

24. Freeth D, Hammick M, Reeves S, Koppel I, Barr H. Effective interprofessional education: development, delivery & evaluation. Oxford: Blackwell Publishing Ltd; 2005.

25. Interprofessional Education and Healthcare Simulation Collaborative (IPEHCS-C). A consensus report from the 2012 interprofessional education and healthcare simulation collaborative. Cincinatti: Society for Simulation in Healthcare; 2012.

26. Knowles M. The modern practice of adult education: from pedagogy to andragogy. Wilton: Association Press; 1980.

27. Kolb D. Experiential learning. Experience as the source of learning and development. Englewood Cliffs: Prentice-Hall; 1984.

28. Kolb D, Fry R. Toward an applied theory of experiential learning. In: Cooper C, editor. Theories of group process. London: Wiley; 1975.

29. Lave D, Wenger E. Situated learning: legitimate peripheral participation. New York: Cambridge University Press; 2008.

30. Schon D. The reflective practitioner. New York: Basic Books; 1983.

31. Thompson N, Pascal J. Developing critically reflective practice. Reflect Pract Int Multidiscip Perspect. 2012;13(2):311–25.

32. Ericsson A, Krampe RT, Tesch-Romer C. The role of deliberate practice in the acquisition of expert performance. Psychol Rev. 1993;100(3):363–406.

33. Ericsson KA. Deliberate practice and the acquisition and maintenance of expert performance in medicine and related domains. Acad Med. 2004;79(10):70–81.

34. Reeves S, Hean S. Why we need theory to help us better understand the nature of interprofessional education, practice, and care. J Interprof Care. 2013;27:1–3.

35. Morrison JB, Deckers C. Common theories in healthcare simulation. In: Palaganas JC, Maxworthy J, Epps C, Mancini MB, editors. Defining excellence in simulation programs. Philadelphia: Wolters Kluwer Lippincott Williams & Wilkins; 2014.

36. Reeves S, editor. Interprofessional theories [Special Issue]. J Interprof Care. 2013;27:1–90.

37. Bion WR. Experiences in groups and other papers. London: Tavistock Publications; 1961.

38. Allport G. The nature of prejudice. 25th ed. Cambridge: Perseus Books Publishing LLC; 1954.

39. Tajfel H, Turner JC. The social identity theory of intergroup behavior. In: Worchel S, Austin LW, editors. Psychology of intergroup relations. Chicago: Nelson-Hall; 1986.

40. Turner J. Some current issues in research on social identity and self-categorisation theories. In: Ellemers N, Spears R, Doosjie B, editors. Social identity. Oxford: Blackwell; 1999.

41. Brown R, Condor S, Mathews A, Wade G, Williams J. Explaining intergroup differentiation in an industrial organization. J Occup Psych. 1986;59:273–86.

42. Bourdieu P. Outline of a theory of practice. Cambridge: Cambridge University Press; 1977.

43. von Bertalanffy L. General systems theory. London: Penguin Press; 1971.

44. Senge PM. The fifth discipline the art and practice of the learning organization. 1st ed. New York: Doubleday/Currency; 1990.

45. Engestrom Y. Expansive theory at work: towards and activity theoretical reconceptualization. J Educ Work. 2001;14:133–56.

46. Fraser SW, Greenhalgh T. Coping with complexity: education for capability. BMJ. 2001;323:799–803.

47. Mezirow J. Perspective transformation. Adult Educ. 1978;28:100–10.

48. Palaganas J, Andersen J, Wilhaus J. Results from the 2012 interprofessional education and healthcare simulation survey. Proceedings of the Interprofessional Education and Healthcare Simulation Symposium; 2012 Jan; San Diego, CA (USA).

49. Interprofessional Education Collaborative Expert Panel. Team-based competencies: building a shared foundation for education and clinical practice. Washington, DC: Interprofessional Education Collaborative; 2011.

50. Interprofessional Education Collaborative Expert Panel. Core competencies for interprofessional collaborative practice: report of an expert panel. Washington, DC: Interprofessional Education Collaborative; 2011.

51. Canadian Interprofessional Health Collaborative. A national interprofessional competency framework. 2010. http://www.cihc.ca/resources/publications.

52. Institute of Medicine. Interprofessional education for collaboration: learning how to improve health from interprofessional models across the continuum of education to practice—workshop summary. Washington, D.C.: IOM; 2013.

53. Institute of Medicine. Measuring the Impact of interprofessional education on collaborative practice and patient outcomes consensus study. Washington, D.C.: IOM; 2014.

54. Rudolph JW, Raemer DB, Simon R. Establishing a safe container for learning in simulation: the role of the presimulation debriefing. Simul Healthc; 2014.

55. Edmondson AC, Roloff KS. Overcoming barriers to collaboration: psychological safety and learning in diverse teams. In: Salas E, Goodwin GF, Burke CS, editors. Team effectiveness in complex organizations: cross-disciplinary perspectives and approaches. New York: Routledge/Taylor & Francis Group; 2009.

56. Palaganas J, Brunette V, Winslow B. Simulation-enhanced interprofessional education: a review of the research literature. Simul Healthc. Submitted for review.

57. Zhang C, Thompson S, Miller C. A review of simulation-based interprofessional education. Clin Simul Nurs. 2011;7:117–26.

58. Sigalet E, Donnon TL, Grant V. Insight into team competence in medical, nursing and respiratory therapy students. J Interprof Care. 29:62–7.doi:10.3109/13561820.2014.940416. (Early Online: 1–6)

59. Sigalet E, Donnon T, Grant V. Undergraduate students' perceptions of and attitudes toward a simulation-based interprofessional curriculum: the KidSIM attitudes questionnaire. Simul Healthc. 2012;7:353–8.

60. Kane L. Educators, learners and active learning methodologies. Int J lifelong Educ. 2004;23(3):275–86.

61. Sigalet E, Donnon T, Cheng A, Cooke S, Robinson, T, Bissett W, Grant V. Development of a team performance scale to assess undergraduate health professionals. Acad Med. 2013;88:989–96.

62. Salas E, Cannon-Bowers JA. The science of training: a decade of progress. Annu Rev Psychol. 2001;52:471–99.

63. Buckley S, Hensman M, Thomas S, Dudley R, Nevin G, Coleman J. Developing interprofessional simulation in the undergraduate setting: experience with five different professional groups. J Interprof Care. 2012;26:362–9.

64. Navedo D, Simon R. Specialized courses in simulation. In: Levine A, DeMaria S, Schwartz A, Sim A, editors. Comprehensive textbook of healthcare simulation. New York: Springer; 2013.

65. Stewart M, Kennedy N, Cuene-Grandidier H. Undergraduate Interprofessional education using high-fidelity paediatric simulation. Clin Teach. 2010;7:90–6.

66. Scott E, Maclean R, Morris A, Cheetham V, Worthington R, Lester Smith D, Hatton L, Gunaskera H, Nerminathan A. Interprofessional practice; developing a program for medical, nursing and allied heath disciplines proceedings from the 6th IPSSW 2014 23rd–25th April; Vienna, Austria.

67. Buckley S, Hensman M, Thomas S, Dudley R, Nevin G, Coleman J. Developing interprofessional simulation in the undergraduate setting: experience with five different professional groups. J Interprof Care. 2012;26:362–9.

Part IV

Pediatric Simulation Specialties

Simulation for Pediatric Hospital Medicine

Lindsay Long and Suzette Cooke

Simulation Pearls

1. Keep it small at first. Start with a pilot.
2. Identify all your stakeholders and engage early adopters at the beginning. Stakeholders may include simulation leaders, pediatric hospitalists, residents, residency program directors, nursing educators, nursing managers, respiratory therapy managers, hospital administrators, and others. Their ongoing support will help to maintain momentum and overcome obstacles in the long run.
3. Interprofessional collaboration is essential to identifying key problems, performing root cause analysis, and determining systems-based solutions.

Introduction

The field of pediatric hospital medicine (PHM) is growing at an accelerated rate. The inpatient clinical environment is dynamic and challenges practitioners to meet not only clinical needs but also demonstrate excellence in medical education, quality improvement, research, and leadership. Simulation education can play a key role in enabling pediatric hospitalists and the interprofessional inpatient teams to provide the highest standard of inpatient care and contribute to improving health outcomes.

Drivers for Simulation Programs in PHM

There are many factors driving simulation programs in PHM. First, there is a need for practitioners to meet core competencies in PHM [1]. Most physicians entering the field come directly out of residency [2]. However, residency training alone is insufficient to prepare a physician to fulfill all core competencies. Studies have shown most pediatric residents complete their training without obtaining sufficient experience in the care of critically ill children and critical care procedural skills [3, 4].

Pediatric hospitalists are expected to care for an inpatient population that is growing in volume, acuity, and medical complexity. The fastest-growing inpatient cohort are those with chronic multisystem, complex, or progressive conditions [5]. In addition, some pediatric hospitalists are taking on roles in sedation, medical transport, and central line placement. They may also be co-managers with surgical specialties, code team leaders, and provide service in the intensive care unit.

This expanding list of roles and services requires that both pediatric hospitalists and the inpatient interprofessional team have a common understanding and achieve competency within their scope of practice. This requires regular, ongoing practice of events that are (i) frequent yet challenging and (ii) rare and critical. Simulation is an educational modality that has the potential to support the interprofessional team to practice these events in a context that is real and relevant. In the sections to follow, we will describe how simulation education can be implemented for inpatient care teams.

Curriculum Development, Design, and Implementation

A common misconception is that scenarios should all be based on urgent *code* situations. However, it is also valuable to simulate less acute scenarios as these are more likely to be encountered on the inpatient wards. The focus may be to optimize *precode* care or rehearse a challenging situation such as disclosure of a medical error. When scenarios are closer to the scope of participants' usual practice, the debriefing tends to be a practical and meaningful learning experience.

L. Long (✉) · S. Cooke
Department of Pediatrics, University of Calgary, Calgary, AB, Canada
e-mail: Lindsay.Long@ahs.ca; c.long@gmail.com

S. Cooke
e-mail: Suzette.Cooke@ahs.ca

© Springer International Publishing Switzerland 2016
V. J. Grant, A. Cheng (eds.), *Comprehensive Healthcare Simulation: Pediatrics*,
Comprehensive Healthcare Simulation, DOI 10.1007/978-3-319-24187-6_16

We will present three models for simulation programs that are contextualized to the inpatient environment. For each, we will describe strengths and challenges, along with suggestions for implementation. We hope this will give a framework for developing a simulation program that best matches a center's needs and available resources.

Just-in-Time Simulation

Just-in-time (JIT) simulation is a novel yet impactful simulation program that can be implemented on a small or large scale. The purpose of JIT is to identify a patient at high risk for deterioration and develop a scenario based on the most likely way this patient may evolve. This enables the actual interprofessional team to rehearse the care they would deliver to this patient. When conducted in situ, simulation is brought to the point of care (see Chap. 12).

Acute Care and Resuscitation

If an interdisciplinary team can practice specific management strategies in advance, there is potential to improve that patient's outcomes. JIT simulation has been shown to improve quality of cardiopulmonary resuscitation (CPR) among intensive care unit staff [6], increase resident participation in orotracheal intubations [7], and decrease the rates of central-lineassociated blood infections [8].

JIT is a particularly feasible modality to teach acute care skills to medical students and residents. One example is a JIT mock code program developed for pediatric residents to complement a modular curriculum focused on acute care [9]. JIT sessions were run one to two times per month. The pediatric chief resident selected one of the sickest patients on the ward earlier that day and created a scenario where that patient acutely deteriorated. The participants included the actual residents and nurses who would be the initial responders in real life, with progressive involvement of respiratory therapists and the intensive care code team. Scenarios were short (approximately 20 min) and were immediately followed by a 10-min debriefing session. In this study, JIT mock codes increased hands-on practice of core resuscitation skills and primed the code team to identify real-life obstacles to care. If scenarios are realistic and predictive of patient deterioration, there is potential to improve pediatric resuscitation outcomes.

In our experience, we have found that a 10–15 min scenario focused at the *precode level* is another effective approach to ward-based JIT simulation. The medical students, residents, and bedside nurse(s) are expected to manage the critical first 10 minutes. The most important elements are prioritized and discussed in the 15-min debriefing session that follows. This allows for a regularly occurring, high-yield learning experience that causes less disruption to the clinical

work day. In order to heighten the realism of the scenario, the JIT session is conducted in an inpatient room whenever possible *(just-in-place)*. Details such as the patient's current medications, intravenous access, level of monitoring, medical devices, and care plans are all incorporated into the scenario. Since the learners are already familiar with the patient, their level of engagement tends to be consistently high, and they are more likely to act as they would in real life.

JIT and Procedures/Psychomotor Skills

The medical literature describes considerable skill decay for procedures requiring complex psychomotor skills and those that are practiced infrequently [6, 7, 10] (see Chap. 11). JIT simulation is well suited for refreshing these skills and has been associated with improved patient outcomes [8].

A compelling example of how regular JIT sessions can improve providers' skills is illustrated in a study on CPR effectiveness in the pediatric intensive care unit [6]. Each day, five of the most critically ill patients were identified. The multidisciplinary teams caring for these patients were given a brief (5 min) refresher simulation on CPR. A portable mannequin/defibrillator system was brought to the bedside to minimize disruption in clinical care *(just-in-place)*. Individuals who participated in two or more sessions per month achieved effective CPR more quickly than those who did fewer sessions (21 vs. 67 s).

As the above example illustrates, the simulation setup should be simple and portable to enable participants to quickly refresh before performing the actual procedure. Some procedures specific to the inpatient population include lumbar puncture, tracheostomy tube changes, and managing chest tubes. Since procedures should be subject to little variability and are based around a well-defined set of knowledge, specific performance objectives and checklists can be easily developed to evaluate learners, both formally and informally.

Challenges of Conducting a JIT Program

The initial challenges of starting JIT programs are issues associated with recruiting and funding skilled simulation education leaders, ensuring availability of sufficient space and equipment, and getting engagement and commitment from all stakeholders including the medical teaching unit, nursing staff, and other health professionals as needed. Other human resource challenges include coverage for bedside nurses to enable them to be released for the JIT session, and maintaining ongoing engagement, commitment, and remuneration of clinical preceptors. Because actual bedside staff are participating in these JIT sessions, punctuality and attendance of learners can also be variable as sessions may compete with clinical care responsibilities. Curricular challenges include supporting integration of objectives suited to various types of learners (inclusive of medicine, nursing, and allied health), limiting the number of learning objectives to fit the

Table 16.1 Points to consider when implementing a just-in-time simulation program

Strengths	Challenges	Solutions
High relevance—scenario, context, and healthcare team are all real	Inconsistent participant availability and punctuality—sessions occur during their clinical work day	In situ simulation makes it easier for learners to attend. Send reminder pages 30 min prior to the start of the session. Make sessions mandatory. A website is helpful to coordinate people and resources
Scenarios are easy to construct as they are based on a real patient	Limited number of learning objectives makes it challenging to meet all learners' needs	Seek nursing input early in the scenario design process to identify relevant learning objectives
Well suited for rehearsing procedural and complex psychomotor skills	Availability of space and equipment	Plan to run in situ simulation but book backup simulation space in case clinical space not available
Potential to improve patient outcomes	Supporting and reimbursing debriefers and educators	Provide simulation educator training. Schedule periodic meetings with all stakeholders to troubleshoot issues regularly

allotted time frame, ensuring some diversity in cases (i.e., selecting some non-respiratory cases during bronchiolitis season), and ensuring adequate training of the debriefers. Space and equipment challenges include inpatient room availability and availability of mannequins and equipment. Table 16.1 describes these challenges of implementing a JIT simulation program and offers solutions to each of these problems.

Residents as JIT Simulation Educators

One further option is to offer JIT sessions as an educational opportunity for senior or chief residents whereby they create and deliver JIT simulations. There are both advantages and challenges to having trainees in this role. To be successful, the basic principles of simulation education and debriefing must be taught beforehand. A physician preceptor and an educator with expertise in simulation provide support to the resident. The major benefit is for residents to learn how to lead a simulation session and to collaborate with an interdisciplinary leadership team. The challenges include the need to coordinate more people and resources, ensuring expectations and roles are communicated clearly, and ensuring that the needs of non-physician learners are met. In our experience, communication of the program, its mission and objectives, and clear up-to-date scheduling are critical to the success of the program. A website can be helpful to communicate these items and share resources such as blank scenario templates and case adjuncts (Fig. 16.1).

Fig. 16.1 Screenshot of a sample website that can be helpful to coordinate people and share resources. (Photo by Lindsay Long)

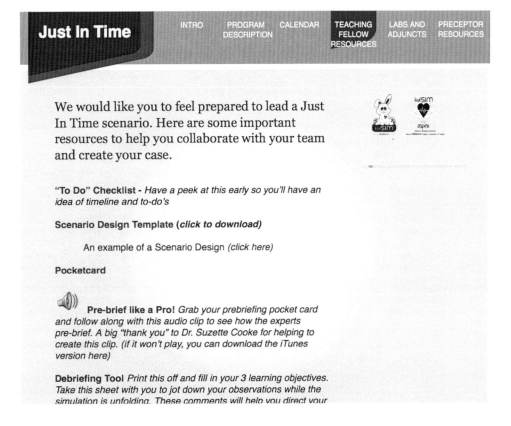

Mock Codes in the Inpatient Setting

Mock codes are designed to support the practice of emergent or code scenarios based on the patient population (inpatients or outpatients) and medical conditions characteristic of the local hospital. Mock codes involve members of the hospital code team—typically the clinical inpatient team including the medical house staff, nurses, respiratory therapists, intensive care staff and/or rapid response team (where available), and relevant subspecialists. Interdisciplinary and interprofessional participation is paramount in mock codes as this allows for full identification of complex medical issues and system-based problems that might not be apparent within the context of a single discipline [11].

Each individual who provides care to inpatients must maintain a subset of core acute care competencies. This can be challenging because life-threatening cardiorespiratory events are relatively uncommon on pediatric inpatient wards. Traditionally, resuscitation skills are taught in didactic courses such as the Pediatric Advanced Life Support (PALS) course. However, many studies have shown that PALS knowledge and skills decay rapidly in the 6–12 months following the course [10]. Mock codes are one modality that may help healthcare team members to reinforce and retain PALS knowledge and skills. Mock code programs have been shown to improve patient outcomes. In a landmark study, implementation of in situ simulation-based interdisciplinary pediatric mock code training was associated with improved patient survival-to-discharge rates following in-hospital cardiac arrest [12].

Similar to JIT sessions, mock codes are preferentially conducted in any potential location a patient may be found including inpatient wards, diagnostic imaging, outpatient clinics, cafeteria, hallway, or therapy pool, among others. Mock codes can also be used to test overcapacity plans for safety and feasibility, such as when patients are placed in designated overflow spaces. In this way, mock codes test the hospital response system and allow learners to discuss best strategies to deliver care to a patient beyond the usual settings.

Challenges of Conducting a Mock Code Program

Many of the challenges of initiating and maintaining a mock code program are similar to JIT programs. However, an additional challenge associated with mock code programs is recruiting and maintaining the engagement of the broader hospital community. Mock codes are usually done spontaneously (i.e., no set day or time). Although this randomization is helpful in testing the system, it can also be disruptive to patient care teams, especially if a sensitive patient care activity is occurring at that time (e.g., performing a lumbar puncture or chairing a multidisciplinary meeting). In our experience, when the mock code team leaders communicate a set day and time, the vast majority of mock code objectives can still be achieved and learner/staff engagement and respect are maintained. We suggest that *random* mock codes contain objectives that require randomness to be a feature. Such objectives may include time to initiate CPR, time to arrival of the inpatient team, time to arrival of the crash cart/PICU team, or how the team/system performs when under a different stress (e.g., middle of the night vs. middle of the day). If randomness is not a critical feature, then scheduled mock codes can achieve most core objectives.

A second unique challenge of mock codes is related to the provision of feedback to both staff and trainees. Since prebriefing is not usually conducted just prior to a mock code, leaders of simulation must carefully create and maintain a culture of learning and support throughout the session. Effective, constructive, and supportive debriefing are essential to creating a positive learning experience.

Other challenges of conducting mock codes relate to management of who shows up, who become the active participants in managing the patient, and who is in the audience. Mock codes can be particularly intimidating for less experienced participants and those who feel stressed in perceived *fish bowl* situations. Ward-based staff may quickly defer to the intensive care team; this behavior may limit their own engagement and learning. It is important for the mock code program leader to communicate to participants well in advance who the intended participant(s) are and to ensure awareness of the objective of these sessions. Table 16.2

Table 16.2 Points to consider when implementing a mock code training program for inpatients

Strengths	Challenges	Solutions
Practice and rehearsal of acute care knowledge, skills, and behaviors	May be disruptive to patient care if mock codes are called at random	Consider announcing dates/times for mock codes ahead of time if randomness is not a critical feature
Systems testing by an interdisciplinary team can identify problems and solution	Can be a stressful learning environment	Establish clarity around the purpose of the session and the intended participants. Create a supportive yet constructive debriefing environment
Potential to improve patient outcomes	Support to sustain a regularly occurring mock code curriculum	Support at least two simulation leaders per domain to help achieve program stability
Facilitates the development of teamwork within a clinical unit	Confusion around roles between inpatient unit staff and code team	Clarify inpatient unit roles and effective transitioning to code team members. Highlight mock codes as an ideal opportunity to practice this

outlines some of the challenges and solutions associated with implementing a simulation-based mock code program on the inpatient ward.

Inpatient Simulation Continuing Professional Development Programs

The majority of simulation education programs are designed for trainees. However, the value of simulation is gaining momentum among staff providers across many healthcare professions. Simulation is particularly beneficial as a way of refreshing and practicing previously learned information and skills. It also has unlimited potential to support the acquisition of new knowledge and skills. A planned continuing professional development (CPD) simulation program can provide a guaranteed curriculum for the inpatient staff team, which is otherwise difficult to achieve via the intermittent JIT and mock code programs.

Some CPD programs start as domain-specific programs (e.g., nursing or physician groups independently) and evolve into interprofessional staff simulation programs (see Chap. 16). Other CPD programs remain domain specific either intentionally (to concentrate on domain-specific objectives) or due to resource limitations. Both models have their own inherent purpose and strengths. The key is to select a program design that best meets the needs of the participants and can be realistically implemented and sustained with the available resources. Interprofessional learning groups are preferable wherever possible because actual patient care is delivered in teams, and participants can thus behave as they would in real life (see Chap. 15). This allows learners to reflect on strategies that specifically allow for most effective teamwork. Such strategies may include leveraging each other's professional skills, honing of team communication, group problem-solving, and sharing knowledge and experience of inpatient systems (e.g., algorithms, access to resources and equipment, congruencies of professional policy and practice, etc.).

The KidSIM Pediatric Simulation Program at Alberta Children's Hospital runs CPD staff simulation sessions that are scheduled well in advance to accommodate clinical work schedules. Sessions can be variable in length but generally last between 1 and 3.5 h. All sessions begin with an orientation and pre-briefing to establish a safe learning environment. This is followed by an orientation to the mannequin(s), space, and equipment as required. Scenarios typically run 20–30 min. Scenarios are followed immediately by debriefing lasting approximately as long as the scenario itself. In a typical 3.5-h interprofessional CPD session, three inpatient scenarios can be run and discussed. Though the debriefing may be led by a domain-specific leader, a co-debriefing model with interprofessional facilitators can lead to a richer discussion that draws upon expertise across several domains.

Ideally, inpatient simulation objectives are based on a comprehensive needs assessment and may include input from participants, clinical and educational inpatient leaders, quality improvement leaders, and code team committees. Scenarios reflect the full spectrum of pediatric inpatients (including both acutely ill and medically complex patients) as well as the continuum of patient stabilities from the more common urgent pre-code situations to the less frequent, life-threatening types of deterioration (e.g., respiratory arrest, septic shock, anaphylaxis).

Curricular emphasis is broad and reflects the full breadth of inpatient medicine. It may include technical skills, practical application of clinical care guidelines and protocols, orientation to new medical equipment, quality improvement initiatives, patient safety issues, response to communication challenges (including delivery of bad news and disclosure of adverse events), and interprofessional team building. Integration of several curricular goals into a single scenario is common. For example, a scenario based on a child with moderate to severe asthma can highlight important practice points from a clinical practice guideline. It could also lead to discussions around techniques to deliver optimal administration of treatment (such as a non-rebreather bag) or how to ensure safe administration of intravenous magnesium sulfate. The same scenario could include a confederate acting as a parent who becomes anxious and requires support and education from the healthcare team to cope with the stress and assist treatment by helping the child remain calm and compliant. Ultimately, inpatient scenarios are designed to facilitate relevant high-quality practice and learning for all members of the inpatient healthcare team.

Challenges of Conducting a CPD Simulation Program

Most CPD simulation programs find that their most significant initial challenges are associated with achieving buy-in from staff members. There are several factors which may contribute to this including lack of time and competing priorities, financial remuneration or credit for attendance (e.g., professional continuing medical education (CME) credits), fear of performance expectations (especially in interprofessional settings), or lack of support from clinical administrative leaders. Although it is ideal for simulation education to be remunerated and incorporated into daily clinical roles and expectations, many programs are unable to achieve this goal. Despite this, successful CPD simulation programs have managed to obtain buy-in from clinical administrators, simulation leaders, and staff participants secondary to the realization of the quality, relevance, and value of CPD simulation

Table 16.3 Points to consider when implementing a continuing professional development program

Strengths	Challenges	Solutions
Dedicated learning time that is protected from clinical duties	Participant availability, particularly if on a volunteer basis	Make attendance a mandatory requirement. Create a culture of learning. Learners build upon success through a mastery learning process
Scenarios are contextualized to the ward setting. All participants are inpatient care providers working through realistic and relevant cases	Need for ongoing curriculum development including creation of new cases that address the needs of an interdisciplinary team	Engage interprofessional educators to assist with new scenario development. Seek collaboration with other simulation educators and share resources and scenarios
Strengthens interprofessional relationships and teamwork	Program sustainability during periods of transition in leadership	Obtain funding for at least two simulation leaders per domain to help achieve program stability

sessions for their staff members. Competency-based assessments may play a greater role in the future to formally demonstrate accountability and assure quality of care in hospital settings.

Staff participants may understandably have a fear of performance expectations when asked to participate in a simulation session with their colleagues. Generally, this can be overcome by carefully creating and maintaining a psychologically safe learning environment. The principles of this (and notably as important for staff as for trainees) include an explicit statement of the assumption that all participants are competent, well intended, trying their best, and interested in learning and self-improvement [13]. It is the simulation leaders' responsibility to ensure that participant integrity is respected and maintained. These principles require a clear introduction prior to starting a program, regular reinforcement during the orientation to every simulation session as well as skill and sensitivity in debriefing fellow staff members. When such a learning environment is created, learning can be safe, meaningful, and productive.

Subsequent challenges of established CPD simulation programs are typically associated with sustainability. In our experience, CPD staff programs require at least two simulation leaders *per domain* in order to maintain program stability. If a simulation leader takes a leave of absence or moves into other career roles, this model allows for continuity while a new facilitator is identified and oriented. Other challenges include limited staff availability during seasonal surges where the need to provide clinical care supersedes staff educational sessions. Established programs may be challenged by sheer numbers of participants and limitations on resources (time, space, equipment, leaders). Finally, to ensure CPD programs remain relevant for participants, simulation leaders must ensure ongoing curriculum development including conducting regular needs assessments, identifying relevant multidisciplinary objectives, creating new scenarios regularly, implementing a curriculum, and conducting periodic program evaluations. Table 16.3 outlines some of the challenges and solutions associated with implementing a CPD simulation program for inpatient providers.

Future Directions

There are many novel applications of simulation that could enhance the delivery of inpatient care. Some applications may have a narrow focus to target situations associated with high rates of medical error or harm. Such examples include delivering an effective handover, rehearsing procedures following child abduction, or the safe use of 4-point physical restraints. Other novel applications may take a broader approach. For example, *extended duration simulation* involves a simulated patient added to the ward to mimic either a real patient or a typical case for that time of year. Nursing staff are assigned to this simulated patient and standardized actors play the role of parents. It is a resource-intensive simulation program that can test systemic issues and highlight error-prone times during the day. One other innovative use of simulation is as an adjunct for teaching acute care skills to families.

There are numerous priorities for inpatient simulation research. As much of the existing literature focuses on pediatric trainees, more studies are needed to evaluate the impact of simulation education on staff healthcare providers. Rigorous evaluation of simulation programs with a focus on clinically significant endpoints would help create transferable knowledge for guiding future program development. Also, as skill decay for acute care procedures remains an ongoing challenge, studies addressing the optimum frequency and method for refresher simulation could lead to improved retention for inpatient care providers. As always, the impact of simulation interventions on patient outcomes and real-life team performance using validated scoring systems should remain the focus of future simulation research.

References

1. Stucky ER, Maniscalco J, Ottolini MC, editors. The pediatric hospital medicine core competencies: a framework for curriculum development. Vol. 5. Hoboken: Wiley; 2010.
2. American Board of Pediatrics. Workforce Data 2013–2014. https://www.abp.org/abpwebsite/stats/wrkfrc/workforcebook.pdf (2014). Accessed 14 Aug 2014.

3. Mills DM, Williams DC, Dobson JV. Simulation training as a mechanism for procedural and resuscitation education for pediatric residents: a systematic review. Hosp Pediatr. 2013;3:167–76.

4. Heydarian C, Maniscalco J. Pediatric hospitalists in medical education: current roles and future directions. Curr Probl Pediatr Adolesc Health Care. 2012;42:120–6.

5. Berry JG, Hall M, Hall DE, Kuo DZ, Cohen E, Agrawal R, et al. Inpatient growth and resource use in 28 children's hospitals: a longitudinal, multi-institutional study. JAMA Pediatr. 2013;167:170–7.

6. Niles D, Sutton RM, Donoghue A, Kalsi MS, Roberts K, Boyle L, et al. "Rolling Refreshers": a novel approach to maintain CPR psychomotor skill competence. Resuscitation. 2009;80:909–12.

7. Nishisaki A, Donoghue AJ, Colborn S, Watson C, Meyer A, Brown C, et al. Effect of just-in-time simulation training on tracheal intubation procedure safety in the pediatric intensive care unit. Anesthesiology. 2010;113:214–23.

8. Scholtz AK, Monachino AM, Nishisaki A, Nadkarni VM, Lengetti E. Central venous catheter dress rehearsals: translating simulation training to patient care and outcomes. Simul Healthc. 2013;8:341–9.

9. Sam J, Pierse M, Al-Qahtani A, Cheng A. Implementation and evaluation of a simulation curriculum for paediatric residency programs including just-in-time in situ mock codes. Paediatr Child Health. 2012;17:e16–e20.

10. Grant EC, Marczinski C, Menon K. Using pediatric advanced life support in pediatric residency training: does the curriculum need resuscitation? Pediatr Crit Care Med. 2007;8:433–9.

11. Andreatta P, Marzano D. Healthcare management strategies: interdisciplinary team factors. Curr Opin Obstet Gynecol. 2012;24:445–52.

12. Andreatta P, Saxton E, Thompson M, Annich G. Simulation-based mock codes significantly correlate with improved pediatric patient cardiopulmonary arrest survival rates. Pediatr Crit Care Med. 2011;12:33–8.

13. Rudolph JW, Simon R, Raemer DB, Eppich WJ. Debriefing as formative assessment: closing performance gaps in medical education. Acad Emerg Med. 2008;15:1010–6.

Simulation for Pediatric Emergency Medicine and Trauma

17

Frank L. Overly, Kevin Ching and Garth D. Meckler

Simulation Pearls

1. In situ simulations in the pediatric emergency department (PED) can be extremely valuable on multiple levels. These sessions provide the opportunity for individuals to practice resuscitation and stabilization of critically ill and injured patients. They provide context for interprofessional educational sessions to improve teamwork dynamics. In situ simulation is also a powerful tool for systems testing and identifying latent safety threats to ensure a safer environment for patient care.

2. Developing a data-collecting system for a pediatric emergency medicine (PEM) simulation program is important to ensure institutional support. Examples include recording procedural performance data for residents and fellows in training programs and recording latent safety threats identified during in situ simulation and proposed solutions. Distributing these data to program directors and leaders within the institution (risk management, chief medical officer, etc.) encourages them to view simulation as a valuable asset and not an expendable expense.

3. PEM boot camps can utilize simulation and provide a foundation for new PEM fellows in knowledge, procedural skills, and code management that can facilitate the transition from residency to fellowship. This is becoming increasingly valuable with the fact that residents are reporting decreasing opportunities and less experience during the residency years of training.

Introduction

PEM is a unique subspecialty within pediatrics with some very specific responsibilities placed on the providers that work in this fast-paced clinical arena. The PEM team is challenged with a wide scope of practice ranging from well-appearing infants with concerned parents to critically ill or injured children with the potential for significant morbidity or mortality. Most of these patients are undifferentiated, meaning they do not present with a diagnosis, rather they present with a complaint or abnormal physiologic state. The PEM team needs to be skilled in rapid assessment and stabilization, which requires an appropriate knowledge base, effective communication, and specific procedural skills (e.g., airway management, cardiopulmonary resuscitation (CPR)). Similar to operating rooms and intensive care units, the PED is a clinical environment where low-frequency and high-stakes events occur, and medical simulation has been accepted as a training modality for these types of clinical environments [1, 2]. In addition, simulation-based education (SBE) applications have been shown to be effective for acute care, resuscitation, and other learning objectives including communication and team performance [3–5]. For these reasons, PEM has embraced simulation as an educational tool and leveraged its use in different areas. Specifically, this chapter will review how simulation can be used in PEM with training programs for students, residents, fellows, attending and interprofessional teams. Simulation training programs offer hands-on opportunities for learning and practice, but may also contain assessment tools looking at knowledge, core competencies, and educational milestones. This chapter will also review various drivers behind using simulation in PEM, including, but not limited to, quality measures, improved patient outcomes, and systems testing.

F. L. Overly (✉)
Department of Emergency Medicine and Pediatrics, Alpert Medical School of Brown University, Hasbro Children's Hospital, Providence, RI, USA
e-mail: foverly@lifespan.org

K. Ching
Department of Pediatrics, Weill Cornell Medical College, New York Presbyterian Hospital – Weill Cornell Medical Center, New York, NY, USA
e-mail: kec9012@med.cornell.edu

G. D. Meckler
Department of Pediatrics and Emergency Medicine, University of British Columbia, BC Children's Hospital, Vancouver, BC, Canada
e-mail: Garth.Meckler@cw.bc.ca

© Springer International Publishing Switzerland 2016
V. J. Grant, A. Cheng (eds.), *Comprehensive Healthcare Simulation: Pediatrics*, Comprehensive Healthcare Simulation, DOI 10.1007/978-3-319-24187-6_17

Table 17.1 Topics and scenarios for PEM-based simulation curricula

	Topics	Scenarios
EM residents (Adler et al.)	*Airway and breathing*	Shock: septic, cardiogenic shock/coarctation, or cardiomyopathy
	Breathing	Tachycardia: SVT, tricyclic antidepressant overdose
	Circulation	Altered mental status: DKA, beta-blocker overdose
	Disability	Trauma: non-accidental trauma, motor vehicle collision
	Exposure/Environment	
Pediatric residents (Stone et al.)	Resuscitation basics	Asthma, anaphylaxis
	Airway and breathing	Seizure
	Circulation	Septic shock, hypovolemic shock
	Teamwork	SVT, VFib
	Core topics	Abdominal trauma, closed head injury
PEM fellows (Cheng et al.)	Respiratory	Asthma, aspiration pneumonia, upper airway obstruction, acute chest syndrome
	Cardiac	SVT, unstable ventricular tachycardia, VFib, pulseless electrical activity/asystole
	Shock	Septic, hypovolemic, anaphylactic, cardiogenic
	Blunt trauma	Abdominal, head, orthopedic, thoracic
	Environmental emergencies	Drowning, hypothermia, electrical injury, smoke inhalation, carbon monoxide
	Infant/neonatal	Non-accidental trauma, bronchiolitis, congenital diaphragmatic hernia, congenital heart disease
	Toxicology	Sympathomimetic, anticholinergic, cholinergic, opioid toxidrome
	Endocrinologic	DKA, adrenal crisis, thyroid storm
	Oncologic	Mediastinal mass, hyperleukocytosis/stroke, tumor lysis syndrome
	Nephrologic	Hypertensive emergency, acute renal failure/hyperkalemia, hyponatremia
	Neurologic	Status epilepticus, coma/depressed level of consciousness, combative/encephalopathy
	Penetrating trauma	Thoracic, neck, spinal cord, abdominal

EM emergency medicine, *DKA diabetic ketoacidosis*, *PEM* pediatric emergency medicine, *SVT* supraventricular tachycardia, *VFib* ventricular fibrillation

Simulation-Based Education

Curriculum Development, Design, and Implementation

PEM has taken on the role of training a variety of learners including undergraduate students; residents from pediatrics, emergency medicine (EM), and family medicine, among others; PEM fellows; as well as continuing professional development for nurses, respiratory therapists, attending physicians, and others. Some educational objectives are outlined by overarching medical organizations, such as the Accreditation Council for Graduate Medical Education, The American Board of Pediatrics, and the Royal College of Physicians and Surgeons of Canada, among others. In an attempt to meet these educational needs, multiple groups have developed curricula and several have published information related to development, content, implementation, and outcomes related to their programs and experiences.

Modular and Longitudinal Curriculum

One example of a modular curriculum designed to meet those needs was developed to teach PEM topics to EM residents,

which included six educational cases and three evaluation cases (see Table 17.1; [6]). The curriculum was designed to focus on the *ABCDE* mnemonic to reinforce the Pediatric Advanced Life Support (PALS) systematic approach to Airway, Breathing, Circulation, Disability, and Exposure/Environment. The team used content maps and assessment domains to develop the scenarios and then scripted them carefully to standardize the intervention in an effort to measure the outcomes. The curriculum evaluation phase required the participants to return for a session to run three evaluation scenarios. The evaluations were scored using a critical action checklist and the results from this specific simulation-based curriculum were limited. They found a correlation with performance and postgraduate year, but did not detect a direct improvement in scores related to the educational intervention.

Another example, designed specifically for pediatric residents, involved implementation and evaluation of a PEM-standardized simulation-based curriculum. This curriculum included nine modules, implemented over a 9-month period with weekly 30-min sessions. Following each simulation, the participants were debriefed and provided a summary of the module's learning objectives [7]. The group used a Kern's framework for medical education and a modified Delphi process with ten subject matter experts to refine the curriculum [8]. They then mapped basic resuscitation skills into specific simulations within each module (see Table 17.1). The overall performance of teams was assessed before and after intervention using the simulation team assessment tool (STAT), which assesses basic resuscitation, airway/breathing, circulation, and teamwork [9]. The results showed statistically significant improvement in each domain, except circulation [7].

A Canadian group of PEM physicians have worked towards establishing a national PEM fellowship simulation-based acute care curriculum. The original published curriculum was designed as a 2-year program, with weekly simulation sessions from a library of 43 different PEM-based cases (Table 17.1). The curriculum was divided into Year One with six core modules designed for first-year fellows and Year Two with six subspecialty modules designed for second-year fellows. As fellows rotate in the PED, they attended two of the sessions, and a database tracked the scenarios they participated in to prevent repetition. The curriculum also included advanced training for PEM fellows interested in developing skills as a simulation educator. This curriculum is an excellent example of incorporating knowledge, clinical skills, technical skills, and crew resource management (CRM) skills and provides a good example of how to develop, revise, and implement a standardized curriculum for a PEM fellowship program [10]. A subsequent study, performed using Delphi methodology across Canada, was performed to identify specific content for a simulation-based national curriculum for all Canadian PEM training programs. From an initial list of 306 topics, the process eventually yielded 48 *Key Curriculum Topics* which fell into the category of *can be taught only by simulation* for PEM fellowship programs. One hundred thirty-five topics were eliminated, and the remaining topics were grouped into 85 *can be taught with simulation* and 87 categorized as *should be taught with simulation*. This provides a very comprehensive list of content that will be used as a basis for the development and implementation of a national PEM fellowship simulation curriculum in Canada [11].

Boot Camps

Boot camps are another form of simulation education where trainees attend an intensive educational experience, often at the beginning of a training program, to assist in establishing a foundation of knowledge and skills for specific subspecialties [12–14]. In general, boot camps can be an effective way to pool simulation resources for a region and not duplicate training efforts between multiple institutions. A PEM-specific boot camp entitled BASE camp was recently developed in the USA which provides a 2-day simulation-based learning opportunity for first-year PEM fellows. BASE camp incorporated procedural training with task trainers and cadavers in addition to high-fidelity mannequin-based simulation to create a progressive learning experience, covering topics ranging from teamwork, airway management, and trauma care. This PEM boot camp has also incorporated interprofessional education (IPE) by including an embedded nursing curriculum. Although this PEM boot camp is designed specifically for beginning first-year fellows, an advanced boot camp, designed for second-year and senior fellows, could provide a valuable experience as these learners have different educational needs.

In Situ Simulation

In situ simulation is a technique which has been shown to be effective in pediatric codes and trauma resuscitations in improving care and patient outcomes (see Chap. 12; Fig. 17.1; [3, 15]). PEM can incorporate in situ simulation into simulation-based curriculum to provide opportunities to practice managing critically ill and injured patients in the actual PED resuscitation bays. In particular, this allows the learners the unique ability to find their typical resources in the actual environment where actual patient care takes place. In addition, any physical or space limitations that are encountered in actual clinical space will need to be overcome. However, there are unique logistical challenges associated with in situ simulation related to incorporating training sessions into the working schedule of a busy clinical setting. Acknowledging these potential challenges and not allowing training sessions to affect patient care are important for staff buy-in and long-term success [16].

Just-in-Time Training

Just-in-time (JIT) training is a unique educational modality where the training takes place just prior to actual patient care. An example of this is demonstrated and described by a PEM group that evaluated JIT training around the procedure of infant lumbar punctures (Fig. 17.2; [17]). In this model of training, trainees were given the opportunity to watch a video demonstrating proper lumbar puncture technique and then practice the procedure on a task trainer until they demonstrated mastery as determined by a lumbar puncture checklist (rated by their supervising physician). Although the study demonstrated improved confidence and lumbar puncture success rates, it uncovered challenges that arise when incorporating educational strategies into a busy work environment. In addition to lumbar puncture, airway management skills and CPR are examples of other procedures that have been taught using JIT training formats and could potentially be implemented in the PEM setting to allow providers the opportunity to hone their skills immediately prior to use on real patients [18, 19].

Fig. 17.1 In situ simulation

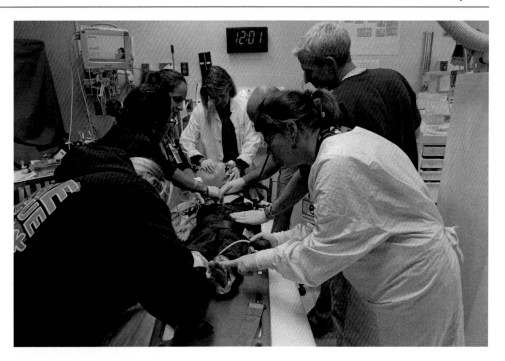

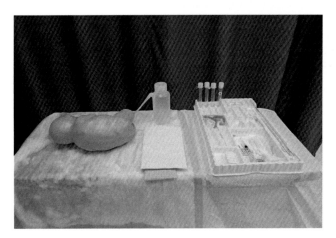

Fig. 17.2 Lumbar puncture task training

Educational Content

Pediatric Trauma

Pediatric trauma patients can be some of the most critical patients cared for in the PED, and simulation-enhanced training has been shown to improve trauma care [15]. One group used simulation to assess pediatric trauma stabilization across 35 different community emergency departments (EDs) and identified deficiencies in systems, equipment, and knowledge [20]. Creating a selection of pediatric trauma scenarios that include blunt trauma, penetrating trauma, isolated head trauma, and non-accidental trauma provides the opportunity for teams to practice the necessary skills required for high-quality and efficient trauma care. These skills include performing the primary and secondary survey and performing a variety of trauma-related procedures (surgical airway, needle decompression of tension pneumothorax, chest thoracostomy tube), some of which occur much more rarely in a PED. In Canada, the Royal College of Physicians and Surgeons of Canada has developed a new pediatric trauma course called *Trauma Resuscitation in Kids (TRIK)*, which incorporates simulation and Web-based learning as key instructional modalities to teach the core knowledge, clinical skills, behavioral skills, and procedural skills required to effectively manage the traumatized pediatric patient [21]. Delivery of courses such as TRIK provides an opportunity for PEM physicians, trauma surgeons, nursing staff, and other allied health professions to hone teamwork and communication skills when managing these critically injured children.

Procedural Skills Training

Incorporated into many of the curricula mentioned previously are specific procedures performed in the PED setting. Procedural training, on either whole-body patient mannequins or specifically designed task trainers, can serve two main purposes. It is a helpful process to allow novice learners to practice certain invasive procedures in a controlled learning environment, promoting patient safety and addressing the ethical issues related to novices practicing procedures on pediatric patients. Procedural training can also be used to allow clinicians the opportunity for training through deliberate practice to maintain or hone certain skills that are not performed routinely (see Chap. 11 for details). The following is a list of the more common procedures performed in the PEM setting which can be simulated:

Vascular Access Intravenous insertion, central venous line insertion, and intraosseous insertion (Fig. 17.3).

Airway Bag-mask ventilation, nasopharyngeal airway, oropharyngeal airway, direct laryngoscopy, video-assisted laryngoscopy, endotracheal intubation, laryngeal mask airway insertion, and difficult airway procedures (use of a gum elastic bougie, needle cricothyroidotomy with transtracheal jet ventilation, surgical airway; Fig. 17.4).

Resuscitation Chest compressions, cardioversion, defibrillation, and pacing (Fig. 17.5).

Trauma Splinting, suturing, needle decompression of tension pneumothorax, chest thoracostomy tube placement, pericardiocentesis, focused assessment with sonography for trauma (FAST) ultrasound, and disaster triage.

Diagnostic/Therapeutic Lumbar puncture, urinary catheterization, and nasal packing for epistaxis.

There have been multiple studies looking at the efficacy of simulation for procedural training. Performing high-quality chest compressions is a procedure that is critical when resuscitating a pulseless patient, and studies have shown that providers demonstrated improved CPR skills during a simulated cardiac arrest following simulation training. Studies have also compared instructor-only training, automated feedback from the task trainer, and a combination of the two. The combined instructor feedback and automated feedback produced the greatest effect, resulting in 100 % compliance with compression rate and depth [22]. The same group also looked at low-dose, high-frequency booster training and found skill retention with compressions was best with the combination of instructor and automated feedback [23].

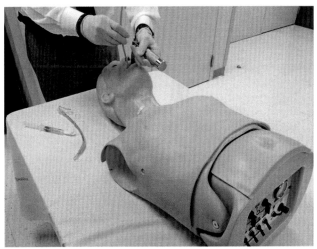

Fig. 17.4 Gum elastic bougie insertion task training. (Photo courtesy of Gaumard Scientific)

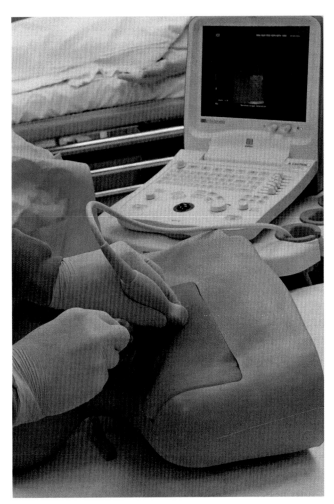

Fig. 17.3 CVL ultrasound-guided task training. *CVL* central venous line. (Photo courtesy of Gaumard Scientific)

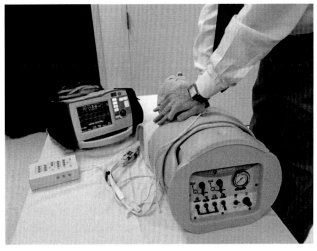

Fig. 17.5 Chest compressions with automated feedback task training. (Photo courtesy of Gaumard Scientific)

Endotracheal intubation is another lifesaving procedure that is not performed daily in PEDs, but a skill that PEM trainees must develop and PEM providers must maintain for the critically ill or injured patient needing emergency airway management. One study assessed transport nurses' and non-anesthesiologist physicians' motor skills related to the procedure of intubation following a refresher training session. The study concluded that brief but frequent (i.e., every 3 months) intubation refresher training sessions were effective in maintaining the psychomotor skills required for pediatric endotracheal intubation [24].

There is a wide variety of commercially available pediatric procedural task trainers for all fields of patient care, including, but not limited to, nursing- and physician-oriented procedures. The driving force behind developing these products is often market based, sometimes with minimal input from the end users, which has resulted in a spectrum of realism ranging from low to high. One study compared commercially available procedural task trainers to homemade task trainers, assessing clinicians' perception of realism. The study included multiple procedures including chest tube insertion, pericardiocentesis, and cricothyroidotomy. The homemade task trainers for chest tube insertion and pericardiocentesis were rated as more realistic than the more expensive commercially available models, but when it came to the surgical airway, the more expensive cricotracheotomy trainer received higher ratings grading realism [25].

Non-technical Skills

The final and overarching areas in PEM where simulation has been incorporated are communication and professionalism. Traditional nursing, respiratory therapy, and medical education had focused a majority of resources on the science related to areas including pathophysiology, pharmacology, and anatomy, but over the past several decades, studies have shown that effective teamwork and communication can reduce medical errors and improve care provided in both the simulated and actual ED settings [4, 26]. Simulation has embraced this, and a critical part of many simulations includes CRM to assist in developing high-functioning teams (see Chap. 4 for details). The concept of effective teams requires and encourages IPE, which is the concept of having learners and professionals from different backgrounds train together. In situ simulation is an excellent example of a type of simulation where nurses, physicians, and respiratory therapists can participate in an IPE session and reflect on team performance after providing care to a simulated pediatric patient in the ED setting. Offering this type of educational experience at the undergraduate level, for nursing, respiratory therapy, and medicine, can help shape students' perceptions and attitudes towards IPE, teamwork, and even their general thoughts and feelings regarding simulation as a learning modality [27].

There are also many unique opportunities using simulation to present clinical situations in the ED whereby difficult discussions occur, ranging from informing a family their child has died to disclosing to a family that a medical error has occurred. Simulation has been used to allow residents and PEM fellows an opportunity to practice difficult discussions and review effective strategies in managing these challenging situations. Other topics with difficult discussions that have been described in simulation literature are non-accidental trauma, domestic violence, and breaking bad news around new diagnoses (see Chap. 23 for details; [28, 29]).

Pediatric Advanced Life Support (PALS)

As detailed previously in this chapter, life-threatening pediatric conditions and events requiring emergency resuscitation are rare. And for pediatric residents in training, the implementation of work-hour restrictions, increasing supervision by attending staff and subspecialty training fellows, and the reduction in time devoted to emergency and critical care training further conspire to restrict these experiences [30]. With few opportunities for physicians, nurses, respiratory therapists, and other health team members to practice and reinforce advanced life support knowledge and skills, many providers charged with caring for critically ill children may have insufficient experience to sustain a high level of proficiency and expertise in PALS [30–32]. Training in PALS is often mandatory among healthcare professionals who have a responsibility for the delivery of pediatric emergency or critical care. According to the American Heart Association (AHA), becoming a certified PALS provider requires the successful completion of a 14-h classroom, video-based, instructor-led course that includes a series of simulated pediatric emergencies [33].

Integration of Simulation into Pediatric Advanced Life Support

The AHA explicitly recommends simulation as a training strategy to enhance performance. As a consequence, more PALS courses are featuring fewer instructor-driven clinical case scenarios and more hands-on experiential learning. When simulation was incorporated into advanced life support training, it was shown to improve knowledge and skills performance in providers tested on simulators [34, 35]. There are currently no data to suggest if adding simulation alters the knowledge decay seen with traditional courses. To address this issue, a novel PALS recertification program that uses immersive high-fidelity in situ simulation scenarios to deliver intermittent modular PALS retraining has been developed [36]. In this program, experienced pediatric critical care nurses and respiratory therapists participated in six 30-min in situ simulation modules consisting of 12 core PALS scenarios and two 15-min automated external defibrillator (AED)/CPR demonstration sessions distributed over 6 months [36]. Although simulation participants spent nearly half the total time they would have spent in a conventional PALS recertification class, their performance in advanced life support skills was superior to their counterparts who were not exposed to simulation.

One simulation-based educational strategy that gives learners more deliberate practice opportunities to improve their resuscitation skills is the principle of rapid cycle deliberate practice (RCDP) [37]. When an error is observed in a simulation, the scenario is interrupted so that instructors can provide expert directed feedback. Learners are then given as many opportunities as necessary to retry the skill or behavior until mastery is achieved. An initial phase of learning is followed by a period of gaining experience where fewer mistakes are committed and the learner is able to perform at a higher level [38]. Pediatric residents who participated in SBE where RCDP was implemented showed sustained improvements in multiple measures of performance for advanced life support skills [37].

Simulation is especially well suited for multidisciplinary teams to participate in advanced life support scenarios. The ability to organize and lead a multidisciplinary team during the resuscitation of a critically ill child requires extensive training and experience. Not surprisingly, while only 44% of pediatric residents felt confident in their ability to lead a resuscitation, a remarkable 44% also graduated without ever having had an opportunity to lead a team [30]. Supervision by fellows and attending staff limits opportunities for residents to develop and practice leadership behaviors in managing code resuscitations. Simulation can be used to bridge this educational gap, and team performance in a resuscitation can be improved when teamwork principles are incorporated into advanced life support training [39–42].

Cardiopulmonary Resuscitation Skills

Without sufficient opportunities for practice, knowledge and skill decay is inevitable [30]. In as little as 6 months after conventional training, proficiency in critical CPR skills such as compression rate and depth may fall dangerously close to pre-training levels [43]. This was demonstrated in pediatric residents' resuscitation skills 6 months after PALS recertification [30, 44]. Even when resuscitation efforts are performed by highly trained healthcare professionals, achieving the AHA's minimum targets for high-quality CPR and providing rapid defibrillation when appropriate are difficult [45–47]. All of these studies support the fact that more frequent refreshers are needed [48, 49].

Even with refresher training sessions, the AHA-defined high-quality CPR is notoriously difficult to achieve and sustain [46, 47]. The AHA's recommended targets for compression depth and rate, as well as emphasis on minimizing

interruptions are demanding. The AHA suggests that CPR prompt/feedback devices may be considered for training and for clinical use to improve the quality of CPR [39, 50]. Multiple human and simulation studies have shown how CPR prompt/feedback devices can help to improve awareness of CPR technique and promote quality improvement [51]. One study reported when real-time CPR feedback was combined with structured debriefing after a simulated arrest, the combined effect on CPR performance was more effective than either intervention alone [52].

Debriefing

Debriefing is a critical component of SBE (see Chap. 3 for details). Acknowledging the value of debriefing as an engine for teams or individuals to reflect on and improve their performance after a simulation scenario, the AHA has recommended that post-scenario debriefing be included in all advanced life support courses [39]. Unlike instructor-driven PALS courses, SBE requires facilitators who are trained in the skill of debriefing [32]. The AHA offers an interactive online *Structured and Supported Debriefing* course to train AHA instructors on how to effectively facilitate a simulation debriefing [53]. An online instructional debriefing module and debriefing tool are included with the 2011 PALS instructor materials to help instructors develop and enhance their debriefing skills [54].

Systems Integration, Quality Improvement, and Patient Safety

In addition to the curricular and team training needs within PEM described in this chapter, various forms of simulation have been used to design, test, and evaluate the pediatric emergency preparedness and response at the departmental, interdepartmental, and systems levels (see Chap. 6 for details). Traditional mannequin-based simulation has been used to improve or maintain staff competence in resuscitation and procedural skills, and foster teamwork and team performance, as discussed below and elsewhere in this textbook. In situ simulation and large-scale exercises have been used to evaluate regional and rural ED performance and identify opportunities for improvement, particularly around trauma. A mixture of simulation strategies has been used to address patient safety in the PED and to promote quality improvement, from identifying potential latent safety risks and testing new equipment or care pathways to enhancing the learning from morbidity and mortality reviews (see Chap. 5 for details). Computer-based simulation and modeling have become important tools to aid in ED design, staffing, and operations, allowing for the evaluation of the impact of operational quality improvement measures on crowding, patient flow, and preparation for pandemic surges.

The use of simulation for emergency systems performance has been well studied in pediatric trauma. Simulation-based individual and team training, including both mannequin-based and virtual reality systems, have also been used to improve pediatric trauma team performance and teach interdisciplinary pediatric trauma skills at the institutional level [55–58]. Simulation has also been used to evaluate larger systems of trauma care at the state level [20]. Thirty-five hospitals in North Carolina were evaluated to assess their ability to assess and stabilize a simulated 3-year-old mock trauma patient according to established PALS and Advanced Trauma Life Support (ATLS) guidelines, including performance on primary and secondary survey as well as procedures and general management. The study, mentioned earlier in this chapter, was able to identify deficiencies in trauma resuscitation of children in EDs throughout the state and, based on the findings, design and implement a simulation-based educational intervention that subsequently improved the trauma system's performance [59].

Simulation has also been used to evaluate and improve patient safety in the PED, both as a tool to identify latent safety threats and test high-risk care models, and as an educational strategy to improve safety through multidisciplinary team training. Mannequin-based mock codes were used in a children's hospital ED to implement and test a quality improvement initiative to replace traditional resuscitation codebooks with a computerized decision support tool. While the goal of the study was to compare decision support tools, the results revealed a concerning gap in participants' ability to recognize and classify life-threatening dysrhythmias, uncovering an important safety threat previously unrecognized [60]. Formal in situ simulation programs (some unannounced) have been used specifically to target latent threats and areas for quality improvement [61]. Following the identification and classification of specific safety threats, simulation-based teamwork training focused on communication to improve quality of care and reduce errors. Provider knowledge and attitudes following the intervention, as well as a decrease in the rate of actual patient safety events within the ED, were demonstrated [62]. Other examples of simulation-based quality and safety improvement strategies in the ED include the use of in situ simulation to test and iteratively improve a protocol-based ED procedural sedation service [63] and the use of high-fidelity mannequin simulations augmented by an audience response system to enhance a case-based morbidity and mortality conference [64].

A computer-based simulation technique known as discrete event simulation (DES), adapted from the field of systems engineering, has been widely used to model complex systems of care in the ED. DES employs an empirically derived probability-based statistical and logical model of complex systems to predict the impact of changes to specific input variables on the larger system performance and allows users to test and analyze outcomes of *what-if* scenarios in a controlled but flexible environment. Examples of the use of DES for ED operations and quality improvement include modeling of patient flow and crowding [65–68]; architectural design and orientation to new ED facilities [69–71]; optimal staffing and resource utilization [72–75]; ED operational unit, interdepartmental, and hospital-wide systems testing and optimization [76–78]; and mass casualty and disaster preparedness through surge capacity planning [79–83].

Strategies for Building a Simulation Program in Pediatric Emergency Medicine

There are several ways to cultivate institutional support for the resources necessary to establish and develop a program in simulation for PEM. Advocates for simulation should consider a range of strategies in building a program, including partnerships with simulation experts and departments outside of PEM. Simulation programs thrive when supported by a diverse constituency. Hospital nursing and physician leadership, patient care and quality control committees, and community advisory groups may be unexpected allies.

Simulation is a relatively low-cost strategy for preventing expensive and potentially catastrophic medical errors. As mentioned in the previous sections, in situ multidisciplinary simulations in the ED permit the testing and assessment of clinical performance, procedures, equipment, and spaces in the department, and could identify complex systems-based failures or simple mechanical malfunctions requiring engineering solutions. Either has the potential for improving the quality of care, reducing preventable medical errors, and saving an institution's money.

PEM simulation programs promote interprofessional training, creating a more robust staff and leading to a spirit of practice and interdependency, self-reflection, and self-improvement, which may have an indirect effect of improving overall morale. The learning objectives are often linked to quality improvement or patient safety initiatives, which create additional value for the department. Promoting simulation's role in providing high-quality medical education activities should also be highlighted whenever possible and can assist in attracting residents, fellows, clinicians, and other healthcare professionals to the institution.

Much like any pediatric simulation program, the resources necessary for a well-rounded program in PEM may include high-, medium-, and low-fidelity simulators to meet the various training objectives. When considering features of high-fidelity pediatric simulators, portability may be just as important as size or age. The capacity to conduct in situ simulations in a busy PED requires a simulator that can be assembled and dismantled quickly to avoid unexpected disruptions in patient care. Consider the training program's priorities for various clinical features such as laryngospasm or the capacity to permit invasive procedures such as cricothyroidotomy when selecting a simulator. There are certainly limitations to fidelity with pediatric simulators, but this is not unique to PEM. Creativity with moulage, props, and well-scripted scenarios allows simulation of a wide variety of clinical scenarios relevant to the PEM setting.

Low-fidelity task trainers for PEM generally address the need to practice skills for managing airway or circulatory emergencies and trauma. They range from simple airway simulators for direct laryngoscopy to ultrasound-compatible torsos for central venous access catheterization. Selecting a task trainer is dependent on curriculum needs (e.g., deficits in emergency trauma procedural skills training), clinical needs (e.g., peripheral intravenous (IV) training for inexperienced nursing staff), and cost.

Simulation programs rely on technology which inevitably includes the requirement for technical support. Having dedicated simulation technicians available allows for greater productivity from simulation faculty who are often busy clinicians, donating time to develop and orchestrate simulation-enhanced sessions. If technical support is not available, tech savvy faculty may be burdened with this responsibility and may look for help from interested PEM fellows, residents, nurses, and students to accomplish the technical tasks associated with running effective simulation programs.

One responsibility that goes along with receiving institutional support from a simulation program in PEM is recording data to show meaningful outcomes. The ultimate outcome is to show improved patient care, but there are additional data that can help to justify a simulation program. Helping graduate medical education programs (pediatric residency, EM residency, and PEM fellowship) with required procedural training and recording data around these procedures is valuable for program directors. Assisting ED administration with tracking attendance when orienting and training novice nurses in resuscitation and trauma can expedite orientation and reduce staffing costs associated with this process. Leveraging simulation through in situ programs to identify latent hazards, develop solutions, test the solutions, and then report this information to administrative leaders and risk management is another meaningful outcome to justify the expense and effort behind a PEM simulation program. Finally, any data that can be gathered demonstrating utilization, improved clinician or team performance, reduction of risk, and improved patient care and outcomes are critical for the sustainment and longevity of PEM simulation.

Conclusions

PEM has been very successful in utilizing simulation in a variety of areas described in this chapter, but there are certainly opportunities for expansion, where simulation can be used in different ways in the future. Educational programs and learners could benefit from more standardized simulation curricula teaching PEM-specific milestones and procedures. Additional simulation-based research can assist with improving care provided to ill and injured children. As PEM simulation matures, it may reach a point where it could be used for measuring and determining competency of critical skills ranging from airway management to trauma resuscitation. There could be a time in the future where simulation may even be part of the interview day for PEM fellow applicants or the certification process for PEM physicians. The field of PEM simulation has come a long way in a short period and promises great things in the future, but there are many areas of investigation where future research needs to be performed. These areas include, but are not limited to: investigating the most effective ways of leveraging simulation, both low and high fidelity, as an educational intervention; the dose needed to see the desired effect; the rate of decay of psychomotor skills after an intervention; and the frequency of maintenance training to maintain a spectrum of critical skills. There is also a need for more realistic pediatric patient simulators to demonstrate finding such as poor perfusion or respiratory distress to assist in educating learners on pediatric assessment. Finally, as better pediatric mannequins and task trainers are developed, it will be important to look for correlation between competency seen on the pediatric simulators and competency with the same procedure on actual pediatric patients. All of these types of research will be critical to justify the significant effort and expense invested in simulation-based training and education in the world of PEM and beyond.

References

1. Allan CK, Thiagarajan RR, Beke D, Imprescia A, Kappus LJ, Garden A, et al. Simulation-based training delivered directly to the pediatric cardiac intensive care unit engenders preparedness, comfort, and decreased anxiety among multidisciplinary resuscitation teams. J Thorac Cardiovasc Surg. 2010;140(3):646–52.
2. Tan SB, Pena G, Altree M, Maddern GJ. Multidisciplinary team simulation for the operating theatre: a review of the literature. ANZ J Surg. 2014;84(7–8):515–22.
3. Andreatta P, Saxton E, Thompson M, Annich G. Simulation-based mock codes significantly correlate with improved pediatric patient cardiopulmonary arrest survival rates. Pediatr Crit Care Med. 2011;12(1):33–8.
4. Morey JC, Simon R, Jay GD, Wears RL, Salisbury M, Dukes KA, et al. Error reduction and performance improvement in the emergency department through formal teamwork training: evaluation results of the MedTeams project. Health Serv Res. 2002;37(6):1553–81.
5. Shapiro MJ, Morey JC, Small SD, Langford V, Kaylor CJ, Jagminas L, et al. Simulation based teamwork training for emergency department staff: does it improve clinical team performance when added to an existing didactic teamwork curriculum? Qual Saf Health Care. 2004;13(6):417–21.
6. Adler MD, Vozenilek JA, Trainor JL, Eppich WJ, Wang EE, Beaumont JL, et al. Development and evaluation of a simulation-based pediatric emergency medicine curriculum. Acad Med. 2009;84(7):935–41.

7. Stone K, Reid J, Caglar D, Christensen A, Strelitz B, Zhou L, et al. Increasing pediatric resident simulated resuscitation performance: a standardized simulation-based curriculum. Resuscitation. 2014;85(8):1099–105.

8. Kern DE, Thomas PA, Hughs MT. Curriculum development for medical education: a six-step approach. 2nd ed. Baltimore: Johns Hopkins University Press; 2009.

9. Reid J, Stone K, Brown J, Caglar D, Kobayashi A, Lewis-Newby M, et al. The simulation team assessment tool (STAT): development, reliability and validation. Resuscitation. 2012;83(7):879–86.

10. Cheng A, Goldman RD, Aish MA, Kissoon N. A simulation-based acute care curriculum for pediatric emergency medicine fellowship training programs. Pediatr Emerg Care. 2010;26(7):475–80.

11. Bank I, Cheng A, McLeod P, Bhanji F. Determining content for a simulation-based curriculum in pediatric emergency medicine: results from a national Delphi process. CJEM. 2015;17(6):662–9. doi: 10.1017/cem.2015.11.

12. Nishisaki A, Hales R, Biagas K, Cheifetz I, Corriveau C, Garber N, et al. A multi-institutional high-fidelity simulation "boot camp" orientation and training program for first year pediatric critical care fellows. Pediatr Crit Care Med. 2009;10(2):157–62.

13. Wayne DB, Cohen ER, Singer BD, Moazed F, Barsuk JH, Lyons EA, et al. Progress toward improving medical school graduates' skills via a "boot camp" curriculum. Simul Healthc. 2014;9(1):33–9.

14. Fernandez GL, Page DW, Coe NP, Lee PC, Patterson LA, Skylizard L, et al. Boot cAMP: educational outcomes after 4 successive years of preparatory simulation-based training at onset of internship. J Surg Educ. 2012;69(2):242–8.

15. Steinemann S, Berg B, Skinner A, DiTulio A, Anzelon K, Terada K, et al. In situ, multidisciplinary, simulation-based teamwork training improves early trauma care. J Surg Educ. 2011;68(6):472–7.

16. Patterson MD, Blike GT, Nadkarni VM. Advances in patient safety in situ simulation: challenges and results. In: Henriksen K, Battles JB, Keyes MA, Grady ML, editors. Advances in patient safety: new directions and alternative approaches (Vol 3: performance and tools). Rockville: Agency for Healthcare Research and Quality (US); 2008.

17. Kamdar G, Kessler DO, Tilt L, Srivastava G, Khanna K, Chang TP, et al. Qualitative evaluation of just-in-time simulation-based learning: the learners' perspective. Simul Healthc. 2013;8(1):43–8.

18. Nishisaki A, Donoghue AJ, Colborn S, Watson C, Meyer A, Brown CA 3rd, et al. Effect of just-in-time simulation training on tracheal intubation procedure safety in the pediatric intensive care unit. Anesthesiology. 2010;113(1):214–23.

19. Niles D, Sutton RM, Donoghue A, Kalsi MS, Roberts K, Boyle L, et al. "Rolling Refreshers": a novel approach to maintain CPR psychomotor skill competence. Resuscitation. 2009;80(8):909–12.

20. Hunt EA, Hohenhaus SM, Luo X, Frush KS. Simulation of pediatric trauma stabilization in 35 North Carolina emergency departments: identification of targets for performance improvement. Pediatrics. 2006;117(3):641–8.

21. TRIK Course. http://www.royalcollege.ca/portal/page/portal/rc/resources/ppi/trik_course.

22. Sutton RM, Niles D, Meaney PA, Aplenc R, French B, Abella BS, et al. "Booster" training: evaluation of instructor-led bedside cardiopulmonary resuscitation skill training and automated corrective feedback to improve cardiopulmonary resuscitation compliance of pediatric basic life support providers during simulated cardiac arrest. Pediatr Crit Care Med. 2011;12(3):e116–21.

23. Sutton RM, Niles D, Meaney PA, Aplenc R, French B, Abella BS, et al. Low-dose, high-frequency CPR training improves skill retention of in-hospital pediatric providers. Pediatrics. 2011;128(1):e145–51.

24. Nishisaki A, Scrattish L, Boulet J, Kalsi M, Maltese M, Castner T, et al. Advances in patient safety effect of recent refresher training on in situ simulated pediatric tracheal intubation psychomotor skill performance. In: Henriksen K, Battles JB, Keyes MA, Grady ML, editors. Advances in patient safety: new directions and alternative approaches (Vol 3: performance and tools). Rockville: Agency for Healthcare Research and Quality (US); 2008.

25. Shefrin A, Khazei A, Cheng A. HYPERLINK "http://www.ncbi.nlm.nih.gov/pubmed/26451232"Realism of procedural task trainers in a pediatric emergency medicine procedures course. Can Med Educ J. 2015;6(1):e68–73.

26. Sigalet E, Donnon T, Cheng A, Cooke S, Robinson T, Bissett W, et al. Development of a team performance scale to assess undergraduate health professionals. Acad Med. 2013;88(7):989–96.

27. Sigalet E, Donnon T, Grant V. Undergraduate students' perceptions of and attitudes toward a simulation-based interprofessional curriculum: the KidSIM ATTITUDES questionnaire. Simul Healthc. 2012;7(6):353–8.

28. Overly FL, Sudikoff SN, Duffy S, Anderson A, Kobayashi L. Three scenarios to teach difficult discussions in pediatric emergency medicine: sudden infant death, child abuse with domestic violence, and medication error. Simul Healthc. 2009;4(2):114–30.

29. Tobler K, Grant E, Marczinski C. Evaluation of the impact of a simulation-enhanced breaking bad news workshop in pediatrics. Simul Healthc. 2014;9(4):213–9.

30. Nadel FM, Lavelle JM, Fein JA, Giardino AP, Decker JM, Durbin DR. Assessing pediatric senior residents' training in resuscitation: fund of knowledge, technical skills, and perception of confidence. Pediatr Emerg Care. 2000;16(2):73–6.

31. Hamilton R. Nurses' knowledge and skill retention following cardiopulmonary resuscitation training: a review of the literature. J Adv Nurs. 2005;51(3):288–97.

32. Schoenfeld PS, Baker MD. Management of cardiopulmonary and trauma resuscitation in the pediatric emergency department. Pediatrics. 1993;91(4):726–9.

33. Association AH. Pediatric advanced life support. [Internet] 2014.

34. Donoghue AJ, Durbin DR, Nadel FM, Stryjewski GR, Kost SI, Nadkarni VM. Effect of high-fidelity simulation on Pediatric Advanced Life Support training in pediatric house staff: a randomized trial. Pediatr Emerg Care. 2009;25(3):139–44.

35. Wayne DB, Butter J, Siddall VJ, Fudala MJ, Linquist LA, Feinglass J, et al. Simulation-based training of internal medicine residents in advanced cardiac life support protocols: a randomized trial. Teach Learn Med. 2005;17(3):210–6.

36. Kurosawa H, Ikeyama T, Achuff P, Perkel M, Watson C, Monachino A, et al. A randomized, controlled trial of in situ pediatric advanced life support recertification ("pediatric advanced life support reconstructed") compared with standard pediatric advanced life support recertification for ICU frontline providers*. Crit Care Med. 2014;42(3):610–8.

37. Hunt EA, Duval-Arnould JM, Nelson-McMillan KL, Bradshaw JH, Diener-West M, Perretta JS, et al. Pediatric resident resuscitation skills improve after "rapid cycle deliberate practice" training. Resuscitation. 2014;85(7):945–51.

38. Ericsson KA. Deliberate practice and the acquisition and maintenance of expert performance in medicine and related domains. Acad Med. 2004;79(Suppl 10):70–81.

39. Bhanji F, Mancini ME, Sinz E, Rodgers DL, McNeil MA, Hoadley TA, et al. Part 16: education, implementation, and teams: 2010 American Heart Association guidelines for cardiopulmonary resuscitation and emergency cardiovascular care. Circulation. 2010;122(18 Suppl 3):920–33.

40. Cooper S. Developing leaders for advanced life support: evaluation of a training programme. Resuscitation. 2001;49(1):33–8.

41. Gilfoyle E, Gottesman R, Razack S. Development of a leadership skills workshop in paediatric advanced resuscitation. Med Teach. 2007;29(9):276–83.

42. DeVita MA, Schaefer J, Lutz J, Wang H, Dongilli T. Improving medical emergency team (MET) performance using a novel curriculum and a computerized human patient simulator. Qual Saf Health Care. 2005;14(5):326–31.

43. Wik L, Myklebust H, Auestad BH, Steen PA. Retention of basic life support skills 6 months after training with an automated voice advisory manikin system without instructor involvement. Resuscitation. 2002;52(3):273–9.

44. Grant EC, Marczinski CA, Menon K. Using pediatric advanced life support in pediatric residency training: does the curriculum need resuscitation? Pediatr Crit Care Med. 2007;8(5):433–9.

45. Hunt EA, Vera K, Diener-West M, Haggerty JA, Nelson KL, Shaffner DH, et al. Delays and errors in cardiopulmonary resuscitation and defibrillation by pediatric residents during simulated cardiopulmonary arrests. Resuscitation. 2009;80(7):819–25.

46. Abella BS, Alvarado JP, Myklebust H, Edelson DP, Barry A, O'Hearn N, et al. Quality of cardiopulmonary resuscitation during in-hospital cardiac arrest. JAMA. 2005;293(3):305–10.

47. Sutton RM, Wolfe H, Nishisaki A, Leffelman J, Niles D, Meaney PA, et al. Pushing harder, pushing faster, minimizing interruptions … but falling short of 2010 cardiopulmonary resuscitation targets during in-hospital pediatric and adolescent resuscitation. Resuscitation. 2013;84(12):1680–4.

48. Makker R, Gray-Siracusa K, Evers M. Evaluation of advanced cardiac life support in a community teaching hospital by use of actual cardiac arrests. Heart Lung. 1995;24(2):116–20.

49. Kaye W. Research on ACLS training—which methods improve skill & knowledge retention? Respir Care. 1995;40(5):538–46. (discussion 46–9).

50. Mancini ME, Soar J, Bhanji F, Billi JE, Dennett J, Finn J, et al. Part 12: education, implementation, and teams: 2010 International Consensus on Cardiopulmonary Resuscitation and Emergency Cardiovascular Care Science With Treatment Recommendations. Circulation. 2010;122(16 Suppl 2):S539–81.

51. Yeung J, Meeks R, Edelson D, Gao F, Soar J, Perkins GD. The use of CPR feedback/prompt devices during training and CPR performance: a systematic review. Resuscitation. 2009;80(7):743–51.

52. Dine CJ, Gersh RE, Leary M, Riegel BJ, Bellini LM, Abella BS. Improving cardiopulmonary resuscitation quality and resuscitation training by combining audiovisual feedback and debriefing. Crit Care Med. 2008;36(10):2817–22.

53. Chamberlain DA, Hazinski MF. Education in resuscitation: an IL-COR symposium: Utstein Abbey: stavanger, Norway: june 22–24, 2001. Circulation. 2003;108(20):2575–94.

54. Cheng A, Rodgers DL, van der Jagt E, Eppich W, O'Donnell J. Evolution of the pediatric advanced life support course: enhanced learning with a new debriefing tool and Web-based module for pediatric advanced life support instructors. Pediatr Crit Care Med. 2012;13(5):589–95.

55. Youngblood P, Harter PM, Srivastava S, Moffett S, Heinrichs WL, Dev P. Design, development, and evaluation of an online virtual emergency department for training trauma teams. Simul Healthc. 2008;3(3):146–53.

56. Mikrogianakis A, Osmond MH, Nuth JE, Shephard A, Gaboury I, Jabbour M. Evaluation of a multidisciplinary pediatric mock trauma code educational initiative: a pilot study. J Trauma. 2008;64(3):761–7.

57. Falcone RA Jr, Daugherty M, Schweer L, Patterson M, Brown RL, Garcia VF. Multidisciplinary pediatric trauma team training using high-fidelity trauma simulation. J Pediatr Surg. 2008;43(6):1065–71.

58. Cherry RA, Ali J. Current concepts in simulation-based trauma education. J Trauma. 2008;65(5):1186–93.

59. Hunt EA, Heine M, Hohenhaus SM, Luo X, Frush KS. Simulated pediatric trauma team management: assessment of an educational intervention. Pediatr Emerg Care. 2007;23(11):796–804.

60. Spanos SL, Patterson M. An unexpected diagnosis: simulation reveals unanticipated deficiencies in resident physician dysrhythmia knowledge. Simul Healthc. 2010;5(1):21–3.

61. O'Leary F, McGarvey K, Christoff A, Major J, Lockie F, Chayen G, et al. Identifying incidents of suboptimal care during paediatric emergencies-an observational study utilising in situ and simulation centre scenarios. Resuscitation. 2014;85(3):431–6.

62. Patterson MD, Geis GL, LeMaster T, Wears RL. Impact of multidisciplinary simulation-based training on patient safety in a paediatric emergency department. BMJ Qual Saf. 2013;22(5):383–93.

63. Kobayashi L, Dunbar-Viveiros JA, Devine J, Jones MS, Overly FL, Gosbee JW, et al. Pilot-phase findings from high-fidelity In Situ medical simulation investigation of emergency department procedural sedation. Simul Healthc. 2012;7(2):81–94.

64. Vozenilek J, Wang E, Kharasch M, Anderson B, Kalaria A. Simulation-based morbidity and mortality conference: new technologies augmenting traditional case-based presentations. Acad Emerg Med. 2006;13(1):48–53.

65. Wiler JL, Griffey RT, Olsen T. Review of modeling approaches for emergency department patient flow and crowding research. Acad Emerg Med. 2011;18(12):1371–9.

66. Eitel DR, Rudkin SE, Malvehy MA, Killeen JP, Pines JM. Improving service quality by understanding emergency department flow: a White Paper and position statement prepared for the American Academy of Emergency Medicine. J Emerg Med. 2010;38(1):70–9.

67. Hoot NR, LeBlanc LJ, Jones I, Levin SR, Zhou C, Gadd CS, et al. Forecasting emergency department crowding: a discrete event simulation. Ann Emerg Med. 2008;52(2):116–25.

68. Hung GR, Whitehouse SR, O'Neill C, Gray AP, Kissoon N. Computer modeling of patient flow in a pediatric emergency department using discrete event simulation. Pediatr Emerg Care. 2007;23(1):5–10.

69. Kobayashi L, Shapiro MJ, Sucov A, Woolard R, Boss RM 3rd, Dunbar J, et al. Portable advanced medical simulation for new emergency department testing and orientation. Acad Emerg Med. 2006;13(6):691–5.

70. Wiinamaki A, Dronzek R. Using simulation in the architectural concept phase of an emergency department design. Proceedings of the 2003 Winter, Simulation Conference 2003; 2003. Vol. 2, pp. 1912.

71. Geis GL, Pio B, Pendergrass TL, Moyer MR, Patterson MD. Simulation to assess the safety of new healthcare teams and new facilities. Simul Healthc. 2011;6(3):125–33.

72. Chin L, Fleisher G. Planning model of resource utilization in an academic pediatric emergency department. Pediatr Emerg Care. 1998;14(1):4–9.

73. Draeger MA. An emergency department simulation model used to evaluate alternative nurse staffing and patient population scenarios. Proceedings of the 24th conference on Winter simulation; 1992. pp. 1057–64.

74. Evans GW, Tesham BG, Unger E. A simulation model for evaluating personnel schedules in a hospital emergency department. Proceedings of the 28th conference on Winter Simulation IEEE Computer Society; 1996.

75. Centeno MA, et al. Emergency departments II: a simulation-ilp based tool for scheduling ER staff. Proceedings of the 35th conference on Winter simulation: driving innovation Winter Simulation Conference; 2003.

76. Hung GR, Kissoon N. Impact of an observation unit and an emergency department-admitted patient transfer mandate in decreasing overcrowding in a pediatric emergency department: a discrete event simulation exercise. Pediatr Emerg Care. 2009;25(3):160–3.

77. Blasak RE, Starks DW, Armel WS, Hayduk MC. The use of simulation to evaluate hospital operations between the emergency department and a medical telemetry unit. Proceedings of the 2003 Winter Simulation Conference 2003; 2003. p. 1887.

78. Ahmed MA, Alkamis TM. Simulation optimization for an emergency department healthcare unit in Kuwait. Eur J Oper Res. 2009;198:936.

79. Kobayashi L, Shapiro MJ, Gutman DC, Jay G. Multiple encounter simulation for high-acuity multipatient environment training. Acad Emerg Med. 2007;14(12):1141–8.

80. Kanter RK, Moran JR. Pediatric hospital and intensive care unit capacity in regional disasters: expanding capacity by altering standards of care. Pediatrics. 2007;119(1):94–100.

81. Kaji AH, Bair A, Okuda Y, Kobayashi L, Khare R, Vozenilek J. Defining systems expertise: effective simulation at the organizational level–implications for patient safety, disaster surge capacity, and facilitating the systems interface. Acad Emerg Med. 2008;15(11):1098–103.

82. Patrick J, Puterman ML. Reducing wait times through operations research: optimizing the use of surge capacity. Healthc Policy (Politiques de sante). 2008;3(3):75–88.

83. McCarthy ML, Aronsky D, Kelen GD. The measurement of daily surge and its relevance to disaster preparedness. Acad Emerg Med. 2006;13(11):1138–41.

Simulation for Neonatal Care

18

Lindsay Callahan Johnston, Douglas Campbell and Deepak Manhas

Simulation Pearls

1. Simulation is an invaluable tool for the neonatal clinician. Individual skill development and teamwork training are crucial elements in which simulation can be used in order to develop competence, improve on patient outcomes, and promote quality and safety as guiding principles.
2. Simulation can be used in preparation for complex clinical or interprofessional situations, such as an extracorporeal membrane oxygenation (ECMO) cannulation or delivery of an infant with a rare congenital anomaly, as well as to identify latent safety threats.
3. Established neonatal resuscitation and stabilization programs such as Neonatal Resuscitation Program (NRP), the **S**ugar & Safe care, **T**emperature, **A**irway, **B**lood pressure, **L**ab work and **E**motional support (S.T.A.B.L.E.) program, and Acute Care of at Risk Newborns (ACoRN) provide frameworks and algorithms that can easily be incorporated into effective critical event simulations.
4. The use of simulation is a key quality improvement tool in improving neonatal intensive care unit (NICU) design, latent hazard identification, and improvement of patient safety.

L. C. Johnston (✉)
Department of Pediatrics, Yale School of Medicine,
New Haven, CT, USA
e-mail: Lindsay.johnston@yale.edu

D. Campbell
Department of Pediatrics, University of Toronto, Toronto, ON, Canada
e-mail: campbelld@smh.ca

D. Manhas
Department of Pediatrics, Department of Neonatal Intensive Care,
University of British Columbia, British Columbia Children's &
Women's Hospital, Vancouver, BC, Canada
e-mail: dmanhas@cw.bc.ca

Introduction

Practitioners in neonatology have been at the forefront of healthcare simulation training since its inception. Obstetrical, neonatal, and anesthesia colleagues were amongst the first to utilize high-fidelity simulation to replicate the delivery room environment to study and optimize human performance [1]. Subsequently, in the 1990s, neonatal high-fidelity and high-technology simulation programs adopted facilitated debriefing for training individual neonatal clinicians and interprofessional teams [2]. Given the unpredictable need for neonatal resuscitation [3] and the high-stakes environment of the NICU, it is critical to ensure that all team members are provided with opportunities to learn and refine medical decision-making, procedural skills, and teamwork prior to caring for patients at risk.

Perhaps even more important, by taking part in interprofessional, multidisciplinary simulations, all members of the neonatal care team are able to optimize their skills in communicating clearly and utilizing effective team strategies to optimize and improve performance. A root cause analysis (RCA) of over 100 sentinel perinatal and neonatal events in 2004 was reported by the Joint Commission of Healthcare Organizations. Of 93 reported neonatal deaths and 16 survivors with severe morbidities, communication failure amongst team members played a role in 72% of cases, while 40% involved orientation and training issues. All of these negative outcomes were felt to be potentially preventable, and recommendations included practice drills with interprofessional team members [4].

Participation in simulation is beneficial for both novices and established care teams and providers. Compared with learners in previous eras, even senior trainees now have more limited exposure to real-life delivery room resuscitations and codes [5, 6]. Opportunities for procedures may be decreased, and rates of success are often suboptimal [5, 7, 8]. Adhering to best practices in adult education [9], current medical, nursing, and allied health professional students more frequently participate in simulation as a standard part of their training. Simulation may offer one solution to allow

© Springer International Publishing Switzerland 2016
V. J. Grant, A. Cheng (eds.), *Comprehensive Healthcare Simulation: Pediatrics,*
Comprehensive Healthcare Simulation, DOI 10.1007/978-3-319-24187-6_18

these novice clinicians to establish competency in medical decision-making and effective team behaviors and communication, and may become more integral in assessing provider's competency for the purposes of certification [10].

In addition to education, the potential role for simulation in the NICU continues to expand through applications such as workflow analysis, facilities planning, device implementation, and quality improvement processes. Video recording of actual neonatal resuscitations has been used to improve educational programming and team training [11]. Simulation has been integral to improving NICU design and as a hazard detection tool when building and moving into newly constructed units [12]. As quality improvement and patient safety continue to be a priority for our healthcare institutions, simulation is a method by which we strive to discover gaps in provider knowledge and skills or the clinical environment, improve skills of all levels of practitioners, and test new educational modalities and devices.

Simulation Education

Scenario Design Considerations for Neonatology

When designing a simulation, several questions must be considered. Who are the targeted learners? What are the objectives of the session? What degree of mannequin realism, or fidelity, is required? How important is standardization in scenario design? (See Chap. 2 for details.)

Participants

Most healthcare professionals have received training amongst peers within their profession, so-called uniprofessional training. Deliberate practice using simulation has been associated with improvements in neonatal resuscitation performance amongst uniprofessional teams [13]. However, interprofessional teams care for patients in the clinical environment. Neonatal team-training utilizing simulation has been shown to improve behavioral skills including leadership, communication, and collaboration [14]. The learning objectives used to design the simulation-based educational experience should be tailored to the level and composition of the learner group in order to best optimize learning outcomes.

Fidelity

Immersion of the learner within a realistic simulated environment enhances adult engagement and learning [9]. A large variety of simulation options exist for use in the education of trainees and staff (Table 18.1) [15]. Low-fidelity simulators offer many advantages since they are less expensive and can be enhanced by the surrounding environment to create high psychological and environmental fidelity [16]. Research comparing neonatal resuscitation education has failed to show a consistent educational advantage in performance when using high- versus low-fidelity mannequins [17, 18]. This may be due to the fact that the mannequin represents only one portion of the simulated learning environment.

Moulage can be used to assist in the replication of a realistic environment. There are commercially available moulage applications designed specifically for neonatal mannequins, including cystic hygroma, cleft lip, forceps scalp markings, myelomeningocele, omphalocele, gastroschesis, polycystic kidneys, and congenital hip dislocations. Other moulage items, such as artificial blood and meconium, can be purchased. Online recipes for these substances are also available, and serve as simple, economical alternatives (e.g., mixing water and red food coloring for blood; using split pea soup or green baby food for meconium). Integrating

Table 18.1 Advantages and disadvantages of different types of simulation equipment

Type of simulator/trainer	Advantages	Disadvantages	Examples for use
Partial task trainer	Less expensive	Dedicated to defined procedures	Airway management
	Portable		Intravenous access
Animal/human tissues	Realistic anatomy	Difficult to obtain	Chest tube insertion
	Compliance of tissues	Potential for infection transmission	Umbilical line insertion
Low-fidelity patient mannequin	Portable	Does not replicate physiologic changes	Resuscitation training
	No need for power source, technical support	Prompts required from instructors to change status	Umbilical line insertion
			Chest compressions
			Chest-tube insertion
High-fidelity patient mannequin	Able to simulate real-time clinical changes	Need for technical support	Resuscitation training for advanced learners/teams
		Most expensive	Cardioversion/defibrillation training
		Programming helpful	

moulage with the most appropriate type of mannequin for the learners' needs should remain a focus for all educators in neonatal resuscitation. These strategies may assist learners in suspending their disbelief, contributing to an optimal environment from which learners can improve skills.

The equipment necessary to complete simulation-based procedural training in neonatology varies significantly. Table 18.2 lists several currently available types of neonatal high-fidelity simulators, their included features, and options for procedural skills training [15]. The type of simulator selected for simulation training should be matched to the educational needs and learning objectives. Obstetrical simulators also have a role to play in the training of neonatal healthcare teams and their environments but are outside the scope of this review.

Standardization

Standardization of a simulated experience is critical to ensuring maximal value as an educational experience and includes a uniform approach to simulation design, formatting and structure of scenarios, and debriefing and reflection [9]. Standardization of the simulated educational experience allows educators to ensure that learners are receiving the same type of session, regardless of when it is delivered or who it is taught by.

Instructional Design Considerations for Neonatology

In Situ Versus Simulation Lab Training

Training in a simulation lab allows for relatively easy access to equipment and standardized audio-visual (AV) setup. Learners and instructors can be scheduled for a dedicated session that will be free of distraction. Advantages include maintaining privacy for participants, facilitating obtaining consent or providing evaluations, and delivering standardized curricula to multiple learners. However, given limited hours of operation and physical distance from the work environment, this option may not be feasible for all learners.

In situ simulation allows teams to practice in their actual clinical environment, and may be used to identify gaps in the team's knowledge or skills as well as to detect latent hazards attributable to the environment or institutional policies and procedures (see Chap. 12) [19]. Numerous advantages for learners and instructors using in situ simulation have been described and include optimal environmental fidelity, quick access to appropriate learners (often minimizing costs), identification of gaps in training, and detection of problems/hazards in the environment which could interfere with patient care [19]. The use of in situ simulation for neonatal resuscitation has recently been associated with improved technical ability and teamwork in simulated resuscitations [20].

Disadvantages for in situ simulation include restricted availability of simulator and AV equipment, availability of space in the clinical area, and labor to set up and remove the equipment. One should also be mindful of increasing anxiety and privacy concerns of both learners and nearby patients and their families.

Boot Camp

Trainees entering neonatal fellowship are less skilled than their attending physician counterparts and, as such, there exists an urgency to begin procedural training at the very beginning of fellowship. Regional neonatal *boot camps* have become common, providing an opportunity for several programs to collaborate and share resources and educational expertise. Robust educational programs can be developed, with a focus on potentially life-saving procedural skills. During these sessions, a larger number of trainees can be instructed on various procedures in a standardized manner over a 1- to 2-day program. Procedural skills are practiced and trainees receive individualized, real-time, formative feedback on their technique. Trainees then continue to develop their skills at their home institution [15]. Boot camps are quickly becoming the norm for ensuring a basic common set of skills for new trainees, but effects on competence in the clinical domain for neonatal-specific skills and behaviors remain unclear.

Procedural Skills Training

In the NICU, a patient's stability may depend upon the successful completion of an invasive procedure, including (but not limited to) endotracheal intubation, umbilical line insertion, thoracentesis, chest tube placement, paracentesis, and exchange transfusion. The baseline level of difficulty of these procedures may be increased exponentially by the hemodynamic instability of the patient, technical challenges of working with a tiny, fragile preterm infant, and the pressure to complete the procedure in a timely manner.

Unfortunately, recent graduates of pediatric postgraduate training programs have demonstrated poor proficiency in neonatal procedural skills [21–23]. For example, a recent multicenter study evaluating success rates in neonatal intubation at five level III academic NICUs found that only 44 % of all attempts were successful and the likelihood of success depended mostly on level of training. Pediatric interns had the lowest success rates at 19 %, and no significant improvement was noted for senior residents [21]. These success rates are lower than those reported prior to the implementation of the Accreditation Council for Graduate Medical Education (ACGME) duty hour restrictions [7, 22, 23], highlighting the need to identify effective and efficient methods to train learners in proper procedural technique to preserve future patient safety.

Table 18.2 Comparison of available high-technology newborn and infant simulators

	Included features													Medical procedures				
Mannequin	Price (USD)[a]	Age	Size (weight and length)	Cyanosis	Breath sounds	Heart sounds	Chest movement	Umbilical pulse	Tone	Vocal sounds	Seizure	Wireless	Intubation	Umbilical catheterization	Needle thoracentesis	IO access	Cardioversion/defibrillation
Premie HAL S3009 (Gaumard Medical)	16,000	Preterm (30 wk) newborn	1.3 kg, 40 cm	✓	✓	✓	✓	✓		✓		✓	✓ (2.5 ETT)	✓		✓	
Newborn HAL S3010 (Gaumard Medical)	19,000	Term newborn	2.3 kg, 53 cm	✓	✓	✓	✓	✓	✓	✓	✓	✓	✓ (3.0 ETT)	✓		✓	
SimNewB (Laerdal Medical)	24,000	Term newborn	3.5 kg, 51 cm	✓	✓	✓	✓	✓	✓	✓	✓		✓ (3.5 ETT)	✓	✓ (Mid-axillary)	✓	
SimBaby (Laerdal Medical)	37,000	6-month infant	4 kg, 63.5 cm	✓	✓	✓	✓		✓	✓			✓ (4.0 ETT)		✓ (Anterior chest, 2nd intercostal, and chest tube insertion mid-axillary)	✓	✓
BabySIM (CAE Healthcare)	45,400	6–9-month infant	7.4 kg, 65 cm	✓	✓	✓	✓			✓			✓ (4.0 ETT)		✓ (anterior chest, 2nd intercostal, and chest tube insertion mid-axillary)	✓	✓

ETT endotracheal tube, *IO* intraosseous

[a] Prices reflect manufacturer quotes received by the authors in September 2013, rounded to the nearest US$100. Actual prices may vary. Prices reflect those of the mannequins and required peripheral devices (control module/laptop, compressors, etc.). Additional options (display monitors, simulation scenario packages, on-site instructions, etc.), and extended warranties can be purchased at additional cost

Fig. 18.1 Umbilical venous catheter (UVC) and med line skills station. (Courtesy of Dr. Deepak Manhas)

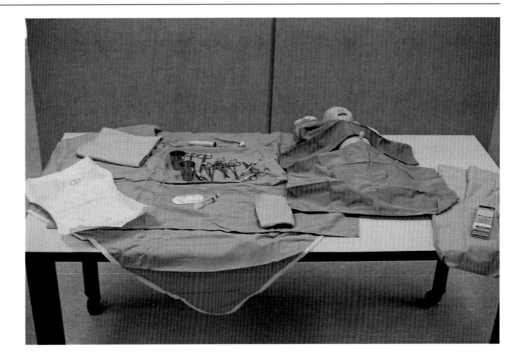

Given growing concern about learning and practicing procedures on patients, alternate techniques have been utilized. Some educators use animals or human tissue, such as the use of ferrets or cats for intubation training, or using fresh umbilical cords to practice umbilical line insertion. Others have recommended requesting parental permission for trainees to practice procedures on deceased infants [24]. The logistics and ethics of these techniques create barriers to achieving procedural competency. Simulation has been utilized increasingly in procedural training instead and is now frequently included in neonatology educational programs. Figure 18.1 shows a skills station for umbilical line placement and emergency medicine administration at an NRP course.

Assessment of Procedural Skills

One challenge in developing a procedural training session is identifying the ideal or best way to perform a particular skill. In the absence of a clearly defined standard, experienced providers often perform procedures slightly differently, and these inconsistencies may confuse trainees. One potential solution is to attempt to develop a consensus on best practices for each relevant procedure [25]. The development and validation of procedural skills checklists has been more extensively reported outside of pediatrics [26, 27]. There are validated procedural checklists for a limited number of procedures in neonatology [28, 29], but these do not cover the full scope of practice (see Chap. 7 for details on assessment). An effort is currently underway through the International Network for Simulation-Based Pediatric Innovation, Research, and Education (INSPIRE) to develop procedural checklists for common procedures in pediatrics, including

several procedures utilized in neonatology, such as intubation, chest tube placement, and umbilical line placement.

Considerations for Implementation

Simulation plays an important role throughout the learning process for procedural skills. This is especially true in the NICU, where patients may not tolerate the multiple, or prolonged, procedural attempts necessary to establish proper psychomotor technique. When learning a new procedure, a trainee should learn the cognitive information about the procedure prior to hands-on practice using a simulator/task trainer. In order to preserve patient safety, prior to performing procedural attempts on patients (under direct supervision), it is essential to ensure that the learner has had the opportunity for deliberate practice [9, 30] on a simulator and has been deemed competent in their simulated performance. Once a trainee has then been successful in clinical procedural performance, they should participate in regular maintenance training sessions on a simulator to prevent decay in their skills. A group of pediatric and neonatal educators have developed an evidence-based framework for procedural skills training utilizing simulation for initial learning and maintenance of skills [31].

Interprofessional Team Training

Patients in a NICU are cared for by both multidisciplinary and interprofessional teams. Traditionally, each group has been trained in silos, independent of the other groups, and learners do not typically receive specific instruction on how to work as a member of a team. Optimal communication amongst providers is not innate; it is a skill that must be learned and practiced. Effective communication and team behaviors are absolutely essential during the perinatal period and in the NICU as they have been correlated with the quality of neonatal resuscitation [32] and have been implicated in RCAs in approximately three quarters of perinatal morbidities and mortalities [33].

After the issue of medical errors was brought to public attention in the 1999 publication *To Err is Human* [34], adoption of human factors training was recommended to improve the performance of healthcare teams. Programs such as MedTeams and TeamSTEPPS™ were developed to apply principles of crew resource management (CRM) from the military and aviation industries to health care [35–39]. There are many studies and publications that support the use of team training in the perinatal and neonatal environments [40–43]. In the obstetrical environment, team training has resulted in the improvement of the Adverse Outcomes Index, [40] decrease in time to emergency cesarean delivery for cord prolapse [41], and decreased incidence of low Apgar scores (<6) and hypoxic-ischemic encephalopathy [41]. A reduction in adverse outcomes in preterm infants was also noted with use of team training [43] (see Chap. 4 for details on team training).

Team Training for Neonatology

Team training has been shown to improve teamwork behaviors amongst neonatal teams in simulated resuscitations [44–46]. Fifty-one interns who were enrolled in an NRP course participated in a 2.5-h course on teamwork and errors, including lecture, role play, video clips and discussion. Following this session, the trainees proceeded through the standard NRP course. Trainees were randomized to practice the team behaviors during the skills stations (as prompted by their instructors) in the intervention group, while control group subjects did not have opportunities to rehearse these skills. During the mock resuscitations at the end of the class, learners served as team leader for a simulated resuscitation on a low-fidelity mannequin. Intervention group trainees were noted to have more frequently demonstrated team behaviors (scored as the number of observed episodes per minute), including information sharing and assertion, than the control subjects. Vigilance and workload management were noted in 100 and 88 % of the intervention group, respectively, while the control group was only noted to have 53 and 20 %. Intervention subjects demonstrated any team behavior an average of 3.34 times per minute, compared to control subjects at 1.03 times per minute. A significant limitation of this study was that only physicians were included, so interprofessional interactions were unable to be assessed [45].

As technology improved, high-fidelity mannequins were found to be very effective in replicating trainee responses from the actual delivery room. In a subsequent investigation,

98 pediatrics interns who were participating in NRP courses were randomized to utilize high-fidelity simulators (intervention HF group), low-fidelity simulators (intervention LF group), and a control group. The resulting simulations were recorded and were rated by blinded, trained observers to evaluate for effective teamwork behaviors and resuscitation quality. Compared to the control group, the intervention groups were noted to have a higher frequency of teamwork behaviors (12.8 vs 9.0 behaviors per minute), improved workload management, and decreased duration of resuscitations. Additionally, these skills were maintained for a longer duration of time, as the intervention groups continued to have more frequently noted teamwork behaviors upon 6-month repeat evaluation (intervention 11.8 vs control 10.0 events per minute) [46]. Since simulation with both low-fidelity and high-fidelity mannequins was shown to improve decision-making and technical skills over time, [46] it follows that training in these behaviors should translate into improved performance during actual resuscitations, although specific evidence supporting this for neonatal resuscitation teams is lacking.

The most recent version of the NRP's training course was revised to promote interprofessional training and now includes mandatory simulation with debriefing. This allows learners to integrate cognitive and technical abilities from the self-study and skills stations with effective communication and behavioral skills, which are vitally important in the effective delivery of resuscitation. Some of the key behavioral skills that have been identified include familiarity with the environment/equipment, anticipation of and planning for potential complications, effective leadership and communication skills, delegation of workload, utilization of information and resources, and calling for assistance in a timely manner [3]. Figure 18.2 shows an interprofessional team participating in simulation training.

There are many types of providers who may benefit from interprofessional team training including obstetrical providers, pediatricians, anesthesiologists, nursing staff, respira-

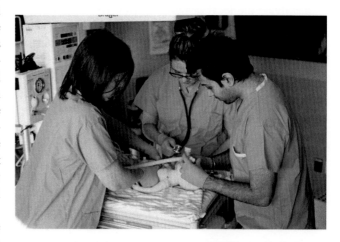

Fig. 18.2 Interprofessional team in a simulation. (Courtesy of Dr. Deepak Manhas)

Table 18.3 Neonatal morbidity associated with shoulder dystocia. (Adapted from [50])

	Incidence (%)		
	Pre-training (n=324)	Post-training (n=262)	Relative risk (95% CI)
Birth-related neonatal injury	30 (9.3)	6 (2.3)	0.25 (0.11–0.57)
Birth-related brachial plexus injury	24 (7.4)	6 (2.3)	0.31 (0.13–0.72)
Brachial plexus injury remaining at 6 months	9 (2.8)	2 (0.8)	0.28 (0.07–1.13)
Brachial plexus injury remaining at 12 months	6 (1.9)	2 (0.8)	0.41 (0.1–1.77)
Fractured clavicle or humerus	6 (1.9)	2 (0.8)	0.41 (0.1–1.77)
Apgar score <7 at 5 min	12 (3.7)	6 (2.3)	0.61 (0.24–1.57)

CI confidence interval

tory therapists, patient care technicians, administrative support personnel, and blood bank personnel as well as their respective trainees [47]. The implementation of an interprofessional team training program for NICU providers at one institution was adapted from TeamSTEPPS™ and included two simulations to allow an opportunity to practice various communication and teamwork skills presented in the course. Some logistical challenges were noted, including high unit census, preventing some sessions from being held in situ, and scheduling sessions during providers' work shifts, resulting in occasional conflicts with patient care. Overall, providers did find the session to be useful and applicable to their practice. Additionally, some items raised by participants as points for improvement had been subsequently implemented. This framework could be utilized to conduct large-scale team training in other units [48]. Education of providers and teams has been shown to improve confidence and simulated performance [49]. Demonstration of efficacy in preventing morbidity and mortality is more challenging. One example of success in this area was the introduction of a PROMPT birthing trainer simulator program in the UK, which resulted in a significant reduction in birth injuries from shoulder dystocia (Table 18.3) [50].

Extracorporeal Membrane Oxygenation and Other Content

In addition to neonatal providers, other professionals are frequently involved in the care of critically ill neonates. Infants requiring extracorporeal membrane oxygenation (ECMO) are amongst the most complicated in a NICU setting and require care by specific specialists who manage the ECMO pump solely, along with other members of the

medical team who are responsible for the care of the patient. Simulation provides an excellent format to review and solidify the proper approach to routine ECMO management as well as ECMO emergencies, which require timely, correct interventions to prevent significant morbidities or mortality. More importantly, cannulations or codes on ECMO require high-level team behaviors and communication between the event leader, the team managing the patient, and the team managing the pump. Simulations can provide opportunities for teams to interact and optimize their communication. Figure 18.3 shows an interprofessional team participating in an ECMO simulation session.

Through participation in ECMO simulation, all providers have the opportunity to take part in a standardized experience and review their performance to ensure that vital concepts are understood [51, 52]. ECMO simulation has been used for introductory training of ECMO providers as well as for ongoing maintenance of ECMO skills for interprofessional ECMO teams [53, 54] Participants in ECMO training programs incorporating simulation were found to spend a significantly greater time spent in active learning compared to traditional training programs (78% vs 14%) [51]. These providers were also noted to more frequently perform key

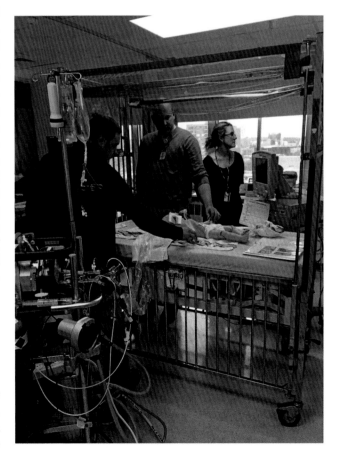

Fig. 18.3 ECMO simulation. (Courtesy of SYN:APSE Simulation Center)

technical skills to resolve ECMO emergencies (i.e., coming off ECMO for emergency, increasing ventilator support when off ECMO), and response times to these actions were improved (average time difference was 27 s). Upon blinded evaluation of video recordings by masked reviewers, behavioral skills improved after simulation-based training [52]. In a study of simulated ECMO cannulations, cardiothoracic surgery trainees were found to have a significant decrease in median time to cannulation and improvement in a validated global rating scale and a Composite ECMO Cannulation Score (CECS) after participating in a simulation-based cannulation curriculum [55].

Simulation also provides a format for practice of many other complex and rare interprofessional scenarios, examples of which include ex utero intrapartum therapy (EXIT) procedures, delivery of infants with congenital anomalies (e.g., conjoined twins, critical congenital heart disease, airway malformations), neonatal transports, or extramural deliveries. In each of these situations, teams can rehearse prior to the actual event, and in so doing, review the ideal sequence of events, identify additional staff members to be present, troubleshoot new equipment, and identify potential latent safety threats. Reviewing these complex interactions could potentially have very positive effects towards optimizing the care provided and preserving patient safety.

Simulation in Established Neonatal Training Organizations

Several neonatal educational programs have incorporated simulation into their curricula including Neonatal Resuscitation Program (NRP), Acute Care of at-Risk Newborns (ACoRN), **S**ugar & **S**afe care, **T**emperature, **A**irway, **B**lood pressure, **L**ab work and **E**motional support (S.T.A.B.L.E.), and Helping Babies Breathe (HBB). While these education programs have designed scenarios of their own, new scenarios can easily be developed to represent a variety of clinical situations. Figure 18.4 provides a template for constructing neonatal simulation scenarios.

Scenario	
Learners	
Scenario Setup	
Confederate Roles	
Mannequin	
Equipment	

Learning Objectives:	**Debriefing Notes:**
Cognitive: 1. 2. 3.	
Behavioral: 1. 2. 3.	
Technical: 1. 2. 3.	

Scenario Description:	

Maternal History		
Age	BMI	Pregnancy
Medical/Surgical history		
Labs		
Medication/Other		

Infant History			
Gestation	CGA	Weight	Apgars
Birth History			
Hospital Course			
Medications			
Others			

A. Initial State (vitals):	
B. Expected Actions (Progression):	
C. Likely Progression (Decompensation):	
D. Expected Actions (Progression)	
E. Expected Endpoint (Outcome):	
F. Potential Distractors:	

Comments:

Fig. 18.4 Design scenario (see text). *BMI* body mass index, *CGA* corrected gestational age. (Created by the authors with the assistance of Nikki Wiggins))

Neonatal Resuscitation Program

The American Academy of Pediatrics (AAP) and the American Heart Association first developed a NRP in 1985 [56]. However, the cognitive and technical skills learned in these courses have been shown to decay as early as 6 months following the course [57]. There have been five revised editions of NRP since the original course to ensure that evidence-based practice is distributed to learners in a timely fashion. Recommendations from the International Liaison Committee on Resuscitation (ILCOR) in 2010 emphasize the use of simulation as a key educational modality in teaching learners at all levels of ability [58, 59]. In the most recent edition, cognitive and technical skills are learned and integrated during the self-study, procedural skills stations, and integrated skills station [3]. The use of simulation and debriefing is now mandated in all NRP courses so that non-technical skills and teamwork are also emphasized as key learning points [3]. Existing NRP instructors have perceived that including simulation and debriefing in NRP instruction is extremely worthwhile [60]. Whether this new instructional framework will change the ability of learners to perform NRP better has yet to be determined. Figure 18.5 shows learners participating in a simulated neonatal resuscitation on a high-fidelity mannequin.

S.T.A.B.L.E

The S.T.A.B.L.E. program (**S**ugar & Safe care, **T**emperature, **A**irway, **B**lood pressure, **L**ab work and **E**motional support) is based upon the six assessment and care modules in the program. It was designed to assist practitioners in post-resuscitation and pre-transport care of critically ill newborns. The S.T.A.B.L.E simulations are validated scenarios that are constructed in a graduated approach. There are four separate neonatal scenarios, each with three separate encounters that gradually progress in difficulty level. These scenarios work as a bridge between NRP and Pediatric Advanced Life Support (PALS) by incorporating initial stabilization with other complications such as hypovolemic shock, arrhythmias, and seizures. Each scenario also stresses interprofessional participation and incorporates the use of medical staff providers (physician, nurse practitioner, or physician assistant), nurses, respiratory therapists, and backup team members [61]. One small study showed an improvement in neonatal admission body temperature, improvement in blood glucose levels, and mortality during hospitalization following the introduction of the S.T.A.B.L.E. program [62].

Fig. 18.5 Simulated neonatal resuscitation on a high-fidelity mannequin. (Courtesy of Dr. Douglas Campbell)

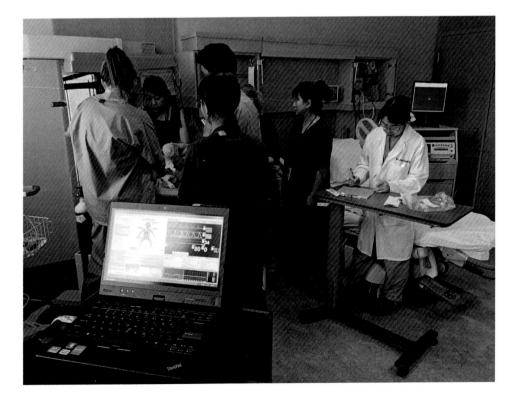

Acute Care of at-Risk Newborns

The Acute Care of the at-Risk Newborn, or ACoRN program, was established in 1995 to provide a systematic approach to recognizing and managing babies that require stabilization, including those requiring assistance with transition from in utero life as well as those who become unwell shortly after birth. The focus is a risk prioritization that integrates assessment, monitoring, diagnostic evaluation, intervention, and ongoing management for this patient population. Through multiple high- and low-fidelity simulations, participants work through the eight steps of the ACoRN process: (1) identifying babies at risk; (2) identifying need for resuscitation; (3) primary survey (respiratory, cardiovascular, neurology, surgical conditions, fluid and glucose management, and thermoregulation); (4) infection; (5) generation of a problem list; (6) ACoRN sequences for the identified problems; (7) consider transport to a regional center for higher level of care; and (8) support for the baby, family, and healthcare team [63]. Following the ACoRN workshops, participants have demonstrated improved confidence and knowledge relating to neonatal stabilization [64].

Helping Babies Breathe

Every year, an estimated 814,000 neonatal deaths are attributed to intrapartum hypoxic events in term infants [65]. In low-income countries, especially those in South Asia and sub-Saharan Africa, they are responsible for two thirds of the world's neonatal deaths and are out of proportion to the world population [66]. The goal of the Helping Babies Breathe (HBB) program is to reduce neonatal mortality due to birth asphyxia in United Nations Millennium Development Goals countries. HBB is an initiative developed by a consortium of partners including the AAP, with input from the World Health Organization (WHO) to improve neonatal resuscitation in resource-limited environments. HBB requires minimal equipment: an *Action Plan* algorithm, a facilitator flipchart, a low-cost low-fidelity simulator, a self-inflating bag and mask, a suction bulb, a stethoscope, and a learner workbook. With visual aids, the *Action Plan* demonstrates a simplified NRP algorithm including warming, drying, clearing the airway, stimulating, ventilating, requesting assistance, and monitoring the baby. The participants review the *Action Plan*, practice the steps on the mannequin, perform an observed structured clinical assessment, and receive feedback on their performance. Since its initiation, HBB has been shown to decrease the number of deaths at 24 h for infants not breathing at birth in Tanzania, while there was no change in the rates of stillbirths [67]. However, research done in India showed a decrease in the number of stillbirths but no change in neonatal deaths [68].

Quality Improvement, Systems Integration, and Patient Safety

Simulation has been recognized by national safety bodies as a training option to allow multidisciplinary and interprofessional teams to practice in an interactive environment while facing lifelike clinical scenarios. It can be used to develop and hone teamwork and communication skills across disciplines, especially for complex scenarios [69]. As with any educational modality, for simulation to be most effective in improving patient safety, a needs assessment or gap analysis is important so that specific skills or learning points can be targeted (see Chap. 5 for details). Various domains of patient safety specific to neonatology have recently been reviewed, with specific knowledge gaps clearly identified, through which simulation has been identified as playing a key role moving forward [70]. Errors in administration of human milk or diagnostic tests being performed on the wrong infant due to incorrect patient identification are common clinical occurrences, but they are rarely studied in a proactive way [70]. Collaboration with obstetrical colleagues within one or more institutions is starting to occur, whereby simulated scenarios serve as a training tool designed in an effort to improve system issues. More work is clearly needed on this type of scale before system changes can occur [71].

Video Recording and Video Review

Neonatology has been one of the first disciplines to use actual video-recorded neonatal resuscitations in order to improve NRP and neonatal curriculum development [33, 72–75]. In over 50% of recordings from actual resuscitations, there are clear deviations from the current NRP guidelines and recurrent errors in skills and communication strategies used [72–75]. Although video analysis has identified gaps in both technical and non-technical skills and helped inform local curriculum development, [75] its systemic use has yet to demonstrate change in culture or improvement in patient outcome.

NICU Design and Workplace Improvement

Proactive use of simulation to improve the workplace and prevent the occurrence of adverse events is clearly appealing for healthcare providers and administrators alike. The use of simulation to detect latent hazards or environmental threats is increasingly being reported and can be utilized in both new and existing NICU space [76]. Prior to building new facilities, healthcare organizations have simulated the drafted proposals in order to identify problems and resolve them before the facilities are actually constructed. In one study, 93 % of the latent safety hazards that were identified were resolved at the time of transition to the new unit [76]. Optimizing the resuscitation bed and using the most appropriate cognitive aids are also excellent situations in which simulation technology can be used, rather than implementing interventions and hoping that the desired clinical effect occurs [77].

Future Directions

Workflow Analysis

Simulation has recently gained wide acceptance in the field of neonatology, but new uses for this modality continue to be identified. Several centers have been running simulations for workflow analysis, for example, in the rollout of a new electronic health record. This has supported *LEAN thinking*, an approach which encourages improvements in efficiency, reduction of medical errors, and minimization of healthcare costs through the elimination of waste [17, 78, 79].

New Technologies

New technology and available devices are rapidly evolving. Several newborn and premature mannequins are currently available on the market. High-fidelity mannequins have appreciable heart and lung sounds, spontaneous chest rise, palpable pulses as well as spontaneous vocalizations and movements. There are models that have realistic airways allowing for intubation and ventilation, and umbilical cords that permit venous and arterial catheterization. Some models allow for intravenous (IV), intraosseous (IO), and peripheral arterial access with palpable pulses and blood return. These models allow trainees to practice technical skills on anatomically correct models, and features such as blood return allow the trainee to monitor success of the skill.

Looking Ahead

Augmentation of the educational experience with immediate visual and/or feedback is a key indicator of fidelity. Integration of mannequins with virtual reality (VR) training (hybrid simulation) has been demonstrated to improve trainees' competency in adult surgical procedures [80]. VR training in neonatology is in its infancy. Current VR models used to

enhance neonatal intubation skill training, although promising, are not of sufficient appeal that they would replace low-fidelity mannequin intubation heads [81].

Optimal practices for the care of the sick neonate, as in other fields of intensive care medicine, change frequently. Simulation is now clearly a valuable educational and research tool in this field, but many challenges lie ahead. It can be time and resource-intensive, so curricula which seek to incorporate the use of simulation should have solid evidence in support of it. Reducing latent hazards and improving team function with in situ simulation seems logical, but evidence supporting this in the clinical environment is lacking. The use of video recording and team training are helpful tools in identifying learning gaps, but more work is needed to demonstrate improvement in patient outcome and actual team performance prior to widespread adoption in healthcare settings.

Conclusions

Simulation has become a vital part of training for neonatal care providers. Simulation has been included as a major component of training in a number of standardized neonatal educational programs, including the NRP, S.T.A.B.L.E, ACoRN, and HBB. Through these efforts, learners across the globe will be ensured training experiences that include opportunities for hands-on practice of procedural skills and incorporation of key behavioral skills, along with learning the requisite medical knowledge and resuscitation algorithms.

The use of simulation also enhances the quality and safety of the care provided to the smallest patients. These include areas such as quality assurance/quality improvement (QA/QI), where a complicated case with a negative outcome could be *animated*. Conversely, the use of simulation can be proactive for unusual complicated cases that have yet to happen. In designing a new NICU or understanding the risks to patient and team with a challenging transport, simulation can be used to identify latent safety threats and hazards. Once identified, these environmental risks and knowledge gaps can be addressed. Similarly, through the use of simulation in workflow analysis, facilities planning, and device implementation, patient care can be continuously improved and optimized.

Through these efforts, the likelihood that the smallest, most critically ill patients may survive and thrive will hopefully continue to improve. Although much progress has been made, a determination of which simulation methods are most effective for improving clinical performance remains elusive, and this should remain the focus of future research efforts.

References

1. Halamek LP, Howard SK, Smith BE, Smith BC, Gaba DM. Development of a simulated delivery room for the study of human performance during neonatal resuscitation. Pediatrics. 1997;100:513–4.

2. Halamek LP, Kaegi DM, Gaba DM, Sowb YA, Smith BC, Smith BE, et al. Time for a new paradigm in pediatric medical education: teaching neonatal resuscitation in a simulated delivery room environment. Pediatrics. 2000;106:45–53.

3. Kattwinkle J, editor. Textbook of neonatal resuscitation. 6th ed. Elk Grove Village: American Academy of Pediatrics and the American Heart Association; 2011.

4. The Joint Commission on Accrediation of Healthcare Organizations (JCAHO). Sentinel event alert. 2004. Issue 30. http:www. jcaho.org/about+us/news+letters/sentinel+event+alert/print/ sea_30.htm.

5. Lee HC, Rhee CJ, Sectish TC, Hintz SR. Changes in attendance at deliveries by pediatric residents 2000–2005. Am J Perinatol. 2009;26(2):129–34.

6. Nadel FM, Lavelle JM, Fein JA, Giardino AP, Decker JM, Durbin DR. Assessing pediatric senior resident' training in resuscitation: fund of knowledge, technical skills and perception of confidence. Pediatr Emerg Care. 2000;16:73–6.

7. Leone TA, Rich W, Finer NN. Neonatal intubation: success of pediatric trainees. J Pediatr. 2005;146:638–41.

8. Bismilla Z, Finan E, McNamara PJ, LeBlanc V, Jefferies A, Whyte H. Failure of pediatric and neonatal trainees to meet Canadian neonatal resuscitation program standards for neonatal intubation. J Perinatol. 2010;30(3):182–7.

9. Issenberg SB, McGaghie WC, Petrusa ER, Lee Gordon D, Scalese RJ. Features and uses of high-fidelity medical simulations that lead to effective learning: a BEME systematic review. Med Teach. 2005;27(1):10–28.

10. McGaghie WC, Issenberg SB. Simulations in assessment. In: Downing SM, Yudkowsky R, editors. Assessment in health professions education. New York: Routledge; 2009. pp. 245–68.

11. Wade DR, Leone T, Finer NN. Delivery room interventions. Clin Perinatol. 2010;3791:189–202.

12. Bender GJ. In situ simulation for systems testing in newly constructed perinatal facilities. Semin Perinatol. 2011;35(2):45–96.

13. Sawyer T, Sierocka-Castaneda A, Chan D, Berg B, Lustik M, Thompson M. Deliberate practice using simulation improves neonatal resuscitation performance. Simul Healthc. 2011;6(6):327–36.

14. Sawyer T, Laubach VA, Hudak J, Yamamura K, Pocrnich A. Improvements in teamwork during neonatal resuscitation after interprofessional Team STEPPS training. Neonatal Netw. 2013;32(1):26–33.

15. Sawyer T, French H, Soghier, Barry J, Johnston L, Anderson J, Ades A. Educational perspectives: boot camps for neonatal-perinatal medicine fellows. NeoReviews. 2014;15:e46–56.

16. Bradley P. The history of simulation in medical education and possible future directions. Med Educ. 2006;40(3):254–62.

17. Campbell DM, Barozzino T, Farrugia M, Sgro M. High-fidelity simulation in neonatal resuscitation. Paediatr Child Health. 2009;14(1):19–23.

18. Finan E, Bismilla Z, Whyte HE, Leblanc V, McNamara PJ. High-fidelity simulator technology may not be superior to traditional low-fidelity equipment for neonatal resuscitation training. J Perinatol. 2012;32(4):287–92.

19. Patterson MD, Blike GT, Nadkarni VM. In Situ Simulation: challenges and results. In: Henriksen K, Battles JB, Keyes MA, Grady ML, editors. Advances in patient safety: new directions and alternative approaches (Vol 3 Performance and Tools). Rockville: Agency for Healthcare Research and Quality; 2008. pp 1–18.

20. Rubio-Gurung S, Putet G, Touzet S, Gauthier-Moulinier H, Jordan I, Beissel A, et al. Simulation training for neonatal resuscitation: an RCT. Pediatrics. 2014;134(3):e790–7.

21. Haubner L, Johnston L, Barry J, Soghier L, Tatum P, Kessler D, et al. Neonatal intubation performance: room for improvement in tertiary neonatal intensive care units. Resuscitation. 2013;84(10):1359–64.

22. Falck AJ, Escobedo MB, Baillargeon JG, Villard LG, Gunkel JH. Proficiency of pediatric residents in performing neonatal endotracheal intubation. Pediatrics. 2003;112:1242–7.

23. O'Donnell CP, Kamlin CO, Davis PG, Morley CJ. Endotracheal intubation attempts during neonatal resuscitation: success rates, duration and adverse effects. Pediatrics. 2006;117:e16–21.

24. Mercurio MR. Teaching intubation with cadavers: generosity at a time of loss. Hastings Cent Rep. 2009;39(4):7–8.

25. Schmutz J, Eppich W, Hoffmann F, Heimberg E, Manser T. Five steps to develop checklists for evaluating clinical performance: an integrative approach. Acad Med. 2014;89(7):1–10.

26. Berg D, Berg K, Riesenberg LA, Weber D, King D, Mealey K, Justice EM, Geffe K, Tinkoff G. The development of a validated checklist for thoracentesis: preliminary results. Am J Med Qual. 2013;28(3):220–6.

27. Berg K, Riesenberg LA, Berg D, Schaeffer A, Davis J, Justice EM, Tinkoff G, Jasper E. The development of a validated checklist for radial arterial line placement: preliminary results. Am J Med Qual. 2013;29(3):242–6.

28. Finan E, Bismilla Z, Campbell C, Leblanc V, Jefferies A, Whyte HE. Improved procedural performance following a simulation training session may not be transferable to the clinical environment. J Perinatol. 2012;32(7):539–44.

29. Shefrin AE, Khazei A, Hung GR, Odendal LT, Cheng A. The TACTIC: development and validation of the tool for assessing chest tube insertion competency. CJEM. 2014: 1–8.

30. Ericsson KA. Deliberate practice and the acquisition and maintenance of expert performance in medicine and related domains. Acad Med. 2004;79(10):70–81.

31. Sawyer T, White M, Zaveri P, Chang T, Ades A, French H, et al. "Learn, See, Practice, Prove, Do Maintain": An evidence-based pedagogical framework for procedural skill training in medicine. Academic Medicine, accepted for publication pending revisions.

32. Thomas EJ, Sexton JB, Lasky RE, Helmreich RL, Crandell S, Tyson J. Teamwork and quality during neonatal care in the delivery room. J Perinatol. 2006;26:163–9.

33. The Joint Commission. Sentinel event alert. Issue 44, January 26 2010. http://www.jointcommission.org/SentinelEvents/ SentinelEventAlert/sea_44.htm. Accessed 30 Aug 2014.

34. Kohn LT, Corrigan JM, Donaldson MS. To err is human: building a safer health care system. Washington, DC: National Academies Press; 2000.

35. Morey JC, Simon RJ, Jay GD, Wears RL, Salisbury M, Dukes KA, et al. Error reduction and performance improvement in the emergency department through formal teamwork training: evaluation results of the MedTeams Project. Health Serv Res. 2002;37(6):1553–81.

36. Morey JC, Simon R, Jay GD, Rice MAA. Transition from aviation crew resource management to hospital emergency department: the MedTeams story. Proceedings of the 12th International Symposium on Aviation Psychology; 2003 Apr 14; Dayton, OH. Wright State University Press; 2003.

37. Baker DP, Gustafson S, Beaubien JM, Salas E, Barach P. Medical team training programs in health care. 2005 Feb. AHRQ Publication No. 05-0021-4.

38. Baker DP, Gustafson S, Beaubien JM, Salas E. Medical teamwork and patient safety: the evidence-based relation. 2005 Apr. AHRQ Publication No. 05-0053.

39. Baker DB, Beaubien JM, Holtzman AK. DoD medical team training programs: an independent case study analysis. Rockville: Agency for Healthcare Research and Quality; 2006. (Contract No. 282-98-0029).

40. Pettker CM, Thung SF, Norwitz ER, Norwitz ER, Buhimschi CS, Raab CA, et al. Impact of a comprehensive patient safety strategy on obstetric adverse events. Am J Obstet Gynecol. 2009;200:e1492.e8.

41. Siassakos D, Hasafa Z, Sibanda T, Fox R, Donald F, Winter C, et al. Retrospective cohort study of diagnosis-delivery interval with umbilical cord prolapse: the effect of team training. Br J Obstet Gynaecol. 2009;116(8):1089–96.

42. Merien AE, van de Ven J, Mol BW, Houterman S, Oei SG. Multidisciplinary team training in a simulation setting for acute obstetrical emergencies: a systematic review. Obstet Gynecol. 2010;115(5):1021–31.

43. Leape LL, Berwick DM. Five years after to err is human: what have we learned? JAMA. 2005;293:2384–90.

44. Grogan EL, Stiles RA, France DJ, Speroff T, Morris JA Jr, Nixon B, et al. The impact of aviation-based teamwork training on the attitudes of healthcare professionals. J Am Coll Surg. 2004;199(6):843–8.

45. Thomas EJ, Taggart B, Crandell S, Lasky RE, Williams AL, Love LJ, et al. Teaching teamwork during the neonatal resuscitation program: a randomized trial. J Perinatol. 2007;27:409–14.

46. Thomas EJ, Williams AL, Reichman EF, Lasky RE, Crandell S, Taggart WR. Team training in the neonatal resuscitation program for interns: teamwork and quality of resuscitation. Pediatrics. 2010;125:539–46.

47. Deering S, Johnston LC, Colacchio K. Multidisciplinary teamwork and communication training. Semin Perinatol. 2011;35(2):89–96.

48. Colacchio K, Johnston LC, Zigmont J, Kappus L, Sudikoff SN. An approach to unit-based team training with simulation in a neonatal intensive care unit. JNPM. 2012;5(3):213–9.

49. Cook DA, Hatala R, Brydges R, Zendejas B, Szostek JH, Wang AT, et al. Technology-enhanced simulation for health professions education: a systematic review and meta-analysis. JAMA. 2011;306:978–88.

50. Draycott TJ, Crofts JF, Ash JP, Wilson LV, Yard E, Sibanda T, et al. Improving neonatal outcome through practical shoulder dystocia training. Obstet Gynecol. 2008;112(1):14–20.

51. Anderson JM, Murphy AA, Boyle KB, Yaeger KA, LeFlore JL, Halamek LP. Simulating extracorporeal membrane oxygenation (ECMO) emergencies to improve human performance, Part I: methodologic and technologic innovations. Simul Healthc. 2006;1:4.

52. Anderson JM, Murphy AA, Boyle KB, Yaeger KA, Halamek LP. Simulating extracorporeal membrane oxygenation (ECMO) emergencies to improve human performance, Part II: assessment of technical and behavioral skills. Simul Healthc. 2006;1:4.

53. Johnston LC, Sudikoff SN. Development of an ECMO, simulation program: experience at Yale New Haven Hospital, Part I: logistics. MEdSim. 2012;1(3):12–5.

54. Johnston LC, Sudikoff SN. Development of an ECMO, simulation program: experience at Yale New Haven Hospital, Part II: curriculum of initial and ongoing ECMO education. MEdSim. 2012;1:4.

55. Allan CK, Pigula F, Bacha EA, Emani S, Fynn-Thompson F, Thiagarajan RR, et al. An extracorporeal membrane oxygenation cannulation curriculum featuring a novel integrated skills trainer leads to improved performance among pediatric cardiac surgery trainees. Simul Healthc. 2013;8(4):221–8.

56. Murphy AA, Halamek LP. Simulation-based training in neonatal resuscitation. NeoReviews. 2005;6:e489–e92.

57. Kaczorowski J, Levitt C, Hammond M, Outerbridge E, Grad R, Rothman A, et al. Retention of neonatal resuscitation skills and knowledge: a randomized controlled trial. Fam Med. 1998;30:705–11.

58. Kattwinkel J, Perlman JM, Aziz K, Colby, Fairchild K, Gallagher J, et al. Part 15: neonatal resuscitation: 2010 American Heart association guidelines for cardiopulmonary resuscitation and emergency cardiovascular care. Circulation. 2010;122:S09–19.

59. Bhanji F, Mancini ME, Sinz E, Rodgers DL, McNeil MA, Hoadley TA, et al. Part 16: education, implementation, and teams: 2010 American Heart Association guidelines for cardiopulmonary resuscitation and emergency cardiovascular care. Circulation. 2010;122(3):920–33.

60. Amin H, Aziz K, Halamek LP, Beran TN. Simulation-based learning combined with debriefing: trainers satisfaction with a new approach to training the trainers to teach neonatal resuscitation. BMC Res Notes. 2013;6:251–3.

61. Karlson K. The S.T.A.B.L.E. Program: post-resuscition/pretransport stabilization care of sick infants. 6th ed. Salt Lake City: S.T.A.B.L.E., Inc; 2013.

62. Veronica RM, Gallo LL, Medina DR, Gutiettez MT, Mancilla JLS, Amezcua MM, et al. Safe neonatal transport in the state of Jalisco: impact of the S.T.A.B.L.E. program on morbidity and mortality. Bol Med Hosp Infant Mex. 2011;68(1):31–5.

63. Solimano A, Littleford J, Ling E, O'Flaherty D. ACoRN: acute care of at-risk newborns. 1st ed. Vancouver: ACoRN Neonatal Society; 2012.

64. Singhal N, Lockyer J, Fidler H, Aziz K, McMillan D, Qiu X. et at. Acute care of at-risk newborns (ACoRN): quantitative and qualitative educational evaluation of the program in a region of China. BMC Med Educ. 2012;12(1):44–52.

65. Lawn JE, Lee AC, Kinney M, Sibley L, Carlo W, Paul VK, et al. Two million intrapartum-related stillbirths and neonatal deaths: where, why and what can be done? Int J Gynaecol Obsete. 2009;107(1):5–19.

66. Lawn JE, Cousens S, Zupan J. 4 million neonatal deaths: when? Where? Why? Lancet. 2005;365(9462):891–900.

67. Msema G, Massawe A, Mmbando D, Rusibamayila N, Manji K, Kidanto HL. et al. Newborn mortality and fresh stillbirth rates in Tanzania after helping babies breathe training. Pediatrics. 2013;131:353–60.

68. Goudar SS, Somannavar MS, Clark R, Lockyer JM, Revankar AP, Fidler HM, et al. Stillbirth and newborn mortality in India after helping babies breathe training. Pediatrics. 2013;131:344–52.

69. National Patient Safety Agency—NPSA. Patient safety and simulation: Using learning from national re- view of serious incidents (January 2010). 2012. http://www.nrls.npsa.nhs.uk/resources/type/guidance/?entryid45=74297.

70. Raju TNK, Suresh G, Higgins RD. Patient safety in the context of neonatal intensive care: research and educational opportunities. Pediatr Res. 2011;70(1):109–15.

71. Zabari M, Suresh G, Tomlinson M, Lavin JP, Larison K, Halamek L, Schriefer JA. Implementation and case-study results of potentially better practices for collaboration between obstetrics and neonatology to achieve improved perinatal outcomes. Pediatrics. 2006;118(Suppl 2):S153–8.

72. Carbine DN, Finer NN, Knodel E, Rich W. Video recording as a means of evaluating neonatal resuscitation perfomance. Pediatrics. 2000;106(4):654–8.

73. van der Heide PA, van Toledo-Eppinga L, van der Heide M, van der Lee JH. Assessment of neonatal resuscitation skills: a reliable and valid scoring system. Resuscitation. 2006;71(2):212–21.

74. Layouni I, Danan C, Durrmeyer X, Dassieu G, Azcona B, Decobert F. Video recording of newborn resuscitation in the delivery room: technique and advantages. Arch Pediatr. 2011;18(2):72–8.

75. Gelbart B, Hiscock R, Barfield C. Assessment of neonatal resuscitation performance using video recording in a perinatal centre. J Paediatr Child Health. 2010;46(7–8):378–83.

76. Bender J, Shields R, Kennally K. Transportable enhanced simulation technologies for pre-implementation limited operations testing: neonatal intensive care unit. Simul Healthc. 2011;6(4):204–12.

77. Bould MD, Hayter MA, Campbell DM, Chandra DB, Joo HS, Naik VNA. Cognitive aid for neonatal resuscitation: a prospective single-blinded randomized controlled trial. Br J Anesth. 2009;103(4):570–5.

78. Gruden N. The Pittsburg way to efficient healthcare: improving patient care using Toyota based methods. New York: Productivity Press; 2008.

79. Tsasis P, Bruce-Bennet C. Organizational change through lean thinking. Health Serv Manage Res. 2008 Aug;21(3):192–8.

80. Larsen CR, Soerensen JL, Grantcharov TP. Effect of virtual reality training on laporoscopic surgery: a randomized controlled trial. BMJ. 2009;338:b1802.

81. Campbell D, Johnston LC. Personal communications/experiences with MySmartSimulation.

Simulation for Pediatric Critical Care Medicine and Transport

19

Jonathan P. Duff, Matthew S. Braga, Melinda Fiedor Hamilton and Nancy M. Tofil

Simulation Pearls

1. Simulation-based training is well suited to the education of pediatric intensive care unit (PICU) healthcare providers. Advances in simulation technology allow educators to develop scenarios across the range of complex technologies used in the PICU.
2. Increasing use of in situ simulation can maximize environmental fidelity and realism both in the PICU and in the transport environment.
3. More research is required to examine the use of novel simulation modalities and debriefing strategies (such as extended duration simulations and rapid cycle deliberate practice) in the PICU.

Introduction

The pediatric intensive care unit (PICU) is one of the most complex environments in pediatric medicine. The patients have life-threatening illnesses, the equipment and technology are advanced, and the interface between these elements can

J. P. Duff (✉)
Department of Pediatrics, Department of Pediatric Critical Care, University of Alberta, Stollery Children's Hospital, Edmonton, AB, Canada
e-mail: jduff@ualberta.ca

M. S. Braga
Geisel School of Medicine at Dartmouth, Department of Pediatric Critical Care Medicine, Children's Hospital at Dartmouth, Lebanon, NH, USA
e-mail: Matthew.s.braga@hitchcock.org

M. F. Hamilton
Department of Critical Care Medicine, Children's Hospital of Pittsburgh of UPMC, Pittsburgh, PA, USA
e-mail: fiedml@ccm.upmc.edu

N. M. Tofil
Department of Pediatrics, University of Alabama at Birmingham, Children's of Alabama, Birmingham, AL, USA
e-mail: ntofil@peds.uab.edu

present unique challenges. A recent study reported that 93 % of in-hospital pediatric cardiac arrests occur in the intensive care unit (ICU) setting [1]. Critically ill pediatric patients require rapid diagnosis, complicated management plans, and emergent interventions or procedures. Their physiology can be complex and rapidly changing, requiring practitioners to have excellent assessment and intervention skills.

It is critical that healthcare providers working in this environment are well trained to handle these challenges. Although the stakes in pediatric critical care medicine are high, pediatric resuscitation events remain rare, making on-the-job training difficult. In recent studies of pediatric residents, a number of large knowledge and performance gaps have been identified in the domains of basic life support, defibrillation, and airway management [2–5]. This trend may worsen as trainees' time working with patients in the PICU decreases. Numerous programs across the world are reducing the on-call hours of pediatric trainees, a time when many learning opportunities in the PICU occur.

Simulation is an ideal educational modality for the PICU. A high-realism simulation can immerse a team of PICU practitioners into a scenario of a critically ill child, requiring accurate physical assessment, diagnosis, and treatment. In a simulation scenario, the team can perform a rapid assessment, order vasoactive medications, perform procedures (for example, insertion of a central venous catheter or endotracheal intubation), and evaluate the changing physiology based on the simulator's response to their decisions and actions. This real-time feedback allows for critical analysis of recent management decisions, and continuous evaluation of the simulated patient and modification of the treatment plan.

To improve availability of simulation in critical care, in situ training is becoming more prevalent [6]. The care of an ICU patient involves considerable technology, specialized equipment, and complex resources including medications and specially trained personnel. Familiarity with and the ability to function in this environment is vital to caring for the ICU patient. In situ simulation allows for caregivers to remain in the ICU setting, with the opportunity to utilize actual ICU equipment, supplies, and personnel in the same environment where they provide patient care. This also frees up the simulation program/center from having to purchase and maintain additional pieces of expensive clinical equipment to fill this need. In situ simulation can similarly be used to evaluate hospital systems, such as assessing for preparedness or latent safety threats. For example, an in situ simulation could show that the response time for bringing a defibrillator to the bedside is too lengthy. Changes to resuscitation cart deployment may improve response times prior to an adverse event in a real patient. These latent safety threats can be evaluated using unannounced simulated resuscitations (*mock* codes) in different areas of the healthcare environment.

Multiple healthcare practitioners from different diverse specialties and disciplines are required in the care of a PICU patient. With such a large group of people, effective teamwork and communication is essential. Despite its importance, this can be a challenge in the PICU when both stress levels and stakes are high. These are skills where simulation training can be very useful. Using simulation-based training, team roles and responsibilities in acute crises can be demonstrated and taught, while the highly important tasks of clear, specific communication can also be emphasized (see Chap. 4).

Critical Care Curriculum Development and Implementation

Code and Code Team Training

Cardiopulmonary arrests are rare, especially in pediatrics. With the introduction of rapid response teams, rates of pediatric arrests have decreased further [7]. Cardiopulmonary arrests are complicated high-stakes time-sensitive events where the efficient execution of cardiopulmonary resuscitation (CPR), teamwork, and crisis management skills is required to provide optimal care and optimize morbidity and mortality. Most hospitals have ad hoc interprofessional and multidisciplinary arrest teams that change daily based on call schedules and staffing assignments. These complicating factors make providing ideal care difficult. American Heart Association (AHA) standardized Pediatric Advanced Life Support (PALS) and Neonatal Resuscitation Program (NRP) algorithms attempt to simplify these complex crisis situations. It is clear, however, that retention of these skills is poor, and although certification is required every 2 years, knowledge and performance decline rapidly as early as 6 months following successful course completion [5, 8].

Simulation, especially involving repeated deliberate practice, can improve individual performance during a resuscitation. A retrospective case-control study showed that internal medicine residents who participated in simulation-based Advanced Cardiac Life Support (ACLS) training demonstrated significantly better adherence to ACLS protocols when compared to traditionally trained residents [9]. Specifically, in pediatrics, a "Rapid Cycle Deliberate Practice (RCDP)" model was used to teach junior pediatric residents basic resuscitation skills [10]. They found that use of this technique significantly improved trainees' time to initiation of chest compressions, no-flow fraction, and time to defibrillation. Unlike traditional simulation sessions where each simulation session continues uninterrupted and is followed by a debriefing, RCDP focuses on maximizing learner's time spent deliberately practicing specific skills which help to create overlearning and *automatization*. If a critical error is made, the scenario is paused and immediate feedback is provided. This method may be best suited when the process to care for a disease is highly standardized, with a specific protocol to be followed in a time-sensitive fashion. Similar models are being explored to teach other concepts such as NRP and CPR. Simulation can also be used to familiarize resuscitation teams with specific challenges of real-life resuscitations, such as parental presence [11].

Although technical skills are important in managing a resuscitation successfully, effective teamwork is equally, if not more, important. Interprofessional critical care unit teams have been shown to improve their teamwork through simulation-based learning [12]. Teams of physicians and nurses demonstrated significant improvements in overall teamwork as well as leadership and team coordination and verbalizing situational information. In a pediatric study, residents who participated in a short case-based teamwork training exercise demonstrated better teamwork behaviors and time to critically important maneuvers [13]. In a larger randomized trial, participation in a simulated cardiac arrest scenario followed by a scripted debriefing improved both knowledge and teamwork skills [14]. More research is required to determine the most effective way to teach these skills to cardiopulmonary arrest teams.

The use of unannounced resuscitation simulations (*mock* codes) can be an effective way of teaching pediatric resuscitation. They can be used to identify performance gaps or latent system errors that should be addressed [15]. In a recent study, surprise simulated resuscitations were implemented in a major children's hospital [14]. Over the period of the study, the authors found that patient survival from in-hospital cardiac arrest increased from 33 % to approximately 50 % over 1 year (Fig. 19.1). This increase in survival correlated with the number of mock codes performed. The surprise nature of these drills allows assessment of all aspects of resuscitation including recognition, the mechanics of activating the resuscitation team, and any other latent safety threats that could further compromise the process (e.g., elevator availability).

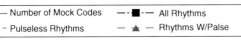

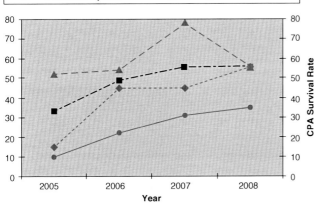

Fig. 19.1 Real pediatric survival rates *(right scale)* related to number of mock codes *(left scale)*. Actual survival rates for pulseless rhythms, rhythms with a pulse, and all rhythms are presented. *CPA* cardiopulmonary arrest. (From Andreatta 2011 (with permission))

Debriefing post-event is a key step in simulation-based training (see Chap. 3). This concept is being adapted to actual patient resuscitations, and the practice of conducting regular post-resuscitation debriefings has also been shown to improve CPR quality and patient outcome [16].

Boot Camps for Critical Care Trainees

As pediatric critical care becomes more complex and duty hour regulations become increasingly restrictive, many training programs are relying on initial supplementary training for the incoming pediatric critical care trainee. Often, these are in the form of an intensive *boot camp*, which uses simulation to augment learning.

In 2009, a descriptive study of the first multi-institutional boot camp for first-year pediatric critical care fellows conducted in the summer of 2006 was published. This study involved 22 fellows from nine institutions with instructors from seven different institutions. This intensive course was organized over 2.5 days for a total of 15.5 h of training, the majority of which was simulation-based pediatric critical care scenarios and complemented by smaller amounts of time participating in task training and didactic sessions (See Table 19.1). Topics included: airway management, vascular access, CPR, shock, sepsis, trauma, and traumatic brain injury. A model of *train to success* utilizing repeated practice until excellent performance is achieved was used. This training method has been shown to be an important aspect of effective use of simulation [17]. Fellows found this course to be highly effective in improving their self-assessed clinical effectiveness and self-confidence both immediately following training as well as after the first 6 months of their

Table 19.1 Agenda for pediatric critical care medicine boot camp. (Akira Nishisaki, personal communication)

Day 1—Afternoon	Airway management scenarios
Day 2—Morning	Central venous catheter training (didactic and skills training)
Day 2—Afternoon	PALS update
	PALS scenarios
Day 3—Morning	Approach to shock (didactic and simulation-based training)
	Trauma

PALS Pediatric Advanced Life Support

fellowship. This course, as well as similar courses in other disciplines, has continued and is growing in trainee numbers yearly [Akira Nishisaki, written communication, September 2014].

Critical Care Nursing Orientation

New nurses can be overwhelmed as they move from school into clinical practice. This transition can be even more daunting for critical care nurses who have to be familiar with different technologies, complex physiology, and rapid-changing patients. Simulation has been used during nursing orientation in critical care environments including the neonatal intensive care unit as well as the cardiac surgery intensive care unit but little exists in the literature on pediatric critical care orientation [18, 19]. These courses focused on high-acuity situations as well as equipment assembly under time pressure. In these studies, learners reported improved confidence and critical thinking skills. They also liked being able to "pause action" to gain clarification on difficult moments during a scenario.

Just-in-Time Training

Just-in-time training (JITT) involves providing training for a critical scenario or procedure in close temporal and physical proximity to when and where it will be performed in the clinical environment. It builds on adult learning theory suggesting that adults are most motivated to learn when immediate application occurs. This technique has been used in a number of different clinical contexts including CPR and intubation [20, 21]. In the PICU, JITT on tracheal intubation has been shown to increase resident participation during actual patient's intubation in the PICU but, unfortunately, was not associated with an improvement of success or a decrease in tracheal intubation-associated events [21]. It is unclear if this is related to the small sample size or suboptimal competence of trainees following the training. It has also been used in providing CPR education at the bedside. JITT

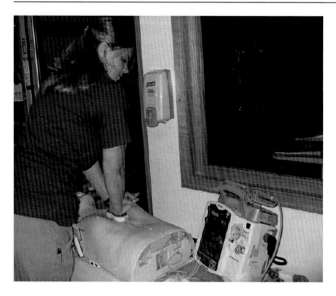

Fig. 19.2 A rolling refresher cart for just-in-time training of cardiopulmonary resuscitation in the pediatric intensive care unit. (From Niles 2009 (with permission))

was shown to improve compliance with chest compression guidelines in pediatric healthcare providers in the PICU [20, 22] (Fig. 19.2). JITT has also been used to train PICU nurses on appropriate central line dressing changes. Post-JITT, the nurses required significantly less corrective prompts. Most importantly, there was a significant decrease in the rate of central line-associated blood stream infections [23].

Skill Acquisition

Airway Management

Pediatric airway management represents a skill that all acute care practitioners must acquire and maintain, given the significant contribution of respiratory failure leading to cardiac arrest in children. As such, appropriate and timely airway management can avert circulatory collapse. Delayed or difficult airway management can lead to significant morbidity and mortality. Although it is an important skill, there is a wide range in the experience of providers who may be required to manage a pediatric airway. In pediatric residents, during simulated airway management scenarios, a number of critical performance gaps were noted [24]. Thus, airway management represents a high-stakes and high-risk skill that for some providers is an infrequent occurrence, yet a skill that is required of them.

As mentioned, simulation has been used for JITT for intubation in the PICU [21]. Learners that had participated in a simulation-based training program demonstrated improved performance in actual intubations in the PICU [25]. A recent systematic review and meta-analysis has also described the current landscape of simulation training for airway management. The type of training described in the meta-analysis

included direct endotracheal intubation, fiber-optic intubation, supraglottic airway insertion, blind intubation, and surgical airway management. This meta-analysis concluded that simulation training for airway management is associated with improved outcomes in terms of participant knowledge and skills performed in a simulated environment. Effects on actual patient outcomes were mixed, but when simulation training was compared to other teaching modalities, simulation was found to be superior [26].

Central Venous Catheter Placement

Central venous catheter placement is often necessary in critically ill children to ensure adequate and stable intravenous access for medications, fluids, nutrition, monitoring as well as advanced therapies including plasmapheresis and dialysis. Thus, central venous line placement represents a life-saving, but complex, bedside procedure that is routinely performed by intensive care physicians, anesthesiologists, emergency department physicians, and surgeons in various stages of their training.

The complexity and nuances of this procedure, a growing culture of patient safety, and the unpredictability of opportunities for trainees to gain experience have all led to substantial interest in using simulation training for central line placement. Many of the described training efforts have focused not only on the technical aspects of the actual procedure but also on strict sterile techniques in attempts to decrease infections. Bedsides, ultrasound is often used to assist with central line placement, and this additional technical aspect has also been featured in simulation training.

There is a growing body of literature describing the benefits on actual patients both in terms of performance with the actual procedure as well as subsequent decreased central line infections associated with simulation-based training. A recent meta-analysis concluded that residents who received simulation training for central venous line placement had greater success rates and required fewer attempts on actual patients [27]. Care bundles including simulation-based training have been associated with a reduction in central line-related infections in several studies [28, 29]. In pediatrics, a simulation-based intervention in ultrasound-guided central venous catheter insertion was effective in improving initial performance [30]. However, more work is required to determine the effect of these types of interventions on actual patient outcomes.

Bronchoscopy

Bronchoscopy is a complex bedside procedure that is routinely used for evaluation and therapy of congenital and acquired airway anomalies of both the upper and lower airways, diagnosis and management of airway and pulmonary infections, transbronchial biopsies post-lung transplantation, and foreign body removal. Providers performing bronchoscopy include pulmonologists, intensive care physicians, and surgeons in various stages of training. A recent meta-analysis concluded that simulation-based training was associated with improved learning outcomes when compared with traditional teaching [31]. This meta-analysis was limited as very few pediatric studies were included and few studies measured outcomes on actual patients.

Difficult Conversations

While simulation in the PICU often focuses on mannequin-based simulation and technical skills, an equally important skill in the PICU is the ability to have difficult conversations with families around bad prognoses, difficult decisions, and end-of-life care. Simulation-based workshops, using standardized patients as parents, have been shown to be effective in improving the ability of pediatric trainees to have these conversations [32] (See Chap. 23, "Communication").

Special Circumstances

Extracorporeal Membrane Oxygenation

Extracorporeal membrane oxygenation (ECMO) is a technique to support pediatric patients with severe cardiorespiratory failure in the PICU. Catheters are placed in the venous system (for respiratory support or veno-venous ECMO) or both the arterial and venous systems (for cardiopulmonary support or venoarterial ECMO). Blood from the patient is pumped through an oxygenator in which oxygen and car-

bon dioxide are exchanged, heated, and then pumped back into the patient. ECMO is technically complex and challenging, and requires the coordination of different groups of providers including PICU physicians and nurses, surgeons, anesthetists, respiratory therapists, operating room staff, and ECMO specialists or perfusionists. Simulation has emerged as a useful technique to educate teams on how to initiate ECMO, how to support a patient on ECMO, and to troubleshoot problems during an ECMO run.

Surgical task trainers have been developed to facilitate training in the procedure of ECMO cannulation resulting in improved time to cannulation [33]. Once the simulated patient is on ECMO, a number of techniques have been used to simulate various ECMO-related problems such as hypovolemia, tamponade, and pump failure. These systems often rely on a system of clamps and access points to infuse or remove volume to simulate different physiological conditions (Fig. 19.3). The advantage of these types of systems is that the team's real ECMO setup can be used to maximize equipment fidelity. These types of systems have shown to improve various technical skills of ECMO teams such as urgently removing a patient from the circuit in the event of a mechanical failure [34, 35]. Simulation can also be used to identify latent safety threats present in these complicated situations [36]. More recently, the use of a simulation-based education ECMO program has been associated with improved times to ECMO cannulation during CPR and compliance with initiation checklists [36, 37].

Ventricular Assist Device

The management of patients on a ventricular assist device (VAD) also requires a dedicated team with specific technical and cognitive skills. Although some VAD simulators exist,

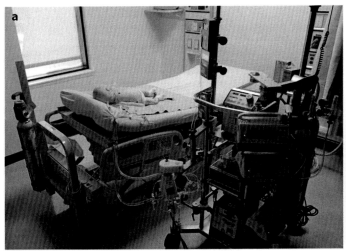
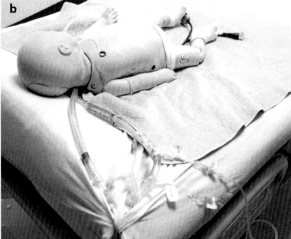

Fig. 19.3 ECMO simulation setup (**a**). The arterial and venous cannula are connected together either under or inside the mannequin (**b**, close-up)

they have typically been used to assess VAD performance in a variety of simulated clinical conditions [38]. In an adult study, a VAD simulator was used with paramedics to assess how easy the various VADs were to use in an emergency situation [39]. More work is required to demonstrate their effectiveness in education.

Continuous Renal Replacement Therapy

Simulation has been used to train PICU staff in the use of continuous renal replacement therapy (CRRT). A simulation-based training program has been shown to improve cognitive skills in CRRT therapy [40]. More importantly, These training programs have been shown to improve CRRT circuit lifespan when used on real patients in the PICU [41].

Pediatric Cardiac Intensive Care

The pediatric cardiac intensive care unit (PCICU) represents another specialized environment in which simulation can play an important role in education. Emergencies in the PCICU often involve multiple practitioners from different subspecialties (such as surgery, anesthesia, and neonatology) caring for patients with complex physiology. The use of simulation-based team training in this environment has resulted in improved confidence and teamwork [42, 43]. Simulation can also be effective in teaching skills commonly used in the PCICU such as echocardiography and emergent sternotomy [44, 45].

Transport Medicine

Pediatric transport services are responsible for transferring acutely ill patients both within and between health centers. These transfers are often long, occur in environments not well suited to patient care, and bring with them specific challenges. Caring for patients in the back of a moving ambulance or helicopter, when space is tight and access to the patient is limited, is a challenge. The transport environment is often noisy, making patient assessment (such as auscultation) difficult to impossible.

Simulation-based curricula can be used to practice the assessment, triage, and initial management of patients. Pediatric transport teams often comprise healthcare providers practicing in extended roles; simulation can be used to educate transport providers in these new roles. Specific challenges of the transport environment (such as the effect of altitude, noise, or specialized equipment) can be highlighted. In addition, with the development of more portable mannequins, teams can practice moving patients through various environ-

ments, so challenges of each environment can be better appreciated (e.g., moving an unstable patient into an elevator only to realize that a critically important piece of equipment has been left behind). This type of simulation brings its own challenges, such as confidentiality as teams move through public spaces, the use of wireless technology, and how details of the case can be appreciated by a facilitator as the teams move through different hospital environments.

Integrating Simulation into the PICU

Although there are clearly good reasons why simulation should be used in pediatric critical care education, there are some barriers that need to be overcome. As mentioned above, the provision of pediatric critical care relies on specialized personnel and equipment. Unfortunately, it can be a challenge to combine current simulator technology and equipment in the PICU. For example, while most mannequins can be ventilated with a PICU ventilator, generating a level of realism to satisfy experienced critical care providers is difficult. Moving or obtaining authentic and current PICU equipment to simulation centers is also a challenge. In situ simulation can help with the equipment issue, though it is often a challenge in a busy PICU to find bed space for simulation that is not already being used for direct patient care. Creative solutions are often required, such as using procedure rooms or nearby classrooms.

Conclusions

Simulation-based education to date has focused largely on the management of a crisis, whether that is the acute resuscitation of a critically ill patient with sepsis or the cannulation of a child onto ECMO. However, simulation has the possibility of being used for more mundane tasks. Instead of running a 10-min scenario on the acute resuscitation of the patient with septic shock, an extended duration simulation can be run allowing for a more realistic experience. In this type of scenario, the mannequin can be set up and then run for 30 min or more. The admitting nurse may be required to perform an initial assessment, chart that assessment, prioritize the tasks required, and then monitor the patient for any deterioration. The physicians looking after the patient can be paged as they would for a real patient, forcing them to perform their own assessments of the patient's status. These types of simulation are more realistic by allowing events to occur in real time, not artificially forced into a 10-min scenario. Even longer simulation events involving multiple simulated patients and healthcare providers have also been done to assess latent safety threats or to evaluate new critical care environments (e.g., prior to the opening of a new ICU).

In critical care, simulation-based training has also largely focused on learners, especially physician trainees and nurses. However, given its power to assess knowledge and skills in a realistic environment, it may have a larger role to play in the continuing education of licensed professionals, including attending physicians. Currently, critical care simulation relies highly on mannequin-based simulation. Improvements in mannequin technology are critical to allow better interfaces with PICU equipment. As other techniques become more sophisticated, such as virtual reality, they may partially address some of the challenges addressed above. However, it is critically important that future research in simulation in the PICU examine the effect of these interventions on patient outcomes. Studies should attempt to address the question of what components of simulation-based training are the most effective in different contexts and what are the effects of patient outcomes in the PICU.

References

1. Berg RA, Sutton RM, Holubkov R, Nicholson CE, Dean JM, Harrison R, et al. Ratio of PICU versus ward cardiopulmonary resuscitation events is increasing. Crit Care Med. 2013;41(10):2292–7.
2. Hunt EA, Patel S, Vera K, Shaffner DH, Pronovost PJ. Survey of pediatric resident experiences with resuscitation training and attendance at actual cardiopulmonary arrests. Pediatr Crit Care Med. 2009;10(1):96–105.
3. Hunt EA, Vera K, Diener-West M, Haggerty JA, Nelson KL, Shaffner DH, et al. Delays and errors in cardiopulmonary resuscitation and defibrillation by pediatric residents during simulated cardiopulmonary arrests. Resuscitation. 2009;80(7):819–25.
4. White JR, Shugerman R, Brownlee C, Quan L. Performance of advanced resuscitation skills by pediatric housestaff. Arch Pediatr Adolesc Med. 1998;152(12):1232–5.
5. Roy KM, Miller MP, Schmidt K, Sagy M. Pediatric residents experience a significant decline in their response capabilities to simulated life-threatening events as their training frequency in cardiopulmonary resuscitation decreases. Pediatr Crit Care Med. 2011;12(3):e141–4
6. Weinstock PH, Kappus LJ, Garden A, Burns JP. Simulation at the point-of-care: reduced-cost, in situ training via a mobile cart. Pediatr Crit Care Med. 2009;10(2):176–81
7. Sharek PJ, Parast LM, Leong K, Coombs J, Earnest K, Sullivan J, et al. Effect of a rapid response team on hospital-wide mortality and code rates outside the ICU in a children's hospital. JAMA. 2007;298(19):2267–74.
8. Grant EC, Marczinski CA, Menon K. Using pediatric advanced life support in pediatric residency training: does the curriculum need resuscitation? Pediatr Crit Care Med. 2007;8(5):433–9.
9. Wayne DB, Didwania A, Feinglass J, Fudala MJ, Barsuk JH, McGaghie WC. Simulation-based education improves quality of care during cardiac arrest team responses at an academic teaching hospital: a case-control study. Chest. 2008;133(1):56–61.
10. Hunt EA, Duval-Arnould JM, Nelson-McMillan KL, Bradshaw JH, Diener-West M, Perretta JS, et al. Pediatric resident resuscitation skills improve after "rapid cycle deliberate practice" training. Resuscitation. 2014;85(7):945–51.
11. Pye S, Kane J, Jones A. Parental presence during pediatric resuscitation: the use of simulation training for cardiac intensive care nurses. J Spec Pediatr Nurs. 2010;15(2):172–5.
12. Frengley RW, Weller JM, Torrie J, Dzendrowskyj P, Yee B, Paul AM, et al. The effect of a simulation-based training intervention on the performance of established critical care unit teams. Crit Care Med. 2011;39(12):2605–11.
13. Blackwood J, Duff JP, Nettel-Aguirre A, Djogovic D, Joynt C. Does teaching crisis resource management skills improve resuscitation performance in pediatric residents? Pediatr Crit Care Med. 2014;15(4):e168–74.
14. Cheng A, Hunt EA, Donoghue A, Nelson-McMillan K, Nishisaki A, Leflore J, et al. Examining pediatric resuscitation education using simulation and scripted debriefing: a multicenter randomized trial. JAMA Pediatr. 2013;167(6):528–36.
15. Tofil NM, Lee White M, Manzella B, McGill D, Zinkan L. Initiation of a pediatric mock code program at a children's hospital. Med Teach. 2009;31(6):e241–7.
16. Wolfe H, Zebuhr C, Topjian AA, Nishisaki A, Niles DE, Meaney PA, et al. Interdisciplinary ICU cardiac arrest debriefing improves survival outcomes*. Crit Care Med. 2014;42(7):1688–95.
17. Issenberg SB, McGaghie WC, Petrusa ER, Lee Gordon D, Scalese RJ. Features and uses of high-fidelity medical simulations that lead to effective learning: a BEME systematic review. Med Teach. 2005;27(1):10–28.
18. Pilcher J, Goodall H, Jensen C, Huwe V, Jewell C, Reynolds R, et al. Special focus on simulation: educational strategies in the NICU: simulation-based learning: it's not just for NRP. Neonatal Netw. 2012;31(5):281–7.
19. Rauen CA. Simulation as a teaching strategy for nursing education and orientation in cardiac surgery. Crit Care Nurse. 2004;24(3):46–51.
20. Niles D, Sutton RM, Donoghue A, Kalsi MS, Roberts K, Boyle L, et al. "Rolling Refreshers": a novel approach to maintain CPR psychomotor skill competence. Resuscitation. 2009;80(8):909–12.
21. Nishisaki A, Donoghue AJ, Colborn S, Watson C, Meyer A, Brown CA 3rd, et al. Effect of just-in-time simulation training on tracheal intubation procedure safety in the pediatric intensive care unit. Anesthesiology. 2010;113(1):214–23.
22. Sutton RM, Niles D, Meaney PA, Aplenc R, French B, Abella BS, et al. "Booster" training: evaluation of instructor-led bedside cardiopulmonary resuscitation skill training and automated corrective feedback to improve cardiopulmonary resuscitation compliance of Pediatric Basic Life Support providers during simulated cardiac arrest. Pediatr Crit Care Med. 2011;12(3):e116–21.
23. Scholtz AK, Monachino AM, Nishisaki A, Nadkarni VM, Lengetti E. Central venous catheter dress rehearsals: translating simulation training to patient care and outcomes. Simul Healthc. 2013;8(5):341–9.
24. Overly FL, Sudikoff SN, Shapiro MJ. High-fidelity medical simulation as an assessment tool for pediatric residents' airway management skills. Pediatr Emerg Care. 2007;23(1):11–5.
25. Nishisaki A, Nguyen J, Colborn S, Watson C, Niles D, Hales R, et al. Evaluation of multidisciplinary simulation training on clinical performance and team behavior during tracheal intubation procedures in a pediatric intensive care unit. Pediatr Crit Care Med. 2011;12(4):406–14.
26. Kennedy CC, Cannon EK, Warner DO, Cook DA. Advanced airway management simulation training in medical education: a systematic review and meta-analysis. Crit Care Med. 2014;42(1):169–78.
27. Madenci AL, Solis CV, de Moya MA. Central venous access by trainees: a systematic review and meta-analysis of the use of simulation to improve success rate on patients. Simul Healthc. 2014;9(1):7–14.
28. Cherry RA, West CE, Hamilton MC, Rafferty CM, Hollenbeak CS, Caputo GM. Reduction of central venous catheter associated blood stream infections following implementation of a resident oversight and credentialing policy. Patient Saf Surg. 2011;5(1):15.
29. Allen GB, Miller V, Nicholas C, Hess S, Cordes MK, Fortune JB, et al. A multiered strategy of simulation training, kit consolida-

tion, and electronic documentation is associated with a reduction in central line-associated bloodstream infections. Am J Infect Control. 2014;42(6):643–8.

30. Thomas SM, Burch W, Kuehnle SE, Flood RG, Scalzo AJ, Gerard JM. Simulation training for pediatric residents on central venous catheter placement: a pilot study. Pediatr Crit Care Med. 2013;14(9):e416–23.

31. Kennedy CC, Maldonado F, Cook DA. Simulation-based bronchoscopy training: systematic review and meta-analysis. Chest. 2013;144(1):183–92.

32. Tobler K, Grant E, Marczinski C. Evaluation of the impact of a simulation-enhanced breaking bad news workshop in pediatrics. Simul Healthc. 2014;9(4):213–9.

33. Allan CK, Pigula F, Bacha EA, Emani S, Fynn-Thompson F, Thiagarajan RR, et al. An extracorporeal membrane oxygenation cannulation curriculum featuring a novel integrated skills trainer leads to improved performance among pediatric cardiac surgery trainees. Simul Healthc. 2013;8(4):221–8.

34. Anderson JM, Murphy AA, Boyle KB, Yaeger KA, Halamek LP. Simulating extracorporeal membrane oxygenation emergencies to improve human performance. Part II: assessment of technical and behavioral skills. Simul Healthc. 2006;1(4):228–32.

35. Chan SY, Figueroa M, Spentzas T, Powell A, Holloway R, Shah S. Prospective assessment of novice learners in a simulation-based extracorporeal membrane oxygenation (ECMO) education program. Pediatr Cardiol. 2013;34(3):543–52.

36. Burton KS, Pendergrass TL, Byczkowski TL, Taylor RG, Moyer MR, Falcone RA, et al. Impact of simulation-based extracorporeal membrane oxygenation training in the simulation laboratory and clinical environment. Simul Healthc. 2011;6(5):284–91.

37. Su L, Spaeder MC, Jones MB, Sinha P, Nath DS, Jain PN, et al. Implementation of an extracorporeal cardiopulmonary resuscita-tion simulation program reduces extracorporeal cardiopulmonary resuscitation times in real patients. Pediatr Crit Care Med. 2014;15(9):856–60.

38. Vandenberghe S, Shu F, Arnold DK, Antaki JF. A simple, economical, and effective portable paediatric mock circulatory system. ProcInst Mech Eng H. 2011;225(7):648–56.

39. Geidl L, Deckert Z, Zrunek P, Gottardi R, Sterz F, Wieselthaler G, et al. Intuitive use and usability of ventricular assist device peripheral components in simulated emergency conditions. Artif Organs. 2011;35(8):773–80.

40. Lopez-Herce J, Ferrero L, Mencia S, Anton M, Rodriguez-Nunez A, Rey C, et al. Teaching and training acute renal replacement therapy in children. Nephrol Dial Transplant. 2012;27(5):1807–11.

41. Mottes T, Owens T, Niedner M, Juno J, Shanley TP, Heung M. Improving delivery of continuous renal replacement therapy: impact of a simulation-based educational intervention. Pediatr Crit Care Med. 2013;14(8):747–54.

42. Allan CK, Thiagarajan RR, Beke D, Imprescia A, Kappus LJ, Garden A, et al. Simulation-based training delivered directly to the pediatric cardiac intensive care unit engenders preparedness, comfort, and decreased anxiety among multidisciplinary resuscitation teams. J Thorac Cardiovasc Surg. 2010;140(3):646–52.

43. Figueroa MI, Sepanski R, Goldberg SP, Shah S. Improving teamwork, confidence, and collaboration among members of a pediatric cardiovascular intensive care unit multidisciplinary team using simulation-based team training. Pediatr Cardiol. 2013;34(3):612–9.

44. Weidenbach M, Razek V, Wild F, Khambadkone S, Berlage T, Janousek J, et al. Simulation of congenital heart defects: a novel way of training in echocardiography. Heart. 2009;95(8):636–41.

45. Lo T, Morrison R, Atkins K, Reynolds F. Novel manikin for chest re-opening simulation training. Intensive Care Med. 2009;35(6):1143–4.

Simulation for Pediatric Disaster and Multiple Casualty Incident Training

20

Mark X. Cicero and Debra L. Weiner

Simulation Pearls

1. Disasters overwhelm healthcare resources. Multiple casualty incidents (MCIs) strain resources. Simulated disasters and MCIs should steer healthcare workers to make decisions about resource allocation.

2. Hospitals can prepare for events such as multiple vehicle crashes and school shootings by testing their healthcare systems with simulation. Systems testing is crucial, not only for hospital providers and personnel, but also for prehospital emergency services, such as emergency medical technicians, paramedics, and firefighters.

3. Simulation provides the opportunity to create the disaster and/or MCI in local or remote environments.

4. Effective disaster and MCI preparedness and response training combine classroom and screen-based didactics with low- and high-fidelity simulation in the form of tabletop exercises, virtual reality, and live drill simulation.

5. Children are vulnerable and impacted by disasters in ways that are different from how adults are impacted. Disaster training must address pediatric-specific evaluation and management of physical and psychosocial manifestations of pediatric disaster victims as well as family and community-related considerations.

Introduction

By definition, disasters and multiple casualty incidents (MCIs) are infrequent events that involve numerous victims. In the case of disasters, medical resources are overwhelmed, while MCIs strain but do not necessarily overwhelm resources [1]. Several reviews describing the epidemiology of disasters exist. One Korean study showed that over a 10-year period, the crude mortality rates for disasters and MCIs were 2.36 deaths per 100,000 persons and 6.78 deaths per 100,000 persons, respectively. The crude injury incidence rates for disasters and MCIs were 25.47 injuries per 100,000 persons and 152 injuries per 100,000 persons, respectively [2]. Further, the report showed human-caused disasters were over ten times more common than natural disasters, and the authors speculated that South Korea has relatively few disasters and MCIs than other nations.

Pediatric Considerations for Disaster and MCI Simulation

Factors that make pediatric disaster and MCI unique include: (1) the etiology and types of injury and illness; (2) the number and demographics of victims; (3) the anticipated duration; (4) available resources of the community; and (5) the unique vulnerabilities of children. When planning disaster and MCI simulation for the purposes of training, systems testing or research, it is advisable to consider all of these factors.

Etiology of the Disaster or MCI

One of the fundamental ways in which disasters and MCIs vary is their cause. Disaster/MCI events may be categorized into (1) natural events, such as tornadoes and earthquakes; (2) accidents and errors, such as the Bhopal, India, gas explosion disaster of 1984; and (3) man-made, or intentional

M. X. Cicero (✉)
Department of Pediatrics, Yale University School of Medicine, Yale-New Haven's Children's Hospital, New Haven, CT 06511, USA
e-mail: Mark.cicero@yale.edu

D. L. Weiner
Department of Pediatrics, Department of Emergency Medicine, Harvard Medical School, Boston Children's Hospital, Boston, MA 02115, USA
e-mail: weiner_d@tch.harvard.edu

© Springer International Publishing Switzerland 2016
V. J. Grant, A. Cheng (eds.), *Comprehensive Healthcare Simulation: Pediatrics*,
Comprehensive Healthcare Simulation, DOI 10.1007/978-3-319-24187-6_20

253

events, such as the Aurora, Colorado, theater shooting of 2012 or the World Trade Centre disaster of 2001. A disaster or MCI's etiology will impact the kinds of injuries and illness at the scene and in hospitals. The etiology will also influence the duration of the event and the likelihood that healthcare workers will be willing and able to respond and provide care to victims [3–5].

Planning for a simulated disaster/MCI should consider the etiology and the types of illness and injury with which patients will present. Other considerations include whether there is an ongoing hazard that endangers healthcare workers, such as a chemical, biological, radiological, or nuclear event, and the hazard vulnerability analysis of the community where the simulation is conducted [6, 7]. For example, healthcare communities in the American Midwest may choose to simulate a response to a tornado, while communities on a coast might simulate a hurricane or cyclone. Both landlocked and coastal communities might be equally likely to respond to a mass shooting or a school bus crash.

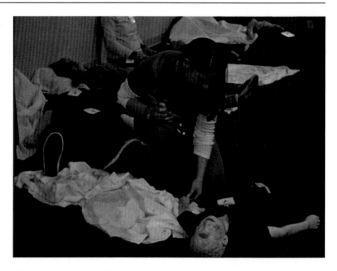

Fig. 20.1 A paramedic performs disaster triage in a mixed-modal simulation. (Photo courtesy of Mark Cicero)

Number of Victims

There is a balance between the number of victims that need assessment and care in a disaster or MCI, the severity of illness and/or injury of individual patients, the age distribution of pediatric victims, whether adults accompanying them also require care, and the healthcare resources of the community (discussed later). The number of simulated victims in an event that overwhelms medical resources impacts how the simulation is conducted. Simulation for events with 10–50 victims can be conducted with standardized patients, child and adult volunteers, and simulation mannequins [8]. Larger events may be difficult to depict and may require tabletop exercises or computer simulation. Additionally, the needs of individual disaster/MCI victims can vary significantly. Mixed-modal simulation allows a means to portray multiple patients and their medical needs [3], as shown in Fig. 20.1. For example, simulation mannequins may portray patients who have extensive injuries or severe illness, or who require invasive procedures (Fig. 20.2), while confederates or standardized actors portray ambulatory and conversant patients (Fig. 20.3). In some cases, hybrids of confederates and manikins or task trainers are used.

Duration

The duration of a disaster or MCI may range from brief and punctuated events, such as the 2013 bombings at the Bos-

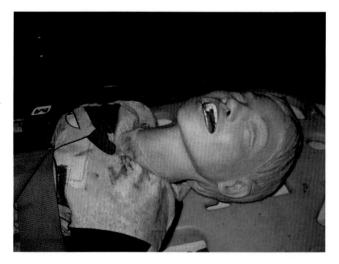

Fig. 20.2 A mannequin portrays a residential fire victim who has succumbed to smoke inhalation. (Photo courtesy of Mark Cicero)

ton marathon finish line, to protracted events, such as the influenza pandemics of 1918 and 2009 [9, 10]. Simulation of such events should include plans for whether patients present in rapid succession over a short period of time, in a protracted, steady stream for hours or days, or a combination of the two temporal patterns (Fig. 20.4) [11]. If the simulated event occurs over the course of hours, such as a mass shooting at a school, simulation may be synchronous, and follow victims for all or any portion of their time in the prehospital setting to emergency departments (EDs) and other receiving facilities, and even definitive care, including hospital admission and the operating room. For practical reasons, protracted events are simulated in an asynchronous manner and divided into scenes.

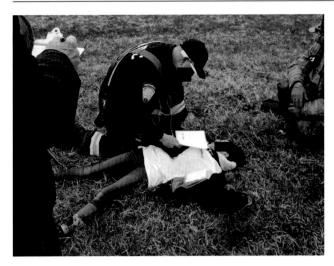

Fig. 20.3 An actor portrays a victim during an aircraft crash simulation. (Photo courtesy of Mark Cicero)

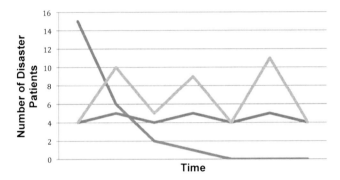

Fig. 20.4 Timing of patient presentation in disasters. Patients may appear in punctuated bursts, as a mass that declines over time, or in a steady flow. (Photo courtesy of Mark Cicero)

Available Resources of the Community

An event with similar etiology, number of patients, and patient acuity may be a disaster in one community and readily addressed in another with more extensive resources. For example, a bus crash with eight injured children in rural Vermont would likely overwhelm resources, with few basic life support ambulances within a 20-minute radius and a critical access hospital as the closest receiving facility [12]. The same event in a large city with robust emergency medical services (EMS) and numerous hospitals might be managed with relative ease. Another consideration for simulation educators and emergency event planners regarding available resources is whether the disaster is occurring in an industrialized country or the developing world [13]. For disasters that overwhelm the resources of a community, disaster response may be augmented by the inclusion of local or remote government agencies or non-government disaster response organizations as well as organizations functioning locally with disaster response capabilities.

Vulnerabilities of Children to Disaster/MCI

Children are more vulnerable to disasters and MCIs than able-bodied adults for several reasons, including cognitive, emotional, and physical vulnerabilities [14]. Inclusion of these vulnerabilities in simulation promotes familiarity with caring for child victims and allows more realistic tests of disaster and MCI response systems.

Cognitively, children are less likely to understand the ongoing threat of a disaster/MCI or to seek shelter. Further, children may lack the problem-solving skills to find responsible caregivers in an ongoing disaster/MCI. When children are separated from adult caretakers, there is a need for a reliable reunification method [15]. When planning a simulation of a disaster/MCI, it is crucial to add elements of patient tracking, family reunification, and the anxiety caregivers feel when children may be injured, and the anxiety children feel when separated from their caregivers. *Emotionally*, children are likely to take their cues from adults during a disaster or MCI. Therefore, when parents and other caregivers respond with anxiety and fear, children are likely to experience similar emotions. In fact, witnessing caregiver stress during an MCI is associated with post-traumatic stress disorder in children [16]. Children have a number of *physical* vulnerabilities in disasters and MCIs. They may be less mobile than adults and less able to seek shelter. They have a greater respiratory rate, therefore toxic gases and aerosolized toxins are inspired in higher doses more quickly than in adults. Regarding radiological and nuclear exposures, children have more rapidly dividing cells and a longer life expectancy than adults [17]. Therefore, they are at greater risk of developing neoplasms due to exposures. Another physical vulnerability is the relative discomfort many EMS providers and general emergency medicine physicians feel when caring for ill and injured children compared to adults [18].

How Disasters and MCIs Differ from Individual Patient Emergencies

In single-patient emergencies, healthcare systems and providers are able to expend personnel time and whatever resources are necessary to attempt to resuscitate a critically ill patient. During a disaster when resources are strained or overwhelmed, the situation (and ethics) are very different [19]. The healthcare team holds the goal of doing the most good, for the most patients, with the most judicious use of resources [20]. Lifeless patients and patients who are unlikely to survive, given the available resources, may be afforded less care, so that other patients who are more likely to survive may receive attention. Initially, it may be difficult to determine whether an event will overwhelm or just strain the response system. Unless it is clear that the event will not overwhelm resources, criteria to rapidly initiate disaster activation should be established, plans for allocation of resources generated, and available responders identified.

During disasters and MCIs, the interface of pre-hospital and hospital care should be robust and well coordinated. Preexisting, offline policies determine where patients are transported. Online medical direction may be required for decisions about non-provision or cessation of resuscitation efforts. Fire personnel, pre-hospital care providers, and/or hazmat teams perform decontamination when chemical, biological, or radiological agents are suspected [21]. Though public health agencies and clinical organizations interact frequently, in disasters and MCIs, there is a particular need to work in concert. Public health efforts include the recognition of index cases, protection of healthcare workers and non-disaster, MCI patients already in the hospital, and distribution of immunizations and medication.

Disasters and MCIs cause anxiety and a demand for information. When disasters or MCIs impact children, family members and other caregivers, members of the community, and media personnel may add to the complexity of response. Family members may present to a disaster/MCI site or ED seeking reunification with their child. Reunification strategies may be tested and refined with simulation [22]. Community members may converge on the event site(s) or a hospital(s) intending to volunteer. Reporters and other media agents will be present, and law enforcement officials may be present. Though none of these groups are patients, all require provisions in a disaster/MCI response plan. Simulations may include a mechanism for reunification of patients with family members, crowd control, and proper interface with the media and law enforcement.

Disaster/MCI Training Principles

Preparation for disaster and MCI responses should be ongoing and iterative, follow an all-hazards approach, engage all potential constituencies, and provide training for knowledge, skills, and team building. Training for disaster and MCI response differs from that for other medical situations in that, in addition to preparing for injuries and illnesses rarely seen in children and providing care for adults victims accompanying pediatric patients, training must also address policies and protocols for activation, utilization of physical and personnel resources, psychosocial issues unique to disaster, MCI, patient volume, impact of disaster/MCI on environmental infrastructure, and healthcare systems and structures. Training

should recognize that non-routine situations, such as disasters and MCIs, particularly those that result in high uncertainty and disrupt the usual practice environment, increase stress, fixation, and loss of situational awareness. For remote disaster response, particularly to austere environments, training must also include situational awareness regarding the location, its infrastructure, weather, regional medical conditions, potentially relevant cultural norms, socioeconomic and political factors, government and nongovernment options for deployment, requirements for personal preparedness, and roles in, and responsibilities and risks of deployment.

Effective and efficient training combines classroom and screen-based didactics with low- and high-fidelity simulation that includes tabletop exercises, virtual reality (VR), and live drill simulation. Classroom and screen-based multimedia interactive didactics and exercises can be effective and efficient for introducing principles of disaster and MCI, pediatric vulnerabilities to and consequences of different types of disasters, MCIs, considerations regarding evaluation and management of pediatric victims, hospital policies and practices for disaster, MCI response, and concepts and specifics of situational awareness.

Tabletop exercises are ideally suited for focus on specific aspects of planning, policies and logistics of disaster, and MCI response, particularly across groups of key personnel with different roles and perspectives. Tabletop exercises can also be effective for training when live drills are impractical and/or too costly, such as for high patient volume disasters, and/or training in low-resource settings. Tabletop exercises may be used in conjunction with live drills to achieve complementary learning objectives. Pediatric disaster educators and planners are advised to consider tabletop exercises as a useful tool in the simulation armamentarium.

VR systems, currently in early-stage development for disaster, MCI preparedness and response training, range from low-fidelity screen-based software intended for individual learners and/or teams to high-fidelity 3D immersion into controlled environments and situations, and may be customizable for individuals and facilities, agencies and/or organizations. The Ready.gov website has a screen-based disaster game for children, as shown in Fig. 20.5. For many disaster learners, especial paramedics and emergency medical technicians, the accessibility of VR disaster/MCI training may be more appealing than the spatial and temporal confines of a live simulation drill.

High-fidelity simulation that uses a combination of mannequins and/or actors is particularly ideal for disaster and MCI response training because it affords opportunities to create environments and situations unique to disasters and MCIs, specifically for each individual facility, agency and/or organization. Simulation must include evaluation and debriefing. Evaluation should be ideally performed by observers not running the simulation using available and applicable

Fig. 20.5 Disaster Master screen-based training for young people (available at www.ready. gov/kids)

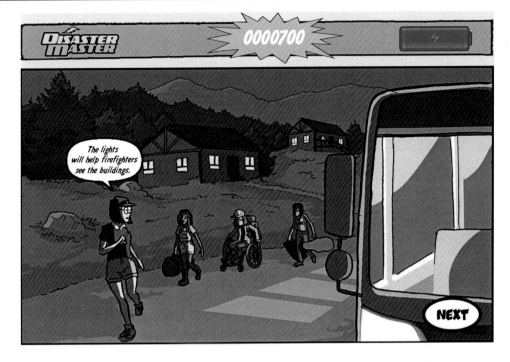

Table 20.1 Best uses of disaster, MCI training modalities

	Classroom, Screen-Based	Tabletop Exercises	Virtual Reality	Live Drill
Disaster Principles, Practice				
Activation				
Patient Care				
Systems Testing, Teamwork				

Darker color indicates greater value. Modalities should be combined iteratively.

Disaster Principles and Practice: Disaster, Multiple casualty incident (MCI) definitions, types; pediatric vulnerabilities, injuries, illnesses; knowledge, skills; crisis resource management; incident command; disaster and site specifics

Activation: Plan elements; staffing; space allocation; equipment,supplies; setup

Patient Care: Transport; decontamination; triage; registration, tracking, documentation; patient trauma, medical care; reunification; disposition; evacuation

Systems Testing, Teamwork: Animating reality; testing environment and systems readiness; teamwork; communication

checklists. Debriefing should be guided by trained facilitators, focus on a limited number of topics, and should engage all participants.

The US Homeland Security Exercise and Evaluation Program (HSEEP) provides guidance for the development and evaluation of disaster training exercises, including simulations [23]. The HSEEP includes guidance for developing disaster training, evaluating learners as well as the training intervention, and methods for improving practice based on gaps revealed in simulation and subsequent debriefing. As with any simulation, it is important to identify overarching goals and specific objectives for simulated disasters and MCIs. The range of educational interventions, including

simulations, and the potential application of those interventions for training and testing the capacity and efficacy of disaster plans are shown in Table 20.1. Specifics of the use of simulation for disaster/MCI education and systems testing are discussed as follows, and a template for creating disaster/MCI simulations is shown in Fig. 20.6.

Use of Simulation in Disaster/MCI Preparedness Education

Simulation is a well-established means of disaster and MCI response education [24–28]. Simulation is used to aid learners' acquisition of disaster- and MCI-specific knowledge and

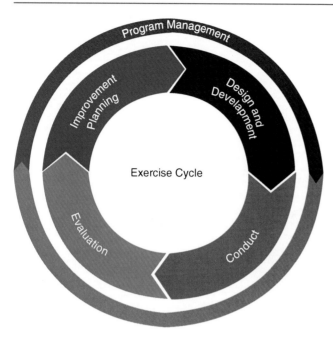

Fig. 20.6 Template for the creation of disaster/MCI

skills for team training and formative evaluation. Knowledge and skills training, in addition to focusing on injury and illness not routinely seen, and care of patients without known identity or caregivers, should incorporate the disaster response ethic of allocating resources to do the most good for the greatest number of patients. Simulation may focus on specific elements of response, engage single or multiple groups of hospital and prehospital providers, and involve one or more subspecialties, healthcare facilities, local, national or international organizations and/or agencies. Disaster and MCI response simulation should transport participants out of their routine environment and practice to the disrupted, chaotic environment created by damage, which locally may include their own healthcare facility, or in the remote austere environment may be superimposed on an already resource-limited setting. Simulation should highlight differences from the routine in the environment, the demographics of victims, their injuries and illnesses, and how providers perform in this environment, as well as emphasize accepted disaster/MCI-specific principles and practices. Performance evaluation and debriefing should focus on knowledge and skills of individuals and the team and on interactions as a team. Debriefing may include, in addition to discussion regarding evaluation and management of disaster, MCI-related injuries and illnesses, thoughts and feelings about the disrupted environment, successes and challenges, and opportunities for improvement (see Chap. 3 for details).

The potential emotional impact of participating in disaster/MCI simulation must be considered when planning educational interventions. Simulations of many ill and injured children, some of whom have horrific injuries or are dead,

can precipitate post-traumatic stress disorder, especially in learners with risk factors for the disorder. A sophisticated debriefing with probes for detecting those who are acutely impacted by the simulation and offering follow-up to assess for sleep disturbance, intrusive thoughts, and other symptoms is advisable. A sample debriefing script is shown in Fig. 20.7.

Simulation Modalities for Disaster/MCI Training

Classroom and screen-based didactics, and high- and low-fidelity simulation, should be combined strategically to provide effective, cost- and time-efficient training.

Tabletop Simulation

Tabletop exercises provide an excellent opportunity to use and reinforce classroom and screen-based didactics to evaluate disaster/MCI plans as well as logistics and resources within and across hospitals and the community. Sessions that present a scenario, divide participants into multidisciplinary and interprofessional groups to work through assigned tasks applying knowledge gained from classroom and screen-based didactics, and then have each group present their strategy are valuable for identifying gaps and opportunities for improvement. Tabletop simulation is also helpful for planning the logistics of full-scale exercises, identifying training agendas, scenarios, and debriefing topics [25, 29]. Tabletop exercises may be the best option for planning for large-scale disasters, disasters in environments that cannot easily be animated by high-fidelity simulation live drills, and/or disasters in low-resource environments [30]. Exercises similar to tabletop exercises and drills can be performed within the routine work environment by posing scenarios or using actual notification of potential low-volume event not expected to require disaster or MCI response to discuss and practice elements of response such as activation, space allocation, staffing, equipment, supplies, incident command, triage, disposition of current patients, and patients expected from the event.

VR Simulation

VR-based disaster and MCI preparedness and response training can contextualize concepts, plans, knowledge and skills gained from classroom and screen-based didactics, as well as tabletop exercises, into a simulated disaster/MCI environment and scenario [31]. VR apps are available that offer the opportunity to customize disaster, MCI type and specifics, the environment as well as the responding facility, organization, and agency roles and resources. A few cities have created virtual versions of their city for this purpose. VR can provide training for individuals' training independently, teaming with virtual responders or actual responders participating from their own or other environments. Interactions can include virtual patients and those accompanying

PRIDE
DISASTER DEBRIEFING SCRIPT–
APPLICATION OF TRIAGE STRATEGY CARD

Learner Code*(Example: First Pet, First Street, State, eg. FluffyElmCT):* _____ Date: _____ On

Day #1 Only: Viewed didactic video before debrief? (Circle one)   Yes   No

Instructions:
1. For each of the seven tasks listed below, check whether the task was <u>PERFORMED WELL</u> vs. <u>NEEDS WORK</u>.
2. Select **AT LEAST FIVE** of the tasks below to debrief. Limit discussion to **TWO MINUTES** only for each task.
3. For each of the five tasks you selected, follow the scripted debriefing in the row that corresponds.

Task	Team Assessment	What I observed or noticed	Why this is important / a concern	Inquiry
1–Identification of Disaster Conditions and Articulation of Disaster Triage Designation	Performed Well □	*It looked to me like you immediately identified that this was a disaster scenario and made that clear to everyone involved.*	*This is great because recognizing that local resources are overwhelmed changes the triage strategy in important ways and it is important that the entire response team operates under the same assumptions.*	*What are some of the fundamental differences between triage strategies in disasters as opposed to individual patient emergencies?*
	Needs Work □	*It wasn't clear to me that this scenario was designated a disaster.*	*This concerns me because recognition that local resources are overwhelmed has important consequences for the triage strategy and it is crucial that all members of the response team are operating under the same assumptions.*	*I was wondering what could be done differently during the initial assessment? What can be done to ensure triage principles are being used consistently?*
2 Communication with Medical Control About Disaster Resources and Coordination	Performed Well □	*After you assessed the scene and determined a disaster existed, I heard you notify medical control.*	*This is great because it allows coordination of multiple resources.*	*Please summarize the important information that should be conveyed to medical control?*
	Needs Work □	*Though it appeared that you recognized that a disaster existed, I didn't hear this communicated to medical control.*	*This is great because it allows coordination of multiple resources.*	*What information do you think is most important to convey to medical control?*
3 Triage of Moribund (Black / Blue) Patients	Performed Well □	*It looked to me like you did a great job recognizing those patients who were moribund.*	*This is great because the patient was pulseless and apneic and under disaster tri21age rules, should not consume limited resources.*	*Can you summarize what criteria you used to designate this patientmoribund?*
	Needs Work □	*It looked to me like you spent quite a bit of time attempting to resuscitate a patient who was unlikely to survive.*	*This concerns me because I worry that the time and resources spent on this patient may take away from those who are more likely to benefit from immediate care.*	*I was wondering if we can review the role of resuscitation (CPR) in a disaster situation? ,*
4–Triage of Immediate (Red) Patients	Performed Well □	*It looked to me like you accurately identified the critical patients in need of immediate medical care.*	*This is great because the patients with the most serious injuries but greatest chance of survival received care first.*	*I was wondering we could review the criteria for designation of critical patients under the (XX) triage algorithm?*
	Needs Work □	*It looked to me like there was some difficulty deciding whether a patient required immediate vs. delayed care.*	*This concerns me because the patient had critical physiology that required immediate intervention and I'm concerned that a delay in care could cause further decompensation.*	*I was wondering what parameters you used in triaging this patient?*
5 – Triage of Delayed (Yellow) Patients	Performed Well □	*It looked to me like you accurately identified the delayed patients in need of further medical care but whose physiology and injuries justified a delay.*	*This is great because this allows expenditure of resources on those requiring most immediate care.*	*I was wondering if we could review the criteria for designation of delayed patients under the (XX) triage algorithm?*
	Needs Work □	*It looked to me like there was some difficulty deciding whether a patient required immediate vs. delayed care*	*This concerns me because the patient utilized critical resources that might have been better spent on more critically ill patients in need of more immediate care.*	*I was wondering what parameters you used in triaging this patient?*
6 – Triage of Minor (Green) Patients	Performed Well □	*It looked to me like you accurately identified the minor patients who did not require further medical attention.*	*This is great because this allows expenditure of resources on those requiring most immediate care.*	*I was wondering if wecould review the criteria for designation of minorpatients under the (XX) triage algorithm?*
	Needs Work □	*It looked to me like there was some difficulty deciding whether a patient required further medical attention or not.*	*This concerns me because of the limited resources available and I'm concerned that some of those resources were allocated to a patient without significant injury.*	*I was wondering what parameters you used in triaging this patient?*

Fig. 20.7 Debriefing script used in a pediatric disaster triage curriculum for paramedics and emergency medical technicians (EMTs). (Image courtesy: Debra Wiener and Mark Cicero)

7 – Triage of Children with Special Health Care Needs	Performed Well ☐	*I was impressed at how you handled the patient with special healthcare needs.*	*It can be challenging to determine whether a patient with deficits is acutely injured as opposed to demonstrating baseline deficits but without acute injury.*	*I was wondering if you could explain your decision making in triaging this patient?*
	Nee Needs Work ds Work ☐	*It looked to me like patient with special health care needs presented a triage challenge in this scenario.*		
Overall Performance	Performed Well ☐	*You did an excellent job of sorting multiple patients efficiently.*	*It is important to limit the field triage to sorting of patients which is the primary role of the scene commander at a disaster.*	*I am wondering what the biggest challenge was in trying to move through all 10 patients in 7 minutes?*
	Needs Work ☐ NeedsWork	*It seemed to take a bit more time than expected to triage all of the patients in this scenario.*		

At conclusion of this section, please summarize by stating:

In summary, the key learning points for this scenario are:

1. *Assessing the scene before beginning triage, determining the existence of a disaster situation that may overwhelm local resources, and communicating this clearly to medical control.*
2. *Rapidly sorting patients into those who require immediate vs. delayed care, those who are dead or moribund, and those who have minor injuries that do not require further medical care.*
3. *Since our state utilizes the XX triage algorithm, lets briefly summarize the key points to each triage designation....*
4. *Recognizing the challenges posed by children with special health care needs, including separating baseline deficits from acute injury requiring medical attention.*

Any final comments or questions?

Fig. 20.7 (Continuation)

the patient. Game apps are a form of VR that involve two or more teams, usually in competition, using rules, data, and procedures to manage disaster/MCI situations. VR allows specifics of the disasters/MCIs or the environment in which they occur to be changed easily to provide training for different types of events, in different environments with different resources. VR training can be repeated at intervals deemed appropriate based on the individual or group, and for just-in-time training based on risk of a specific disaster or MCI, given factors such as local environment and/or time of year.

Live Simulation

High-fidelity simulation drills conducted within or across EMS, other community organizations, and/or hospitals provide the opportunity to test any or all elements from a single operation or function within a group or division to a multidisciplinary, multiagency community-wide test of personnel, environment, and system readiness and performance for disaster or MCI response. While the drill will center on a particular event, an all-hazard approaches should be emphasized. The expense and time that full-scale drills require limit

the frequency with which they can be conducted. It is therefore important that high-fidelity live simulation drills maintain focus on elements specific to disaster, MCI preparedness and response, and to the extent possible, are conducted after potential system weaknesses have been addressed rather than for the purpose of identifying them.

Live simulation with high-fidelity simulation mannequins and standardized patients provides an efficacious means for prehospital and hospital providers to learn principles of disaster/MCI triage and become facile with use of available triage tools appropriate for pediatric disasters and MCI victims [3, 24]. As part of triage training, healthcare providers can be challenged to decide where and in what order the patients should be transported as well as which patients are prioritized for other limited resources (e.g., diagnostic imaging, blood products, operating rooms, etc). Hospital providers should understand that, particularly with scoop and run transport, often by EMS providers with limited pediatric experience, re-triage of victims on arrival to the healthcare facility is valuable for assessing and prioritizing patient needs and allocating patient care resources. Through simulation, retention of triage skills can be assessed, and educators can determine the effectiveness of just-in-time training [25].

Simulation of disaster/MCI situations allows EMS and hospital providers, including physicians, nurses, social workers, mental health providers, unit coordinators, emergency management personnel, security, and others to learn how to decontaminate, triage, register, track, and provide and document care for child disaster victims. For example, learners can encounter multiple simulated victims of traumatic events [32], chemical attacks [33], or bombings [16]. For basic and intermediate learners, simulation educators are urged to focus on a few goals, such as decontamination of patients, the administration of pralidoxime and atropine in an organophosphate poisoning event, or lifesaving interventions like airway maneuvers and tourniquets. Advanced and experienced learners may benefit from multiple types of injury distributed across the patients, and focus on rapid stabilization, prioritization of care, and disposition within or outside the hospital. Multimodal simulation with both mannequins and patient actors may be necessary to depict a full range of injuries, illnesses, mental health manifestations, and social issues.

Team Training

Aspects of simulation-based team training unique to disaster/MCI response should highlight the incident command system that recognizes chain of command, closed-loop communication, and crisis resource management principles and practice (see Chap. 4 for details). Simulation scenarios for in-hospital response should stress that, as much as possible, providers assume their usual patient care roles unless assigned to do otherwise. For remote disaster response, scenarios should address practice based on knowledge and skills rather than titles, the possibility that providers may need to perform evaluation and management tasks that they perform rarely in children, and/or are outside of their routine scope of practice, and the likelihood that providers may never have worked together or even know each other. Performance evaluation and debriefing should focus on team performance. Debriefing focused on teamwork should include defining and performing roles, communication, and team dynamics (see Chap. 3).

Another consideration for disaster and MCI simulation-based training is mental health response and psychological first aid [34]. The inclusion of anxious, scared, or angry children and caregivers increases the reality of simulation and presses learners to employ field techniques to address the acute psychological impact of disaster/MCIs [35]. Responders should also be trained to expect that the situation might impose considerable stress for themselves as individuals due to the chaotic environment, severity of injury and illness of victims, uncertainty about the event that has taken place, and concerns about the safety of one's own family and friends who may also be victims. As discussed earlier, careful follow-up of participants may be warranted.

Just-in-Time Training

Just-in-time training is training that is conducted immediately before an anticipated event, and preferably in the same clinical environment where the event is likely to occur. When healthcare personnel are preparing for imminent response to a disaster/MCI, just-in-time simulation provides a means for review of the kinds of patients and variety of illnesses and injuries that will be encountered, a review of activation, decontamination, registration and triage protocols, resource allocation, and specific disaster/MCI-related patient care. For deployment to remote disaster, national or international, just-in-time training in addition to information about the disaster itself and its impact on people and infrastructure should also include information regarding the geography, weather, culture, economics, and politics of the region as relevant to disaster response and requirements for personnel preparedness and safety. The efficacy of simulation for healthcare worker's disaster preparation has been established for domestic and international response [36].

Use of Simulation in Disaster and MCI Systems Testing

Disasters and MCIs are unpredictable, in that when and where they will occur are difficult to predict. As part of planning, simulation can be used to assess the number of patients an EMS system or hospital can reasonably treat, strategies for allocation of hospital space, staff, equipment and supplies, and to compare the relative efficacy of response strategies under different circumstances. Perhaps, the first simulation in which a person participates happens long before professional education. School disaster drills provide a means for determining the speed of building evacuation and to test student tracking [37]. In full-scale exercises, a school disaster drill can be the starting point for an evaluation of EMS and hospital response.

Exercises for EMS providers combine infrequent events (disasters/MCIs) with relatively infrequent patients (children). Simulation disaster/MCI response testing for EMS systems can reveal gaps between ideal care for individual patients and the population of casualties, and also gaps in disaster and MCI response efficacy [38]. Debriefing the learners, evaluating the exercise, generating a list of specific actions to be taken to improve future performance, and setting a date for a follow-up exercise increase the likelihood that an EMS system will improve its ability to provide care to child disaster/MCI victims [39]. The HSEEP system, shown in Fig. 20.6, provides a model for integrating simulation into continuous systems evaluation and improvement.

There are many strategies for triaging child disaster/MCI victims [40, 41]. Whether it works best to (1) identify children with the most acute illness or injury or (2) to improve outcomes for the population of disaster victims will depend on the specifics of each disaster and the resources available for response. Simulation offers a means to compare outcomes when existing triage systems are used and a means for comparing novel systems to existing methods [42, 43].

The extent to which existing ED resources, which are already chronically taxed in some EDs, will be stressed or overwhelmed will also depend on the specifics of the disaster/MCI and on triage strategies and practice. Simulation in the ED and hospital setting allows for testing of disaster/MCI plans [44, 45]. Again, following an HSEEP-based evaluation system and setting measurable post-simulation objectives are key to improving the response plan. Full-scale exercises integrate the prehospital response with the response of the receiving facility.

Chemical, biological, and radiological incidents, whether they are natural or intentional in origin, create an ongoing hazard for healthcare workers and patients alike. Live simulation is the best way to experience what it feels like to don a hazmat suit and deliver care and communicate while wearing the suit. The importance of personal protective equipment has been underscored by the Ebola pandemic of 2014 which began in West Africa (Fig. 20.8). Furthermore, live simulation may reveal bottlenecks and challenges in on-scene and hospital decontamination practices [46], including setting up and using decontamination equipment, disrobing and washing children with soap and water and passing off to providers for further triage, evaluation, and management. The US Government Agency for Healthcare Research and Quality provides a video detailing pediatric decontamination (Fig. 20.9). Pediatric considerations for decontamination include the risk of hypothermia, modesty issues, holding slippery, nonambulatory children, patient identification, addressing fears, and the need to decontaminate special equipment, such as wheelchairs [47].

Another practical test of disaster/MCI response systems, both on-scene and in the hospital, is patient registration, tracking, documentation, and reunification. Patient registration strategies that allow creation of medical records prior to or immediately on victim arrival without dependence on knowing victim identity have been developed. Patient tracking in disasters/MCIs is facilitated by simple wristbands, barcode, and GPS tracking [48]. Facial recognition technology and digital images may be used to expedite and increase the likelihood of safe, secure reunification of children with their caregivers [49, 50]. Simulations involving minors, including nonverbal children, separated from their parents can be used to test patient tracking and reunification plans.

Simulation also provides an opportunity to test hospital back-up systems to mitigate internal infrastructure compromise and hospital evacuation with patient transfer if disaster/MCI results in an inadequately functioning or unsafe structural environment. Simulation for response in austere environments may be used to test systems to mobilize team members, set up and functioning of mobile healthcare facility structures, equipment and supplies, and communication systems.

Future Directions

There are several important directions for mass casualty and disaster research over the next decade. First, efforts will be made to test the disaster readiness of larger systems, such as the interaction of fire services, EMS, and hospitals, with public health services. Next, researchers will focus their efforts on the efficacy of just-in-time training, and the frequency of educational reinoculation needed to maintain readiness in health systems. Additionally, simulation will be used to test the relative efficacy of pediatric disaster protocols, including triage methodologies.

Fig. 20.8 Healthcare workers don personal protective equipment in Liberia during the West African Ebola epidemic. (Source: www.usaid.gov)

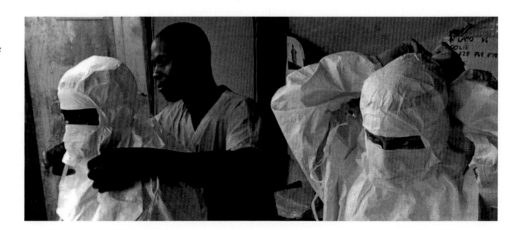

Fig. 20.9 During decontamination, the *hot zone* is where contaminated patients enter the facility, the *warm zone* is the area where the decontamination process occurs, and the *cold zone* is the where clean patients enter the hospital property. (Source: www.ahrq.gov)

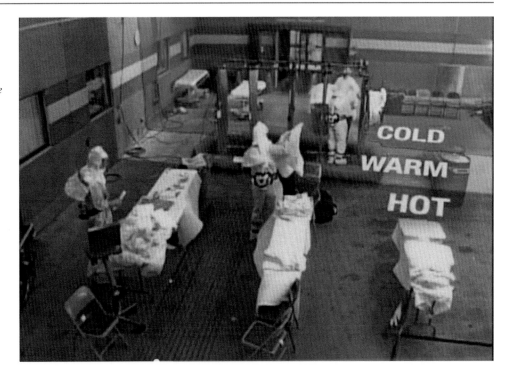

Conclusions

Simulation is ideal for disaster and MCI response training, particularly in pediatrics. An understanding of the elements of disasters/MCIs and preparedness and response for them is important for developing and delivering appropriate training. Classroom and screen-based didactics and high- and low-fidelity mannequin-based simulation, including tabletop exercises, VR, and live drills as needed, should be combined strategically to provide effective and efficient training. Simulation should focus on principles, situations, and practices unique to disasters and MCIs.

References

1. American Academy of Pediatrics Committee on Pediatric Emergency Medicine, American Academy of Pediatrics Committee on Medical Liability, Task Force on Terrorism. The pediatrician and disaster preparedness. Pediatrics. 2006;117:560–5.
2. Kim SJ, Kim CH, Shin SD, Lee SC, Park JO, Sung J. Incidence and mortality rates of disasters and mass casualty incidents in Korea: a population-based cross-sectional study, 2000–2009. J Korean Med Sci. 2013;28:658–66.
3. Cicero MX, Brown L, Overly F, et al. Creation and Delphi-method refinement of pediatric disaster triage simulations. Prehosp Emerg Care. 2014;18(2):282–9.
4. Connor SB. When and why health care personnel respond to a disaster: the state of the science. Prehosp Disaster Med. 2014;29:270–4.
5. Cone DC, Cummings BA. Hospital disaster staffing: if you call, will they come? Am J Disaster Med. 2006;1:28–36.
6. Thomalla F, Downing T, Spanger-Siegfried E, Han G, Rockström J. Reducing hazard vulnerability: towards a common approach between disaster risk reduction and climate adaptation. Disasters. 2006;30:39–48.
7. Arnold JL. Disaster medicine in the 21st century: future hazards, vulnerabilities, and risk. Prehosp Disaster Med. 2002;17:3–11.
8. Lerner E, Schwartz R, Coule P, Pirrallo R. Use of SALT triage in a simulated mass-casualty incident. Prehosp Emerg Care. 2010;14:21–5.
9. D'Andrea SM, Goralnick E, Kayden SR. Boston Marathon bombings: overview of an emergency department response to a mass casualty incident. Disaster Med Public Health Prep. 2013;7:118–21.
10. Bulut Y, Güven M, Otlu B, et al. Acute otitis media and respiratory viruses. Eur J Pediatr. 2007;166:223–8.
11. Guha-Sapir D, van Panhuis WG, Lagoutte J. Short communication: patterns of chronic and acute diseases after natural disasters—a study from the International Committee of the Red Cross field hospital in Banda Aceh after the 2004 Indian Ocean tsunami. Trop Med Int Health. 2007;12:1338–41.
12. Brantley MD, Lu H, Barfield WD, Holt JB, Williams A. Mapping US pediatric hospitals and subspecialty critical care for public health preparedness and disaster response, 2008. Disaster Med Public Health Prep. 2012;6:117–25.
13. Rubinson L, Hick JL, Hanfling DG, et al. Definitive care for the critically ill during a disaster: a framework for optimizing critical care surge capacity: from a Task Force for Mass Critical Care summit meeting, January 26–27, 2007, Chicago, IL. Chest. 2008;133:18S–31S.
14. Kollek D, Karwowska A, Neto G, Sandvik H, Lyons S, Spivey J, et al. Pediatrics in disasters. In: Kollek D, editor. Disaster preparedness for healthcare facilities. Shelton: People's Medical Publishing House-USA; 2013.
15. Brandenburg MA, Arneson WL. Pediatric disaster response in developed countries: ten guiding principles. Am J Disaster Med. 2007;2:151–62.
16. Kerns CE, Elkins RM, Carpenter AL, Chou T, Green JG, Comer JS. Caregiver distress, shared traumatic exposure, and child ad-

justment among area youth following the 2013 Boston Marathon bombing. J Affect Disord. 2014;167:50–5.

17. Kollek D, Karwowska A. Populations at risk-paediatrics. Radiat Prot Dosimetry. 2009;134:191–2.

18. Langhan M, Keshavarz R, Richardson LD. How comfortable are emergency physicians with pediatric patients? J Emerg Med. 2004;26:465–9.

19. Berger JT. Resource stewardship in disasters: alone at the bedside. J Clin Ethics. 2012;23:336–7.

20. Hick JL, Hanfling D, Cantrill SV. Allocating scarce resources in disasters: emergency department principles. Ann Emerg Med. 2012;59:177–87.

21. Timm N, Reeves S. A mass casualty incident involving children and chemical decontamination. Disaster Manag Response. 2007;5:49–55.

22. Chung S, Shannon M. Reuniting children with their families during disasters: a proposed plan for greater success. Am J Disaster Med. 2007;2:113–7.

23. McCormick LC, Hites L, Wakelee JF, Rucks AC, Ginter PM. Planning and executing complex large-scale exercises. J Public Health Manag Pract. 2014;20(Suppl 5):S37–43.

24. Cicero MX, Auerbach MA, Zigmont J, Riera A, Ching K, Baum CR. Simulation training with structured debriefing improves residents' pediatric disaster triage performance. Prehosp Disaster Med. 2012;27:239–44.

25. Franc-Law J, Ingrassia P, Ragazzoni L, Corte F. The effectiveness of training with an emergency department simulator on medical student performance in a simulated disaster. CJEM. 2010;12:27–32.

26. Silenas R, Akins R, Parrish A, Edwards J. Developing disaster preparedness competence: an experiential learning exercise for multiprofessional education. Teach Learn Med. 2008;20:62–8.

27. Scott JA, Miller GT, Issenberg SB, et al. Skill improvement during emergency response to terrorism training. Prehosp Emerg Care. 2006;10:507–14.

28. Kotora JG, Clancy T, Manzon L, Malik V, Louden RJ, Merlin MA. Active shooter in the emergency department: a scenario-based training approach for healthcare workers. Am J Disaster Med. 2014;9:39–51.

29. Dausey DJ, Buehler JW, Lurie N. Designing and conducting tabletop exercises to assess public health preparedness for man-made and naturally occurring biological threats. BMC Public Health. 2007;7:92.

30. Leow JJ, Brundage SI, Kushner AL, et al. Mass casualty incident training in a resource-limited environment. Br J Surg. 2012;99:356–61.

31. Hsu EB, Li Y, Bayram JD, Levinson D, Yang S, Monahan C. State of virtual reality based disaster preparedness and response training. PLoS Curr. 2013;5:p ii.

32. Lowe C. Pediatric prehospital medicine in mass casualty incidents. J Trauma. 2009;67:S161–7.

33. Foltin G, Tunik M, Curran J, et al. Pediatric nerve agent poisoning: medical and operational considerations for emergency medical services in a large American city. Pediatr Emerg Care. 2006;22:239–44.

34. Gold J, Montano Z, Shields S, et al. Pediatric disaster preparedness in the medical setting: integrating mental health. Am J Disaster Med. 2009;4:137–46.

35. Pfefferbaum B, Newman E, Nelson SD. Mental health interventions for children exposed to disasters and terrorism. J Child Adolesc Psychopharmacol. 2014;24:24–31.

36. Vincent DS, Berg BW, Ikegami K. Mass-casualty triage training for international healthcare workers in the Asia-Pacific region using manikin-based simulations. Prehosp Disaster Med. 2009;24:206–13.

37. Ramirez M, Kubicek K, Peek-Asa C, Wong M. Accountability and assessment of emergency drill performance at schools. Fam Community Health. 2009;32:105–14.

38. Nathawad R, Roblin PM, Pruitt D, Arquilla B. Addressing the gaps in preparation for quarantine. Prehosp Disaster Med. 2013;28:132–8.

39. Savoia E, Preston J, Biddinger PD. A consensus process on the use of exercises and after action reports to assess and improve public health emergency preparedness and response. Prehosp Disaster Med. 2013;28:305–8.

40. Wallis LA, Carley S. Comparison of paediatric major incident primary triage tools. Emerg Med J. 2006;23:475–8.

41. Cross KP, Cicero MX. Head-to-Head comparison of disaster triage methods in pediatric, adult, and geriatric patients. Ann Emerg Med. 2013;61:668–76.e667.

42. Cone DC, Serra J, Kurland L. Comparison of the SALT and Smart triage systems using a virtual reality simulator with paramedic students. Eur J Emerg Med. 2011;18(6):314–21.

43. Vincent D, Sherstyuk A, Burgess L, Connolly K. Teaching mass casualty triage skills using immersive three-dimensional virtual reality. Acad Emerg Med. 2008;15:1160–5.

44. Ballow S, Behar S, Claudius I, Stevenson K, Neches R, Upperman J. Hospital-based disaster preparedness for pediatric patients: how to design a realistic set of drill victims. Am J Disaster Med. 2008;3:171–80.

45. Nager A, Khanna K. Emergency department surge: models and practical implications. J Trauma. 2009;67:S96–9.

46. Fertel B, Kohlhoff S, Roblin P, Arquilla B. Lessons from the "Clean Baby 2007" pediatric decontamination drill. Am J Disaster Med. 2009;4:77–85.

47. Freyberg C, Arquilla B, Fertel B, et al. Disaster preparedness: hospital decontamination and the pediatric patient–guidelines for hospitals and emergency planners. Prehosp Disaster Med. 2008;23:166–73.

48. Cole SL, Siddiqui J, Harry DJ, Sandrock CE. WiFi RFID demonstration for resource tracking in a statewide disaster drill. Am J Disaster Med. 2011;6:155–62.

49. Chung S, Shannon M. Reuniting children with their families during disasters: a proposed plan for greater success. Am J Disaster Med. 2007;2:113–7.

50. Brandenburg MA, Watkins SM, Brandenburg KL, Schieche C. Operation Child-ID: reunifying children with their legal guardians after Hurricane Katrina. Disasters. 2007;31:277–87.

Simulation for Pediatric Anesthesia

Tobias Everett, John Zhong and M. Dylan Bould

Simulation Pearls

1. Pediatric anesthesia is a multidisciplinary team pursuit—consider interprofessional simulation where possible.
2. Full-body mannequin simulation is not the panacea in pediatric anesthesia simulation—do not overlook screen-based simulation for teaching in the operating room or standardized parents for perioperative communication challenges.
3. Procedures in pediatric anesthesia rarely translate seamlessly from adult anesthesia—use appropriately-sized task trainers prior to attempting procedures on children.
4. Simulation-based refreshers and updates are useful for anesthesiologists practicing in community settings with occasional responsibility for pediatric anesthesia or resuscitation.

Introduction

The earliest documented use of pediatric anesthesia was in 1842 [1]. From the outset, it was recognized that pediatric patients reacted differently to anesthesia than adults. William Morton, one of the earliest proponents of ether anesthesia, was reluctant to use it in children due to more frequent nausea and vomiting compared to adults [2]. Interestingly, the first documented death attributable to anesthesia was in 1848—a 15-year-old named Hannah Greener who was anesthetized with chloroform for ingrown toenail removal [3].

With the first pediatric anesthesia textbook by Dr. Morton Digby-Leigh in 1948 [4] and pediatric anesthesia training programs established by Dr. Robert Smith in the 1950s [5], pediatric anesthesia emerged as a distinct specialty. Pediatric anesthesia fellowship training has been available since the 1970s, but the Accreditation Council for Graduate Medical Education (ACGME) officially recognized pediatric anesthesia subspecialty training only in 1997. Some programs offer 2-year advanced pediatric anesthesia fellowships providing additional training in cardiac anesthesia, education, pain management, palliative care, research, and quality improvement [6].

In the UK, The Royal College of Anaesthetists (RCoA) has actively promoted pediatric anesthesia as a distinct specialty, periodically publishing guidelines on pediatric anesthesia services. Its most recent guidelines recommend annual multidisciplinary scenario-based training as part of the process of physician revalidation [7]. Many countries in continental Europe have adopted the Recommendations on Training in Pediatric Anesthesia by the European Federation of Associations of Pediatric Anesthesia [8]. In Japan, by contrast, a survey of members of the Japanese Society of Anesthesiologists published in 2006 revealed that most members felt it was premature to subspecialize in pediatric anesthesia [9].

Since the introduction of the first pediatric computerized mannequin in 1999, there are now several commercially available mannequins, of various ages/sizes, suitable for pediatric anesthesia simulation. Anesthesiologists have been early adopters of simulation as a teaching aid and pediatric anesthesiologists are no exception [10]. Simulation-based pediatric anesthesia training offers an opportunity for the rehearsal of clinical skills and judgment required to provide anesthesia to children, without the risk of patient detriment.

T. Everett (✉)
Department of Anesthesia and Pain Medicine, The Hospital for Sick Children, University of Toronto, Toronto, ON, Canada
e-mail: tobias.everett@sickkids.ca

J. Zhong
Department of Anesthesiology and Pain Management, UTSW Medical Center, Children's Medical Center of Dallas, Dallas, TX, USA
e-mail: John.zhong@childrens.com

M. D. Bould
Department of Anesthesiology, University of Ottawa, Children's Hospital of Eastern Ontario, Ottawa, Canada

© Springer International Publishing Switzerland 2016
V. J. Grant, A. Cheng (eds.), *Comprehensive Healthcare Simulation: Pediatrics,*
Comprehensive Healthcare Simulation, DOI 10.1007/978-3-319-24187-6_21

Simulation-Based Education for Pediatric Anesthesia

Despite recent significant advances in the other areas of pediatric anesthesia simulation discussed here, the discipline remains predominantly used for the purpose of education. There are a number of considerations particular to pediatric anesthesia simulation-based education that distinguish it from adult anesthesia simulation and pediatric simulation in related specialties (e.g., Pediatric Emergency Medicine or Pediatric Critical Care). In this section, we will discuss those considerations under the themes of type of learners, focus of learning objectives, learning environment, and mode of simulation. We will then describe some task trainers specific to pediatric anesthesia and finish the section with an example of a pediatric anesthesia curriculum.

Type of Learners

Pediatric anesthesia simulation programs must be learner focused and designed and delivered sensitive to the nature of the intended learners. Depending on the context, anesthesia may be delivered by a variety of practitioners, assisted by other practitioners with a variable level of specific training and experience. For example, independent anesthesiologists may practice full-time in a tertiary level pediatric hospital or conversely may have an occasional commitment to anesthetizing children in a community or general hospital. The nature of their day-to-day pediatric anesthesia challenges will vary in intensity, as will their comfort level with certain adverse events. These must be considered and accommodated in the curriculum construction. In teaching hospitals, house staff (residents, registrars, etc.) form part of the anesthesia care team, whereas in a community hospital, the team will be leaner, without the second anesthesiologist immediately available. If trainee anesthesiologists are among the learner group, then consideration should be given to their level of training in both anesthesia generally and specifically in pediatric anesthesia.

In most developed world contexts, the principal anesthesia provider will be a medical doctor (MD) with a proportion of their responsibilities delegated to a qualified deputy. However, it is important to recall that the majority of anesthesia delivered worldwide is done so by non-physician anesthetists or nursepractitioner anesthetists (NPAs), and if they are to be included in a learner group, the content should be adjusted accordingly. The nature of the trained assistance available to the anesthesia provider is country specific and should also receive attention. As is clear, the delivery of anesthesia to children can involve a range of healthcare providers, and, consequently, the simulation of pediatric anesthesia should be sensitive to which of that range will be constituents of the learner group.

Combinations of Learners Types—Pediatric Anesthesia Interprofessional Education (IPE)

The pediatric anesthesiologist does not function in isolation but alongside multiple other disciplines and specialties. IPE offers benefits in terms of team building, sharing mental models and decision-making priorities, and understanding the agenda and motivations of coworkers (see Chap. 15). The simulated clinical environment is the ideal place to explore these issues and confer insight into the thought processes of other team members.

From a logistical perspective, coordinating multiple healthcare providers simultaneously to free themselves from a busy clinical workload is a significant challenge. The alternative is to create a uniprofessional session targeted at anesthesiologists and script confederates to act out the roles of the other team members, accepting the increased faculty requirement. The selecting, briefing, and scripting of faculty confederates or actors (sometimes termed Embedded Simulation Personnel, ESP) is important to consider and is covered elsewhere in this book (see Chaps. 2 and 8). In overview, the confederates are scripted such that they are helpful but do not show initiative, and their responses should not be expansive such that they lead the primary learner. There is sometimes a temptation for the confederate to deliver excessive quantities of information or assistance (perhaps to demonstrate their own competence) but in doing so reduce the impact for the primary learner. Conversely, if the confederate is determined that the learner should figure it out for themselves, this can result in them adopting an unrealistically unhelpful or even obstructive stance. This is also undesirable and may lead to poor learning outcomes. For these reasons, using actual care providers would be preferable to ESP, especially when evaluating interprofessional team-based skills.

Focus of Learning Objectives

As in other acute care specialties, the clinical challenges encountered in pediatric anesthesia may be categorized into medical management, technical skills, and nontechnical skills (variably termed human factors or crisis resource management). It is clear that these are analogous to the three realms of knowledge, skills, and attitudes that so frequently arise in competence assessments. Each is amenable to simulation-based learning, but the nature of the simulation session constructed must be sensitive to the focus of the learning objectives. There is often some overlap of these realms and scenarios with combinations of learning objectives being common.

Medical Management Learning Objectives

Simulation sessions aimed at imparting knowledge and experience of the management of medical crises in pediatric anesthesia are well suited to computerized mannequin-based simulation, with anesthesiologists as the participants and faculty confederates playing the roles of other practitioners present in the scenario. These scenarios present an opportunity for the anesthesiologist to rehearse the management strategies of various low-frequency, high-stakes events that might be considered the fundamentals of pediatric anesthesia emergencies. When the focus of the learning objectives is medical management, faculty as confederates can standardize the responses of the other practitioners, thereby controlling for human factors (i.e., conflict resolution, prioritization, resource utilization, etc.), especially if the scenario is designed to achieve a combination of medical management and non-technical objectives (see Chap. 2).

Human Factors Learning Objectives

Simulated operating room crises with a focus on non-technical skills (or human factors) are well suited to IPE. In this context, challenges are written into the scenario which obliges the interprofessional team to tackle issues such as task management, decision-making, conflicting priorities, and leadership (see Chap. 4). While interprofessional scenarios involving anesthesiologists might have an element of anesthesia-specific content, each of the disciplines involved in IPE should stand to derive an equal benefit from the exercise.

Table 21.1 lists some potential participants for an interprofessional exercise involving anesthesia.

Technical Skills Learning Objectives

There are many skills specific to pediatric anesthesia where simulation is a suitable training tool but for which computerized mannequin whole-body simulation is unnecessary. Part-task trainers are available to conduct deliberate practice or mastery learning exercises before exposing a child to a novice anesthesiologist. The portability of the devices means the context of this learning may be with multiple learners at a scheduled session, or *just-in-time* training for a single learner immediately before undertaking the real-life procedure. The following section describes some part-task trainers specific to pediatric anesthesia as well as the notion of *hybrid* simulation involving the combination of multiple simulation modalities.

Environments for Pediatric Anesthesia Simulation

The range of procedures for which children require anesthesia is more extensive and diverse than in the adult population. As a pediatric anesthesiologist may deliver patient care in multiple locations around the hospital, it follows that simulation activities should mirror this diversity. Any clinical area where an anesthesiologist provides patient care may also host an in situ session or be recreated in a simulation laboratory. There are a few nuances to be considered with each location.

Operating Room

The majority of anesthesia simulations will be staged in the operating room. Environmental realism is achieved if the anesthesia workstation is the same make and model as in the learners' home institution. Where this is not possible, a thorough orientation to the anesthesia machine is required during the introduction of the simulation session. Similarly, learners should be oriented to the other equipment and disposables and informed which may be opened, manipulated, drawn-up, injected, etc. Operating room furniture, sets, trays, and disposables can be acquired to augment the realism of the simulated environment. Supply carts should be stocked with the complete range of disposables for every size of pediatric patient. Even if the same-sized mannequin is used for all simulations, the learners should still be exposed to the challenge of selecting appropriately sized equipment. Confederates are required to take the role of other operating room team members. This should include a trained assistant (e.g., induction nurse or anesthesia assistant) and usually a surgeon. Whether there will be a second anesthesiologist available should be considered. In the context of interprofessional operating room simulation, fewer confederates are necessary as the whole team is represented by the learners. The operating room is a good setting for crisis scenarios, human factor scenarios, interprofessional team training, and testing feasibility and utility of algorithms and checklists. Furthermore, in situ operating room scenarios are useful for trialing novel

Table 21.1 Example of potential participants for an anesthesia-focused IPE session

Anesthesiologist	Anesthesia assistant	Nursing	Proceduralist	Other Specialties	Other support staff
Staff/attending/consultant	Induction nurse	Operating room	Surgeon(s)	Intensive care staff	Operating room aides
Fellow/senior trainee	Anesthesia assistant	Diagnostic imaging	Endoscopist	Emergency room staff	Blood bank
Resident/registrar	Nurse practitioner	Emergency room	Oncologist	Radiology staff	Transport
Medical student	Respiratory therapist		Cardiologist		
	Operating department practitioner		Interventional radiologist		

IPE interprofessional education

Fig. 21.1 Otolaryngology operating room in situ interprofessional simulation. (Author's image, with permission)

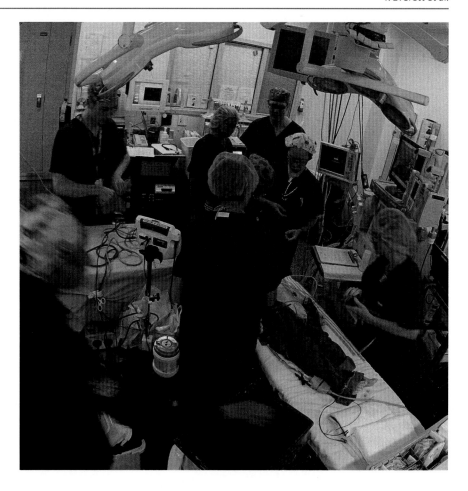

operating room processes or equipment (e.g., introduction of new anesthesia workstations) or for exposing latent safety threats (see Fig. 21.1; see Chap. 5).

Cardiac Operating Room

The complex interprofessional processes involved in cardiac surgery that include the interplay of surgeons, anesthesiologists, perfusionists, and nurses are ideal for rehearsal or *drilling* in a simulated context. The Orpheus Perfusion Simulator® (Terumo, Ann Arbor, MI) [11] has allowed for the creation of in situ hybrid simulation team training programs, where the perfusion simulator is used alongside other simulation modalities in whole-team exercises [12, 13].

Perioperative Medicine

Simulation is a useful modality for exploring preoperative and postoperative issues. Assessing a child's readiness for general anesthesia or preparing for emergency anesthesia is perhaps overlooked as an application for simulation. On occasion, the best decision an anesthesiologist can make is *not* to anesthetize the patient at that given point—this can be simulated by creating scenarios in the preoperative phase where the anesthesiologist must collect information, assess the patient, and prepare prior to an urgent surgery. They must also make a judgment regarding how best to proceed safely, whether to summon assistance, selection, and preparation of

Table 21.2 Pediatric anesthesia standardized patient/parent scenarios

History taking or examination
Seeking consent for procedures
Disclosing an adverse event (e.g., medication error, intraoperative complication, or emergence delirium)
Communication challenges (e.g., dissatisfied parent who witnessed a combative induction)
Explaining the conduct of anesthesia in lay terms to an anxious parent or adolescent

emergency medications, etc. This can all be accomplished with the added time pressure of a mannequin with deteriorating vital signs. Other perioperative scenarios can include classroom-based communication stations where a learner must conduct a difficult conversation with a standardized parent or patient. Table 21.2 gives some examples of these.

Postoperative complications in the post-anesthesia care unit are another topic amenable to simulation, where compromise of the airway, ventilation, hemodynamics, or mental status can require rapid assessment and intervention. Emergence delirium is a pediatric anesthesia situation that is more challenging to simulate acutely, but explaining an episode of emergence delirium to an anxious parent (i.e., confederate) makes a useful postoperative communication, disclosure, and professionalism station (see Chap. 23 for details).

Trauma Room, Emergency Department

Pediatric anesthesiologists are pivotal members of the trauma team. Simulations conducted in situ in the trauma room have the potential to address multiple issues simultaneously. They can cover topics of medical management and human factors, but also expose latent errors in the complex processes necessary to coordinate all team members in the cooperative delivery of care. Consideration must be given to how simulation will disrupt care of real patients, and a contingency plan must be formulated in the event when the trauma room is suddenly needed for real patient care. Commonly, the imminent arrival of a real trauma case is flagged in advance by the paramedic team, such that the simulation paraphernalia can be uninstalled in sufficient time to allow admission of the real patient. Feasibility of this approach has to be judged based on the frequency of trauma calls in a given center. Faculty should agree in advance the extent to which participants are expected to seek and open equipment and disposables. To access everything as they would in reality increases environmental and conceptual realism but depletes stock and mandates rigorous restocking and checking of carts as after a real patient encounter.

Off-Site Pediatric Anesthesia

Pediatric anesthesia is employed for much more than surgical operations. Painful or unpleasant procedures are conducted in multiple locations around the children's hospital that require the services of an anesthesiologist. Examples include magnetic resonance imaging, image-guided therapy, cardiac catheterization laboratory, hematology/oncology ward (e.g., for bone marrow aspirations and lumbar punctures), gastrointestinal endoscopy unit, and burns wards (e.g., for dressing changes). It is of particular benefit to run simulations in these areas that are rarely challenged by adverse events.

Modes of Pediatric Anesthesia Simulation

Full-Body Computerized Mannequin

Many medical simulation companies now make pediatric versions of their simulation mannequins. Neonate, infant, and child mannequins are available with varying levels of functionality. These are described further in a separate section of this book (Chap. 10). They each have their strengths and weaknesses, but these are not specific to pediatric anesthesia and, as such, there is not one mannequin that stands out as particularly well-suited to pediatric anesthesia simulation. If the purchase of a new mannequin is being considered, it is crucial that educators from all the services who will use the mannequin are invited to the product demonstrations provided by the industry representatives. This gives the opportunity prior to purchase for end users to inspect the product for suitability in their specialty. Most of the mainstream high-fidelity mannequins can be intubated and ventilated via a manual ventilation device, anesthesia workstation, or standalone ventilator. They exhibit realistic airway pressures which can usually be manipulated (depending on the mannequin in question). Of note is that some infant mannequins have lungs that are undersized for the size of the patient, so that when mechanically ventilated, the tidal volumes accommodated are in the order or 2 mL/kg. Although this is unrealistically low, the learner can be oriented to this at the start of the session. If it is important to the anesthesia educator to achieve realism in this regard, then that specification should be sought and confirmed prior to purchase (see Fig. 21.2; Chap. 10 for details).

Fig. 21.2 Uniprofessional full-body computerized mannequin simulation in a simulation laboratory. (Author's image, used with permission)

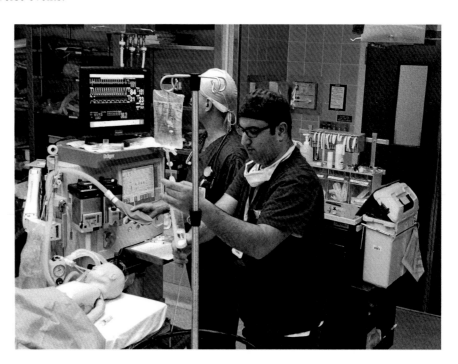

Simulated Parents or Patients

Standardized patients and parents (actors) are probably underused in pediatric anesthesia simulation but are powerful tools and, aside from organizing the actor and script, require the least administration/set-up. As described earlier, standardized parents and patients are useful for re-creating the perioperative communication challenges and difficult discussions that arise in pediatric anesthesia. Some examples are given in Table 21.2 (see Chap. 8 for details).

Screen-Based Simulation

Many of the decision-making challenges in pediatric anesthesia can be simulated at a desk, using software installed on a personal computer or mobile device. Virtual patients can be introduced and a scenario played out on-screen with opportunities for the participants to direct the management by selecting predefined options with the simulation storyboard unfolding accordingly (see Chap. 9). Examples of these facilities include the Virtual Interactive Case System (VICS) (Toronto, ON, Canada) [14] and Anesoft (Laguna Niguel, CA, USA) [15]. Screen-based simulations have been shown to be associated with improved performance on subsequent mannequin-based scenarios [16]. There are numerous mobile device applications that apply to pediatric anesthesia [17], but among those which have a simulation education angle is ET-Yale, an infant endotracheal intubation trainer [18] (MySmartSimulations®, Saratoga Springs, NY, USA; see Fig. 21.3). There are other screen-based anesthesia simulators that may be configured (by age, weight, and other variables) to run pediatric cases. GasMan software (San Ramon, CA, USA) [19], which allows trainers and trainees to run volatile anesthesia simulations, and another example is iTIVA [20], which allows a total intravenous anesthesia regimen to be entered before the simulation is run and the pharmacokinetic data for that simulation displayed graphically. The medication regimen can then be manipulated and the impact on plasma and effect-site concentration observed.

Pediatric Anesthesia Task Training

In general, task trainers that are specific to pediatric anesthesia are sparse. There are useful task trainers for anesthesia, but these are often not available in pediatric versions. There are other task trainers for pediatrics, but these are not anesthesia specific (e.g., venous cannulation and lumbar puncture). There are many examples, both published and anecdotal, of pediatric anesthesiologists improvising task trainers to fill a gap in the commercial market. Generic pediatric task trainers are considered elsewhere in this book. What follows is a description of task trainers that are specific to pediatric anesthesia.

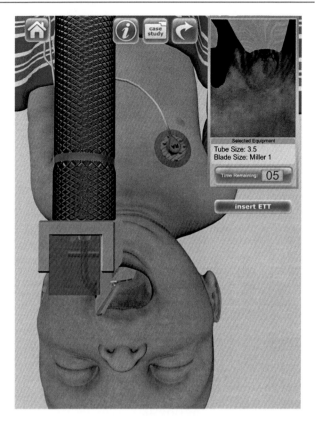

Fig. 21.3 Screenshot of ET-Yale screen-based intubation trainer. (Used with permission of Marc Auerbach, Yale University, New Haven, Connecticut, USA, and mySmartSimulations, Inc.)

Pediatric Airway Trainers

Many manufacturers carry baby, infant, and child head and neck airway trainers in their product line. They can be used for bag-mask ventilation and for the sizing and insertion of oropharyngeal, nasopharyngeal, and other supraglottic airways. At most, the learner can perform direct laryngoscopy and endotracheal intubation, although this is not universal to all head and neck task trainers, so faculty should be clear on the specifications before purchase (see Chap. 10). Similarly, some airway task trainers have a realistic nasal cavity and nasopharynx, for the nasal approach to fiberoptic intubation, whereas others do not. Also available are abnormal airway task trainers. For example, AirSim Pierre Robin® (TruCorp, Belfast, UK; Fig. 21.4) features the airway morphology of a baby with Pierre Robin sequence and allows for the simulation and deliberate practice of difficult airway solutions. A few manufacturers also produce pediatric cricothyrotomy simulators (e.g., Simulaids, Saugerties, NY, USA) which are particularly useful for running hybrid simulations involving a pediatric *can't intubate, can't oxygenate* scenario.

An important component of pediatric anesthesia is the selection of age/size-appropriate airway devices. Whether these are laryngoscope blades (sizes or designs), video laryngoscopes, fiberoptic bronchoscopes, endotracheal tubes, or all manner of supraglottic devices, the devices will not

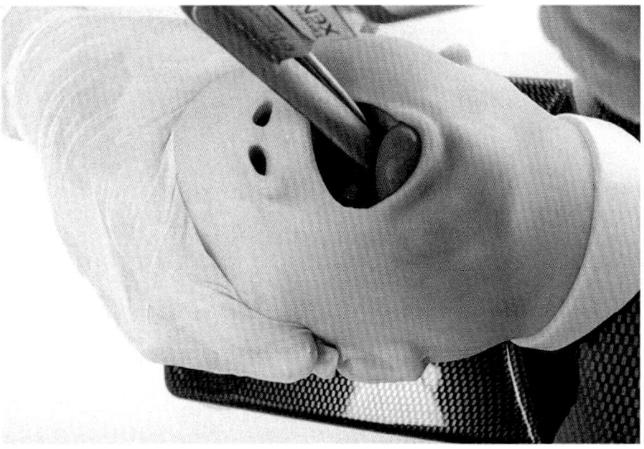

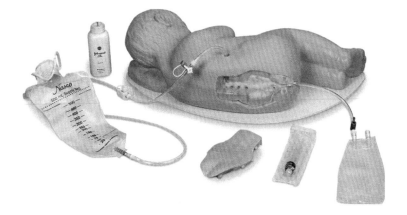

Fig. 21.4 TruCorp AirSim Pierre Robin airway task trainer. (Used with permission of TruCorp Ltd.)

function as planned if incorrectly sized. The simulation laboratory is a good context in which to encounter these challenges and practice using these devices. The limited physical realism of the airway trainers does not negatively impact the benefit to the trainee of handling and manipulating the various difficult airway devices. Indeed, in some airway training courses, the task trainer does not even resemble an airway, instead being a black-box obstacle course through which the trainee can manipulate the fiberoptic bronchoscope to visualize a target at the end.

Pediatric Regional Anesthesia Trainers

Simulation-based pediatric regional anesthesia training programs have been shown to be associated with an increase and retention of cognitive and technical skills in the techniques [21]. Due to its crossover applications, pediatric lumbar puncture task trainers are commonplace. They permit intrathecal injection so as to allow the simulation-based mastery learning of spinal anesthetic administration and all the associated procedures (aseptic technique, skin preparation, draping, etc.). Task trainers for other types of pediatric regional anesthesia are less common, although are available.

The Pediatric Caudal Injection Simulator (eNasco, Fort Atkinson WI, USA; Fig. 21.5) is one such example that allows learners to practice the commonest of pediatric regional anesthetic techniques [22]. There is a gap in the market when it comes to other approaches to the epidural space in children (e.g., percutaneous lumbar or thoracic epidural catheter placement). The simulation of these other pediatric regional anesthesia techniques at this stage relies on utilization of adult size commercially available phantoms, or anesthesia educators improvising smaller sized solutions. Phantoms that can be imaged with ultrasound and needled as for an ultrasound-guided regional anesthetic technique can be manufactured by simulation educators. There are various recipes available that involve embedding objects in a suspension of hypoechoic media that range from gelatin [23] to tofu [24] to multiple other solutions [25]. These can be created in sizes appropriate for simulating pediatric procedures.

Pediatric Vascular Access Trainers

Many manufacturers offer pediatric peripheral venous cannulation task trainers. Some of these task trainers are amenable to ultrasound scanning so as to simulate the *difficult i.v.*, where learners can perform an ultrasound-guided peripheral intravenous cannulation. An example of a pediatric central venous access trainer is the VascularAccessChild System (Simulab Corporation, Seattle, WA, USA). Central line trainers are commonly ultrasound compatible and often have a hand bulb to create an arterial pulsation during the procedure. There is convincing evidence that simulation-based mastery learning of central venous access procedures is associated with better adherence to key steps [26], increased success rates [26], fewer complications [27], and even cost saving [15] (when the cost of the education program is balanced against the healthcare costs saved). Pediatric arterial cannulation is a skill that frustrates many novices in pediatric anesthesia. Perhaps surprisingly then, pediatric-sized arterial cannulation task trainers are currently only in development phase [28]. Educators must therefore decide whether they

Fig. 21.5 Life/form® Pediatric Caudal Injection Simulator. (Used with permission of Nasco Healthcare)

Fig. 21.6 *Homemade* pediatric size arterial cannulation task trainer. (Image courtesy: Katherine Taylor, The Hospital for Sick Children, Toronto, ON, Canada, and Tracy Tan, Kandang Kerbau Hospital, Singapore)

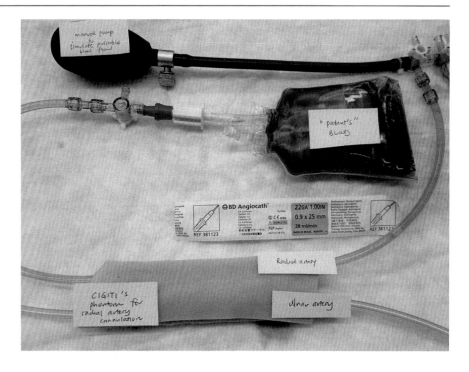

will have trainees practice on adult-sized task trainers or manufacture their own smaller version. Figure 21.6 shows a homemade version which has a palpable pulse and blood reservoir such that the learners will see the characteristic flashback in the cannula.

Just-in-Time Training in Pediatric Anesthesia

Just-in-time training refers to engagement in learning activities immediately before performing that procedure in real life. In the context of pediatric anesthesia, this might be on a task trainer (e.g., demonstrating safe technique for central venous catheterization on a task trainer, before performing it on a real patient) or a full-body computerized mannequin (e.g., rehearsing the induction of anesthesia of an infant with Tetralogy of Fallot immediately before inducing a similar patient in the operating room).

Hybrid Simulation in Pediatric Anesthesia

Hybrid simulation refers to the combination of multiple simulation modalities in one, usually complex, scenario. An example of operating room hybrid simulation might be a *can't intubate, can't oxygenate* scenario that could be started on a computerized mannequin, but when the participant reaches the point of a front-of-neck procedure, they perform the procedure on a part-task trainer (which is until that point concealed nearby).

Example of a Pediatric Anesthesia Curriculum

As for any process of educational curriculum design, a pre-established framework should be followed to ensure that the

process is robust, transparent, and can be evaluated and refined. One such framework is the six-step approach advocated by Kern et al. [29] (Table 21.3).

The sources of information to satisfy step one include liaison with the country-specific licensing authority, college, or board that would be able to indicate what would be considered key competencies and whether they have any data on whether these are achievable within a pediatric anesthesia rotation. Learners' needs (step 2) can be ascertained by surveying learners and their trainers and discovering if the learning objectives mandated by their licensing authority are currently achieved by existing training in pediatric anesthesia. Goals and objectives must be specific and measurable in order that the success of the program can subsequently be evaluated. In step four, educators must ask themselves if simulation is even the most suitable modality for addressing the identified needs. Description of the implementation phase of a new pediatric anesthesia simulation curriculum is beyond the scope of this discussion, but included in table 21.4 is a list of potential pediatric anesthesia scenarios that could be included in a course.

An example of one such pediatric anesthesia curriculum that underwent this rigorous process of curriculum design is

Table 21.3 Kern's six steps of curriculum design

1. Problem identification and needs assessment
2. Learners' needs assessment
3. Goals and objectives
4. Educational strategies
5. Implementation
6. Evaluation and feedback

Table 21.4 Potential scenarios for a pediatric anesthesia curriculum

Hypovolemia/dehydration (recognition preinduction)
Anesthesia machine failure
Laryngospasm
Can't intubate, can't oxygenate
Venous air embolism
Hyperkalemia
Massive hemorrhage
Local anesthetic toxicity
Intraoperative bronchospasm
Ventilator-associated tension pneumothorax
Severe post-intubation stridor
Anaphylaxis
Neonatal laparotomy
ICP control during craniotomy
Malignant hyperthermia
Pediatric Trauma
Retained throat pack in PACU
Arrhythmia in PACU
Bleeding post-op tonsillectomy
Post-appendectomy systemic sepsis
ICP intracranial pressure, PACU post-anesthesia care unit

the Managing Emergencies in Pediatric Anesthesia (MEPA) course [10, 30]. The MEPA course has been the basis of an international network of pediatric anesthesia educators and the focus of simulation research, as discussed below.

Research

The evolution of research in pediatric anesthesia simulation is relatively recent. Cook has described a framework for classifying medical education research as description research (*what was done?*), justification research (*did it work?*) and clarification research (*why or how did it work?*) [31]. To date, much of research in pediatric anesthesia simulation has been at the description stage [32, 33]. Justification research can be classified according to the level of outcome that is considered. The Kirkpatrick classification [34] is often used to categorize research. Level 1 refers to the reaction of learners, for instance whether learners feel that the simulation experience was effective [35], or as Berlacu and colleagues found that simulation increases confidence in trainee pediatric anesthesiologists [36]. Kirkpatrick level 2 refers to the demonstration of learning after training and there is little work at this level in pediatric anesthesiology training [37], although its effectiveness at this level is also supported by the literature in adult anesthesia simulation [38, 39] and in other acutecare specialties in pediatrics [40]. Kirkpatrick level 3 refers to actual changes in practice in the workplace,

and although this has been demonstrated in adult anesthesia [41], we know of no studies that have examined this level of outcome in pediatric anesthesia. The highest level, Kirkpatrick 4, describes patient level outcomes from simulation training, and although this has been shown in other medical [42, 43] and surgical [44] specialties, including pediatric cardiac arrest [45], there is currently no evidence at this level for simulation in anesthesia. It may prove challenging to establish this kind of evidence for simulation in the specialty of anesthesia, in part due to the high level of patient safety and low incidence of negative outcomes in anesthesia care. Cost has been described as the *missing outcome* in simulation research [46] and few studies have described this aspect of pediatric anesthesia simulation [47], with no evaluations to date of return on investment in terms of educational outcomes per dollar spent.

Assessment

Simulation shows promise for competence assessment in pediatric anesthesia. It has been demonstrated that anesthesia trainees who perform well in oral exams cannot necessarily translate that performance to simulation scenarios [48]. Pediatric anesthesiologists may be assessed using workplace-based assessments for routine cases [49], but this is not possible for crisis situations which occur relatively infrequently and where it would be ethically unacceptable to allow poor performance in order to assess an individual's competence [50].

Computerized mannequin-based simulation has been evaluated for the assessment of pediatric anesthesiology skills using many scenarios including bronchospasm, malignant hyperthermia, venous air embolus, laryngospasm, appendicitis with sepsis, airway foreign body, newborn resuscitation, infant seizure, postoperative apnea, accidental extubation, anaphylaxis, machine failure, hypovolemia, pulseless electrical activity, ventricular fibrillation, and local anesthetic toxicity [51–54]. Outcome measures have included time taken to critical interventions [51], scenario-specific checklists [52–54], and the MEPA Global Rating Scale [52] which is an overall assessment of competence applicable to any scenario. Simulation-based assessment has been found to be reliable in pediatric anesthesia [52, 53], and there is also some limited evidence for validity (meaning that the test is measuring what is intended to be measured) [55] in terms of relationships to other variables: More experienced residents perform better on pediatric anesthesia simulations than more junior trainees [53]. However, as is also found in the simulation literature more generally [56], there is still much work to be done in terms of the validation of simulation for pediatric anesthesiology for high-stakes purposes, in particular establishing the relationship between performance in the simulator and performance in actual clinical practice, and also consequential validity, that is, what are the intended and unintended consequences of introducing high-stakes simulation-based assessment [57]. In the USA, The American Board of Anesthesiology (ABA) has made simulation a component of the Maintenance of Certification in Anesthesiology (MOCA) process [58], although it is important to note that it is currently simply participation that is recognized and candidates are not actually assessed [59]. The process of incorporating pediatric aspects into the MOCA has begun [60]. Pediatric-specific MOCA courses are already available. A similar system in the UK involves physicians taking responsibility for a continuous revalidation, whereby all aspects of practice are updated and documented compliant with a practice matrix. Although anesthesia simulation potentially satisfies a number of the items in the matrix, simulation-based assessments are not mandated. In Canada, three times the quantity of continuing medical education credit per hour is awarded for simulation-based activities, highlighting its value in maintenance of skills [61].

Other tools have been used to assess nontechnical skills in anesthesia, such as situation awareness, decision-making, task management, and teamwork, and notably the Anaesthetists' Non-Technical Skills (ANTS) Framework from the University of Aberdeen [62]. The use of simulation to test competence in pediatric anesthesia non-technical skills is appealing as they have been found to contribute to patient level outcomes [63, 64], and teaching these skills has been shown to improve patient outcomes including mortality [65].

Quality Assurance/Patient Safety

Simulation can be used to stress a system beyond its business-as-usual function without the risk of patient detriment. It allows for the repeated rehearsal (or *drilling*) of complex interprofessional protocols with the potential for revealing process deficiencies or latent safety threats—deficits in the system or patient care pathways that have the potential to cause patient harm. Simulation can also be used to evaluate new patient care environments, as described in the evaluation of a pediatric emergency department of a new hospital facility [66]. Based on the findings, the authors were able to make policy recommendations, refine patient care pathways, and customize environments to optimize patient safety. As simulation-based examinations of patient care areas become mainstream, there are numerous (unpublished) examples of new or renovated operating rooms or anesthesia areas in pediatric emergency rooms being tested with simulations prior to introduction of real patients and real clinical care.

Environments, facilities, equipment, and policies can only go so far to ensure patient safety. Ultimately, the well-being of a child under anesthesia relies on the knowledge,

judgment, and skills of the individual practitioner. Evidence was recently published for the reliability and validity of behaviorally anchored assessment instruments for "identifying gaps in the competency of anesthesia residents ... critical to patient safety" [67]. It could be argued that any simulation-based assessment of anesthesiologist competence ultimately benefits patient safety.

Globalization of Pediatric Anesthesia Simulation

The MEPA International collaborative [68] is an internationally renowned network of pediatric anesthesia simulation educators. The network evolved from the expansion of a local course in Bristol, UK, in 2006 [10] and has grown rapidly to now becoming available in multiple centers on four continents [30, 69]. The MEPA course is also at the foundation of ongoing multicenter simulation research studies [52]. There are other international organizations to which pediatric anesthesia simulation educators may want to subscribe. The INSPIRE network [70] has a substantial representation of pediatric anesthesiologists. The Society for Simulation in Health care has special interest groups in anesthesia and pediatrics, although at this time it does not have a dedicated subgroup for pediatric anesthesia.

Conclusions

The evolution of pediatric anesthesia has coincided with the residency duty hour restrictions (USA) and the European working time directive, which have limited exposure to pediatric anesthesia for anesthesia trainees. In the UK, this has meant achievement of the RCoA-recommended minimum numbers for advanced training is jeopardized [71]. Not surprisingly, simulation has been identified as one of a range of solutions to address this shortfall. As described above, simulation is already a mandatory component of an anesthesiologist's maintenance of certification, and this is only likely to extend across more jurisdictions. Several studies have shown that an anesthesia team with pediatric experience can significantly lower perioperative mortality and morbidity in children [72, 73]. One prominent study analyzing data on perioperative deaths concluded that anesthesiologists should avoid occasional pediatric practice [74]. From a practical perspective, rural or remote hospital practice means that this recommendation is unfeasible. This is another opportunity for simulation-based maintenance of knowledge and skills. This could involve anesthesiologists with occasional commitment to pediatric anesthesia travelling to tertiary centers for center-based courses or pediatric anesthesia *outreach*, where the tertiary center brings a travelling road show of mobile in situ simulation to the host hospital. There are successful precedents for both models. While much pediatric anesthesia simulation research to date has been investigating simulation as a modality, it is likely that we will witness the increasing use of simulation as the tool by which some other aspect of pediatric anesthesia is evaluated, be it new facilities, patient care pathways, or critical event preparedness.

References

1. Long CW. An account of the first use of sulphuric ether by inhalation as an anesthetic in surgical operations. South Med J. 1849;5:705–13.
2. Bigelow HJ. Insensibility during surgical operations produced by inhalation. Boston Med Surg J. 1846;35(16):309–17.
3. Lyman HM. Artificial anaesthesia and anaesthetics. New York: W. Wood; 1881.
4. Mai CL, Cote CJ. A history of pediatric anesthesia: a tale of pioneers and equipment. Paediatr Anaesth. 2012;22(6):511–20. Epub 2012/03/27.
5. Holzman RS. An appreciation of Robert Moors Smith MD, an icon of pediatric anesthesiology. Paediatr Anaesth. 2010;20(8):767–70. Epub 2010/07/31.
6. Viola L, Clay S, Samuels P. Education in pediatric anesthesiology: competency, innovation, and professionalism in the 21st century. Int Anesthesiol Clin. 2012;50(4):1–12.
7. Anaesthetists RCo. Sub-specialty training programmes—Training requirements. 2014. http://www.rcoa.ac.uk/system/files/TRG-PICM-Subspecialty.pdf. Accessed 19 Sept 2014.
8. Astuto M, Lauretta D, Minardi C, Disma N, Salvo I, Gullo A Does the Italian pediatric anesthesia training program adequately prepare residents for future clinical practice? What should be done? Pediatr Anesth. 2008;18:172–5.
9. Shimata Y. Pediatric anesthesia practice and training in Japan: a survey. Paediatr Anaesth. 2006;16(5):543–7.
10. Molyneux M, Lauder G. A national collaborative simulation project: paediatric anaesthetic emergencies. Pediatr Anesth. 2006;16(12):1302.
11. Morris RW, Pybus DA. "Orpheus" cardiopulmonary bypass simulation system. J Extra Corpor Technol. 2007;39(4):228–33.
12. Lansdowne W, Machin D, Grant D. Development of the orpheus perfusion simulator for use in high-fidelity extracorporeal membrane oxygenation simulation. J Extra Corpor Technol. 2012;44(4):250–5.
13. Sistino J, Michaud N, Sievert A, Shackelford A. Incorporating high fidelity simulation into perfusion education. Perfusion. 2011;26(5):390–4.
14. Wayne DB, Barsuk JH, McGaghie WC. Procedural training at a crossroads: striking a balance between education, patient safety, and quality. J Hosp Med. 2007;2(3):123.
15. Cohen ER, Feinglass J, Barsuk JH, Barnard C, O'Donnell A, McGaghie WC, et al. Cost savings from reduced catheter-related bloodstream infection after simulation-based education for residents in a medical intensive care unit. Simul Healthc. 2010;5(2):98–102.
16. Schwid HA, Rooke GA, Michalowski P, Ross BK. Screen-based anesthesia simulation with debriefing improves performance in a mannequin-based anesthesia simulator. Teach Learn Med. 2001;13(2):92–6.
17. Bhansali R, Armstrong J. Smartphone applications for pediatric anesthesia. Pediatr Anesth. 2012;22(4):400–4.
18. mySmartSimulations. Infant Endotracheal Intubation (Ipad App). Saratoga Springs, NY, USA.
19. MedMan Simulations Inc. GasMan Volatile Anesthesia Simulator. San Ramon, CA, USA. http://www.gasmanweb.com/.
20. RamirezMD. iTIVA (Android App).
21. Moore DL, Ding L, Sadhasivam S. Novel real-time feedback and integrated simulation model for teaching and evaluating ultrasound-guided regional anesthesia skills in pediatric anesthesia trainees. Paediatr Anaesth. 2012;22(9):847–53.
22. Polaner DM, Taenzer AH, Walker BJ, Bosenberg A, Krane EJ, Suresh S, et al. Pediatric regional anesthesia network (PRAN): a multi-institutional study of the use and incidence of complications of pediatric regional anesthesia. Anesth Analg. 2012;115(6):1353–64.
23. Gibson KI. A home-made phantom for learning ultrasound-guided invasive techniques. Australas Radiol. 1995;39(4):356–7.
24. Pollard BA. New model for learning ultrasound-guided needle to target localization. Reg Anesth Pain Med. 2008;33(4):360–2.
25. Sultan SF, Shorten G, Iohom G. Simulators for training in ultrasound guided procedures. Med Ultrason. 2013;15(2):125–31.
26. Barsuk JH, McGaghie WC, Cohen ER, Balachandran JS, Wayne DB. Use of simulation based mastery learning to improve the quality of central venous catheter placement in a medical intensive care unit. J Hosp Med. 2009;4(7):397–403.
27. Barsuk JH, Cohen ER, Feinglass J, McGaghie WC, Wayne DB. Use of simulation-based education to reduce catheter-related bloodstream infections. Arch Intern Med. 2009;169(15):1420.
28. Whiteside G, Limbs and Things. Personal communication. 2014.
29. Kern DE, Thomas PA, Hughes MT. Curriculum development for medical education: a six-step approach. Baltimore, ML, USA: JHU Press; 2010.
30. Everett T, Bould D, Ng E, Taylor M, de Beer D, Doherty C, et al. Transcontinental telesimulation: the global proliferation of the managing emergencies in paediatric anaesthesia (MEPA) Course. Simul Healthc. 2013;8(6):433.
31. Cook DA, Bordage G, Schmidt HG. Description, justification and clarification: a framework for classifying the purposes of research in medical education. Med Educ. 2008;42(2):128–33.
32. Nargozian C. Teaching consultants airway management skills. Paediatr Anaesth. 2004;14(1):24–7. Epub 2004/01/14.
33. Schaefer JJ 3rd. Simulators and difficult airway management skills. Paediatr Anaesth. 2004;14(1):28–37. Epub 2004/01/14.
34. Kirkpatrick D. Evaluating training programs: the four levels. San Francisco: Barrett-Koehler; 1997.
35. Edler AA, Chen M, Honkanen A, Hackel A, Golianu B. Affordable simulation for small-scale training and assessment. Simul Healthc. 2010;5(2):112–5. Epub 2010/07/28.
36. Burlacu CL, Chin C. Effect of pediatric simulation training on candidate's confidence. Paediatr Anaesth. 2008;18(6):566–7. Epub 2008/05/01.
37. Moore DL, Ding L, Sadhasivam S. Novel real-time feedback and integrated simulation model for teaching and evaluating ultrasound-guided regional anesthesia skills in pediatric anesthesia trainees. Paediatr Anaesth. 2012;22(9):847–53. Epub 2012/05/23.
38. Yee B, Naik VN, Joo HS, Savoldelli GL, Chung DY, Houston PL, et al. Nontechnical skills in anesthesia crisis management with repeated exposure to simulation-based education. Anesthesiology. 2005;103(2):241–8.
39. Savoldelli GL, Naik VN, Park J, Joo HS, Chow R, Hamstra SJ. Value of debriefing during simulated crisis management: oral versus video-assisted oral feedback. Anesthesiology. 2006;105(2):279–85.
40. Nishisaki A, Hales R, Biagas K, Cheifetz I, Corriveau C, Garber N, et al. A multi-institutional high-fidelity simulation "boot camp" orientation and training program for first year pediatric critical care fellows. Pediatr Crit Care Med. 2009;10(2):157–62.
41. Bruppacher HR, Alam SK, LeBlanc VR, Latter D, Naik VN, Savoldelli GL, et al. Simulation-based training improves physicians' performance in patient care in high-stakes clinical setting of cardiac surgery. Anesthesiology. 2010;112(4):985–92.

42. Barsuk JH, Cohen ER, Feinglass J, McGaghie WC, Wayne DB. Use of simulation-based education to reduce catheter-related bloodstream infections. Arch Intern Med. 2009;169(15):1420–3.

43. Barsuk JH, McGaghie WC, Cohen ER, O,ÄôLeary KJ, Wayne DB. Simulation-based mastery learning reduces complications during central venous catheter insertion in a medical intensive care unit. Crit Care Med. 2009;37(10):2697–701.

44. Ahlberg G, Enochsson L, Gallagher AG, Hedman L, Hogman C, McClusky DA III, et al. Proficiency-based virtual reality training significantly reduces the error rate for residents during their first 10 laparoscopic cholecystectomies. Am J Surg. 2007;193(6):797–804.

45. Andreatta P, Saxton E, Thompson M, Annich G. Simulation-based mock codes significantly correlate with improved pediatric patient cardiopulmonary arrest survival rates. Pediatr Crit Care Med. 2011;12(1):33–8.

46. Zendejas B, Wang AT, Brydges R, Hamstra SJ, Cook DA. Cost: the missing outcome in simulation-based medical education research: a systematic review. Surgery. 2013;153(2):160–76.

47. Weinstock PH, Kappus LJ, Kleinman ME, Grenier B, Hickey P, Burns JP. Toward a new paradigm in hospital-based pediatric education: the development of an onsite simulator program. Pediatr Crit Care Med. 2005;6(6):635–41. Epub 2005/11/09.

48. Savoldelli GL, Naik VN, Joo HS, Houston PL, Graham M, Yee B, et al. Evaluation of patient simulator performance as an adjunct to the oral examination for senior anesthesia residents. Anesthesiology. 2006;104(3):475–81.

49. Boulet JR, Murray D. Review article: assessment in anesthesiology education. Can J Anesth. 2012;59(2):182–92.

50. Ziv A, Wolpe PR, Small SD, Glick S. Simulation-based medical education: an ethical imperative. Acad Med. 2003;78(8):783–8.

51. Tofil NM, Dollar J, Zinkan L, Youngblood AQ, Peterson DT, White ML, et al. Performance of anesthesia residents during a simulated prone ventricular fibrillation arrest in an anesthetized pediatric patient. Paediatr Anaesth. 2014;24(9):940–4. Epub 2014/04/15.

52. Everett TC, Ng E, Power D, Marsh C, Tolchard S, Shadrina A, et al. The managing emergencies in paediatric anaesthesia global rating scale is a reliable tool for simulation-based assessment in pediatric anesthesia crisis management. Pediatr Anesth. 2013;23(12):1117–23.

53. Fehr JJ, Boulet JR, Waldrop WB, Snider R, Brockel M, Murray DJ. Simulation-based assessment of pediatric anesthesia skills. Anesthesiology. 2011;115(6):1308–15. Epub 2011/11/01.

54. Howard-Quijano KJ, Stiegler MA, Huang YM, Canales C, Steadman RH. Anesthesiology residents' performance of pediatric resuscitation during a simulated hyperkalemic cardiac arrest. Anesthesiology. 2010;112(4):993–7. Epub 2010/03/18.

55. Bould M, Crabtree N, Naik V. Assessment of procedural skills in anaesthesia. Br J Anaesth. 2009;103(4):472–83.

56. Cook DA, Brydges R, Zendejas B, Hamstra SJ, Hatala R. Technology-enhanced simulation to assess health professionals: a systematic review of validity evidence, research methods, and reporting quality. Acad Med. 2013;88(6):872–83.

57. Kane MT. Validating the interpretations and uses of test scores. J Educ Meas. 2013;50(1):1–73.

58. Maintenance of Certification in Anesthesiology. http://www.theaba.org/Home/anesthesiology_maintenance. Accessed 2 Sept 2014.

59. Weinger MB, Burden AR, Steadman RH, Gaba DM. This is, not a test!: misconceptions surrounding the maintenance of certification in anesthesiology simulation course. Anesthesiology. 2014;121(3):655–9.

60. Fehr JJ, Honkanen A, Murray DJ. Simulation in pediatric anesthesiology. Paediatr Anaesth. 2012;22(10):988–94. Epub 2012/09/13.

61. Canada TRCoPaSo. Maintenance of certification. http://www.royalcollege.ca/portal/page/portal/rc/members/moc. Accessed 3 Dec 2014.

62. Fletcher G, Flin R, McGeorge P, Glavin R, Maran N, Patey R. Anaesthetists' non-technical skills (ANTS): evaluation of a behavioural marker system. Br J Anaesth. 2003;90(5):580–8.

63. Eppich WJ, Brannen M, Hunt EA. Team training: implications for emergency and critical care pediatrics. Curr Opin Pediatr. 2008;20(3):255–60.

64. Williams A, Lasky R, Dannemiller J, Andrei A, Thomas E. Teamwork behaviours and errors during neonatal resuscitation. Qual Saf Health Care. 2010;19(1):60–4.

65. Neily J, Mills PD, Young-Xu Y, Carney BT, West P, Berger DH, et al. Association between implementation of a medical team training program and surgical mortality. JAMA. 2010;304(15):1693–700.

66. Geis GL, Pio B, Pendergrass TL, Moyer MR, Patterson MD. Simulation to assess the safety of new healthcare teams and new facilities. Simul Healthc. 2011;6(3):125–33.

67. Blum RH, Boulet JR, Cooper JB, Muret-Wagstaff SL, Group HAoARPR. Simulation-based assessment to identify critical gaps in safe anesthesia resident performance. Anesthesiology. 2014;120(1):129–41.

68. Managing Emergencies in Pediatric Anesthesia (MEPA). [cited 2014 16 September]. https://mepa.org.uk/.

69. Taylor M, Everett T, De Beer D, Mackinnon R. Managing emergencies in pediatric anesthesia (MEPA): evolution of an international simulation training collaboration to improve the management of pediatric anesthetic emergencies. Eur J Anaesthesiol. 2014;31:168–9.

70. Cheng A, Auerbach M, Hunt E, Kessler D, Pusic M, Chang T, et al. The international network for simulation-based pediatric innovation, research and education (INSPIRE): collaboration to enhance the impact of simulation-based research. Simul Healthc. 2013;8(6):418.

71. Fernandez E, Williams D. Training and the European working time directive: a 7 year review of paediatric anaesthetic trainee caseload data. Br J Anaesth. 2009;103(4):566–9.

72. Auroy Y, Ecoffey C, Messiah A, Rouvier B. Relationship between complications of pediatric anesthesia and volume of pediatric anesthetics. Anesth Analg. 84(1):234–5.

73. Lunn J. Implications of the national confidential inquiry into perioperative deaths for paediatric anaesthesia. Paediatr Anaesth. 1992;2:69–72.

74. Campling EA, Devlin HB, Deaths NCEiP, Lunn JN, Hoile RW, Cepod. The report of the national confidential enquiry into perioperative Deaths 1992/1993: (1 April 1992 to 31 March 1993): National confidential enquiry into perioperative Deaths; 1995.

Steven R. Lopushinsky and Guy F. Brisseau

Simulation Pearls

1. Simulation in pediatric surgery is an educational tool that can be used within the context of a greater surgical educational curriculum.
2. The growing availability of pediatric task trainers and procedure-specific trainers allows for dedicated practice outside of the operating room to achieve and maintain clinical competency.
3. Target learner-specific needs when choosing type and fidelity of simulation modality for training.

Introduction

Giving consent to the assault of surgery—the cutting of flesh and manipulation of organs—trusts at the most basic level that your surgeon is capable. Yet, there is a list of assumptions that the naive patient must make, including but not limited to, graduation from a surgical residency informs competency, passing board exams demonstrates adequate knowledge and judgment, and the referral process is based on reputation and expertise. Training a surgeon initially to achieve competency, and subsequently maintaining competency, poses a unique set of problems and ethical dilemmas. At many steps in training we must appreciate the learning curve and recognize potential pitfalls for the patient. Preventable harm can occur to a patient unless proper measures are taken during skill development and gaining of expertise.

S. R. Lopushinsky (✉)
Section of Pediatric Surgery, Cumming School of Medicine, University of Calgary, Alberta Children's Hospital, Calgary, AB, Canada
e-mail: steven.lopushinsky@albertahealthservices.ca

G. F. Brisseau
Department of Pediatric Surgery, Sidra Medical & Research Center, Doha, Qatar
e-mail: gbrisseau@sidra.org

Unlike professional sports, we do not publicly debate the merits of surgeon qualities or breakdown performance after each procedure. After a poor showing, a surgeon generally risks no demotion to the *minor leagues* or worse yet being let go completely. This assumes of course that a tragic outcome has not occurred—rather than a game lost—a patient dies or suffers a debilitating injury prompting suffering for both the patient and the family, as well as potential legal action and physician delicensing. The practicing surgeon does not work under the public spotlight but is somehow trusted to perform competently. Perhaps this is even more relevant when the patients are children, judged to be the most vulnerable in society, and seemingly deserving of only top performers. The aim of this chapter is to explore the role of simulation in training pediatric surgeons and maintaining their surgical skillset.

Deliberate Practice in Surgical Education

It has been recognized in medicine and across other professional domains that experience is not necessarily tied to objective performance. According to Eriksson, consistent improvement towards superior performance can be achieved through a combination of setting task-specific goals, timely feedback, and opportunity for repetitive performance [1]. Such scheduled activity is termed deliberate practice (DP). Developing expert surgical competencies goes beyond achieving automaticity in movement but ability to evaluate, problem-solve, and adapt to a changing and challenging environment. From an ethical perspective, can we accept the notion that it takes 10 years plus or 10,000 hours to achieve expertise while simultaneously credentialing fresh new surgeons to manage rare and complex pediatric surgical diseases? In the current apprenticeship model of surgical training in North America, there are evolving barriers to safe and efficient training. Program directors somehow must address declining case exposure and independence secondary to restricted work hours [2–4] and perceived litigious risk. The threat to repetitive exposure, and

© Springer International Publishing Switzerland 2016
V. J. Grant, A. Cheng (eds.), *Comprehensive Healthcare Simulation: Pediatrics,*
Comprehensive Healthcare Simulation, DOI 10.1007/978-3-319-24187-6_22

opportunity for DP, goes beyond training given the evidence of declining case volume to surgeon ratios once in practice [5, 6]. Pediatric surgery is perhaps at greatest risk of these challenges given the smaller population demographic and rarity of index pediatric surgical diseases. Junior attending surgeons are performing less than four cases per year respectively for gastroschisis/omphalocele, anorectal malformation, congenital diaphragmatic hernia (CDH), esophageal atresia, and Hirschprung disease [6]. Median experience for choledochal cyst, portoenterostomy, sacrococcygeal tertaoma, laparotomy for trauma, and others was zero.

Operative case volume of graduating pediatric surgery residents at first glance has changed little over the past decade [7]. Despite a documented increase in the number of graduating pediatric surgical trainees in North America, mean case volumes remain intact but with significant variability in operative experience. We are witness to many residents/fellows graduating with one or fewer specialty-defining cases. Findings show that the average pediatric surgery resident completes less than five and in some cases zero esophageal atresia repairs, choledochal cyst excisions, portoenterostomies, or resections of sacrococcyceal teratoma [7, 8]. Of further concern is that general surgery residents, many of whom will care for children at significant geographic distance from major pediatric centers, seem to be doing fewer pediatric cases [9]. It is not known what factor is driving this trend, but the decline in operative exposure does not appear related to classified index cases, considered the domain of fellows or more senior trainees. Cases appropriate for a community institution such as inguinal and umbilical hernia repair dropped from 26.7 cases per North American general surgery resident to 18.5, a 30.7% drop from the 1989–1990 academic year through 2007–2008 [9]. Since volume–outcome relationships are a well-described phenomenon across multiple surgical specialties, a drop in cases gives pause for concern. Indeed superior outcomes have been demonstrated in association with volume or specialty training for pediatric extracorporeal membrane oxygenation (ECMO) [10, 11], pyloromyotomy [12, 13], appendectomy [14], urology [15, 16], and cardiac surgery [17].

In a 1974 editorial, William Tunell wrote:

> The dilemma for pediatric surgeons is to meaningfully supplement and influence the education of general and thoracic surgical residents, anticipating that general and specialty surgeons will continue to provide most of the surgical care to children, while at the same time maintain an elitist view of neonatal and uncommon children's surgery as the province of the pediatric surgeon [18].

While there has been an explosion of pediatric surgeons in North America, much of the dilemma remains the same. If there is an expectation for our general surgery trained surgeons to be performing less complex procedures, then we must consider methods for replacing these diminishing cases. Further, if the *province* of the pediatric surgeon is to perform neonatal and uncommon surgery, in the presence of a growing pediatric surgery workforce, we must consider replacing real-life experience with some alternative. Simulation represents a viable option for not only training these techniques but also for ongoing maintenance of skills.

Evolution of Simulation in Pediatric Surgery

The steep advancement of technology, specifically tools making minimally invasive surgery (MIS) a reality, represents a major change in the delivery of surgical care over the past 20 years. The potential patient-level benefits, primarily lessened pain, fewer wound complications, and improved cosmesis, are now rarely debated. Innovation continues with the development of high-definition equipment, single-port and endoluminal surgery. Of the surgical specialties, pediatric surgery is somewhat unique in that all trainees will have completed adult residency programs. Knowledge and surgical techniques learned in adult training are leveraged to expand the skillset of the pediatric subspecialist. The curriculum of most generalist training programs provides exposure to realistic models (low- and high-fidelity trainers), virtual reality trainers (computer based), and scenario-based training [19].

Widely recognized and adopted at many levels is the Fundamentals of Laparoscopic Surgery (FLS) program developed by the Society of American Gastrointestinal and Endoscopic Surgeons (SAGES) based on the McGill experience [20]. Here, surgeons are exposed to a web-based curriculum plus basic manual skills in peg transfer, cutting, suturing, and intracorporeal knot tying. Construct validity has been demonstrated in its ability to make distinction between novice and experienced operators with some evidence of concurrence validity in its ability to transfer skills to the operating room (OR) [21]. Successful completion of the FLS program is now embedded in adult general surgery training programs and is an eligibility requirement prior to writing the American Board of Surgery (ABS) exams.

Pediatric surgeons further expand on this skillset to perform such tasks as delicate dissection, suturing, and intracorporeal knot tying in a much smaller domain and limited field of vision. For example, the technical demand of a thoracoscopic tracheoesophageal fistula (TEF) repair is clearly an advanced skillset but is absolutely rooted in generalist training principles. Using a computer simulation model, Hamilton et al. demonstrate that space limitations distinguish the adult and pediatric surgeon [22].

The impact on training is not as well understood. Many surgical educators are themselves early in the MIS learning curve, and only when expertise is achieved will there be a shift downward to junior trainees. As one example, general

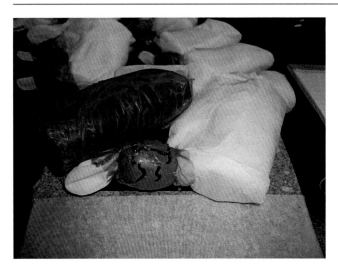

Fig. 22.1 Pyloric stenosis model. Using simple materials a hypertrophied pylorus can be mass produced. The inanimate structure can then be placed into a standard task trainer for dedicated practice of performing an appropriate pyloromyotomy. Trainees can then practice (1) a linear cut in the serosa, (2) *crack* the muscle, and (3) complete the myotomy with adequate spreading until the respective limbs move independently. (Provided by: Dr. Joseph A. Iocono, M.D. Associate Professor of Surgery and Pediatrics, Division Chief, Pediatric Surgery, Kentucky Children's Hospital. University of Kentucky. Reproduced with permission)

surgery residents are doing fewer pyloromyotomy procedures in association with greater adoption of the laparoscopic technique [23]. Certainly there is evidence that involving residents in MIS procedures increases operative time and perhaps morbidity [24]. The opportunity for DP outside of the OR has the potential to decrease the technical learning curve with improved patient outcomes and OR efficiency. In fact, one of the first pediatric surgery simulators described in the literature is for the laparoscopic pyloromyotomy (Fig. 22.1, [25]). The adoption of MIS for pyloric stenosis is not alone, with techniques exploding for gastroesophageal reflux disease [26], intussusception [27], intestinal atresia [28], and CDH [29].

Scaffolding on previous training is instrumental for the ability to take on more difficult tasks, but there is potential for unintended consequences. In the North American context, individuals entering a pediatric surgery residency do so having minimum 5 years of prior training and thus come with an already heightened expectation of performance. Instead they are respectively met with new physiology, unique disease patterns, and distinct surgical requirements, putting performance at risk. Preventable errors, particularly in surgical patients, occur more frequently in pediatric academic centers compared to community institutions [30], although the relationship to trainees is not well elucidated.

Not surprising, pediatric surgeons and residents alike perceive simulation as beneficial to training [31]. Only half of those surveyed, however, had regular access to pediatric simulators and even fewer identified self-improvement with

Table 22.1 ACGME core competencies

Patient care
Medical knowledge
Practice-based learning
Interpersonal and communication skills
Professionalism
Systems-based practice

ACGME Accreditation Council for Graduate Medical Education

Table 22.2 CanMEDS competencies (2005) [33]

Medical expert
Professional
Communicator
Collaborator
Manager
Health advocate
Scholar

such training. The implication for educators is multifold: There is an apparent lack of appropriate pediatric simulators, there is a lack of DP on simulators, and hypothetically, incorporated simulation curriculum represents untapped potential to improve skills more efficiently.

Incorporating Simulation into a Pediatric Surgery Curriculum

The development of simulation programs and centers is a daunting task and requires much time and effort. Often the role of the simulation program in the overall educational enterprise can be overlooked. Simulation is a powerful educational tool for teaching and assessment. However, it remains a tool. As a simulation program becomes integrated within the overall educational enterprise, its true potential is fully realized. Modern surgical training programs are a complex enterprise with many educational activities culminating in a competent graduate who, depending on the program, is independent practice ready. The plan that guides this educational enterprise is the curriculum.

The curriculum identifies the components of education that are necessary for the learner. These components are distributed across all skill domains including cognitive, technical, and behavioral. Accrediting bodies have attempted to capture these components in various models, including the Accreditation Council for Graduate Medical Education (ACGME) core competencies (Table 22.1, [32]) and the Royal College of Physicians and Surgeons of Canada (RCPSC) Canadian Medical Education Direction For Specialists (CanMEDS) competencies (Table 22.2,

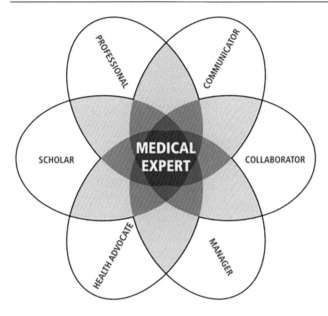

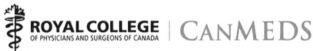

Fig. 22.2 The CanMEDS physician competency framework describes the knowledge, skills, and abilities that specialist physicians need for better patient outcomes. (Copyright © 2005 The Royal College of Physicians and Surgeons of Canada. http://rcpsc.medical.org/canmeds. Reproduced with permission)

Fig. 22.2, [33]). These frameworks continue to evolve with the ACGME adopting milestones effective July 1, 2014 [34] and the RCPSC developing CanMEDS 2015 [35]. Moving forward, trainees will progress on the basis of prescribed competency milestones. Conversely, accreditation of programs will be dependent on a structured curriculum that supports this comprehensive skill acquisition. Table 22.3 contains an abbreviated *milestones* document that guides curriculum for the topic of Hirschprung's disease at the author's institution.

These overarching competencies have had a profound effect in shaping current training paradigms. Each program however must develop its own unique curriculum to teach and assess these overarching competencies. This curriculum is what guides the learner's education and is what the simulation program must be guided by. In order to meet the overall objectives, learners will undertake a number of educational activities. These include mandatory clinical rotations, electives, academic half-days, grand rounds, as well as a plethora of other undertakings, including simulation. Each of these activities should be guided by clear and measurable objectives. The following example further illustrates this point.

An example of key surgical objectives would include:

Describe the characteristics and use of commonly used sutures in General Surgery

or

Demonstrate efficient and consistent closure of the fascia with a running suture.

The first objective is clearly cognitive and a necessary objective for the surgical learner. The second is more technical. While both are related, they can be taught and assessed together or separately. The program must teach and assess these objectives for each learner. Each program should choose the best teaching and assessment modality for these objectives. There is no prescriptive best method of teaching and indeed each program may have a different but equally acceptable approach. One program may choose a didactic or e-learning methodology for the cognitive objective while the other may do this integrated in the technical teaching in the simulation program. Similarly, assessment of a cognitive objective could be by written assessment (MCQ, short answer, etc.) or as part of the skills assessment.

While the description given above infers that the teaching and assessment are done once and in isolation, this is not true. Important teaching points must be revisited at an ever-escalating sophistication throughout the overall curriculum. This spiral curriculum, where key learning is revisited and enhanced, is part of a modern curriculum that needs an overarching master plan. This planned repetition is beneficial.

As such, all simulation activities must have objectives that are guided by the program's curriculum and objectives. These objectives should be mapped directly back to the program objectives. Making these links clear in all documentation and descriptions for simulation events inform our teachers and learners as to how the simulation activities are integrated into the overarching educational program. This documentation of the linkage is called a *curricular map* or *blueprint*. This blueprint is a characteristic of a very mature program.

As previously mentioned, simulation can be used to teach virtually any aspect of the curriculum across all of the competencies and in any domain (cognitive, technical, and behavioral). The key is that the objectives of the simulation activity be clearly defined and guided by the program curriculum. This can be difficult, particularly when a simulation curriculum has been developed outside of the program curriculum. Furthermore, many educational activities have multiple learners. These can involve different levels (medical students, residents, and practicing physicians) or disciplines. If disparate learners are involved the objectives should map back to all of their respective curricula. This further enables the concept of learner-specific objectives and is a powerful way to further define and refine the objectives for each learner.

Table 22.3 Example of building milestones into a pediatric surgery curriculum (Hirschprung's disease educational milestones at the University of Calgary, AB, Canada)

Learning context	CanMEDs role(s)	Learning outcomes: goals/objectives	Source doc(s)	Specific competencies	Learning/teaching Strategies	Evaluation method or tools
The goal of this module will be for the trainee to diagnose and to develop a treatment plan for patients with *H.D.* Also to be able to perform appropriate surgical procedures for the condition. All CanMED competencies will be incorporated in ongoing treatment and advise to the patient's family	*Medical expert* *Scholar* *Manager* *Collaborator* *Communicator* *Professional* *Health advocate*	*Orientation* Knowledge of anatomy, embryology and assessment of risk of H.D. including family history and trisomy 21 Knowledge of presentation and differential diagnosis of neonatal distal intestinal obstruction including H.D. Knowledge of different types of motility disorders Knowledge of diagnostic plan minimizing invasive procedures Knowledge of physiology in H.D. to include rectal manometry to evaluate rectoanal inhibitory reflex Knowledge of medical and surgical causes of chronic constipation	Pediatric Surgery Seventh Edition (2012) Editors: Coran et al. *Elsevier* *Score* modules Pediatric Surgery (Fellowship) Operative Pediatric Surgery Second Edition (2014) Editors: Ziegler et al. McGraw-Hill	Competent in: Embryology anatomy and assessment of child with delayed passage of meconium including risk of H.D. Presentation and differential of a child with neonatal distal intestinal obstruction to include H.D. Salient features from history and PE Different types of motility disorders Development of investigations to diagnose H.D. minimizing invasive procedures including rectal biopsy Evaluation of recto-anal inhibitory reflex Diagnosis of older child with chronic constipation to include medical and surgical causes includes variant Hirschsprung's disease	Review source documentation/ literature Case-based learning, bedside teaching with the opportunity to discuss Observation and opportunity to ask questions and discuss in clinical settings Case presentations and reviews during team rounds and presentations Individual supervision with opportunities to discuss diagnosis and evidence-based treatments Direct observation of supervisory surgeon(s) modeling all of the specific competencies with the opportunity for questions and discussions afterwards	Observe History (Hx) and Physical Exam (PE) exams Written and MCQ exams to assess cognitive knowledge Structured orals to assess applied knowledge Throughout the module the trainee will receive informal summative and formative feedback from attendings and other associated health professionals Evaluation from attending/allied health professionals during course of treatment in various CanMEDs roles: *Scholar* *Manager* *Professional* *Collaborator* *Communication* *Health Advocate* *Medical Expert* Multisource feedback (360°) from allied health professionals Review surgical log

Table 22.3 (continued)

Learning context	CanMEDs role(s)	Learning outcomes: goals/objectives	Source doc(s)	Specific competencies	Learning/teaching Strategies	Evaluation method or tools
	Medical Expert *Manager* *Collaborator* *Communicator*	*Orientation* Knowledge of workup plan to determine length of aganglionic segment from preoperative imaging and intraoperative biopsy Knowledge of refractory constipation with the presence of ganglion cells in the rectum including variant Hirschsprung's disease Knowledge of indications and contraindications for nonoperative versus operative procedure in H.D. Knowledge of child with H.D. requiring urgent management	Pediatric Surgery Seventh Edition (2012) Editors: Coran et al. *Elsevier* *Score* modules Pediatric Surgery (Fellowship) Operative Pediatric Surgery Second Edition (2014) Editors: Ziegler et al. McGraw-Hill	Development of plan to diagnose length of aganglionic segment by preoperative and operative methods Ability to develop alternative diagnosis and potential nonoperative approaches from results of biopsies, manometry, radiology imaging, and biochemical tests Ability to develop a treatment protocol dependent of clinical condition and length of aganglionic segment Ability of develop a treatment protocol in a neonate with bowel obstruction, bowel perforation, or enterocolitis in H.D.	Observe attending during perioperative surgical setup and surgical exposure	Structured orals to assess applied knowledge during course of treatment in various CanMEDS roles: *Medical Expert* *Professional* *Manager* *Collaborator* *Communicator* Multisource feedback (360°) from allied health professionals

H.D. Hirschprung's disease

Simulation and Evaluation

Simulation has been well established as an educational modality, particularly as a tool to provide feedback (typically formative) to the learner. However, another area that is rapidly emerging is the use of simulation for high stakes summative assessment (see Chap. 7). An example of this is the use of Objectively Structured Clinical Examinations in the United States Medical Licensing Exam and the Canadian Medical Licensing exams.

The use of simulation has further been studied and validated in the assessment of technical skills . Various tools such as the Objective Structured Evaluation of Technical Skills (OSATS) have been developed to assess technical skills [36]. These tools can be used by simulation programs to assess learner competence [37]. Building on this work, validated assessment programs have been developed, such as the aforementioned FLS Program [38]. The value of this program is best demonstrated by its use in surgeon certification. FLS has been adopted by the ABS, and successful completion is now a requirement for all individuals before eligibility to take the ABS examination.

Individual programs have used simulation to a varying extent as an assessment tool. However, this is increasing as simulation programs further develop and mature. As with teaching, the assessment program using simulation must be mapped to the educational curriculum of the learner. An exemplary program will have an assessment as well as a teaching map or blueprint that clearly demonstrates where all assessment activities take place and the specific modalities used. One specific example of the need to tailor simulation to the needs of the learner is evidenced by the findings of some early adopters in pediatric surgery simulation [39]. A relatively unsophisticated program was developed to mimic pediatric-specific activities in which a small box was used for peg transfer and pattern cutting in a see-through environment. Peg transfer, clip application, and wire twisting in a standard laparoscopy trainer followed these tasks. The authors found no improvement for individuals with prior laparoscopic experience (defined as > 10 cases) but closed the gap for those surgeons with no previous experience. In the context of today's learner, only medical students or the very junior surgical resident is likely to benefit from this type of activity.

Another group evaluated a hybrid curriculum consisting of task trainer exercises plus time on a virtual reality (computer-based) trainer for MIS-inexperienced pediatric surgeons [40]. At baseline, performance of the pediatric surgeon was weaker compared to the adult surgeon with respect to the number of completed sutures and time to complete suturing tasks. However, following the training program the gap was essentially eliminated, albeit at the consequence of an increased number of errors. Specifically, there was an increase in the number of suture deviations from the intended target, an increase in the number of injuries to the task sheet materials, and a greater number of loose sutures. Given that the study was done on an adult model, it does not begin to address advanced skills or pediatric-specific issues but does demonstrate potential for learning. Conversely, there is the suggestion that simulation models may also teach short cuts, perhaps gaming to method of evaluation (time) and thereby improving scores, but at potential risk of good technique.

Nearly all residents/fellows in accredited pediatric surgery training programs in North America incorporate a series of postgraduate courses into their respective curricula. For example, senior fellows now travel for a hands-on advanced MIS course that uses a variety of models (both low- and high-fidelity task-trainers as well as animal models) to practice advanced MIS techniques with significant mentoring. Initially held for first-year fellows, only recently has it moved to a second-year course with a higher degree of difficulty given the progression of baseline skills coming out of surgical residency.

Simulators in Pediatric Surgery

The core skills of a surgeon are those that enable safe, efficient, and reproducible outcomes in the OR. Training for high-level performance is certainly more complex as lofty competencies in decision-making and adaptability become increasingly important. How best then to train a pediatric surgeon novice in a given skillset, technique, or procedure? Can this be done outside of the OR where patient risk is avoided and OR efficiency is unaffected?

There are two competing, yet complementary, approaches to teaching surgical skills using simulation. First is to teach and practice specific skills that can then be transferred into the OR environment. Second is to recreate or mimic entire operations from start to finish. There is growing evidence that the level of fidelity required is dependent on the level of the learner [41]. Lower fidelity platforms are perhaps more appropriate for the novice learner to develop such skills as cutting, suturing, and intra-corporeal knot tying. Higher fidelity simulators represent an opportunity to develop procedure-specific skills such as incision and port placement, anatomical dissection, tissue manipulation, and intraoperative decision-making. The general thinking is that the higher-level learner will benefit more from an immersive experience that essentially replicates an operation [41–43]. Interestingly, this is somewhat in conflict with the findings of medical-based simulation research where in resuscitation-based scenarios the trueness of physical exam findings do not necessarily impact the perceived realism by the learner [44].

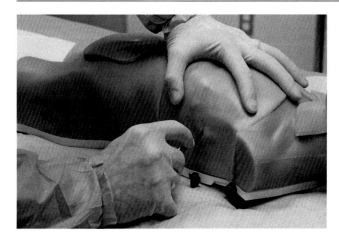

Fig. 22.3 TraumaChild (Simulab, Seattle, WA, US) models a 5-year-old body and allows trainees to practice chest tube insertion (as pictured with blood loss), cricothryoidotomy, percutaneous tracheostomy, pericardiocentesis, and diagnostic peritoneal lavage. (Reproduced with permission of Simulab)

To this end, there are a number of part-task trainers designed to recreate pediatric anatomy and allow training in emergency airway management, vascular access, chest tube insertion, and point of care ultrasound use. Examples of these products include: TraumaChild (Fig. 22.3) and VascularAccessChild System (Simulab, Seattle, WA, USA), AirSim Baby, AirSim Child, and Pediatric FAST/Acute Abdomen Phantom (Limbs and Things, Bristol, UK), Pediatric 4 Vessel Ultrasound Training Block Model (Blue Phantom,

Redmond, WA, USA), and SimJunior (Laerdal, Wappingers Falls, NY, USA) (See Chap. 10 for details).

The first validated pediatric laparoscopic task trainer was developed at The Hospital for Sick Children in Toronto, Canada [45, 46]. The pediatric laparoscopic surgery (PLS) simulator is similar to the SAGES/FLS adult trainer but reduced in dimension by a factor of 20 (Fig. 22.4). The authors took measurements of infants over the course of a year to determine the appropriate dimensions. Like the FLS program, the PLS simulator has been shown to discriminate between less- and more-experienced MIS surgeons suggesting construct validity. Data is still lacking as to whether it actually improves intraoperative efficiency or more importantly superior patient-level outcomes.

Procedure-specific simulators are slowly becoming available in pediatric surgery but have not yet become mainstream. Drawing from the experience of bile duct injuries in the early days of laparoscopic cholecystectomy, it is recognized that the surgeon learning curve may adversely affect outcomes. Surgeon specialty (pediatric surgeon vs general surgeon; [12, 47]) and surgical volume [48] impacts quality of pyloromyotomy reflected in higher mucosal perforation rates or inadequate muscle split even in the open surgical experience. Similarly, there is evidence that laparoscopic pyloromyotomy has a higher rate of complications when performed by less-experienced trainees. Haricharan et al. showed that general surgery residents (postgraduate year; PGY 3–4) had a 5.4-fold increased risk of causing a

Fig. 22.4 A comparison of the adult FLS simulator to the PLS system. The pediatric simulator is smaller than the adult simulator by a factor of 20. *PLS* pediatric laparoscopic surgery, *FLS* fundamentals of laparoscopic surgery. (Image provided by: Dr. Georges Azzie MD, Assistant Professor, Sick Kids Hospital, University of Toronto, Toronto, Ontario, Canada. Reproduced with permission)

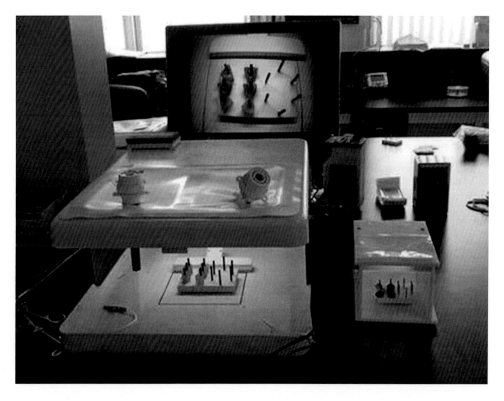

mucosal perforation during the procedure compared to a pediatric surgery resident (PGY 6–7) even when supervised by an experienced attending surgeon [49]. Such data not only further discriminates the need for subspecialist care but also suggests that those less experienced may benefit from practice before actually performing on a live infant. Indeed, this learner could be a surgical resident new to pediatric surgery, as described, or perhaps a senior pediatric surgeon new to the MIS technique. A number of models for laparoscopic pyloromyotomy have been described in pediatric surgery circles, but only one has been published to date [25]. In this model, a surgical glove is pulled through the lumen of an olive to recreate the force characteristics of a hypertrophied pylorus. The benefit of such a model is that it is easily reproducible and inexpensive.

The role of thoracoscopy and laparoscopy in the neonate is controversial [50] but is being attempted for such diseases as CDH, esophageal atresia with TEF, and congenital intestinal atresias. The description of simulators for these disease entities is limited but evolving. A group in the USA has led the way in developing an innovative neonatal thoracic model combining a 3D-printed plastic thorax and bovine mediastinal tissues ([43, 51]; Fig. 22.5). The esophagus and trachea are surgically altered to create a proximal esophageal atresia and a distal TEF, representing the most common variation of TEF. When used by pediatric surgery residents, the model performed well on initial validation studies scoring high in the domains of relevance, physical realism, realism of experience, realism of materials, and overall value. The same group has modified the simulator to create a construct for CDH and duodenal atresia.

Another technique for replicating the surgical anatomical environment is the use of animal models. Animal models of TEF are described [52], although work is ongoing to replace the need for bovine or other animal components with synthetic materials to improve availability, avoid the intrinsic ethical difficulties, and potentially reduce cost [51]. It remains to be seen if MIS will supplant traditional open surgery for TEF given concerns of intraoperative carbon dioxide retention and potential for higher anastamotic complications. It is the opinion of these authors that given the infrequency of these cases and the technical demand, dedicated practice is clearly indicated.

One specific challenge to surgical educators with the explosion of MIS technique may be the lack of available open procedures in surgical training. The surgical decision to convert a laparoscopic case back to a traditional open operation may actually be impaired or limited by the lack of case exposure. At this point, the authors are unaware of any open abdominal surgery pediatric simulator. An excellent example of a program designed to maintain exposure to traditional open surgery is the American College of Surgery (ACS)-based Advanced Trauma Operative Management (ATOM)

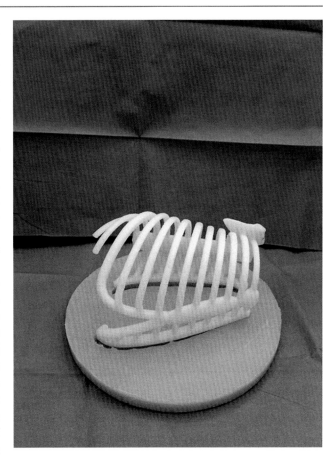

Fig. 22.5 Neonatal thoracic cage model created through 3D printing technology. (Reprinted with permission from Elsevier [43])

course, which requires participants to identify and surgically repair traumatic injuries in an animal (porcine) model. Trauma surgery principles remain the same regardless of patient age and certainly a smaller animal model could be used to specifically mimic a pediatric setting. The limitations of the development of such models remain ethics, cost, and availability. The American College of Surgery Advanced Trauma Life Support (ATLS) course has transitioned its use of animal models to mannequin-based ones for such skills as chest tube insertion and surgical airways. Open models, both synthetic and animal, have been described for dedicated Extra Corporeal Life Support (ECLS) cannulation [53–56]. As part of a structured curriculum consisting of cannula insertion through multidisciplinary resuscitative simulations, improvements in individual knowledge and skill have been demonstrated, as has team functioning as a whole [53, 57]. At our institution, a combination of animal labs, high-fidelity vascular access mannequins, and scenario-based simulations were used to bring online a successful ECLS program despite widespread prior inexperience [57]. Figure 22.6 demonstrates how dedicated practice on lifelike mannequins can result in successful patient outcomes.

Fig. 22.6 a Modified mannequin to practice neck cannulation
for extra corporeal life support
(ECLS). **b** First patient undergoing cannulation following a dedicated curriculum to introduce an
ECLS program. (Photo courtesy
of KidSIM Pediatric Simulation
Program, Alberta Children's
Hospital)

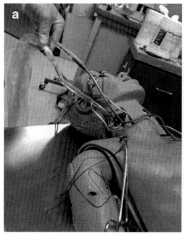
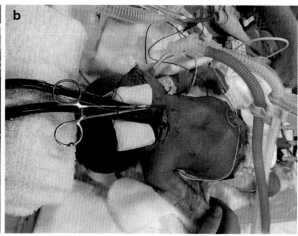

The reality is that the evidence to support simulation in pediatric surgery is minimal. Beyond the data mentioned above where some simulators seem to have content valid- ity (judged to be realistic by its users) and construct validity (ability to measure differences in skill), there is little to no data to suggest actual improvements in outcome. Fortunate- ly, the results of investigation in this area are forthcoming. Subsequent to their early work developing the PLS system, Nasr and Azzie are using motion and force analysis to ana- lyze an individual's movements, hopefully targeting specific skills and educational interventions in real time [58]. Wheth- er surgical simulation is worth the buzz remains to be shown but we are likely to see a proliferation of literature to this point in the near future.

Scenario-Based Team Training in Pediatric Surgery

Training a surgeon in the twenty-first century is certainly more than just training one individual in a procedural skill. The expectation is that surgeons are contributing members of a team, able to effectively communicate with patients and colleagues, and become advocates in the community. Com- petency-based frameworks in surgical education now reflect these expectations with significant weighting to non-medical expert domains. Indeed, the expectation of such skills may be higher and more demanding in the pediatric population, especially with the addition of an alternate caregiver (i.e., parent) in the equation. Many of the concepts for team-based training and crisis resource management are discussed else- where in this book (see Chap. 4). In the surgical realm, a number of non-pediatric-specific courses are offered such as the ACS Leadership course. ATLS, which combines didac- tic lecture with skill practice and case-based simulation, has been shown to improve trauma resuscitation skill and confi- dence but the greatest improvement may be in team behav- ior [59]. A new simulation-based course in pediatric trauma,

Trauma Resuscitation in Kids (TRIK, RCPSC) is likely to have a similar effect. Refer to the RCPSC website for more details [60].

Greater attention is certainly being paid to the role of the interprofessional team in preventing adverse events. Simula- tion training in the OR is often centered around emergent scenarios with the aim to improve team communication and efficiency. Despite barriers to implementation such as staff recruitment and cost, it has been shown to be both feasible and have favorable outcomes, such as increased knowledge, confidence, and team communication [61–63].

The Global Perspective

Barriers to subspecialty pediatric surgery access include geographic distance and resource-limited environments (see Chap. 25) [64]. In developing countries, the ratio of practic- ing pediatric surgeons to population size is alarmingly small. Techniques considered standard of care in much of the world are less available due to economic limitations and lack of expertise. As resources allow, there has been an increased interest in learning these techniques. A 3-day FLS course run in Botswana, Africa, was able to significantly improve the technical skill of surgeons [65]. Of the 20 surgeons partici- pating, the median laparoscopy exposure prior to the course was only 4.5 cases, likely contributing to the 10% overall pass rate. Participants however did significantly improve on each of the FLS tasks as well as the total FLS simulator score. In a setting of limited resources, 11 surgeons reached adequate competency to pass the manual skills portion in just 3 days. Assuming that the advantages of MIS will also ben- efit patients in these developing countries, how best to train surgeons in these techniques? It is clear that compact courses may improve skill but do not replace ongoing learning, ex- perience, and mentorship. In addition, the cost and human resources required to deliver these courses are prohibitive. Telesimulation, a teaching method in which simulators are linked between instructor and trainee in different locations, is a promising alternative [66, 67]. Using the Internet so that teachers and trainees can see each other as well as their respective laparoscopy simulators has been shown to be superior to self-practice [66]. This fits the Eriksson model of DP, where constructive feedback in the setting of practice speeds development of performance. Applied to pediatric resuscitation and procedural skills, telesimulation has been shown effective for teaching intraosseous insertion techniques across great distances [67].

New Technologies and the Future of Simulation in Pediatric Surgery

Innovation and technology continue to advance at an incredibly fast rate. It would be foolish to predict the appearance of surgery in the generations to come. Already, advances in medical imaging and interventional radiology techniques are changing the surgical landscape. Three-dimensional printers are being used to develop high-fidelity simulators but could one day be developed for patient-specific planning and surgical *dry-runs*. Animal models continue to be phased out, replaced by synthetic models, and perhaps one day completely by virtual reality. In the OR, 3D-MIS is in its infancy and will likely require expansion of skill prior to hitting primetime. Most of all, we must remember that simulation is merely a tool and needs to be kept within the context of a planned curriculum. To do this, we must involve our learners as well as our patients in terms of expectations and maintaining our contract with society. One example is the use of social media to broadcast surgical procedures around the world with the ability for live interaction with the surgical team. The potential reach to learners is tremendous so long as the risk to patients is mitigated.

Conclusions

Simulation in pediatric surgery is in its infancy. Dedicated surgical educators continue to build the literature, but to date there is little hard evidence linking surgical simulation to an improvement in actual patient outcomes. Simulation however likely represents the most promising educational intervention to combat declining case exposure and independence for learners of all levels.

References

1. Ericsson KA. Deliberate practice and acquisition of expert performance: a general overview. Acad Emerg Med. 2008;15(11):988–94.
2. Drake FT, Horvath KD, Goldin AB, Gow KW. The general surgery chief resident operative experience: 23 years of national ACGME case logs. JAMA Surg. 2013;148(9):841–7.
3. Drolet BC, Sangisetty S, Tracy TF, Cioffi WG. Surgical residents' perceptions of 2011 accreditation council for graduate medical education duty hour regulations. JAMA Surg. 2013;148(5):427–33.
4. Antiel RM, Reed DA, Van Arendonk KJ, Wightman SC, Hall DE, Porterfield JR, et al. Effects of duty hour restrictions on core competencies, education, quality of life, and burnout among general surgery interns. JAMA Surg. 2013;148(5):448–55.
5. Somme S, Bronsert M, Kempe A, Morrato EH, Ziegler M. Alignment of training curriculum and surgical practice: implications for competency, manpower, and practice modeling. Eur J Pediatr Surg. 2012;22(1):74–9.
6. Behr CA, Hesketh AJ, Akerman M, Dolgin SE, Cowles RA. Recent trends in the operative experience of junior pediatric surgical attendings: a study of APSA applicant case logs. J Pediatr Surg. 2015;50(1):186–90.
7. Fingeret AL, Stolar CJH, Cowles RA. Trends in operative experience of pediatric surgical residents in the United States and Canada. J Pediatr Surg. 2013;48(1):88–94.
8. Rowe MI, Courcoulas A, Reblock K. An analysis of the operative experience of North American pediatric surgical training programs and residents. J Pediatr Surg. 1997;32(2):184–91.
9. Gow KW, Drake FT, Aarabi S, Waldhausen JH. The ACGME case log: general surgery resident experience in pediatric surgery. J Pediatr Surg. 2013;48(8):1643–9.
10. Freeman CL, Bennett TD, Casper TC, Larsen GY, Hubbard A, Wilkes J, Bratton S. Pediatric and neonatal extracorporeal membrane oxygenation: does center volume impact mortality? Crit Care Med. 2014;42(3):512–9.
11. Karamlou T, Vafaeezadeh M, Parrish AM, Cohen GA, Welke KF, Permut L, McMullan DM. Increased extracorporeal membrane oxygenation center case volume is associated with improved extracorporeal membrane oxygenation survival among pediatric patients. J Thorac Cardiovasc Surg. 2013;145(2):470–5.
12. Langer JC, To T. Does pediatric surgical specialty training affect outcome after Ramstedt pyloromyotomy? A population-based study. Pediatrics. 2004;113(5):1342–7.
13. Brain AJ, Roberts DS. Who should treat pyloric stenosis: the general or specialist pediatric surgeon? J Pediatr Surg. 1996;31(11):1535–7.
14. Wei P-L, et al. Volume-outcome relation for acute appendicitis: evidence from a nationwide population-based study. PLoS ONE [Electronic Resource]. 2012;7(12):e52539.
15. Tasian GE, Wiebe DJ, Casale P. Learning curve of robotic assisted pyeloplasty for pediatric urology fellows. J Urol. 2013;190(4 Suppl):1622–6.
16. Nelson CP, Dunn RL, Wei JT, Gearhart JP. Surgical repair of bladder exstrophy in the modern era: contemporary practice patterns and the role of hospital case volume. J Urol. 2005;174(3):1099–102.
17. Allen SW, Gauvreau K, Bloom BT, Jenkins KJ. Evidence-based referral results in significantly reduced mortality after congenital heart surgery. Pediatrics. 2003;112(1 Pt 1):24–8.
18. Tunell WP. The role of pediatric surgery in general surgical education. J Pediatr Surg. 1974;9(5):743–7.
19. Stefanidis D, Colavita PD. Simulation in general surgery. In A. I. Levine et al., editors. The comprehensive textbook of healthcare simulation. New York: Springer Science; 2013. p. 353–66.
20. Derossis AM, Fried GM, Abrahamowicz M, Sigman HH, Barkun JS, Meakins JL. Development of a model for training and evaluation of laparoscopic skills. Am J Surg. 1998;175(6):482–7.
21. McCluney AL, Vassiliou MC, Kaneva PA, Cao J, Stanbride DD, Feldman LS, et al. FLS simulator performance predicts intraoperative laparoscopic skill. Surg Endosc. 2007;21(11):1991–5.
22. Hamilton JM, Kahol K, Vankiuram M, Ashby A, Notrica DM, Ferrara JJ. Toward effective pediatric minimally invasive surgical simulation. J Pediatr Surg. 2011;46(1):138–44.
23. Cosper GH, Menon R, Hamann MS, Nakayama DK. Residency training in pyloromyotomy: a survey of 331 pediatric surgeons. J Pediatr Surg. 2008;43(1):102–8.

24. Davis SS Jr, Husain FA, Lin E, Nandipati KC, Perez S, Sweeney JF. Resident participation in index laparoscopic general surgical cases: impact of the learning environment on surgical outcomes. [Erratum appears in J Am Coll Surg. 2013 May;216(5):1034]. J Am Coll Surg. 2013;216(1):96–104.

25. Plymale M, Ruzic A, Hoskins J, French J, Skinner SC, Yuhas M, et al. A middle fidelity model is effective in teaching and retaining skill set needed to perform a laparoscopic pyloromyotomy. J Laparoendosc Adv Surg Tech Part A. 2010;20(6):569–73.

26. Peter SD St, Barnhart DC, Ostlie DJ, Tsao K, Leys CM, Sharp SW, et al. Minimal vs extensive esophageal mobilization during laparoscopic fundoplication: a prospective randomized trial. J Pediatr Surg. 2011;46(1):163–8.

27. Apelt N, Featherstone N, Giuliani S. Laparoscopic treatment of intussusception in children: a systematic review. J Pediatr Surg. 2013;48(8):1789–93.

28. Li B, Chen W-B, Zhou W-Y. Laparoscopic methods in the treatment of congenital duodenal obstruction for neonates. J Laparoendosc Adv Surg Tech Part A. 2013;23(10):881–4.

29. Becmeur F, Reinberg O, Dimitriu C, Moog R, Philippe P. Thoracoscopic repair of congenital diaphragmatic hernia in children. Semin Pediatr Surg. 2007;16(4):238–44.

30. Matlow AG, Baker GR, Flintoft V, Cochrane D, Coffey M, Cohen E, et al. Adverse events among children in Canadian hospitals: the Canadian paediatric adverse events study. CMAJ Can Med Assoc J. 2012;184(13):E709–18.

31. Lasko D, Zamakhshary M, Gerstle JT. Perception and use of minimal access surgery simulators in pediatric surgery training programs. J Pediatr Surg. 2009;44(5):1009–12.

32. Leach DC. A model for GME: shifting from process to outcomes. A progress report from the accreditation council for graduate medical education. Med Educ. 2004;38(1):12–4.

33. Frank JR, et al. Report of the CanMEDS phase IV working groups. 2005: Ottawa.

34. Hirschl R. The pediatric surgery milestone project: a joint initiative of the accreditation council for graduate medical education and the American board of surgery. 2014. http://acgme.org/acgmeweb/Portals/0/PDFs/Milestones/PediatricSurgeryMilestones.pdf. Accessed 11 Nov 2014.

35. Frank JR, Snell L. Draft CanMEDS 2015 Physician Competency Framework—Series I. 2014, The royal college of physicians and surgeons of Canada: Ottawa.

36. Martin JA, Regehr G, Reznick R, Macrae H, Murnaghan J, Hutchison C, et al. Objective structured assessment of technical skill (OSATS) for surgical residents. Br J Surg. 1997;84(2):273–8.

37. Chipman JG, Schmitz CC. Using objective structured assessment of technical skills to evaluate a basic skills simulation curriculum for first-year surgical residents. J Am Coll Surg. 2009;209(3):364–70.e2.

38. Peters JH, Fried GM, Swanstrom LL, Soper NJ, Sillin LF, Schirmer B. Development and validation of a comprehensive program of education and assessment of the basic fundamentals of laparoscopic surgery. Surgery. 2004;135(1):21–7.

39. Nakajima K, Wasa M, Takuguchi S, Taniguchi E, Soh H, Ohashi S, et al. A modular laparoscopic training program for pediatric surgeons. JSLS. 2003;7(1):33–7.

40. Ieiri S, Nakatsuji T, Higashi M, et al. Effectiveness of basic endoscopic surgical skill training for pediatric surgeons. Pediatr Surg Int. 2010;26(10):947–54.

41. Grober ED, Hamstra S, Wanzel KR, Reznick RK, Matsumoto ED, Sidhu R, et al. The educational impact of bench model fidelity on the acquisition of technical skill: the use of clinically relevant outcome measures. Ann Surg. 2004;240(2):374–81.

42. Matsumoto ED, Hamstra SJ, Radomski SB, Cusimano MD. The effect of bench model fidelity on endourological skills: a randomized controlled study. J Urol. 2002;167(3):1243–7.

43. Barsness KA, Rooney DM, Davis LM. Collaboration in simulation: the development and initial validation of a novel thoracoscopic neonatal simulator. J Pediatr Surg. 2013;48(6):1232–8.

44. Donoghue AJ, Durbin DR, Nadel FM, Stryjewski GR, Kost SI, Nadkarni VM. Perception of realism during mock resuscitations by pediatric housestaff: the impact of simulated physical features. Simul Healthc. 2010;5(1):16–20.

45. Azzie G, Gerstle JT, Nasr A, Lasko D, Green J, Henao O, et al. Development and validation of a pediatric laparoscopic surgery simulator. J Pediatr Surg. 2011;46(5):897–903.

46. Nasr A, Gerstle JT, Carrillo B, Azzie G. The pediatric laparoscopic surgery (PLS) simulator: methodology and results of further validation. J Pediatr Surg. 2013;48(10):2075–7.

47. Pranikoff T, Campbell BT, Travis J, Hirschl RB. Differences in outcome with subspecialty care: pyloromyotomy in North Carolina. J Pediatr Surg. 2002;37(3):352–6.

48. Safford SD, Pietrobon R, Safford KM, Martins H, Skinner MA, Rice HE. A study of 11,003 patients with hypertrophic pyloric stenosis and the association between surgeon and hospital volume and outcomes. J Pediatr Surg. 2005;40(6):967–72; discussion 972–3.

49. Haricharan RN, Aprahamian CH, Celik A, Harmon CM, Georgeson KE, Barnhart DC. Laparoscopic pyloromyotomy: effect of resident training on complications. J Pediatr Surg. 2008;43(1):97–101.

50. McHoney M, Giacomello L, Nah SA, De Coppi P, Kiely EM, Curry JI, et al. Thoracoscopic repair of congenital diaphragmatic hernia: intraoperative ventilation and recurrence. J Pediatr Surg. 2010;45(2):355–9.

51. Hawkinson EK, Davis LM, Barsness KA. Design and development of low-cost tissue replicas for simulation of rare neonatal congenital defects. Stud Health Technol Inform. 2014;196:159–62.

52. Bidarkar SS, Deshpande A, Kaur M, Cohen RC. Porcine models for pediatric minimally invasive surgical training—a template for the future. J Laparoendosc Adv Surg Tech Part A. 2012;22(1):117–22.

53. Allan CK, Pigula F, Bacha EA, Emani S, Fynn-Thompson F, Thiagarajan RR, et al. An extracorporeal membrane oxygenation cannulation curriculum featuring a novel integrated skills trainer leads to improved performance among pediatric cardiac surgery trainees. Simul Healthc. 2013;8(4):221–8.

54. Anderson JM, Boyle KB, Murphy AA, Yaeger KA, LeFlore J, et al. Simulating extracorporeal membrane oxygenation emergencies to improve human performance. Part I: methodologic and technologic innovations. Simul Healthc. 2006;1(4):220–7.

55. Anderson JM, Murphy AA, Boyle KB, Yaeger KA, Halamek LP. Simulating extracorporeal membrane oxygenation emergencies to improve human performance. Part II: assessment of technical and behavioral skills. Simul Healthc. 2006;1(4):228–32.

56. Allan CK, Thiagarajan RR, Beke D, Imprescia A, Kappus LJ, Garden A, et al. Simulation-based training delivered directly to the pediatric cardiac intensive care unit engenders preparedness, comfort, and decreased anxiety among multidisciplinary resuscitation teams. J Thorac Cardiovasc Surg. 2010;140(3):646–52.

57. Sanchez-Glanville C, Brindle ME, Spence T, Blackwood J, Drews T, Menzies S, Lopushinsky SR. The introduction of extracorporeal life support technology to a tertiary-care pediatric institution: smoothing the learning curve through inter-professional simulation training. J Pediatr Surg. 2015;50(5):798–804.

58. Nasr A, Carrillo B, Gerstle JT, Azzie G. Motion analysis in the pediatric laparoscopic surgery (PLS) simulator: validation and potential use in teaching and assessing surgical skills. J Pediatr Surg. 2014;49(5):791–4.

59. Marshall RL, Smith JS, Gorman PJ, Krummel TM, Haluck RS, Cooney RN, et al. Use of a human patient simulator in the development of resident trauma management skills. J Trauma Inj Infect Crit Care. 2001;51(1):17–21.

60. http://www.royalcollege.ca/portal/page/portal/rc/resources/ppi/trik_course.
61. Arriaga AF, Gawande AA, Raemer DB, Jones DB, Smink DS, Weinstock P, et al. Pilot testing of a model for insurer-driven, large-scale multicenter simulation training for operating room teams. Ann Surg. 2014;259(3):403–10.
62. Cumin D, Boyd MJ, Webster CS, Weller JM. A systematic review of simulation for multidisciplinary team training in operating rooms. Simul Healthc. 2013;8(3):171–9.
63. Acero NM, Motuk G, Luba J, Murphy M, McKelvey S, Kolb G, et al. Managing a surgical exsanguination emergency in the operating room through simulation: an interdisciplinary approach. J Surg Educ. 2012;69(6):759–65.
64. Mayer ML, Beil HA, von Allmen D. Distance to care and relative supply among pediatric surgical subspecialties. J Pediatr Surg. 2009;44(3):483–95.
65. Okrainec A, Smith L, Azzie G. Surgical simulation in Africa: the feasibility and impact of a 3-day fundamentals of laparoscopic surgery course. Surg Endosc. 2009;23(11):2493–8.
66. Okrainec A, Henao O, Azzie G. Telesimulation: an effective method for teaching the fundamentals of laparoscopic surgery in resource-restricted countries. Surg Endosc. 2010;24(2):417–22.
67. Mikrogianakis A, Kam A, Silver S, Bakanisi B, Henao O, Ikrainex A, Azzie G. Telesimulation: an innovative and effective tool for teaching novel intraosseous insertion techniques in developing countries. Acad Emerg Med. 2011;18(4):420–7.

Simulation for Teaching Communication Skills

23

Jennifer R. Reid, Kimberly P. Stone and Elaine C. Meyer

Simulation Pearls

1. Communication in healthcare can be as straightforward as a personal introduction to patients/parents or as complex as delivering bad news.
2. Skillfully conveying both factual content and navigating the emotional experience takes skill and practice.
3. Simulation methodology can train healthcare providers to better navigate all healthcare communications.

Introduction

Conversations between healthcare providers, patients, and families unfold constantly across clinical settings. From everyday clinical encounters to challenging situations such as when sharing serious new diagnoses, broaching end-of-life issues, or discussing adverse medical outcomes, these conversations matter [1]. For each test, procedure, or surgery that must be conducted, there are typically one or more accompanying conversations. Care discussions are ubiquitous. To punctuate the point, it is estimated that the average physician will hold between 160,000–300,000 medical interviews and conversations over the course of a 40-year career [2]. The research is convincing that practitioners' communication and relational skills are associated with improved patient health outcomes, better treatment adherence, fewer medication errors, less malpractice litigation, and greater patient and clinician satisfaction [3]. Yet, practitioners often describe minimal training, lack of skillfulness, and diminished confidence when holding these important conversations [4]. Simulation can be part of the solution to address this pressing need.

Conversations in healthcare typically include a combination of factual information and emotional aspects. Factual information may include laboratory results, radiological findings, differential diagnoses, treatment plans, and education about particular diagnoses. The emotional aspects of the communicative encounter include responses such as disbelief, sadness, anxiety, anger, fear, frustration, relief, and confusion, among others. Patients and family members have their emotional responses, as do healthcare providers. For example, factual information of healthcare conversations may be a blood test that suggests a diagnosis of diabetes. The emotional aspects of the conversation, for the patient, family, and provider, are the feelings, memories, and associations these facts may trigger. The child may be fearful and wonder when they will feel better. Parents may be sad and overwhelmed, wondering how the diagnosis will affect the child's daily life, nutrition, friendships, and development. Healthcare providers might experience relief that the tests did not indicate cancer and be confused that the family does not seem relieved. Simulation allows healthcare providers to practice the full spectrum of healthcare conversations, tailored to the learners' needs and course objectives. In this chapter, we will share some examples of the full spectrum of healthcare conversation simulations, progressing from those with greater factual content to those with higher emotional content. Please see also Chap. 4 ("Simulation-based Team Training") for additional discussions about teamwork and communication.

J. R. Reid (✉) · K. P. Stone
Department of Pediatrics, Division of Emergency Medicine, University of Washington School of Medicine, Seattle Children's Hospital, Seattle, WA, USA
e-mail: Jennifer.reid@seattlechildrens.org

K. P. Stone
e-mail: Kimberly.stone@seattlechildrens.org

E. C. Meyer
Department of Psychiatry, Institute for Professionalism and Ethical Practice, Harvard Medical School, Boston Children's Hospital, Boston, MA, USA
e-mail: elaine.meyer@childrens.harvard.edu

© Springer International Publishing Switzerland 2016
V. J. Grant, A. Cheng (eds.), *Comprehensive Healthcare Simulation: Pediatrics,*
Comprehensive Healthcare Simulation, DOI 10.1007/978-3-319-24187-6_23

Introductions and Setting the Stage for the Clinical Encounter

Although seemingly minor, the manner in which healthcare providers introduce themselves, and the message that is conveyed during those first few moments, sets a tone for the clinical encounter and the relationship. As we know, one does not get a second chance to make a first impression. Clinical introductions can range from "Hello, I'm Jennifer" to "I'm Jennifer, part of the pediatric team" to "Hello, I am Doctor Jennifer Reid. I am the resident physician on the pediatric medicine team who will be taking care of your daughter Sarah today." New physicians, for example, can experience discomfort when introducing themselves as *doctor*. It is not unusual for healthcare providers to simply refer to themselves by their subspecialty, such as *renal* or *anesthesia,* which diminishes the personhood of the provider and leaves the family wondering who they are. Another common issue can arise when healthcare providers simply introduce themselves as the *covering* nurse or physician implying only a temporary role that might leave the family worrying about the level of investment in the care and the cohesiveness of the teamwork [5]. This discomfort on the part of healthcare providers can be reflected not only in the words care providers use or do not use when they introduce themselves, but also in their tone of voice, posture, and nonverbal communication.

From the patient and family perspective, "Hello, I'm Jennifer" may seem friendly and welcoming to some, but to others may be viewed as too casual and leave the family uncertain about the person's role or level of experience. Such an introduction could unwittingly undermine the healthcare provider's role and expertise, derail the establishment of the therapeutic relationship, or compromise care. When multiple providers wear scrubs and look the same, it can be understandably hard to distinguish among clinical support staff, nurses, and physicians. Under these circumstances and in busy clinical settings, introductions become even more important. Something as seemingly straightforward as an introduction, that clarifies an individual's name and role within the healthcare team, can benefit from forethought and practice in the context of simulation.

At the Program to Enhance Relational and Communication Skills (PERCS) workshops, offered by the Institute for Professionalism and Ethical Practice at Boston Children's Hospital, realistic enactments with professional actors have been used to help physicians and healthcare staff reflect on, craft, and practice their introductions and the art of holding challenging conversations in healthcare [3, 6, 7]. Is it more comfortable and effective to introduce oneself as "Jennifer" or "Dr. Jennifer Reid"? How does one describe their role and their place on the team, in terms that children and family members can understand? As a respiratory therapist or the unit psychologist, for example, how does one convey the clinical role, describe their part within the team, and instill confidence? Should one shake hands, or not, especially in settings where hand washing is all-important to combat the spread of infection? The process of learning is iterative and includes interprofessional peers, actors, and faculty members, some of whom are patients and family members. Healthcare providers take turns simulating introducing themselves and then hold challenging conversations with simulated patients and their families. After each simulation, providers give and receive feedback from each other, continuing the simulation process until they develop an introduction style that is clear, comfortable, and effective. Throughout the workshops, healthcare providers learn and practice a myriad of communication skills, have the opportunity to observe others, and receive individualized feedback. Interprofessional learners who have participated in the workshops report greater sense of preparation and confidence, greater communicative skills and ability to establish relationships, and reduced anxiety in holding difficult conversations [7, 8]. Examples of difficult conversations are discussed later in this chapter.

Obtaining a History

Simulation has long been used to help medical and nursing students practice taking medical histories. For example, at the University Of Washington School Of Medicine, over the past 15 years, medical students transitioning to clinical rotations simulate conducting medical histories with standardized patients (Jennifer Reid, written communication, September 2014). The simulations are conducted in hospital inpatient rooms and are videorecorded. At the end of the simulation, the standardized patient has the opportunity to provide the student with feedback on their communication style, nonverbal language, and receptivity. The student also has the opportunity to view the videorecording and reflect and discuss the simulation with the standardized patient and with course instructors.

One medical student describes that in medical school students are typically taught a *script* but as so often happens in actual clinical practice, the script *ends* when a patient asks a question or when unexpected information or findings arise [9]. Simulation with improvisational actors enables young and seasoned clinicians alike to continually hone their communication and relational skills, and to be better prepared for, and comfortable with, the unexpected.

Verbal Handoffs

Handoffs in medicine are commonplace: Healthcare providers usually receive and give multiple handoffs each time they work. A number of handoff tools have been developed with similar underlying goals: to create a structured, succinct handoff that addresses pertinent issues, so that critical information is not missed and providers have an opportunity to clarify (see Table 23.1) [10]. Experience from one institution demonstrates that simulation-based handoff training results in increased transfer of critical communication between nurses [11].

Simulation-based training for handoffs need not be complicated. One example could involve residents using a standard verbal handoff checklist for admitting a pediatric patient from the emergency department to the inpatient medical team. The residents can pair up: a first-year resident with a second- or third-year resident. Since these conversations often occur over the phone, the pair can sit back-to-

back. They each read the same patient care summary. For the initial simulation, the more experienced resident uses the handoff checklist to *handoff* the patient. The junior resident then has the opportunity to ask questions, debrief with the senior resident, and provide feedback. The pair then changes roles, with the junior resident providing the verbal handoff on the same patient. Depending on the learners, the same or different handoffs can be repeated until the communication goals are achieved. One could imagine swapping healthcare providers (e.g., nurses, pharmacists, respiratory therapists) to simulate a variety of everyday handoffs (e.g., shift report).

For institutions with greater resources, more comprehensive simulation-based training handoff programs, which may include didactics and computer-based and in-person simulation, can be implemented. Implementation of a comprehensive multi-institutional handoff program was associated with reductions in medical errors, preventable adverse events, and improved communication, without negative effect on workflow [10].

Table 23.1 I-PASS mnemonic elements. The I-PASS mnemonic (Illness severity, Patient Summary, Action items, Situation awareness and contingency planning, Synthesis by receiver) can be used as a way to standardize the verbal (oral) handoff process at shift change during in-person verbal communication. It can also be used as a framework to standardize the written handoff process by integrating the individual mnemonic elements in computerized handoff tools within word processing documents or, ideally, within the electronic medical record where possible. (Reproduced with permission [10])

Mnemonic letter	Description	Key points
I	Illness severity	Identification of patient's level of acuity to focus attention appropriately at the start of the handoff communication
		Suggest classifying each patient using a standardized language such as stable, "watcher" (a patient where any clinician has a concern that a patient is at risk of deterioration), or unstable
		May include code status
		Classification may vary depending on unit acuity, provider type, or institutional culture
P	Patient summary	Describes succinctly the reason for admission, events leading up to admission, hospital course, and plan for hospitalization
		Should reflect global plan for entire hospital stay and avoid "to-do" items for next shift
		Should be maintained and updated regularly with modification of assessment, diagnoses, and changes in treatment plans as necessary
A	Action items	Includes a "to-do" list with specific elements to accomplish over next shift by team assuming care of patient
		Should specify time frame for completion, level of priority, and who is responsible
		Specify "nothing to do" if no action items are anticipated
S	Situation awareness and contingency plans	Situation awareness: knowing what is going on for members of the care team (status of patients, environmental factors, team members) and for each individual patient (status of disease process, progress towards goals for hospitalization)
		Contingency plans: with situation awareness in mind, provide team assuming care of the patient with specific instructions for how to handle anticipated problems
		Typically includes "if/then" statements
		Specify "no contingencies anticipated" for stable patients
		Ensures accepting team is prepared to anticipate changes in patient status and respond to potential events
S	Synthesis by receiver	Provides a brief restatement of essential information in a cogent summary by receiving team
		Demonstrates information is received and understood
		Ensures effective transfer of information and responsibility
		Opportunity for receiver to clarify elements of handoff, ensure clear understanding, and play an active role in handoff process
		Will vary in length and content depending on acuity level of patient
		Should prioritize restatement of key action items and contingency plans: not a restatement of the entire verbal handoff

Consultations

A common challenge for healthcare providers is to succinctly and clearly convey concerns, assessments, and requests to other team members. Many team members express frustration or disappointment in some of their communication interactions because of a seeming lack of understanding or response. When the conversation is analyzed, there is often more than one conversation occurring—based on the eye or ear of the beholder.

Consider this example:

Nurse *says:* "Doctor, the child I just put in room 10 doesn't look good."

Nurse *thinks:* "The child in room 10 looks like he might be septic. His heart rate is too high, despite being afebrile, he seems listless."

Doctor *says:* "I'll go see him as soon as I can."

Doctor *thinks:* "I still need to call the consultant for the patient in room 8, write orders for the patient in room 9, talk to the mom in room 2 and get something to eat…the patient in room 10 just came back…I'll let him wait until I get caught up."

In order to help learn about and practice these conversations, iterative simulations can focus specifically on the communication of concerns and requests. As part of nursing orientation at one institution, all nurses are introduced to the SBAR (Situation, Background, Assessment, Recommendation) format for expressing concerns and requests [12]. See Table 23.2. In a three-part simulation, each nurse cares for a simulated patient, who becomes progressively more ill. The nurse first simulates having a telephone conversation, initially with his or her charge nurse, then with a resident physician, and finally with a member of the rapid response team. In each conversation, the nurse practices using the SBAR format. Both the recipient of the phone call (a confederate who understands the learning objectives) and an instructor provide feedback on the learner's utilization of SBAR and clarity. Participants have the opportunity to try it again and again until they achieve fluency (written communication, Jennifer Reid, September 2014). A recent study of effective SBAR training identified role-play simulation (such as described above) to be a more effective method than traditional didactic methods, such as a lecture, in training nurses to using SBAR as a communication tool [13].

Informed Consent

Ideally, the informed consent process includes a combination of fact sharing regarding procedures, risks, alternatives, responses to questions, and careful attention to emotional responses that may arise. Simulation has been reported in a limited number of publications to assess and develop informed consent communication skills. One study examined how different providers (consultant surgeons vs. senior trainees vs. junior trainees) performed during an informed consent conversation. Assessment focused on the factual content: description of surgical risks [14]. In one educational intervention, anesthesiology trainees simulate interacting with a standardized patient, conducting a history, physical, and obtaining informed consent. The debriefing includes their ability to answer patient questions, use of nonverbal strategies to create an open atmosphere, reflections on posture and mannerisms, and comfort with the interaction overall [15].

Conveying Difficult or Bad News

Conveying bad news to families in pediatrics can be extremely challenging [4, 16, 17] due to both the emotional stress and potential for long-term impact on the family [18, 19]. Although healthcare providers identify the desire to communicate difficult news well [15, 16, 20, 21], parents report high variability in their experience [18]. Simulation has

Table 23.2 SBAR (Situation, Background, Assessment, Recommendation): a framework for team members to effectively communicate information to one another [38]. To incorporate this into a progressive simulation, e.g., where a nurse has the opportunity to *repeat* the SBAR with different members of the healthcare team or as a patient progresses, after the first simulation, you can either have them simulate the SBAR again, with a different member of the healthcare team or provide additional information, e.g., update: another hour has passed, your patient failed to improve, she has ongoing increased work of breathing and more signs of fatigue

Mnemonic letter	Description	Sample scenario: 3-year-old girl with asthma, with ongoing work of breathing, decreasing oxygen saturations, and increasing signs of fatigue, despite 1 hour of ongoing asthma treatment
S	*Situation:* What is going on with the patient?	3-year-old girl with respiratory distress
B	*Background:* What is the clinical background or context?	3-year-old girl with history of asthma, increasing fatigue, ongoing work of breathing, decreasing saturations after 1 hour of asthma treatment
A	*Assessment:* What do I think the problem is?	I think she is in early respiratory failure
R	*Recommendation:* What would I recommend?	Let us reevaluate as a team and escalate her therapy

been used to help healthcare providers practice and be evaluated on their communication skills in delivering bad news. Delivering bad news has also been referred to as *breaking bad news*. However, in our view, when healthcare providers are trained via simulation to have these conversations, nothing should be *broken* and, in fact, these conversations can go well.

A simulation-based workshop focused on conveying difficult news recently published its structure and results. After receiving classroom-based instruction, small groups of residents participated in three scenarios, each starting with a simulated resuscitation and followed by two conversations with an actor portraying a patient's parent, followed by debriefing. Residents self-reported improvement in their ability to deliver bad news and were observed to statistically improve, using an evaluation tool completed by experts and parents [22]. Additional formative interventions describe scenarios where trainees have the opportunity to deliver bad news to standardized patients or actors regarding either patient harm or death, and receive feedback [15, 23, 24].

Disclosure of Medical Errors

Despite improvements in patient safety, medical errors still occur, creating the opportunity for challenging conversations which combine high factual content in addition to high emotional content [25]. Gallagher emphasizes that the most important features of these conversations include an appropriate *apology*, *an explanation* of what care is being provided to remedy and address the harm for the patient, and *assurances* that the situation will be thoroughly investigated and measures implemented to guard against future similar errors [26]. Simulation has the potential to recreate scenarios where medical errors or unavoidable bad outcomes occur, allowing providers to practice disclosure and receive feedback on their disclosures. Communication curricula have been described which include the use of simulation scenarios with a medication error for residents to practice error disclosure to actors playing the role of parents [23]. Another study utilized an error disclosure performance checklist to evaluate residents on the overall quality of their disclosure to a standardized patient [27] (Table 23.3). In this study, two key points stood out: (1) Increased experience with error disclosure alone did not result in higher scores, indicating that dedicated training programs that describe and provide feedback on specific communication skills are required, and (2) standardized patients, independent observers, and the residents disclosing the error all scored the communication similarly. The similarity of their scores adds validity to the checklist, opening up possibilities for broader application.

End-of-Life Discussions

Publications focused on withdrawal of care, disclosing a patient's death, or practicing difficult family interactions in simulation in pediatrics is limited [22, 23]. Most describe formative scenarios, which may or may not provide focused feedback based on communication best practices [22]. The paucity of literature suggests that integration of some of the most factually complex and highly charged emotional content into a standardized communication and simulation curriculum has yet to occur.

Specific Patient Populations

Two specific patient populations deserve special mention: adolescents and mental health patients. These populations represent distinct communication challenges. Much of adolescent medicine focuses on obtaining histories of, and counseling for, risk behaviors and psychosocial issues. The ability to gather and deliver this sensitive information requires the healthcare provider to gain the trust of the adolescent and maintain a therapeutic relationship. Training experiences at the Israel Center for Medical Simulation underscore the uniqueness of this type of communication and the need for simulation-based training [28–31]. One role-play exercise used teen actors from a high school drama department to simulate characteristic adolescent medical problems in a healthcare interaction, including confidentiality issues and both home and school difficulties. Despite the large group format of this training, participants appreciated the need for careful listening, a nonjudgmental approach and the need for confidentiality [28]. Based on their experiences, this group of simulation educators and researchers developed a 1-day course to enhance healthcare providers' communication with adolescents [29]. In addition, they created a simulation-based communication program that is part of a multiyear diploma course in adolescent medicine in Israel [30].

Much of psychiatry revolves around conversations between providers and patients, making the ability to connect even more poignant. In addition, healthcare providers often have anxiety due to lack of experience. Simulation has been used to improve healthcare providers' interview skills with psychiatric patients, promote therapeutic communication, and decrease providers' anxiety [32]. In one study, comparing the use of high-fidelity simulation versus traditional lectures for training senior nursing students in communication skills essential to psychiatric nursing, high-fidelity simulation was more effective in improving nursing student's self-efficacy in communication with mental health patients [33]. A full-scale simulated mental health ward, including stan-

Table 23.3 Items on the Error Disclosure Rating Scale for encounters between standardized patients and 42 postgraduate second-year internal medicine residents used to determine the residents' ability to disclose medical error, University of Toronto, 2005. (Reproduced with permission [27])

Explanation of medical facts regarding error
How did it happen?
Told me what the error was in my care
Explained to me why the error occurred
What are the consequences?
Told me how the error impacted my health
Told me how the consequences of the error will be corrected
Overall impression on explanation of medical facts regarding error
Honesty and truthfulness
Took responsibility for the error
Explained the error to me freely and directly, without me having to ask a litany of probing questions to get the details of the error
Did not keep things from me that I should know
Never avoided my questions (not evasive)
Overall impression on honesty and truthfulness
Empathy
Apology: said he/she was sorry and apologized in a sincere manner. Acknowledgement of feelings
Allowed me to express my emotions regarding this error
Told me that my emotional reaction was understandable
Overall impression of empathy
Prevention of future errors
Told me that an effort will be made to prevent a similar error in the future
Told me what he/she would have done differently
Told me his/her plan for preventing similar errors in the future
Overall impression of prevention of future errors
General communication skills
Degree of coherence in the interview
Verbal expression
Nonverbal expression
Responded to my needs
Checked for my understanding of the information he/she provided
Overall impression on general communication skills

Scoring: each component—1 (not performed), 2 (attempted but incomplete or ineffective), 3 (performed excellently, completely, and effectively); each category—overall, 1–5 (5 high score)

dardized patients, has been created in the US Midwest for nursing students to practice skills, such as nursing assessment and medication administration, along with therapeutic communication with inpatient psychiatric patients [19].

Simulation Approaches and Modalities

Simulation focused on healthcare conversations has employed a variety of modalities, often integrating different types of simulators, to create the highest-fidelity experience. Standardized patients have been used in both research and training programs to ensure consistency in the responses experienced by participants, how participants are evaluated, and feedback [22, 34–36]. Confederates or actors, with variable levels of training and restrictions have been integrated into formative training programs (see Chap. 4) [23]. Simulators have been incorporated, in a mixed-methods approach, for participants to experience a clinical situation (bad out-

come, medical error, or death) which they then had to communicate to either a standardized patient or actor playing the role of a family member. By blending simulation modalities, participants can enter the conversation with emotions elicited from the previous simulation experience, making the conversation more realistic and perhaps more challenging to conduct.

The selection of modalities depends on both learning objectives and resources. The more standardized or structured the responses of those playing the role of the patient or family, the more consistent the learning experience may be for the participants. Enhancing fidelity, by including a human patient simulator prior to disclosure of a bad outcome, can add to the emotional realism and complexity of the scenario for both the instructors and the participants, particularly for more experienced providers. Professional actors, from learner and faculty perspectives, increase realism. They facilitate feedback from non-medical perspectives and allowing improvisation, providing the opportunity to titrate the scenarios to the needs of the learners [37]. Resources may limit what modalities training programs are able to provide. Standardized patients or actors usually require more time for preparation and financial resources, incorporating human patient simulators, and clinical space may require either center-based or in situ simulation space that requires additional funds, time, and physical space that may or may not be available.

Conclusions

Conversations between healthcare providers, patients, and families are ubiquitous. From everyday clinical encounters to challenging situations, these conversations matter [2]. Simulation is only beginning to explore and develop how it can help healthcare providers become more experienced and effective managers of both the factual and emotional content contained in every healthcare conversation. As this field develops, exploring simulation modalities and formats will be critical to helping healthcare providers hone their communication skills.

References

1. Levetown M. Communicating with children and families: from everyday interactions to skill in conveying distressing information. Pediatrics. 2008;121(5):1441–60.
2. Lipkin M Jr. Preface. In: Lipkin M Jr, Putnam SM, Lazare A, editors. The medical interview: clinical care, education and research. New York: Springer; 1995. pp. Ix–Iii.
3. Rosen D. Vital conversations: improving communication between doctors and patients. New York: Columbia University Press; 2014.
4. Orgel E, McCarter R, Jacobs S. A failing medical educational model: a self-assessment by physicians at all levels of training of ability and comfort to deliver bad news. J Palliative Med. 2010;13(6):677–83.
5. Janvier A, Lantos J. Ethics and etiquette in neonatal intensive care. JAMA Pediatr. 2014;168(9):857–8.
6. Browning DM, Meyer EC, Truog RD, Solomon MZ. Difficult conversations in health care: cultivating relational learning to address the hidden curriculum. Acad Med. 2007;82(9):905–13.
7. Meyer EC, Sellers DE, Browning DM, McGuffie K, Solomon MZ, Truog RD. Difficult conversations: improving communication skills and relational abilities in health care. Pediatr Crit Care Med. 2009;10(3):352–9.
8. Meyer EC, Brodsky D, Hansen AR, Lamiani G, Sellers DE, Browning DMA. Interdisciplinary, family-focused approach to relational learning in neonatal intensive care. J Perinatol. 2011;31(3):212–9.
9. Haq C, Steele DJ, Marchand L, Seibert C, Brody D. Integrating the art and science of medical malpractice: innovations in teaching medical communication skills. Fam Med. 2004;36(Suppl):43–50.
10. Starmer AJ, Spector ND, Srivastava R, West DC, Rosenbluth G, Allen AD, Elizabeth L, Noble EL, Tse LL, Dalal AK, Keohane CA, Lipsitz SR, Rothschild JM, Wien MF, Yoon CS, Zigmont KR, Wilson KM, O'Toole JK, Solan LG, Aylor M, Bismilla Z, Coffey M, Mahant S, Blankenburg RL, Destino LA, Everhart JL, Patel SJ, Bale JF, Spackman JB, Stevenson AT, Calaman S, Cole S, Balmer

DF, Hepps JH, Lopreiato JO, Yu CE, Sectish TC, Landrigan CP for the I-PASS Study Group. Changes in medical errors after implementation of a handoff program. NEJM. 2014;371:1803–12.
11. Berkenstadt H, Haviv Y, Tuval A, Shemesh Y, Megrill A, Perry A, et al. Improving handoff communications in critical care: utilizing simulation-based training toward process improvement in managing patient risk. Chest. 2008;134(1):158–62.
12. Haig KM, Sutton S, Whittington J. SBAR: a shared mental model for improving communication between clinicians. Jt Comm J Qual Patient Saf. 2006;32(3):167–75.
13. Chaaharsoughi NT, Ahrari S, Alikhah S. Comparison the effect of teaching of SBAR technique with role play and lecturing of communication skill of nurses. J Caring Sci. 2014;3(2):141–7.
14. Black SA, Nestel D, Tierney T, Amygdalos I, Kneebone R, Wolfe JHN. Gaining consent for carotid surgery: a simulation-based study of vascular surgeons. Eur J Endovasc Surg. 2009;37:134–9.
15. Spofford CM, Szeluga DJ. From beginning to end in anesthesia: a 3 part series on obtaining informed consent, handling a difficult airway and delivering bad news. Simul Healthc. 2013;8(4):262–71.
16. Kolarick RC, Walker G, Arnold RM. Pediatric resident education in palliative care: a needs assessment. Pediatrics. 2006;117:1949–54.
17. Horowitz N, Ellis J. Paediatric SpRs' experiences of breaking bad news. Child Care Health Dev. 2007;33(5):625–30.
18. Fallowfield L, Jenkins V. Communicating sad, bad and difficult news in medicine. Lancet. 2004;363:312–19.
19. Finaly I, Dallimore D. Your child is dead. BMJ. 1991;302:1524–5.
20. Orlander JD, Fincke BG, Hermanns D, Johnson GA. Medical residents' first clearly remembered experiences of giving bad news. J Gen Intern Med. 2002;11:825–31.
21. Colletti L, Gruppen L, Barclay M, Stern D. Teaching students to break bad news. Am J Surg. 2001;182:20–3.
22. Tobler K, Grant E, Marczinski C. Evaluation of the impact of a simulation-enhanced breaking bad news workshop in pediatrics. Simul Healthc. 2014;9:213–19.
23. Overly FL, Sudikoff SN, Duffy S, Anderson A, Kobayashi L. Three scenarios to teach difficult discussions in pediatric emergency medicine: sudden infant death, child abuse with domestic violence and medication error. Simul Healthc. 2009;4:114–30.
24. Park I, Gupta A, Mandani K, Haubner L, Peckler B. Breaking bad news education for emergency medicine residents: a novel training module using simulation with the SPIKES protocol. J Emerg Trauma Shock. 2010;3(4):385–8.
25. Institute of Medicine Committee on Quality of Health Care in America. To err is human: building a safer health system. Washington, D. C.: National Academies Press (US); 2000. (Kohn LT, Corrigan JM, Donaldson MS, editors)
26. Chan DK, Gallagher TH, Reznick R, Levinson W. How surgeons disclose medical errors to patients: a study using standardized patients. Surgery. 2005;138(5):851–8.
27. Stroud L, McIllroy J, Levinson W. Skills of internal medicine residents in disclosing medical errors: a study using standardized patients. Acad Med. 2009;84(12):1803–8.
28. Hardoff D, Schonmann S. Training physicians in communication skills with adolescents using teenage actors as simulated patients. Med Educ. 2001;35(3):206–10.
29. Hardoff D, Benita S, Ziv A. Simulated-patient-based programs for teaching communication with adolescents: the link between guidelines and practice. Georgian Med News. 2008;156:80–3.
30. Hardoff D, Danziger Y, Reisler G, Stoffman N, Ziv A. Minding the gap: training in adolescent medicine when formal training programmes are not available. Arch Dis Child Educ Pract Ed. 2009;94(5):157–60.
31. Beyth Y, Hardoff D, Rom E, Ziv A. A simulated patient-based program for training gynecologists in communication with adolescent girls presenting with gynecological problems. J Pediatr Adolesc Gynecol. 2009;22:79–84.

32. Doolen J, Giddings M, Johnson M, Guizado de Nathan G, O Badia L. An evaluation of mental health simulation with standardized patients. Int J Nurs Educ Scholarsh. 2014;11.

33. Kameg K, Howard VM, Clochesy J, Mitchell AM, Suresky JM. The impact of high fidelity human simulation on self-efficacy of communication skills. Issues Ment Health Nurs. 2010;31(5):315–23.

34. Greenburg L, Ochsenschlager D, O'Donnell R, Mastruserio J, Cohen G. Communicating bad news: a pediatric department's evaluation of a simulated intervention. Pediatrics. 1999;103:1210–17.

35. Schildmann J, Kupfer S, Burchardi N, Vollmann J. Teaching and evaluation of breaking bad news: a pre-post evaluation study of a teaching intervention for medical students and a comparative analysis of different measurement instruments and raters. Patient Educ Couns. 2012;86(2):210–19.

36. Amiel GE, Ungar L, Alperin M, Baharier Z, Cohen R, Reis S. Ability of primary care physicians to break bad news: a performance based assessment of an educational intervention. Patient Educ Couns. 2006;60(1):10–5.

37. Bell SK, Pascucci R, Fancy K, Coleman K, Zurakowski D, Meyere EC. The educational value of improvisational actors to teach communication and relation skills: perspectives of interprofessional learners, faculty and actors. Patient Educ Couns. 2014;96(3):381–8.

38. TeamSTEPPS and SBAR material. http://teamstepps.ahrq.gov.

Simulation for Rural Communities

Linda L. Brown and Ralph James MacKinnon

Simulation Pearls

1. As with any educational endeavor, it is important to clearly identify the objectives before starting a rural simulation program. Is the focus on teamwork and communication, assessment of the systems and processes of care, procedural training, or another topic? Clarifying these objectives will lead to the best methods for training.
2. In situ and mobile simulations are two useful methods for training in rural settings.
3. Consider collaboration with other local or regional centers to further expand your simulation resources.
4. Advance planning and buy-in by both stakeholders and participants are critical for developing and sustaining a successful rural simulation program.

Introduction

The term *rural* is defined by the *Merriam-Webster's Dictionary* as "relating to the country and the people who live there, instead of the city" [1]. In the medical literature, this definition varies and can even be controversial. There is often an attempt to incorporate the population density of the area in question or the proximity to urban centers, but ultimately the definition may be unique to each country or region. The identification of these rural communities is important, however, to allow for discussion of some of the challenges these

L. L. Brown (✉)
Department of Pediatrics and Emergency Medicine, Alpert Medical School of Brown University, Hasbro Children's Hospital, Providence, RI, USA
e-mail: lbrown8@lifespan.org

R. J. MacKinnon
Faculty of Health, Psychology & Social Change, Department of Paediatric Anaesthesia & Paediatric Intensive Care, Manchester Metropolitan University, Royal Manchester Children's Hospital, North West & North Wales Paediatric Transport Service, Manchester, UK
e-mail: ralph.mackinnon@cmft.nhs.uk

areas may face, including the need to provide high-quality health care to ill and injured pediatric patients. In the USA, it is estimated that approximately 20 % of the population live in rural areas, while less than 10 % of physicians practice there [2]. Similar numbers are reported in other countries [3]. In these rural communities, healthcare providers are required to administer care to patients distributed over a broad geographic area, yet are fully integrated into the local community [4]. Hospitals in these areas often have a lower patient census and limited access to subspecialty consultation as compared to larger urban centers, but they are still required to provide safe, effective, equitable, and efficient care to all who enter their doors. For the purposes of this chapter, we will discuss simulation-based education (SBE) and its potential utility and impact on pediatric education and training in these rural communities. Of note, SBE in *resource-limited settings*, areas typically characterized by insufficient healthcare funds resulting in a lack of infrastructure, trained personnel, equipment, supplies, and medications, will be discussed separately in Chap. 25.

The optimal care of acutely ill and injured children requires ongoing education and frequent practice by members of any healthcare team. Many of the children who receive emergency care are seen in community hospitals with relatively low pediatric volumes, rather than larger academic children's hospitals. In fact, it is estimated that 85–90 % of children presenting for emergency care are seen by general emergency medicine physicians in community emergency departments (EDs), while 50 % of EDs in the USA care for fewer than ten pediatric patients per day [5–8]. In the rural setting, the management of critically ill infants and children is a rare event, and the providers often have limited access to pediatric consultants and pediatric-specific continuing education. In 2008, an attempt at mapping the access to pediatric subspecialists and hospitals with pediatric intensive care units in the USA was published. The authors found that overall 64.1 % of the pediatric population lived within 50 miles of a pediatric critical care resource. However, there were multiple states where this number was less than 10 % [9].

Published literature also reports that there is variability in the quality of care delivered to pediatric patients in this lower-volume community setting as compared to higher-volume children's hospitals [10].

In discussing SBE and its use for pediatric education in rural communities, an important component of the review must be focused on why simulation is being considered for use in this setting. As with any educational endeavor, predetermined learning objectives should be set by those responsible for its implementation. Are these objectives related to improving medical knowledge, assessing skills or competencies, practicing interprofessional teamwork and communication, or as a tool for the assessment of the systems and processes of care in this setting? Although these topics will be covered in detail in other chapters, we will discuss each topic to discuss how simulation may be utilized for pediatric education by healthcare providers, administrators, or educators in rural communities, as well as some of the challenges and facilitators to its use in this unique setting.

Assessing and Improving Medical Knowledge

Medical decision-making and clinical reasoning have classically been taught in a lecture-based format, refined at the bedside during training, and maintained through clinical practice. Over the past decade, SBE has been proved to be an engaging and effective method for educating medical professionals and has become an integral component in this process. Not surprisingly, the highest utilization of simulation is often centered in urban, tertiary care teaching hospitals. In this environment, it is frequently used as a method to teach trainees and established healthcare providers the best practices for managing a variety of medical emergencies. In rural communities, where there are low pediatric volumes, pediatric-specific knowledge and skills may deteriorate quickly. Unfortunately, the options for pediatric continuing medical education are also often limited in these areas, and it is here that simulation can play an important role. Even in centers with fewer resources, medical decision-making can be practiced and assessed through the use of screen-based simulation programs, often referred to as online or computer-based simulations or serious gaming. This method of SBE allows for easy access to pediatric-specific scenarios and education. It allows the providers to walk-through their decisions regarding care with infinite possibilities in the patient's progression depending on their interventions, as predetermined by programming in the game's engine. Examples of the use of gaming for rare and acute events include disaster triage and emergency department or Pediatric Advanced Life Support (PALS) scenarios. This time-critical decision-making allows for experiential learning, with the online or computer-based setting allowing for a more readily accessible training opportunity for all healthcare providers. Screen-based simulation is discussed in further detail in Chap. 9.

In Situ and Mobile Simulation

In situ simulation is an event that takes place in the actual clinical environment, allowing the healthcare team to practice caring for patients in their own space, with their own equipment and resources (see Chap. 12 for details). It has been shown to deliver high levels of realism and participant satisfaction [11, 12]. Through observation of the team's performance during a simulation scenario, an expert in debriefing can introduce discussion on published guidelines and updates in the literature on the optimal care of children presenting with a variety of complaints, from pediatric respiratory failure, sepsis, and trauma-related complaints to cardiac arrest.

The use of SBE for pediatric education in Critical Access Hospitals in the USA has been evaluated [10]. Critical Access Hospitals are small-volume rural institutions with no more than 25 inpatient beds but with 24-h, seven-days-a-week emergency care units. These facilities are maintained to provide access to emergency and outpatient care for rural communities, with patients requiring prolonged admission or subspecialty care transferred to other institutions. Not surprisingly, healthcare providers in these settings will infrequently encounter critically ill children. In this study, a high-fidelity in situ curriculum was developed to allow providers to practice the care of such pediatric patients. Although no information has yet been reported on the impact of this intervention on actual clinical care, at the conclusion of the study providers reported significant improvements in their comfort level in taking care of these patients [11]. These findings are supported by other studies with similar programs where healthcare providers have reported increased comfort with these infrequent, high-acuity events at the completion of a simulation-based intervention [13, 14].

Although SBE may be best known for allowing healthcare providers to practice these low-frequency, high-acuity events, for healthcare institutions it may also be used to provide insights into the preparedness of the system to care for these patients. In situ simulation is being increasingly used for this purpose and has been shown to efficiently and effectively assess the systems and processes of care in a variety of settings [15–17]. In 2006, in situ simulation was used to evaluate the care of pediatric trauma patients presenting to a spectrum of EDs in North Carolina. The ability of interprofessional teams to assess and manage a simulated 3-year-old trauma patient after a fall was evaluated. Information on the quality of care delivered was assessed, as well as several system-level issues, including the lack of appropriate-sized equipment (e.g., cervical collars) and inadequate preparation for safe transport to computed tomography (CT) scan [18]. Similar methods have been used to assess the systems and processes of care, and to evaluate for latent safety threats in both established and new clinical environments [15, 17, 19]. In rural institutions, where pediatric-specific systems are rarely tested, this could be an invaluable tool for quality improvement (see Chap. 6 for details).

It is important to acknowledge, however, that there are challenges associated with in situ simulation, particularly in the rural setting. These include the need to provide actual clinical space and equipment. In areas where the space for clinical care may be limited, this will require significant planning on contingencies for what to do when an actual patient arrives. It is very important that discussions prior to the day of the simulation involve administration as well as physician and nursing leadership.

As transporting all rural providers to a distant simulation center for training or developing a local in situ simulation program, as described above, may not be feasible, the use of *mobile* simulation is becoming increasingly utilized. In this method, the simulation-specific resources are brought to the participants. Mobile simulation occurs in one of the two ways. The first way is the transportation of mannequins, equipment, and simulation facilitators to the rural environment for in situ simulation as described above (see Fig. 24.1a, c). The second way includes all of the human and equipment resources listed above, as well as a *mobile patient care space*, often in the form of a repurposed ambulance, recreational vehicle (e.g., motorhome or caravan), van, or bus (see Fig. 24.2a, c). This allows for a standard practice environment, one that is not impacted by actual patient care as seen in in situ simulation. Individuals and interprofessional teams can practice procedures or high-fidelity simulation scenarios without the need for each rural institution to purchase and maintain costly simulation equipment and resources. However, there are specific questions to ask prior to creating, building, or participating in such a program. Important discussion points that should be considered for in situ and mobile simulation space methods are detailed in Table 24.1.

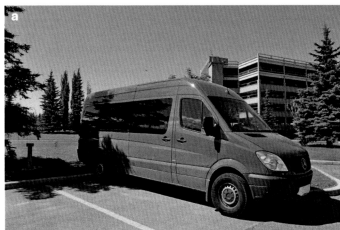
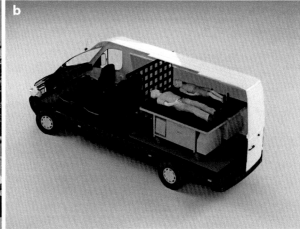
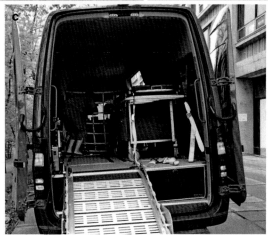

Fig. 24.1 Examples of a *mobile simulation unit* designed to transport in situ stretchers, simulation equipment, clinical equipment, and the education team that will perform the training. (Reproduced with permission of eSIM Provincial Simulation Program, Alberta Health Services)

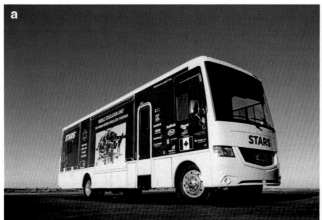
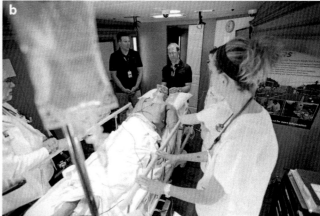
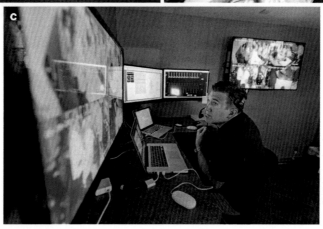

Fig. 24.2 Examples of a mobile simulation unit designed to include a: (a) mobile patient care space; (b) and all associated simulation equipment, clinical equipment, audiovisual equipment; and (c) a control room. The unit is designed to be completely self-dependent for simulation education delivery. (Reproduced with permission of STARS Air Ambulance)

Table 24.1 Questions to consider when planning for in situ or mobile simulation

In situ simulation	
Will we use our own equipment and medications?	This will require thought as to how medications will be accessed, how quickly can the equipment be replaced, and how to cover the costs associated with replacement
If not, how can we be sure that the simulation equipment and medications are not used on actual patients	This will require special labeling and storage, as well as specific checks to confirm that no contamination occurs
If safety threats are identified, how will they be reported?	Immediate safety threats should be reported in real time to physician and nursing leadership. How will these be tracked for resolution?
Will the actual medical team be participating in the simulation? If so, what will happen if a patient arrives for care?	Back-up providers or a plan to halt the simulation based on preset criteria are possible solutions. In addition, how will the costs of additional staffing be covered? What is the optimal number of participants for the simulation? Ideally, this should be representative of actual practice
Where/when will the simulation take place?	Is there a specific resuscitation room we would like to utilize? What is the best time of the day to use this room? Lower volume times are often earlier in the morning. How long do we want the sessions to last? Discuss how long it is possible to use this space without affecting patient care/flow
Mobile simulation space	
Are we interested in assessing our equipment or resources or the processes of caring for pediatric patients?	If so, in situ methods may be more appropriate. If not, how can we be sure that equipment adequately mirrors our own equipment to allow for optimal buy-in by participants?
How will the participants be oriented to the mobile simulation lab?	Time will need to be set aside for an overview of the mobile setting, allowing for hands-on practice with equipment if necessary
How will this be funded and staffed?	Are the participants being paid for their time? What is the optimal number of learners? Does this replicate actual practice? Can we apply for continuing education credits as an incentive for providers?
Where will the mobile simulation lab be located?	Is this location easily accessed by participants and not obstructive to patient care?

It is important to recognize that endeavors such as these require significant simulation resources. Not only do they involve the use of mannequins and the technology to support these simulations, but also the experts available for facilitation and debriefing, arguably the most important component of a successful SBE program. As mentioned previously, acute care pediatric expertise may be limited in rural communities. To address this issue without the expense of mobile simulation, the utilization of telemedicine has been steadily increasing. This technology allows for immediate consultation with subspecialists regarding the care of pediatric patients and has been shown to have a positive impact on the quality of the care delivered [20–22]. Similarly, the use of telemedicine for educational purposes is now being investigated and may allow for remote debriefing and facilitation of simulation scenarios and procedural training when the expertise is not locally available [23].

Interprofessional Teamwork and Communication

For the purposes of interprofessional education, including critically important teamwork and communication skills and behaviors, mannequin-based simulations have long been utilized and found to be both engaging and effective [12, 24, 25]. A number of simulation-based studies have also identified the importance of teamwork, good leadership, and good communication in managing emergency situations and their role in medical error when they are suboptimal [26–28]. Teamwork training has been shown to improve subsequent team performance ([29–31] (see Chaps. 4 and 15 for details). SBE has also produced a host of tools to assess both technical and nontechnical skills, which may also be useful in the rural setting [32–37]. See Chap. 7 for a complete list of assessment tools for pediatrics.

Another area of recent interest that has applicability in the rural domain is that of cognitive aids, including checklists. In other high-reliability professions, such as in the aviation and nuclear power industries, checklists and simulation are used as standard for the management of rare but high-acuity events or stressor situations [38–40]. In the healthcare field, there is evidence supporting improved patient safety outcomes with the use of checklists, including the use of a preoperative checklist that has demonstrated a reduction in communication failures [41–43]. The improvement in the management of operating room crises demonstrated by the use of checklists with training on simulators within a simulation suite may be a step toward improved patient care for rare events in the rural setting using the same checklist approach.

When creating these programs, it is important to recognize that the realism of the scenario can be an important component of the buy-in by the participants, and this knowledge should be considered, along with the predefined learning objectives, during scenario development. Realistic scenarios that are possible encounters in each setting should be carefully planned and piloted prior to their use. This is not the time for rare cases but rather straightforward, plausible cases with well-established guidelines for medical management, such as sepsis, PALS algorithms, and status epilepticus, that allow for not only the building and consolidation of fundamental pediatric acute care knowledge but also the practice and discussion of important teamwork and communication principles. Building fundamental knowledge and skill in the more common pediatric presentations will have the greatest impact on children care for by rural providers, and will likely also provide positive spin-offs when having to care for rare cases. Piloting the scenarios with input from physicians, nurses, and other participating healthcare providers will also allow for problem-solving and amelioration of any possible threats to a successful program.

Collaboration in Simulation-Based Education

Access to simulation technology and expert facilitation and debriefing, which provide much of the learning and mentorship during simulation-based educational programs, is often limited in rural communities. Through collaboration with larger academic centers, however, access to this educational modality may become possible. Each rural community is unique in its objectives. Many site-specific factors can affect the best way to successfully develop and sustain a simulation program, including the location, the patient volume, the diversity of patient complaints and acuity, relevant equipment, and personnel resources. Sites with established affiliations with larger academic institutions may be able to access simulation through this relationship. However, smaller, more isolated sites may have difficulty in accessing these resources. In several areas worldwide, the academic institutions have facilitated this relationship through collaboration with other centers for dissemination of SBE across larger areas and a broader spectrum of institutions.

In 2012, findings from a regional Canadian task force on simulation were published [44]. The British Columbia Simulation Task Force was created "to bring together key academic and health authority stakeholders from across the province to design a comprehensive SBE model…" In this manuscript, methods and findings from a needs assessment are described and an educational model to provide access to SBE for all healthcare providers in British Columbia,

Fig. 24.3 Model of simulation for rural settings. *CPD* continuing professional development. (Used with permission of [44])

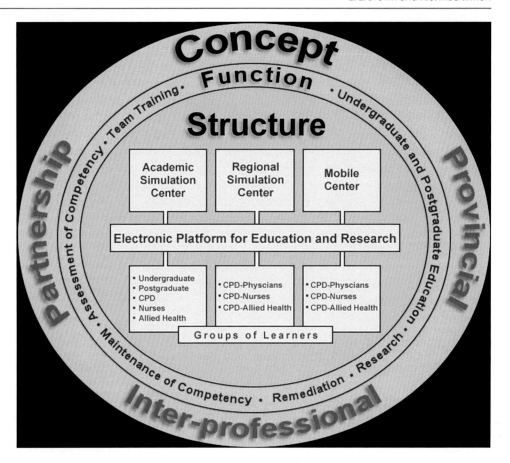

irrespective of their geographic location and/or institutional affiliation, is discussed. They determined that using a combination of online, web-based learning, followed by access to academic and regional simulation centers and mobile simulation centers, utilizing specially designed mobile units with in situ simulations for rural settings, is an optimal model (Fig. 24.3). They report that the implementation of this system is currently underway but stands as a model for collaboration between academic centers and community-based hospitals to provide SBE for all who desire it.

In our experience, building such an outreach program requires mutual trust and respect. Developing this relationship can be markedly different from that of introducing simulation internally to another department in a base hospital. In Table 24.2, we list considerations that may facilitate such relationship building.

As relationships and trust build, broader collaboration within a wider geographic area and standardization of curricula across these centers become possible. The content of the curricula can still contain objectives that are seen as important to the rural centers, while also covering known cases where rural teams have struggled with pediatric care. The KidSIM Pediatric Simulation Program (Alberta Children's Hospital, Calgary, Canada) runs a mobile rural in situ simulation program in Southern Alberta, Canada, that delivers 12 standardized scenarios over a 4-year period (i.e., three scenarios per year). The advantage of the standardized curricula is that they allow the simulation program education team to more intimately learn the three cases for the year and repeat the cases at each of the rural sites for a given year. This is a practical way of ensuring that the cases remain consistent and are of high quality. The main advantage for the rural sites is that they are delivered a consistent set of cases that are felt to be necessary to build fundamental knowledge, clinical and team skills in pediatric acute care driven by objectives developed mutually. In addition, by standardizing the cases (and program), continuing education credits are more easily applied for, which acts as an additional motivation for rural care providers (Vincent Grant, written communication, December 2014). Regional transport teams that support rural or district hospitals, by a rapid response team or telephone advice, may also form an anchor point for collaborative simulation curricula. With knowledge of all the critically ill children presenting to the hospitals within the region, The North West & North Wales Paediatric Transport Team (NWTS, UK) outreach program aims to provide mobile SBE programs responsive to specific educational goals of 28 hospitals each year (Kate Parkins & Kathryn Claydon-Smith,

Table 24.2 Developing a rural simulation outreach program from a base center: relationship building

Key task	Steps for implementation
Introduce the concept to key interprofessional and multidisciplinary stakeholders	Discuss the acceptability of simulation within the rural team setting
	Inquire how simulation may be of the highest value in their setting
	Explain options for education, team training, and process improvements
	Suggest starting based on your own hospital's successes with simulation
	Identify educators within the rural facility to help champion this process
	Talk through the simulation, highlighting plausible scenarios, and debriefing points
	Suggest outcomes and how to track simulation interventions
	Discuss costs of equipment and staff time and the increasing scale of complexity
	Consider applying for continuing education credits for providers
Organize an event to meet as many staff as possible and show the technology	Involve the rural team in a live demo and promote reflection on this
	Develop together a remediation plan for any staff member who may request or require this after completion of the simulations
Establish regular meetings/teleconferences to build relationships further	Discuss progress and challenges
	Plan for new scenarios
	Expand the number of local champions
	Review outcomes
Consider collaboration across a wider geographic area to build a standardized curricula for multiple rural centers	Discuss other potential local or regional collaborators
	Consider potential for sharing resources, curricula

Fig. 24.4 Simulation within an educational area at the base (rural) hospital with permission of The North West & North Wales Paediatric Transport Service (UK)

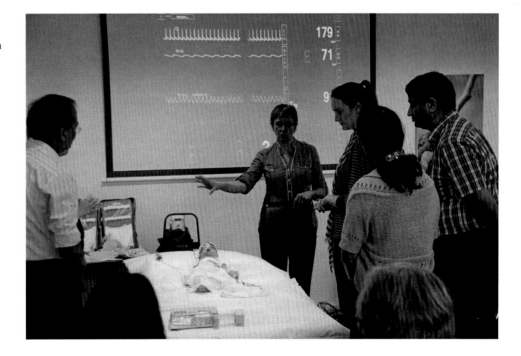

written communication, December 2014). These simulation-based educational programs are planned in advance to occur in either clinical areas or educational areas in base hospitals (Fig. 24.4). A number of differing approaches may be undertaken to achieve collective collaborative educational goals. Different examples of rural simulation-based itineraries are presented in Table 24.3.

Procedural and Skills Training

One of the main objectives when discussing SBE is the acquisition and assessment of infrequently practiced skills and procedures. Simulation has been proven to be an effective tool for teaching and maintaining competencies in a variety of procedures that require refined and practiced

Table 24.3 Examples of collaborative rural simulation-based education itineraries

KidSIM Pediatric Simulation Program (Alberta Children's Hospital, Calgary, Canada)	Morning session
Full-day session	1. Skills station with hands-on practice and mentorship (45 min) for all participants (while other team members set up mannequin-based simulation sessions)
Can be done in clinical space (in situ) or in classroom (if necessary)	
Four facilitators	2. Rotation of groups through three immersive scenario-based simulations with debriefing lasting 45 min (Participants divided into 2–3 groups)
Maximum of 20 interprofessional participants	Afternoon session
	A new set of participants and the above skills station and three scenario-based simulations are repeated
The NWTS (UK) in situ Program 1	Morning session—rotation through:
	1. Difficult actual case discussions (1 h)
Full day session	Two cases—one provided by NWTS and one by base hospital (30 min each), for example, lithium button battery ingestion with catastrophic hemorrhage
Emergency department or ward area available	
Four facilitators	2. Case-based procedural workshops with part task trainers (90 min), for example, intraosseous insertion and fluid management
Approximately 20–30 multidisciplinary participants	Afternoon session
	In situ high-fidelity team-based simulation (45 min; team using own equipment, drawing up medications, etc.)
	Half of participants active in simulation, half observing
	Interactive debrief—all participants involved (1 h), for example, management of meningococcal sepsis
The North West & North Wales Paediatric Transport Service (UK) Program 2	Rotation through two sessions in the morning and two sessions in the afternoon
Full-day session	1. Airway case with part task trainer (1 h), for example, management of unpredicted difficult airway
Educational area only available	
Four facilitators	2. Breathing case with mannequin (1 h), for example, high-flow humidified oxygen and setting up noninvasive ventilation in an asthmatic child
Approximately 20–30 multidisciplinary participants	3. Circulation case—part task trainer (1 h), for example, fluid resuscitation of shocked child with intraosseous insertion
	4. Neurological case with mannequin (1 h), for example, base hospital extubation of a child who had status epilepticus responding to thiopentone

NWTS North West & North Wales Paediatric Transport Team

psychomotor skills. These include central venous access placement, lumbar puncture, and emergency airway management techniques [45–47]. It is therefore another useful option for rural healthcare providers who may not have the volume or variety of patients to allow for maintenance of competency in these procedures. This is also an objective that may be accomplished on a relatively low budget, with options for less-expensive, low-fidelity task trainers available for a variety of procedures. Procedural and skills training is discussed in detail in Chap. 11.

Developing Resilience in Rural Communities Through Simulation

Resilience can be defined as the "long-term capacity of a system or society to deal with change and to continue to develop" [48]. The resilience approach focuses on the dynamic interplay between gradual daily occurrences versus sudden dramatic events, and the change required to optimize the responses to such stressor events. This section aims to explore how different simulation-based educational strategies may improve resilience in the rural setting. We will also discuss the potential role of this educational strategy in rural healthcare facility preparation and in particular assessment, dissemination of learning, and healthcare advocacy.

Although discussed previously, it is worthwhile to examine preparation or readiness in more depth. Rural healthcare systems, including emergency medical/prehospital services and hospitals, provide the first response and care for the clinical needs of the majority of children requiring health care. It has been recognized for decades that healthcare system preparation is vital to meet this challenge, in terms of the provision of appropriate personnel, equipment, protocols, and infrastructure from initial resuscitation to transfer to definitive care [49]. Current strategies to improve the capacity of a healthcare system deal with change, and continue to develop, include reviews of care and regulatory interventions at a national or regional level. Healthcare facility level audit cycles and close inspection of untoward incidents also aim to assess, achieve, and maintain high-quality care for children. One example of a national strategy is the 2001 American Academy of Pediatrics (AAP) and the American College of Emergency Physicians (ACEP) "Care of Children in the Emergency Department: Guidelines for Preparedness" document [50]. These guidelines include recommendations for staff training, an endorsed list of age and size-appropriate equipment and supplies, guidelines for policies, procedures, and support for establishing inter-facility transfer agreements. Subsequent studies indicate that despite a national framework and guideline approach, inconsistencies remain in the preparedness of hospitals to care for emergency pediatric patients [51, 52]. In one US study, factors associated with a lack of readiness to care for pediatric emergencies included the availability of services and equipment in rural and community hospitals [52]. A follow-up report by the Committee on the Future of Emergency Care in the United States Health System (Institute of Medicine of the National Academies) highlighted that a significant number of children are first cared for in the community or rural setting, and re-emphasized the need for such a healthcare system to be prepared to manage all types of cases [50].

As discussed previously, the case mix presenting in the rural setting is a key issue. The understanding that the lack of frequency of challenging pediatric emergencies not only adversely affects the clinical skills of healthcare providers, but also the rural hospital infrastructure, was a driver to the national guideline development. Another driver for the national guideline approach was a perceived lack of appreciation for the severity of injuries, the urgency of clinical scenarios, incorrect clinical decision-making, and a lack of confidence particularly in caring for critically unwell children [50]. Simplistically, one can visualize two strands to developing resilience in rural health settings: one of better preparation of the healthcare facilities and systems, and another of training to and maintaining the excellent performance of healthcare providers (including paramedics, emergency medical service personnel, physicians, nurses, and other allied health professionals). To date, SBE has played an integral role in developing both strands, but one important future direction may be to highlight how interwoven both strands are and how we can build upon this.

This includes using simulation to encourage healthcare advocacy in all personnel involved in the preparation and delivery of care, including the rural environment. The role of healthcare advocates is essential in improving the quality of care provided within a facility. To act effectively, health professionals must be given the tools to capture the intricate interplay between teams of healthcare providers and the facility they work in. One example of such a tool is the Field Assessment Conditioning Tool (FACT). The FACT (Fig. 24.5)

was designed as both a qualitative and quantitative series of evaluations in the context of pediatric trauma in rural hospitals to disseminate both areas of existing excellence in care, as well as areas of focus to further optimize care [53]. The FACT uses SBE as a cornerstone educational intervention and was developed as part of collaborative approach across three continents by the International Network for Simulation-based Pediatric Innovation, Research and Education (http://www.inspiresim.com). The use of simulation-based tools to develop healthcare advocacy and to support decision-making in the rural setting is a potentially fruitful avenue to explore. A current international multisite study aims to determine the effectiveness of such tools, focusing specifically on satellite hospitals geographically linked to major trauma centers in the USA, New Zealand, and the UK [53]. Using high-fidelity simulators as surrogates for traumatically injured children, this study explores the effectiveness of the FACT to empower individuals to invoke clinical management changes within their distinct hospital settings and disseminate the learning across all team members. In the same way that a close clinical relationship between rural and major centers of care is optimal for care provision, it may also be true in terms of education, continued professional development, and process improvement. SBE is therefore a powerful potential conduit to achieve such relationships and provides the opportunity for all of us to learn from one another.

Conclusions

This chapter has described how the spectrum of simulation-based training can provide opportunities for rural practitioners to advance along a novice to expert trajectory, the evidence base behind such a structured simulation approach, the use of simulation in rural EDs to highlight deficiencies and improve performance post-educational interventions, and how in situ simulation could be used to identify latent safety threats in the rural setting [15, 18, 54]. The continual evolution of SBE also provides the platform to address further the challenges of rural healthcare practice, in terms of an effective method of assessing competencies [55–57], the effectiveness of other educational interventions [54, 58], and measuring quality improvement [59]. There are potential barriers to implementing a simulation program within a rural community, including the lack of resources and access to the required simulation-based expertise and equipment. It is therefore important to obtain early buy-in from physician and nursing leadership, as well as hospital administration, as to the objectives of the simulation program. *Is it focused on interprofessional education/teamwork and communication? Procedural skills? Medical decision-making for low-frequency, high-acuity events? Assessment of the systems and processes of care?* Once the objectives for the program

a

Field Assessment Conditioning tool
FACT - Rural Hospital
Readiness to Receive Traumatically injured Children

Positive Elements

Mental
Models
Survey

Comments All potential members of hospital trauma team invited to view a vedio of the primary survey of an injured child & complete an anonymous on-line questionnaire of how they would manage the child with differing vital signs & to evaluate potential team - hospital system delays.

The case: 6 year old boy fallen from tree, unconscious GCS =3, one dilated pupil, breathing face-mask oxygen spontaneously.

The question: the child has normal vital signs for age, what should be done before any CT scan?

The next cases: same child, same history and primary survey findings except differing vital signs on screen.

The question: would you go to a CT scanner without further stabilisation?

The question: What are the team & hospital delays to CT scanning in your institution.

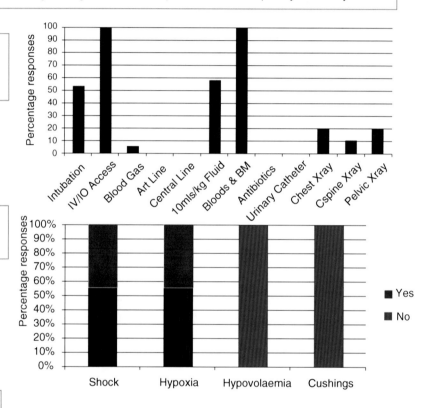

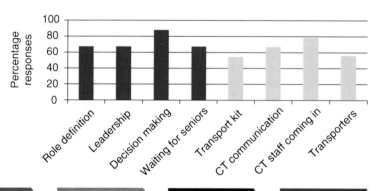

Fig. 24.5 Example of a Field Assessment Conditioning Tool (FACT) report (for hospitals with CT scanning capability)

b   **FACT Positive Elements**

Site Visit

Comments WHO essential trauma care checlist, maximum 3 scored for all components

Basic airway management	External haemorrhage control	Splinting of fractures	Documentation
Advanced airway management	IV access&appropriate fluids	Basic closed fracture management	CME certification
Oxygen	Blood transfusion capabilities	External & Internal fixation	QI program
Chest drains	Wound care	Spinal immobilisation	Trauma Team

Knowledge Test

Comments

50 true/false questions on the management of paediatric trauma completed by a randomly selected trauma team.

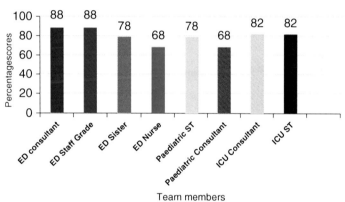

Adherence to Best Practice   ## Key Timings

Comments

2 traumatically injured children (using high fidelity simulators as proxies for patients) presented to the Emergency Dept bays and were managed in trun by trauma call activation and team managemant as per normal care provition.

Best Practice Adhered to:

Primary & secondary survey of Paediatric Advanced Trauma Care Completed.
Immediate life threatening injuries assessed & managed.
On identification of time critical head injury appropriate neuro-protection, planning for transport then imaging & operative intervention under taken at Major Trauma Centre.
Major haemorrhage protocal activated and appropriately managed.

Child One

Time to senior arrival (minutes)	Time to pupil check (minutes)	Time to declaration of dilated pupil	Time to intubation	Time to discussion with major trauma centre
<1	3	4	12	3

Child Tow

Time to senior arrival (minutes)	Time to IV / IO access (minutes)	Time to firstfluid bolus (minutes)	Time to Major Haemorrhage Protocal activation (minutes)
1	2	4	4

Time to Fast Ultrasound Scan of abdomen (minutes)	Time to blood administration (minutes)	Time to discussion with senior surgeon (minutes)
3	15	8

Fig. 24.5b Continued

c

FACT Positive Elements

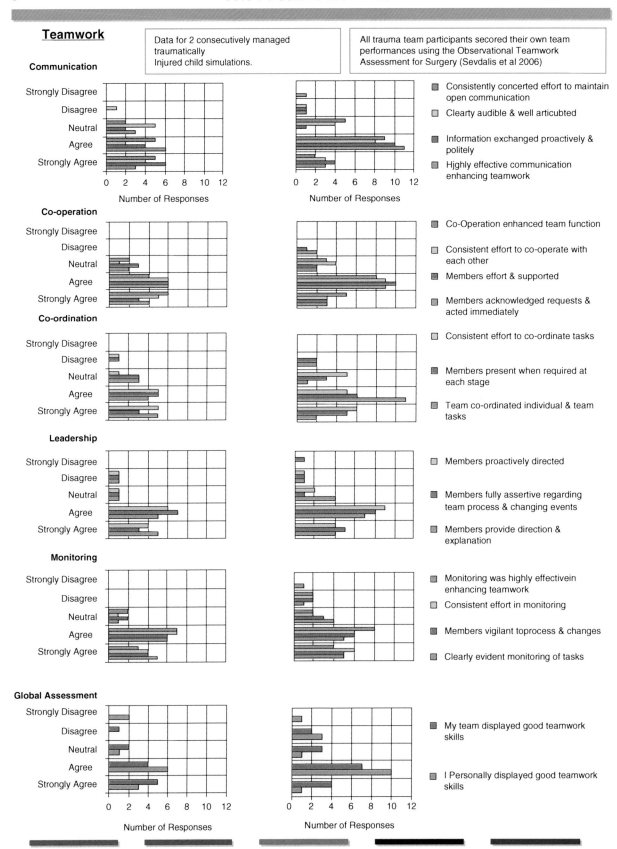

Fig. 24.5c Continued

d

FACT Delta Elements

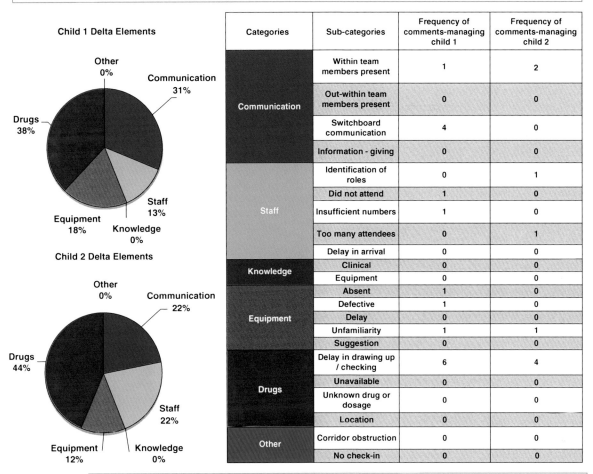

Comments Elements of team-hospital interaction identified by team members as factors that could improve care provision.

Categories	Sub-categories	Frequency of comments-managing child 1	Frequency of comments-managing child 2
Communication	Within team members present	1	2
	Out-within team members present	0	0
	Switchboard communication	4	0
	Information - giving	0	0
Staff	Identification of roles	0	1
	Did not attend	1	0
	Insufficient numbers	1	0
	Too many attendees	0	1
	Delay in arrival	0	0
Knowledge	Clinical	0	0
	Equipment	0	0
Equipment	Absent	1	0
	Defective	1	0
	Delay	0	0
	Unfamiliarity	1	1
	Suggestion	0	0
Drugs	Delay in drawing up / checking	6	4
	Unavailable	0	0
	Unknown drug or dosage	0	0
	Location	0	0
Other	Corridor obstruction	0	0
	No check-in	0	0

Child 1 Delta Elements

Other 0%
Communication 31%
Drugs 38%
Staff 13%
Equipment 18%
Knowledge 0%

Child 2 Delta Elements

Other 0%
Communication 22%
Drugs 44%
Staff 22%
Equipment 12%
Knowledge 0%

Risk **Comments** Delta elements linked to standard risk matrix of Untoward Incident Levels of research base hospital.

Child 1 Team's feedback (one commenttype per person)	Incident Level
"switchboard told me there was no paediatric trauma team" "Bleeped to attend as maternity anaesthetist" "Switchboard unsure abouta paediatric trauma call"	Major
"called urgently to emergency room – not called to paeds trauma"	Minor
"batteries did not work for laryngoscope blade" "paeds trolley lacked masks and circuit"	Moderate
"no orthopaedic attendance"	Low
"Intubation signif. delayed no access to cupboard & fridge" "weren't able to find drugkeys" "did not know who had drugkeys" "difficult to find drugs and equipment to draw up drugs" "nurse as signed to prepare anae sthetic drugs struggled" "ICU nurse would beuseful for RSI drugs/procedure"	Moderate
"not been shown where equipment was so difficult to find"	Low
"critical care consultant dealing with another case"	Low

Child 2 Team's feedback (one comment type per person)	Incident Level
"not enough room for all the bodies"	Minor
"long delay in obtaining crashcall protocols and infusions" "crashcall online calculator slow to access" "clear problem with access to crashcall.net"	Moderate
"A&E bleep was not activated by switchboard" "did not know who was who" "did not know where equipment was"	Low
"blood could have arrived earlier"	Moderate
"delay in asking for blood gas to get Haemoglobin level"	Low

Fig. 24.5d Continued

are clearly defined, the best mechanisms to obtain these goals can then be identified. These include online education, procedural task trainers, and in situ, mobile, or center-based simulation programs. The investigation of remote mechanisms to facilitate and debrief procedural and interprofessional training and the evolving collaborations between institutions across regions and countries are striving to make these resources available for all those who care for infants and children and who strive to deliver safe, high-quality care whenever and wherever it is required.

Moving forward, simulation has a key role to play in both better preparation of the healthcare facilities and systems and training to/maintaining excellent performance of the healthcare providers (including paramedics, emergency medical service personnel, physicians, nurses, and allied health professionals). Accepting the stance that the stabilization of a critically unwell child is a complex interplay between a team of providers and the healthcare facility they are in, one can postulate that the needs of both the healthcare provider and facility are symbiotic. To improve patient care, the rural healthcare system needs the participants, and vice versa. A future direction of simulation may be to explore how learning best occurs in the rural setting, how this learning is best disseminated (whether horizontally across all potential team members and/or vertically through the health facility governance tree), and how patient care is impacted.

References

1. http://www.merriam-webster.com/. Accessed 1 April 2015.
2. Rosenblatt RA, Hart LG. Physicians and rural America. West J Med. 2000;173(5):348–51.
3. Easterbrook M, Godwin M, Wilson R, Hodgetts G, Brown G, Pong R, et al. Rural background and clinical rural rotations during medical training: effect on practice location. CMAJ. 1999;160(8):1159–63.
4. Farmer J, Lauder W, Richards H, Sharkey S. Dr John has gone: assessing health professionals' contribution to remote rural community sustainability in the UK. Soc Sci Med. 2003;57(4):673–86.
5. Pitts SR, Niska RW, Xu J, Burt CW. National Hospital Ambulatory Medical Care Survey: 2006 emergency department summary. Natl Health Stat Report. 2008;(7):1–38.
6. Bourgeois FT, Shannon MW. Emergency care for children in pediatric and general emergency departments. Pediatr Emerg Care. 2007;23(2):94–102.
7. Sacchetti A, Baren J, Carraccio C. The paradox of the nested pediatric emergency department. Acad Emerg Med. 2005;12(12):1236–9.
8. Gausche-Hill M, Schmitz C, Lewis RJ. Pediatric preparedness of US emergency departments: a 2003 survey. Pediatrics. 2007;120(6):1229–37.
9. Brantley MD, Lu H, Barfield WD, Holt JB, Williams A, Mapping US. Pediatric hospitals and subspecialty critical care for public health preparedness and disaster response, 2008. Disaster Med Public Health Prep. 2012;6(2):117–25.
10. Dharmar M, Marcin JP, Romano PS, Andrada ER, Overly F, Valente JH, et al. Quality of care of children in the emergency department:

association with hospital setting and physician training. J Pediatr. 2008;153(6):783–9.
11. Katznelson JH, Mills WA, Forsythe CS, Shaikh S, Tolleson-Rinehart S. Project CAPE: a high-fidelity, in situ simulation program to increase Critical Access Hospital Emergency Department provider comfort with seriously ill pediatric patients. Pediatr Emerg Care. 2014;30(6):397–402.
12. Allan CK, Thiagarajan RR, Beke D, Imprescia A, Kappus LJ, Garden A, et al. Simulation-based training delivered directly to the pediatric cardiac intensive care unit engenders preparedness, comfort, and decreased anxiety among multidisciplinary resuscitation teams. J Thorac Cardiovasc Surg. 2010;140(3):646–52.
13. Mills DM, Wu CL, Williams DC, King L, Dobson JV. High-fidelity simulation enhances pediatric residents' retention, knowledge, procedural proficiency, group resuscitation performance, and experience in pediatric resuscitation. Hosp Pediatr. 2013;3(3):266–75.
14. Rosen MA, Hunt EA, Pronovost PJ, Federowicz MA, Weaver SJ. In situ simulation in continuing education for the health care professions: a systematic review. J Contin Educ Health Prof. 2012;32(4):243–54.
15. Patterson MD, Geis GL, Falcone RA, LeMaster T, Wears RL. In situ simulation: detection of safety threats and teamwork training in a high risk emergency department. BMJ Qual Saf. 2013;22(6):468–77.
16. Patterson MD, Blike GT, Nadkarni VM. Advances in patient safety in situ simulation: challenges and results. In: Henriksen K, Battles JB, Keyes MA, Grady ML, editors. Advances in patient safety: new directions and alternative approaches (vol 3: performance and Tools). Rockville: Agency for Healthcare Research and Quality (US); 2008.
17. Geis GL, Pio B, Pendergrass TL, Moyer MR, Patterson MD. Simulation to assess the safety of new healthcare teams and new facilities. Simul Healthc. 2011;6(3):125–33.
18. Hunt EA, Hohenhaus SM, Luo X, et al. Simulation of pediatric trauma stabilization in 35 North Carolina emergency departments: identification of targets for performance improvement. Pediatrics. 2006;117:641–8.
19. Walker ST, Sevdalis N, McKay A, Lambden S, Gautama S, Aggarwal R, et al. Unannounced in situ simulations: integrating training and clinical practice. BMJ Qual Saf. 2013;22(6):453–8.
20. Dharmar M, Romano PS, Kuppermann N, Nesbitt TS, Cole SL, Andrada ER, et al. Impact of critical care telemedicine consultations on children in rural emergency departments. Crit Care Med. 2013;41(10):2388–95.
21. Heath B, Salerno R, Hopkins A, Hertzig J, Caputo M. Pediatric critical care telemedicine in rural underserved emergency departments. Pediatr Crit Care Med. 2009;10(5):588–91.
22. Marcin JP, Schepps DE, Page KA, Struve SN, Nagrampa E, Dimand RJ. The use of telemedicine to provide pediatric critical care consultations to pediatric trauma patients admitted to a remote trauma intensive care unit: a preliminary report. Pediatr Crit Care Med. 2004;5(3):251–6.
23. Abadia de Barbara AH, Nicholas Iv TA, Del Real Colomo A, Boedeker D, Bernhagen MA, Hillan Garcia L, et al. Virtual simulation training using the Storz C-HUB to support distance airway training for the Spanish Medical Corps and NATO partners. Stud Health Technol Inform. 2012;182:1–9.
24. Merien AE, van de Ven J, Mol BW, Houterman S, Oei SG. Multidisciplinary team training in a simulation setting for acute obstetric emergencies: a systematic review. Obstet Gynecol. 2010;115(5):1021–31.
25. Issenberg SB, McGaghie WC, Petrusa ER, Lee Gordon D, Scalese RJ. Features and uses of high-fidelity medical simulations that lead to effective learning: a BEME systematic review. Med Teach. 2005;27(1):10–28.
26. Schaefer HG, Helmreich RL, Scheidegger D. Human factors and safety in emergency medicine. Resuscitation. 1994;28(3):221–5.

27. Leape LL, Brennan TA, Laird N, Lawthers AG, Localio AR, Barnes BA, et al. The nature of adverse events in hospitalized patients. Results of the Harvard Medical Practice Study II. N Engl J Med. 1991;324(6):377–84.

28. Hunziker S, Johansson AC, Tschan F, et al. Teamwork and leadership in cardiopulmonary resuscitation. J Am Coll Cardiol. 2011;57(24):2381–8.

29. Bhanji F, Mancini ME, Sinz E, Rodgers DL, McNeil MA, Hoadley TA, et al. Part 16: education, implementation, and teams: 2010 American Heart Association Guidelines for Cardiopulmonary Resuscitation and Emergency Cardiovascular Care. Circulation. 2010;122(18 Suppl 3):S920–33.

30. Mancini ME, Soar J, Bhanji F, Billi JE, Dennett J, Finn J, et al. Part 12: education, implementation, and teams: 2010 International Consensus on Cardiopulmonary Resuscitation and Emergency Cardiovascular Care Science with Treatment Recommendations. Circulation. 2010;122(16 Suppl 2):S539–81.

31. Capella J, Smith S, Philp A, Putnam T, Gilbert C, Fry W, et al. Teamwork training improves the clinical care of trauma patients. J Surg Educ. 2010;67(6):439–43.

32. Ahmed K, Miskovic D, Darzi A, Athanasiou T, Hanna GB. Observational tools for assessment of procedural skills: a systematic review. Am J Surg. 2011;202(4):469–80.e6.

33. Steinemann S, Berg B, DiTullio A, Skinner A, Terada K, Anzelon K, et al. Assessing teamwork in the trauma bay: introduction of a modified "NOTECHS" scale for trauma. Am J Surg. 2012;203(1):69–75.

34. Yule S, Rowley D, Flin R, Maran N, Youngson G, Duncan J, et al. Experience matters: comparing novice and expert ratings of non-technical skills using the NOTSS system. ANZ J Surg. 2009;79(3):154–60.

35. Cooper S, Cant R, Porter J, Sellick K, Somers G, Kinsman L, et al. Rating medical emergency teamwork performance: development of the Team Emergency Assessment Measure (TEAM). Resuscitation. 2010;81(4):446–52.

36. Fletcher G, Flin R, McGeorge P, Glavin R, Maran N, Patey R. Anaesthetists' Non-Technical Skills (ANTS): evaluation of a behavioural marker system. Br J Anaesth. 2003;90(5):580–8.

37. Hull L, Arora S, Kassab E, Kneebone R, Sevdalis N. Observational teamwork assessment for surgery: content validation and tool refinement. J Am Coll Surg. 2011;212(2):234–43.e1–5.

38. Karl RC. Aviation. J Gastrointest Surg. 2009;13:6–8.

39. Byrne AJ, Jones JG. Responses to simulated anaesthetic emergencies by anaesthetists with different durations of clinical experience. Br J Anaesth. 1997;78:553–6.

40. Reason J. Human error. Cambridge: Cambridge University Press; 1990.

41. Moorthy KMY, Adams S, et al. Self-assessment of performance among surgical trainees during simulated procedures in a simulated operating theatre. Am J Surg. 2006;192:114–8.

42. Arriaga AFBA, Wong JM, et al. Simulation-based trial of surgical-crisis checklists. N Engl J Med. 2013;368(3):246–53.

43. Lingard L, Regehr G, Orser B, Reznick R, Baker GR, Doran D, et al. Evaluation of a preoperative checklist and team briefing among surgeons, nurses, and anesthesiologists to reduce failures in communication. Arch Surg (Chicago, Ill:. 1960). 2008;143(1):12–7; (discussion 8).

44. Qayumi K, Donn S, Zheng B, Young L, Dutton J, Adamack M, et al. British Columbia interprofessional model for simulation-based education in health care: a network of simulation sites. Simul Healthc. 2012;7(5):295–307.

45. Barsuk JH, Cohen ER, Potts S, Demo H, Gupta S, Feinglass J, et al. Dissemination of a simulation-based mastery learning intervention reduces central line-associated bloodstream infections. BMJ Qual Saf. 2014;23(9):749–56.

46. Barsuk JH, Cohen ER, Caprio T, McGaghie WC, Simuni T, Wayne DB. Simulation-based education with mastery learning improves residents' lumbar puncture skills. Neurology. 2012;79(2):132–7.

47. Donoghue A, Ades A, Nishisaki A, Zhao H, Deutsch E. Assessment of technique during pediatric direct laryngoscopy and tracheal intubation: a simulation-based study. Pediatr Emerg Care. 2013;29(4):440–6.

48. http://www.stockholmresilience.org/21/research/what-is-resilience.html. Accessed 10 Jan 2014

49. Seidel JSHM, Yoshiyama K, et al. Emergency medical services and the pediatric patient: are the needs being met? Pediatrics. 1984;73:769–72.

50. American Academy of Pediatrics, Committee on Pediatric Emergency Medicine and American College of Emergency Physicians, and Pediatric Committee. Care of children in the emergency department: guidelines for preparedness. Pediatrics. 2001;107:777–81.

51. Athey JDJ, Ball J, et al. Ability of hospitals to care for pediatric emergency patients. Pediatr Emerg Care. 2001;17:170–4.

52. Burt CW, Middleton KR. Factors associated with ability to treat pediatric emergencies in US hospitals. Pediatr Emerg Care. 2007;23:681–9.

53. MacKinnon RJ, et al. Research protocol: a fitness for purpose study of the field assessment conditioning tool (FACT). BMJ Open. 2015;5:e006386. doi:10.1136/bmjopen-2014-006386.

54. Hunt EA, Heine M, Hohenhaus SM, et al. Simulated pediatric trauma team management: assessment of an educational intervention. Pediatr Emerg Care. 2007;23:796–804.

55. Brett-Fleegler MB, Vinci RJ, Weiner DL, Harris SK, Shih MC, Kleinman ME. A simulator-based tool that assesses pediatric resident resuscitation competency. Pediatrics. 2008;121(3):e597–603.

56. Hogan MP, Pace DE, Hapgood J, Boone DC. Use of human patient simulation and the situation awareness global assessment technique in practical trauma skills assessment. J Trauma. 2006;61(5):1047–52.

57. Mosley C, Dewhurst C, Molloy S, Shaw BN. What is the impact of structured resuscitation training on healthcare practitioners, their clients and the wider service? A BEME systematic review: BEME Guide No. 20. Med Teach. 2012;34(6):e349–85.

58. Mikrogianakis A, Osmond MH, Nuth JE, Shephard A, Gaboury I, Jabbour M. Evaluation of a multidisciplinary pediatric mock trauma code educational initiative: a pilot study. J Trauma. 2008;64(3):761–7.

59. Gruen RL, Gabbe BJ, Stelfox HT, Cameron PA. Indicators of the quality of trauma care and the performance of trauma systems. Br J Surg. 2012;99(Suppl 1):97–104.

Simulation in Limited-Resource Settings

Nicole Ann Shilkofski and Peter A. Meaney

Simulation Pearls

1. Key elements for successful implementation of simulation programs in limited-resource settings(LRS) must take into account sustainability and dissemination, collaboration with local health authorities and local stakeholders, appropriate mannequin selection, and impact of culture and language on educational methodology.
2. Priority areas for application of simulation-based education (SBE) in limited resource settings (LRS) include patient safety, clinical decision-making, technical skills, teamwork and communication development, and appropriate allocation of resources.
3. Telesimulation may be a method to share resources and educational expertise between more developed simulation programs and those in LRS, while m-Health technologies may be a way forward for data collection to demonstrate clinical impact after simulation program implementation in LRS.
4. Resuscitation training in both trauma and newborn resuscitation in developing countries has been shown in studies to reduce mortality, but this has not been consistently demonstrated with other types of training programs to date.
5. SBE in the form of widely disseminated programs such as Helping Babies Breathe (HBB) has the potential to impact Millennium Development Goal (MDG) #4, to decrease the neonatal morbidity and mortality rates in LRS. Demonstrating efficacy of these types of programs that are being implemented in global settings will be important

in their use as a platform to understand successful and sustainable education and implementation strategies.

Introduction

Uses of Simulation in Limited-Resource Settings

The past few decades have seen major advancements in technology within medicine and nursing, both for clinical care and for educational purposes. As a result, the old adage *see one, do one, teach one* has been largely supplanted by other forms of formative educational strategies that are more in keeping with patient safety priorities. SBE has many uses as a pedagogical strategy in medicine and can enhance the entire spectrum of both care and education, for both novice and expert clinicians. While many of the technological advances in medicine and SBE have had their footholds in the developed world, the idea of *practicing on plastic* has also seen an increase in the developing world, with applications of different types of simulations being implemented in LRS internationally, as part of an encouraging trend toward the globalization of healthcare education.

The need to promote skill development in both medicine and nursing care, in a manner that does not harm patients, has been a primary driver for pedagogical change throughout the world. Development of educational infrastructure and integration of resources (such as simulation) becomes even more salient in the developing world, specifically in LRS. This is due to an epidemiologic mismatch of supply and demand; developing countries often have the highest burden of morbidity and mortality globally, while being under-resourced in the number of practicing clinicians and equipment within the country. Figures 25.1, 25.2, and 25.3 demonstrate this mismatch pictorially in regard to a major worldwide problem, early neonatal mortality, compared to the number of healthcare workers worldwide. SBE programs to address early neonatal mortality on a global scale will be addressed later in this chapter.

N. A. Shilkofski (✉)
Departments of Pediatrics and Anesthesiology/Critical Care Medicine, Johns Hopkins University School of Medicine, Baltimore, Maryland, USA
e-mail: nshilko1@jhmi.edu

P. A. Meaney
Department of Anesthesia and Critical Care, University of Pennsylvania School of Medicine, Children's Hospital of Philadelphia, Philadelphia, PA, USA
e-mail: Meaney@email.chop.edu

© Springer International Publishing Switzerland 2016
V. J. Grant, A. Cheng (eds.), *Comprehensive Healthcare Simulation: Pediatrics*, Comprehensive Healthcare Simulation, DOI 10.1007/978-3-319-24187-6_25

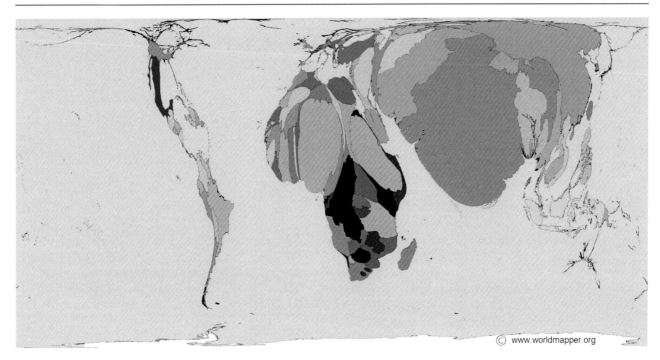

Fig. 25.1 Early neonatal mortality: territory size is proportional to the number of early neonatal deaths in that region, defined as deaths within the first week of life. (Reproduced with permission of www.worldmapper.org)

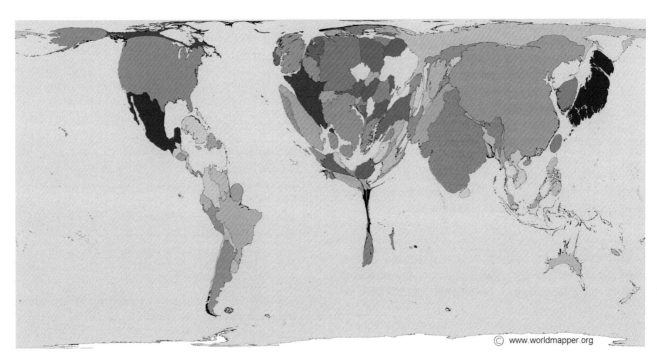

Fig. 25.2 Physicians working worldwide: In 2004, there were 7.7 million physicians working around the world. If physicians were distributed according to population, there would be 124 physicians to every 100,000 people. The most concentrated 50% of physicians live in territories with less than a fifth of the world population. The worst off fifth are served by only 2% of the world's physicians. (Reproduced with permission of www.worldmapper.org)

A World Health Organization (WHO) patient safety study identified ten key health areas where industrialized countries have the most to learn from the developing world; low-technology simulation training was one of these key areas [1]. This chapter describes the various types of SBE in use within LRS, including mannequin-based simulation, partial task trainer models, standardized or simulated patients (SPs), virtual reality simulation, and screen-based or computer

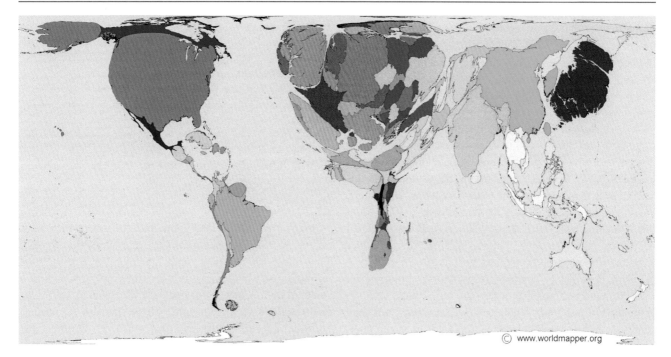

Fig. 25.3 Nurses working worldwide: The USA, China, and the Russian Federation are where the largest number of nurses work. However, the highest numbers of nurses per person can be found in Western European territories such as Finland and Norway. The fewest nurses working per person in the population are in Haiti, Bangladesh, and Bhutan—territories where there is much more need for nurses than is found in many other places. (Reproduced with permission of www.worldmapper.org)

simulation. The chapter will also highlight SBE programs that have been implemented in multiple LRS internationally as an example of attempts to target MDGs established by the United Nations [2].

Pediatric Education for Practitioners and Clinicians in Limited-Resource Settings

Due to a lack of availability of specialist consultants, infants and children in LRS are often cared for by general practitioners. However, many of these practitioners, while often quite skilled and clinically astute, have few formal training opportunities in the care of critically ill or injured children. This can result in a type of *mental paralysis* when confronted with a very sick child. In emergency situations with pediatric patients, *one size does not fit all*. It is well known and recognized that caring for a critically ill child can entail significant cognitive burden when considering clinical elements such as weight-based dosing for fluids and resuscitative medications, age-based consideration of differential diagnoses, and need for different-sized equipment for resuscitation of infants, children, and adolescents [3]. There are a multitude of other physiological, psychological, and psychosocial factors that also impact clinical care for children in these settings [4]. Surveys of practicing clinicians in LRS in parts of Africa and Asia identified significant self-assessed knowledge deficits

in caring for critically ill children and identified skills training and education in this area as a major priority. Practitioners cited lack of knowledge in algorithms/protocols, limited opportunity for hands-on practice, and lack of knowledge in functionality of resuscitative equipment (e.g., defibrillators) as major barriers to caring for critically ill children in their settings [5]. This is where pediatric simulation can play a major role in identifying and seeking closure to these gaps in both knowledge and skills.

Overview of Simulation-Based Education Implementation and Interventions in Limited-Resource Settings

Assessment and evaluation methods in medical education that are used in many settings in North America and Europe can often be inaccurate, expensive, and/or infeasible in many LRS. Therefore, innovative approaches are critical when implementing new assessment methods in these settings. Simulation is one of these creative approaches that can be used in the education and assessment of practicing clinicians in urban and rural settings, including community health workers and traditional birth attendants (TBAs) functioning in LRS. In many of these settings, a country's lack of available trained medical and nursing staff is a major obstacle that impedes progress toward improving healthcare outcomes. In developing countries, inadequate initial assessment, inappropriate treatment, and inadequate monitoring contribute to poor outcomes, in part because in-hospital care providers are frequently undertrained in life support techniques [6–11]. The use of simulation in the creation of a sustainable system to manage emergencies can help to negate these obstacles.

A systematic review of the literature on resuscitation training in developing countries concluded that training in trauma and newborn resuscitation in developing countries has been shown to reduce mortality in some studies, but this has not been demonstrated with other training programs [12]. For example, several studies of trauma resuscitation training in developing countries have demonstrated improvement in survival and reductions in mortality from 3 to 33 % after training of both prehospital and hospital-based providers [13–16]. In terms of newborn resuscitation, improvement in operational performance of hospital-based providers was associated in one study with a decrease in asphyxia-related deaths, while improved performance of TBAs in the community was associated with a decrease in overall mortality in another study [17, 18]. Two studies of newborn resuscitation programs examined effect of training on neonatal (28 days) or early neonatal (7 days) mortality and were able to demonstrate a successful improvement in survival [19, 20]. On the other hand, several studies in LRS involving adult life support training were unable to demonstrate an association between training and improved long-term patient survival [21, 22]. Unfortunately, at the time of the systematic review, there were no studies of pediatric life support training that examined subsequent changes in patient outcomes in the clinical setting in LRS.

Simple, community-based interventions have improved mortality in both developed and developing countries [23–28]. Most studies that reported positive outcomes in knowledge acquisition did so by using differences between cognitive assessments at various time intervals in relation to training intervention, but no studies exist which link cognitive knowledge to patient outcome. Many studies reported psychomotor skills post training, but few used validated scoring systems. Incomplete contextualization of SBE designed originally for resource-rich settings often creates a barrier to effective education. Methods for consideration by educators in order to overcome these barriers in LRS are suggested in Table 25.1.

Other studies have assessed models for the design of training programs in fields beyond resuscitation and acute care, such as surgical training programs in rural locations in Romania and Botswana with demonstration of significant improvement in technical skills [29–32]. Many surgical simulation studies have focused on the feasibility and cost-effectiveness of task trainer simulation in LRS and the use of this type of simulation to develop training programs to address the human resources deficit in developing countries [33–36].

Table 25.1 Considerations to overcome barriers to implementation of simulation-based education (SBE) programs in limited resource settings

Collaborate with local experts to maintain overarching themes while adapting to local cultural and clinical contexts
Create simulation scenarios tailored to the local clinical setting
Track operational performance and evaluate patient outcomes after training
Anticipate higher-than-expected requirements to maintain essential functioning equipment for adequate practice
Increase allotted time for the course to incorporate local cultural norms and to consider language comprehension for non-native speakers

Innovative models and simulators for use in LRS must address portability, sustainability, and cost-effectiveness. They must be simplistic while maintaining fidelity. One example, used in Guyana, is a reusable tool to introduce a standard hollow needle for pediatric intraosseous (IO) infusion designed for use in LRS, where standard IO needles are often unavailable for emergency use [37]. Another example is the development of a low-cost simulator for management of postpartum hemorrhage (PPH) in Africa to train TBAs and nurse midwives in the use of bimanual compression to manage PPH [38]. The assessment of this simulator's efficacy included its use to train illiterate learners, since some TBAs living in rural areas may not be literate. Another example within the field of obstetrics is the creation of an inexpensive low-technology birth simulator that has been successfully used in Mexico and other countries for obstetrical emergency training (Fig. 25.4; [39]). Other studies have

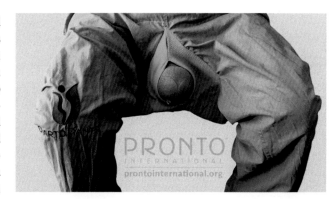

Fig. 25.4 PartoPants™: This simulator is made from a modified pair of surgical scrub pants outfitted with a vagina, a urethra, a rectum, and other anatomical landmarks. It is designed to be worn by an actress or standardized patient who simulates a birth, postpartum hemorrhage, or an eclamptic seizure. This low-technology, low-cost simulator has been used as part of a larger program called PRONTO (Programa de Rescate Obstétrico y Neonatal: Tratamiento Óptimo y Oportuno), focusing on improving the quality of care for women and neonates during obstetric emergencies in response to the WHO Millennium Development Goals 4 and 5. More than 2400 providers have been trained in six countries (Mexico, Guatemala, Kenya, Ethiopia, Namibia, and India) through early 2014 using this simulator. (Figure used with permission from PRONTO International; [86])

discussed the use of this type of low-technology simulator in coordination with an SP as a form of hybrid simulation to enhance realism for learners [40]. All of these simulation models represent creative thinking to overcome cost and access limitations in LRS. Diffusion of these innovations has the potential to benefit health care in both the developed and developing worlds.

Challenges and Barriers in Limited-Resource Settings Simulation with Proposed Methods and Solutions to Overcome Them

Cultural Considerations

The examples above show that simulation is feasible and can be effective in global settings. However, conducting simulation and debriefing in LRS requires consideration of the culture and language of the region in order to be maximally effective. Culture can be conceptualized as shared motives, values, beliefs, identities, and interpretations or meanings of significant events that result from common experiences of members of collectives that are transmitted across generations [41]. There is often a dichotomy between Western and non-Western cultures in ways of learning and conceptualizing entities such as the team construct [42]. This dichotomy can become particularly salient when considering the process of debriefing, discussed further below. With appropriate cultural contextualization, simulation has the potential to improve several areas of team functionality, including membership, role, context, process, and action-taking by focusing intentional learning effort and debriefing on each of these areas [43].

However, in experiential learning, an individual must also engage in reflective practice in the process of debriefing after simulation participation. Most studies of effective debriefing models stem from Western cultures and therefore may not always be generalizable to other cultures and settings. In debriefing, the instructor ideally functions as a facilitator for reflective group discussion by the learners. However, in cultures where *saving face* is important and deference to an instructor or teacher is valued over disclosure of personal viewpoint, a simulation debriefer may find the learner group minimally communicative and seemingly unwilling to engage in reflective practice. This may be due, in part, to the fact that the process of metacommunication (communicating about communication) in non-Western cultures is conceptualized very differently. Participants in a team-based simulation will often be hesitant to reflect on any team performance that seems critical of a team leader, particularly when the team is interprofessional and of mixed gender [43].

Culture also has an impact on conceptualization of different team dynamics, including hierarchy, leadership/followership models, and role delineation within teams. This may be influenced by different cultural interpretation of values, such as the more stereotypically Western *individualism* as compared to the more Eastern *collectivistic* approach to team dynamics and learning [32]. Similarly, there are some cultures that value communal learning and others in which learning is an individual enterprise [41]. In ad hoc teams with members from different cultures and nations, this dichotomy can create barriers to communication and effective patient care and can create problems in SBE ranging from nonacceptance of the *fiction contract* in simulation to unwillingness to engage in an active learning strategy. Simulation itself can often help to improve communication and create a shared mental model that reach beyond cultural bounds for these types of teams [43]. These shared mental models can improve the functionality of medical teams in the care of patients [44].

There is no *one-size-fits-all* solution to these cultural issues that can be barriers to effective implementation of simulation programs. In many ways, broad awareness and recognition of the issues and cultural differences by facilitators can be the first step in overcoming the potential barriers. However, several studies in the literature describe curricular adaptations that have been made for SBE programs in LRS (ranging from virtual patients to computerized patient simulation) to address cultural humility, sociocultural constraints, local epidemiology, and language differences [45–47]. Adaptations of curricula must also consider the influence of culture on assertiveness and leadership styles, uncertainty avoidance, reflective capacity, and individual's degree of introversion/extroversion in order to be successful. Facilitators should incorporate more time than anticipated for teaching and debriefing in order to factor in these considerations.

Impact of Language on Teaching and Comprehension for Learners

Implementation of any new simulation programs internationally will require consideration of cultural sensitivity and linguistic factors if a program is to be successful longitudinally. In a study conducted across medical professionals in different countries in Asia, Africa, and South America, physicians and nurses identified language as a major component for misunderstanding during the conduct of simulation debriefings [43]. Accented speech, methods of pronunciation, differing colloquialisms, or frank language barriers were identified as the origin of misunderstandings and lack of awareness by team members. As a potential solution, the widespread use of skilled interpreters and translation of teaching materials in advance of a planned course or program can be critical to successful implementation of simulation programs in LRS. As mentioned above, facilitators and instructors must also allocate more time than usual for teaching and debriefing when language is a factor, particularly when interpreters are utilized. It can be helpful to use interpreters who have a clinical background, rather than laymen, as this facilitates logical translation of medical terminology in other languages.

Impact of Language on Debriefing Techniques and Strategies

The article *It Is Time to Consider Cultural Differences in Debriefing* discusses the importance for facilitators to understand an individual's frame of reference or mental model in order to optimally structure a debriefing experience [48]. However, this may not be possible when there is a difference in native language between debriefer and learner. In most forms of Western communication, it is the speaker who is expected to communicate ideas without ambiguity, compared with a more *receiver-oriented* culture, in which the listener is responsible to make sense of a communication. Some cultures may value courteous communication over assertive communication and may use mitigated speech when debriefing, so as not to offend the learner or receiver. In the field of medicine, however, this could be a threat to patient safety in the clinical setting, particularly if the mitigated speech does not properly address a knowledge or skill deficiency. These potential barriers make the essential argument for use of interpreters and native speakers as part of the debriefing team. The native speakers should ideally understand the cultural values and linguistic idiosyncrasies in the setting where the debriefing is occurring, thereby serving as a filter and interpreter in order to maximize communication and reflective learning. The barriers discussed above could also potentially be overcome, in part, by wide adoption of the *good judgment* and *advocacy/inquiry* models of debriefing [49, 50]. These models, if taught properly, could appeal to a wide variety of cultures, in that the model acts as a springboard to explore the learner's viewpoints, beliefs, assumptions, and frames of references—all elements that could be a source of cultural misunderstanding between debriefer–learner dyads from different cultures. However, instructors may still find difficulty even when using the *debriefing-with-good-judgment* approach when debriefing learners from cultures in which deference to authority and elders is culturally important since the learners may feel reluctant to express views that seem to contradict the instructor. In this context, the recourse recommended is explicit preparation regarding the goals and norms of the simulation environment, but difficulty may still exist [48].

Other models and techniques of debriefing that promote facilitated discussion, active reflection, and self-discovery may also be helpful in LRS with participants who have language and cultural barriers. When teaching using a train-the-trainer model in LRS, it is crucial for new trainers to explicitly understand and role model the difference between giving *feedback* to learners on their performance and *debriefing* after simulation (see Chap. 3). Some facilitators have anecdotally reported successful use of the structured and supported debriefing *GAS* (Gather–Analyze–Summarize) model with mixed group learners from different linguistic backgrounds, even with clinical bedside teaching and debriefing in international settings [5, 51]. This model, developed in collaboration with the American Heart Association (AHA) for the Advanced Cardiac Life Support (ACLS) and Pediatric Advanced Life Support (PALS) courses, is a learner-centered process that can be rapidly assimilated, is scalable for different levels of learners, and is designed to standardize a debriefing interaction following a simulation scenario, making it ideal for use in LRS and simulation courses utilizing cascade *train the trainer* models. In addition to promoting learner self-reflection and self-discovery, the GAS model promotes closure of performance gaps through discussion and reflection and elicits how learners will change actions in subsequent practice [52]. It can integrate educational objectives for each scenario in the *analysis* phase of the debriefing, thus ensuring that goals for an educational session are achieved and any performance or knowledge gaps are discussed and addressed. The GAS model has already been successfully integrated into debriefing tools for real-time use during PALS to enhance and standardize a scripted debriefing process for PALS instructors [53]. This scripted debriefing process has been shown to be more effective at increasing acquisition of knowledge and team leader behavioral skills than non-scripted debriefing [54]. It is easy to see how these tools could be adapted for use in LRS, both within PALS instruction and other uses of pediatric SBE.

It is also worth considering that there may be a role for both terminal and concurrent debriefing techniques with learners in LRS, depending on the learning goals and objectives. When significant language barriers exist and interpreters are being used, facilitators may find concurrent debriefing to be useful to correct cognitive errors and enhance understanding in real time, particularly when the focus is on skill development. This is an important consideration that should be discussed and agreed upon by facilitators and debriefers in advance when establishing courses and programs in LRS. Some facilitators may also find the incorporation of the *rapid cycle deliberate practice* model to be helpful with learners in LRS when the learning objectives include rapid acquisition of procedural or teamwork skills. This method, which applies concepts of overlearning and automatization to create muscle memory for skill mastery, utilizes more directive feedback and prioritizes opportunities for learners to repeatedly practice skills with *coaching* over lengthy debriefings [55]. This model could be integrated into SBE in LRS when mastery of a skill is a critical learning objective and language differences preclude complex or lengthy debriefings.

Essentially, SBE and debriefing methods that combine opportunities for repetitive practice with reflection and facilitated discussion would be useful when functioning in LRS in order to draw on student's professional experiences and enhance their motivation to assimilate new concepts.

Local Support Considerations

Partnerships with in-country practitioners or stakeholders, ministries of health (MOH), and nongovernmental organizations (NGOs) can help to overcome barriers of competing priorities and potential diversion of resources in LRS. While this is not always an easy task, some groups have found success by partnering with local medical schools, academic institutions, and universities in LRS to establish, develop, and nurture relationships with MOH and ministries of education, but this is of course quite variable from country to country. Some programs such as HBB maintain online lists of country-by-country partnering organizations and academic affiliates working toward program implementation in various LRS. Opportunities for collaborative and cross-disciplinary international projects should be considered in order to promote widespread dissemination of programs and educational interventions. Collaboration with MOH to establish SBE programs is an essential component of program advocacy and realistic potential for widespread acceptance, adoption, and dissemination. When considering implementation and teaching of algorithms in pediatric resuscitation and pediatric acute care, it is critical to ensure that what is taught is consistent with local MOH protocols. These protocols may differ in LRS from traditional algorithms taught in PALS courses due to the types of diseases and comorbidities seen in LRS, such as malnutrition or dengue shock as considerations in fluid resuscitation.

Models for program delivery and dissemination should consider train the trainer paradigms that can also encourage program sustainability and local stakeholder investment. Any individual, team, or organization that endeavors to undertake simulation in LRS should be willing to invest in system strengthening and capacity building within that setting. A plan to demonstrate and measure both short- and long-term impacts is key to obtaining or sustaining funding for educational projects in these settings. The establishment of attainable and realistic educational goals and rigorous research methodology to measure impact are the basis for effecting change. Achievement of pragmatic goals will require interprofessional input from local healthcare providers as partners to incorporate diversity of perspectives and experience.

Program Scalability and Sustainability

It is often the case with pilot education projects that it is initially easier to plan an educational conference or training session outside of the clinical environment. This allows for assurance of quality as well as the ability to teach large numbers of learners rapidly while utilizing the simplest logistics for the intervention. Additionally, the ability to teach at scale allows lowering of direct price per student from the supporting agency. However, these methods often have unanticipated indirect costs on an already limited system. Conference-style educational interventions can require large numbers of personnel to be away from clinical duties, and often there is not enough personnel resource redundancy, leading to significant decrements in clinical staffing during the training. Additionally, large conferences lead to more general and less practical training—leading to a *one size fits none* program. Finally, large group education tends to move toward unidirectional, didactic training and decreases the efficiency of educational transfer associated with SBE. In considering solutions to these potential barriers, it is important in LRS to consider instructor to learner ratios in order to maintain small group learning methodologies that are essential to successful SBE.

Telesimulation and m-Health Technologies

A technological innovation that has advanced the field of international simulation in LRS is the phenomenon of telesimulation. This combines the principles of simulation with remote Internet access to teach procedural skills, conduct simulated resuscitation sessions, or teach other concepts remotely to target learners in LRS. This technology has been used successfully in the field of surgery to teach laparoscopic skills as well as the procedure of IO needle insertion [22, 56]. The utility of telesimulation was also used to conduct pediatric resuscitation training and debriefing sessions between consult and remote hospitals, with a trend toward improved-quality cardiopulmonary resuscitation (CPR) endpoints by practitioners in remote hospitals [57]. Telesimulation may be a way to overcome lack of specialty expertise within LRS, with remote teaching and/or local faculty development by facilitators in developed nations.

Mobile phone messaging applications, such as short message service (SMS) and multimedia message service (MMS), may offer a way to support data collection and reporting in the field of simulation education in LRS. M-Health is the provision of health-related services using mobile communication technology. Many modern information and communication technologies are not yet widely available in LRS. However, the mobile phone is a notable exception that has reached even remote ares in many low- and middle-income countries. M-Health tools have been successfully used as data collection devices, assessment tools, and real-time surveillance techniques and platforms for delivering sustainable interventions [58]. Several investigators have reported on the use of mobile phones to collect data on pregnancy outcomes, PPH rates, and other health outcomes in remote areas of Ghana and Liberia [59–61]. There is great potential for the use of this type of technology to remotely assess both skill retention and actual clinical outcomes after simulation-based training in these settings.

Implementation of Mannequin and Task Trainer Simulation in Limited-Resource Settings

Technology Versus Fidelity and Their Roles in Creating Sustainability in Limited-Resource Settings

The concepts of fidelity and transfer of learning are salient in the developing world when considering sustainability and scalability of a simulation program in LRS. It is often assumed that *high-technology* mannequins or equipments translate to *high-fidelity* environments and transfer of learning to clinical settings. However, this is not always the case, nor is it feasible and sustainable in many LRS, where limitations can range from lack of trained human resources to frequent loss of a consistent electrical power source. The example below of the HBB program demonstrates a large-scale and widespread simulation program initiative in the developing world that utilizes low- to medium-fidelity equipment to create a sustainable educational framework [62].

Mannequin Design Considerations for Limited-Resource Settings

Any health technology or simulator that is developed specifically for LRS must conform to certain considerations that are often unique to these environments. These include:

1. Harsh environmental conditions including temperature extremes, humidity, and dust.
2. Supply chain: Distribution and repair of simulators can be challenging in LRS. Industry support for higher technology simulators in many countries is usually lacking. Therefore, mannequins that require disposables, replacement parts, or frequent servicing are less likely to remain operational.
3. Lack of operator training: Mannequins in LRS generally need to be simple enough that community-level providers with limited training can safely and effectively use them to disseminate teaching programs. Therefore, their design must be relatively simplistic and user-friendly.
4. Cost: Per capita healthcare expenditures in LRS are a small fraction of what they are in the developed world, which results in enormous cost pressures on healthcare products for LRS. Simulation technologies are often unaffordable for both governments and individuals in LRS. This will inevitably result in a lack of supply of healthcare technologies by established manufacturers to LRS markets.
5. Need for quality: Simulation technology for LRS markets need to be of at least as high quality and reliability as those for developed countries to be setting appropriate and achieve impact. A simulator that fails in the developed world can usually be readily replaced or fixed, but that may not be possible in LRS, as discussed above.
6. Paucity of country-specific evidence: Most simulation technology and devices are designed and developed for populations in high-resource countries that typically constitute the primary and most lucrative markets for these products. The vast majority of simulation task trainers have not been evaluated in LRS. This leaves LRS populations vulnerable to suboptimal devices for their educational needs.

MamaNatalie® Birthing Simulator

MamaNatalie® is a simulation device, worn by an SP or facilitator that can simulate PPH, high-risk deliveries, and a wide range of other obstetric complications (see Fig. 25.5a, b).

Fig. 25.5 a MamaNatalie® Birthing Simulator and **b** its use in situ: This simulator is strapped on to the operator who takes the role of the mother and manually controls the training scenario. The simulator has the following features: bleeding to simulate postpartum hemorrhage, positioning and delivery of the baby, delivery of the placenta, fetal heart sounds, cervix landmark, urinary bladder catheterization, uterine massage, and uterine compression. (Photos used with permission from Laerdal Medical)

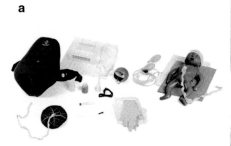

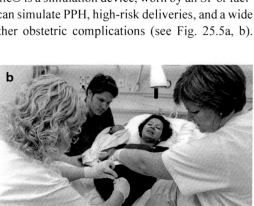

Fig. 25.6 a NeoNatalie®
Newborn Simulator for neonatal
resuscitation and its use in situ in
Senegal: An inflatable, portable
simulator designed to teach basic
neonatal resuscitation skills. The
simulator has a natural weight
when filled with water and includes features such as spontaneous breathing, palpable umbilical
pulse, and crying. It can be used
for role-play scenarios such as
normal post-birth care, standard
resuscitation, positive pressure
ventilation, and chest compressions. Training materials have
been translated into multiple
languages for use in LRS around
the world, as can be seen in **b**.
(Photos used with permission of
Laerdal Medical)

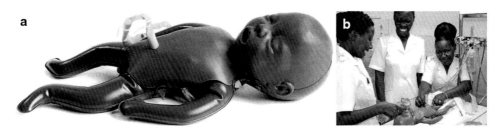

The mannequin was designed to be used in collaboration
with NeoNatalie® for training of TBAs and midwives in
LRS, who may need to manage care of both mother and infant after delivery. The use of this simulator is being increasingly implemented in LRS where emergency obstetric care
may be limited to community health workers and TBAs as
part of the Helping Mothers Survive: Bleeding After Birth
(HMS:BAB) program. This SBE program is aimed at reducing PPH, the leading cause of maternal mortality worldwide
and another target of the WHO MDGs [63, 64].

NeoNatalie® Newborn Simulator

NeoNatalie® is a low-technology inflatable neonatal simulator designed to teach basic neonatal resuscitation skills
(see Fig. 25.6a and b). The simulator's features include
crying, spontaneous breathing, chest wall movement with
bag-mask ventilation, and umbilical cord pulsation. It was
purpose-built for the HBB program and has been used in LRS
for dissemination of the HBB curriculum described below.

Examples of Program Implementation in Limited-Resource Settings Using Mannequin Simulation

Helping Babies Breathe Program

HBB is an initiative of the American Academy of Pediatrics
in collaboration with other partners, developed with curricular input from WHO. It is a neonatal resuscitation curriculum using SBE for resource-limited circumstances [62].
Prior curricular programs in Essential Newborn Care (ENC)
and Neonatal Resuscitation Programs (NRP) with birth attendants in rural communities demonstrated mixed outcomes
[65–67]. Data from observational studies have shown that
community health workers can perform basic resuscitation

skills that have the potential to substantially reduce intrapartum-related neonatal deaths, but that a major gap existed in
terms of strategies to address home births and births in rural
and LRS facilities far from referral institutions [68]. The
HBB program was developed to address these gaps.

The program was piloted in Kenya and Pakistan, where
assessment of participant knowledge and skills pre-/post-
program demonstrated significant gains. Bag-valve-mask
ventilation was identified as a skill that required more active practice and mentoring in order to be mastered by some
participants [69]. The program has subsequently been implemented in several LRS countries, and studies of its efficacy
in these settings are ongoing. In India, a train the trainer
cascade model was used to train almost 600 birth attendants
from rural primary health centers and district and urban hospitals. Investigators examined over 4000 births before and
after implementation of training and were able to demonstrate a significant reduction in stillbirths in the area where
training had been integrated. However, neonatal mortality
rates overall remained unchanged [70].

The HBB strategy was used to train master instructors
in Tanzania, who subsequently delivered the program to regional instructors, who in turn trained health providers in
smaller facilities. Within the 2 years after intervention, there
was a 24 % reduction in the rate of stillbirths and a 47 % reduction in early neonatal mortality, defined as death within
the first 24 h. This program focused on grassroots birth attendants practicing in rural facilities rather than on hospital-
based physicians [71]. HBB program implementation has
also been formally studied in Ethiopia, Rwanda, and Nepal
with promising preliminary results toward the objective of
addressing MDG #4 to reduce child mortality [72–74]. The
preliminary successes of this type of program demonstrate
the feasibility of an evidence-based curriculum utilizing
SBE in LRS.

Saving Children's Lives Program

Saving Children's Lives (SCL) is an initiative of the AHA in collaboration with the Children's Hospital of Philadelphia that aims to reduce under-five mortality rates (UFMR) through a contextualized resuscitation training program utilizing SBE. It is designed to increase healthcare provider competence to treat pneumonia and diarrhea, improve system-level reporting of resource availability, and increase reporting of quality of provider performance. Begun in late 2013, this program has been piloted in Tanzania and Botswana, with early data showing significant improvement in provider confidence and knowledge of correct management of acute pneumonia and diarrhea [75]. The SCL program is also being piloted in Gujarat, India, to train community health workers to coordinate with local emergency response systems to identify and treat children in the community with pneumonia and diarrhea early in their disease course.

Operation Smile—Simulation-Based Education in Perioperative Pediatric Training

SBE has a role in mission-based healthcare delivery as well. Operation Smile, an NGO focused on cleft lip and palate repair, has endeavored to develop increased local capacity in LRS countries where clefts are epidemiologically common. In collaboration with SBE experts, an educational perioperative pediatrician (POP) training program was developed for Operation Smile pediatric volunteers from LRS countries. Based on the AHA PALS course, POP was tailored to the clinical situations commonly presenting during perioperative emergencies in LRS. The program was implemented with clinicians from different cultures and linguistic backgrounds, being piloted with students from nine different countries [76]. High-fidelity simulators and real-time language interpretation were used to enhance active learning. During the 2-day course, over 50 % of the time was spent in hands-on simulation training. The SP scenarios developed for the POP course are also commonly used as preparatory mock codes during missions, which are implemented with the clinical care team prior to the first surgical case during mission-based surgery. These contextualized simulated emergency scenarios serve as a mechanism to enable ad hoc mission teams to discuss threats to patient safety, reinforce emergency protocols, and allocate team roles during emergency situations arising during the surgical missions.

Emergency Triage Assessment and Treatment

Emergency Triage Assessment and Treatment (ETAT) is a three and a half-day course designed by the WHO based on the UK Advanced Pediatric Life Support Training and tailored to LRS. Its simulated scenarios are designed to teach health workers with limited clinical background to triage sick children as well as initiate treatments for airway and breathing, circulation, and neurologic emergencies in children under 5 years of age. Although simulation mannequins are not mandatory, the course utilizes existing resources and equipment to train participants, which increases the relevance to the participants' work environments [77, 78].

Examples of Simulation-Based Education Programs Using Task Trainer Simulation

There are a multitude of studies on CPR training in LRS, but few of these examine comparative SBE teaching modalities with feedback [79, 80]. One study that did so examined whether task trainer CPR mannequins with feedback and lower instructor to student ratios could train learners as well as traditional instructor-led CPR [81]. Baseline performance data were collected on healthcare providers in Botswana using CPR task training mannequins and then prospectively randomized participants to three training groups: instructor-led, limited instructor with mannequin feedback, or self-directed learning. Subsequently, serial examinations on performance were measured after training up until 6 months post training. Excellent CPR skill acquisition was significant and was retained to 3 and 6 months. Novel training with mannequin feedback was not inferior to traditional instructor training [81]. This is encouraging data to support the use of simple task training mannequins with feedback in LRS. The use of feedback mannequins may be more reliable and equally cost-effective to developing and maintaining a large training infrastructure in LRS.

Use of Simulated or Standardized Patients and Hybrid Simulation in Limited-Resource Settings

Simulated or Standardized Patients (SPs) have been used in LRS for both instruction and assessment [82–84]. In LRS that may be remote from tertiary care facilities and therefore may not have access to specialty care patients, SPs can supplement the learner experience by providing a standardized presentation of specific disease processes for both formative and summative learning. SPs also provide psychological safety within the learning environment for novice learners, particularly in the practice of sensitive examinations, such as pelvic breast or rectal examinations, which may be even more critical in certain sociocultural and religious contexts. In some conservative societies, female patients may refuse certain providers and not be willing to allow students to examine them.

Researchers in Myanmar used SPs playing the role of a patient's mother to assess ability of providers to diagnose and treat pediatric malaria [83]. Another development in SP simulation has been in the use of online *virtual patients* for

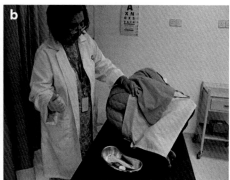

Fig. 25.7 Hybrid simulation for sensitive examinations: The photos (**a, b**) depict combined use of partial task trainers (pelvic exam trainer and rectal exam trainer) in conjunction with a standardized patient to assess both clinical examination skills and patient communication skills. In a multicultural or conservative society, it can be difficult to recruit standardized patients willing to allow novices to perform sensitive examinations such as breast, pelvic, or rectal exams. Hybrid simulation provides a way to circumvent these issues while maintaining a standardized educational experience for novice learners. (Photos used with permission of Perdana University Clinical Skills Unit, Kuala Lumpur, Malaysia)

technological skills instruction and capacity building for healthcare educators in Malawi [85]. These *virtual patients* are designed by teams of healthcare professionals to be contextualized for in-country medical education.

SPs provide a degree of fidelity which is not possible when using mannequins alone. However, partial task trainers and mannequins provide students with the ability to practice invasive procedures such as venous cannulation, urinary catheterization, and sensitive examinations to which SPs may not wish to be subjected. When a partial task trainer (such as a pelvic exam model or rectal model) and an SP are combined, as in the case of a *hybrid* simulation, students are able to participate in a realistic human interaction and practice communication skills while performing basic clinical skills (see Fig. 25.7a and b). Hybrid simulation has also been used in medical and nursing school curricula in the Middle East, where gender and religious preference often limit student exposure to opposite-sex, gender-specific examinations [84]. Investigators have been able to demonstrate improved student confidence in sexual history taking and breast/pelvic examination skills after participation in hybrid simulations designed to teach these skills.

The Future of Simulation-Based Education in Limited-Resource Settings

With the ongoing globalization of medical education, LRS are the next frontier in SBE. If the medical community at large is able to address many of the MDGs, it must be with a platform in mind for global educational reform as a priority to accomplish these goals. Simulation can and should play a major role in this platform. It will be crucial to anticipate and address in advance the many challenges that will be inherent

in this. The importance of program dissemination, sustainability, and local buy-in cannot be understated. The creation of sustainability can be a difficult process, but involving interprofessional local in-country partners is a critical and key component in the process in order to obtain diversity of perspectives and ensure pragmatic applicability of programs. Other challenges will include competing priorities and potential diversion of resources by MOH, Ministries of Education, and other governmental agencies that often govern these types of programs in LRS countries.

Educators must also consider the global epidemiology of disease burden and ensure that SBE programs address this epidemiology in a country-specific or region-specific manner. Essential to this process is the creation of learning objectives and program goals that align with local needs and protocols in order to address pertinent medical issues that are relevant to a particular country or area. Within the field of pediatrics, many platforms for SBE in LRS have already begun, but further demonstration of both short- and long-term impacts of these programs will be the key to sustain funding and interest. As mentioned above, organizations that undertake simulation in LRS must be willing to invest in system strengthening and capacity building in the settings where they establish these programs. It is now incumbent upon the medical education community to ensure that these programs achieve success through the use of rigorous research methodologies, with the ultimate goal being improvement in current and future health care for children on a global scale.

References

1. Syed SB, Dadwal V, Rutter P, Storr J, Hightower JD, Gooden R, et al. Developed-developing country partnerships: benefits to developed countries? Global Health. 2012;8:17.

2. United Nations Millenium Development Goals. United Nations. [cited 2013 July 10]. http://www.un.org/millenniumgoals/.

3. Luten R, Wears R, Broselow J, Croskerry P, Joseph M, Frush K. Managing the unique size-related issues of pediatric resuscitation: reducing cognitive load with resuscitation aids. Acad Emerg Med. 2002;9(2):840–7.

4. Bishop S. Evaluating teams in extreme environments: from issues to answers. Aviat Space Environ Med. 2004;75(7):C14.

5. Shilkofski N, Jung J, Rice J, Crichlow A. Needs assessment for pediatric and neonatal resuscitation program dissemination in low-resource countries. Pediatr Crit Care Med. 2014;15(4):12.

6. Nolan T, Angos P, Cunha AJ, Muhe L, Qazi S, Simoes EA, et al. Quality of hospital care for seriously ill children in less-developed countries. Lancet. 2001;357(9250):106–10.

7. English M, Esamai F, Wasunna A, Were F, Ogutu B, Wamae A, et al. Assessment of inpatient paediatric care in first referral level hospitals in 13 districts in Kenya. Lancet. 2004;363(9425):1948–53.

8. Kandasami P, Inbasegaran K, Lim WL. Perioperative death in Malaysia: the transition phase from a developing nation to a developed one. Med J Malaysia. 2003;58(3):413–9.

9. Jat AA, Khan MR, Zafar H, Raja AJ, Hoda Q, Rehmani R, et al. Asian J Surg. 2004 Jan;27(1):58–64.

10. Khan AN, Rubin DH. International pediatric emergency care: establishment of a new specialty in a developing country. Pediatr Emerg Care. 2003;19(3):181–4.

11. Kapadia FN. Code 99-an international perspective. Chest. 1999;115(5):1483.

12. Meaney PA, Topjian AA, Chandler HK, Botha M, Soar J, Berg RA, et al. Resuscitation training in developing countries: a systematic review. Resuscitation. 2010;81(11):1462–72.

13. Arreola-Risa C, Vargas J, Contreras I, Mock C. Effect of emergency medical technician certification for all prehospital personnel in a Latin American city. J Trauma. 2007;63:914–9.

14. Ali J, Adam RU, Gana TJ, Williams JI. Trauma patient outcome after the pre-hospital trauma life support program. J Trauma. 1997;42:1018–21.

15. Husum H, Gilbert M, Wisborg T, Van Heng Y, Murad M. Rural prehospital trauma systems improve trauma outcome in low-income countries: a prospective study from North Iraq and Cambodia. J Trauma. 2003;54:1188–96.

16. Ali J, Adam R, Butler AK, et al. Trauma outcome improves following the advanced trauma life support program in a developing country. J Trauma. 1993;34:890–8.

17. Deorari AK, Paul VK, Singh M, Vidyasagar D, Medical Colleges Network. Impact of education and training on neonatal resuscitation practices in 14 teaching hospitals in India. Ann Trop Paediatr. 2001;21:29–33.

18. Kumar R. Training traditional birth attendants for resuscitation of newborns. Trop Doct. 1995;25:29–30.

19. Zhu XY, Fang HQ, Zeng SP, Li YM, Lin HL, Shi SZ. The impact of the neonatal resuscitation program guidelines (NRPG) on the neonatal mortality in a hospital in Zhuhai, China. Singapore Med J. 1997;38:485–7.

20. Chomba E, McClure EM, Wright LI, Carlo WA, Chakraborty H, Harris H. Effect of WHO newborn care training on neonatal mortality by education. Ambul Pediatr. 2008;8:300–4.

21. Arreola-Risa C, Mock C, Herrera-Escamilla AJ, Contreras I, Vargas J. Cost-effectiveness and benefit of alternatives to improve training for prehospital trauma care in Mexico. Prehospital Disaster Med. 2004;19:318–25.

22. Moretti MA, Cesar LA, Nusbacher A, Kern KB, Timerman S, Ramires JA. Advanced cardiac life support training and long-term survival from in-hospital cardiac arrest. Resuscitation. 2007;72:458–65.

23. Carcillo JA, Kuch BA, Han YY, Day S, Greenwald BM, McCloskey KA, et al. Mortality and functional morbidity after use of PALS/APLS by community physicians. Pediatrics. 2009;124(2):500–8.

24. Rivers EP, Ahrens T. Improving outcomes for severe sepsis and septic shock: tools for early identification of at-risk patients and treatment protocol implementation. Critical Care Clinics. 2008;24(3 Suppl):S1–47.

25. Carcillo JA, Davis AL, Zaritsky A. Role of early fluid resuscitation in pediatric septic shock. JAMA. 1991;266(9):1242–5.

26. Han YY, Carcillo JA, Dragotta MA, Bills DM, Watson RS, Westerman ME, et al. Early reversal of pediatric-neonatal septic shock by community physicians is associated with improved outcome. Pediatrics. 2003;112(4):793–9.

27. Ngo NT, Cao XT, Kneen R, Wills B, Nguyen VM, Nguyen TQ, et al. Acute management of dengue shock syndrome: a randomized double-blind comparison of 4 intravenous fluid regimens in the first hour. Clin Infect Dis. 2001;32(2):204–13.

28. Oliveira CF, Nogueira de Sa FR, Oliveira DS, Gottschald AF, Moura JD, Shibata AR, et al. Time- and fluid-sensitive resuscitation for hemodynamic support of children in septic shock: barriers to the implementation of the American College of Critical Care Medicine/Pediatric Advanced Life Support Guidelines in a pediatric intensive care unit in a developing world. Pediatr Emerg Care. 2008;24(12):810–5.

29. Mutabdzic D, Bedada AG, Bakanisi B, Motsumi J, Azzie G. Designing a contextually appropriate surgical training program in low-resource settings: the Botswana experience. World J Surg. 2013;37(7):1486–91.

30. Moldovanu R, Tarcoveanu E, Lupascu C, Dimofte G, Filip V, Vlad N, et al. Training on a virtual reality simulator–is it really possible a correct evaluation of the surgeons' experience? Rev Med Chir Soc Med Nat Iasi. 2009;113(3):780–7.

31. Okrainec A, Smith L, Azzie G. Surgical simulation in Africa: the feasibility and impact of a 3-day fundamentals of laparoscopic surgery course. Surg Endosc. 2009;23(11):2493–8.

32. Okrainec A, Henao O, Azzie G. Telesimulation: an effective method for teaching the fundamentals of laparoscopic surgery in resource-restricted countries. Surg Endosc. 2010;24(2):417–22.

33. Dorman K, Satterthwaite L, Howard A, Woodrow S, Derhew M, Reznick R, et al. Addressing the severe shortage of health care providers in ethiopia: bench model teaching of technical skills. Med Educ. 2009;43(7):621–7.

34. Kiely DJ, Stephanson K, Ross S. Assessing image quality of low-cost laparoscopic box trainers: options for residents training at home. Simul Healthc. 2011;6(5):292–8.

35. Kigozi G, Nkale J, Wawer M, Anyokorit M, Watya S, Nalugoda F, et al. Designing and usage of a low-cost penile model for male medical circumcision skills training in Rakai, Uganda. Urology. 2011;77(6):1495–7.

36. Waikakul S, Vanadurongwan B, Chumtup W, Assawamongkolgul A, Chotivichit A, Rojanawanich V. A knee model for arthrocentesis simulation. J Med Assoc Thai. 2003;86(3):282–7.

37. Kalechstein S, Permual A, Cameron BM, Pemberton J, Hollaar G, Duffy D, et al. Evaluation of a new pediatric intraosseous needle insertion device for low-resource settings. J Pediatr Surg. 2012;47(5):974–9.

38. Perosky J, Richter R, Rybak O, Gans-Larty F, Mensah MA, Danguah A, et al. A low-cost simulator for learning to manage postpartum hemorrhage in rural Africa. Simul Healthc. 2011;6(1):42–7.

39. Cohen S, Cragin L, Rizk M, Hanbeg A, Walker D. PartoPants: the high-fidelity, low-tech birth simulator. Clin Simul Nurs. 2010;7(1):e11–18.

40. Walker D, Cohen S, Estrada F, Monterroso M, Jenny A, Fritz J, et al. PRONTO training for obstetric and neonatal emergencies in Mexico. Int J Gynecol Obstet. 2012;116(2):128–33.

41. Yamazaki Y. Learning styles and typologies of cultural differences: a theoretical and empirical comparison. Int J Intercult Relat. 2005;29(5):521–48.

42. Joy S, Kolb D. Are there cultural differences in learning style? Int J Intercult Relat. 2009;33(5):69–85.

43. Shilkofski NA, Hunt EA. Identification of barriers to pediatric care in limited-resource settings: A simulation study. Pediatrics. 2015; doi: 10.1542/peds.2015–2677.

44. Hunt EA, Shilkofski NA, Nelson K, Stavroudis L. Simulation: translation to improved team performance. Anesthesiol Clin North America. 2007;25(2):301–19.

45. Fahey JO, Cohen SR, Holme F, Buttrick ES, Dettinger JC, Kestler E, et al. Promoting cultural humility during labor and birth: putting theory into action during PRONTO obstetric and neonatal emergency training. J Perinat Neonatal Nurs. 2013;27(1):36–42.

46. Bediang G, Bagayoko CO, Raetzo MA, Geissbuhler A. Relevance and usability of a computerized patient simulator for continuous medical education of isolated care professionals in sub-saharan Africa. Stud Health Technol Inform. 2011;169:666–70.

47. Muntean V, Calinici T, Tigan S, Fors UG. Language, culture and international exchange of virtual patients. BMC Med Educ. 2013;13:21.

48. Chung HS, Dieckmann P, Issenberg SB. It is time to consider cultural differences in debriefing. Simul Healthc. 2013;8(3):166–70.

49. Rudolph JW, Simon R, Rivard P, Dufresne RL, Raemer DB. Debriefing with good judgment: combining rigorous feedback with genuine inquiry. Anesthesiol Clin. 2007;25(2):361–76.

50. Rudolph JW, Simon R, Dufresne RL, Raemer DB. There's no such thing as "nonjudgmental" debriefing: a theory and method for debriefing with good judgment. Simul Healthc. 2006;1(1):49–55.

51. Phrampus PE. Clinical bedside teaching can benefit from "Simulation Style Debriefing". Pittsburgh: Paul E. Phrampus- Patient safety, quality, simulation and education expertise. 2014 August- [cited 2014 Dec 9]. http://phrampus.com/Blog.html.

52. Phrampus PE, O'Donnell JM. Debriefing using a structured and supported approach. In: Levine AI, DeMaria S, Schwartz AD, Sim AJ, editors. The comprehensive textbook of healthcare simulation. New York: Springer; 2013. pp. 73–84.

53. Cheng A, Rodgers DL, van der Jagt E, Eppich W, O'Donnell J. Evolution of the Pediatric Advanced Life Support course: enhanced learning with a new debriefing tool and Web-based module for Pediatric Advanced Life Support instructors. Pediatr Crit Care Med. 2012;13:589–95.

54. Cheng A, Hunt E, Donoghue A, et al.; for the EXPRESS pediatric Simulation Collaborative. EXPRESS- Examining Pediatric Resuscitation Education using Simulation and Scripting: the birth of an international pediatric simulation research collaborative- From concept to reality. Simul Healthc. 2011;6:34–41.

55. Hunt EA, Duval-Arnould JM, Nelson-McMillan KL, Bradshaw JH, Perretta JS, Shilkofski NA. Pediatric resident resuscitation skills improve after "Rapid Cycle Deliberate Practice" training. Resuscitation. 2014;85(7):945–51.

56. Mikrogianakis A, Kam A, Silver S, Bakanisi B, Henao O, Okrainec A, et al. Telesimulation: an innovative and effective tool for teaching novel intraosseous insertion techniques in developing countries. Acad Emerg Med. 2011;18(4):420–7.

57. Yang C, Hunt E, Shilkofski N, Dudas R, Schwartz J. Can telemedicine improve adherence to resuscitation guidelines for critically ill children at community hospitals: a randomized controlled trial using high fidelity simulation. Crit Care Med. 2012;40(12):1–328.

58. Krishna S, Boren SA, Balas EA. Healthcare via cell phones: a systematic review. Telemed J E Health. 2009;15(3):231–40.

59. Andreatta P, Debpuur D, Danquah A, Perosky J. Using cell phones to collect postpartum hemorrhage outcome data in rural Ghana. Int J Gynaecol Obstet. 2011;113(2):148–51.

60. Lori JR, Munro ML, Boyd CJ, Andreatta P. Cell phones to collect pregnancy data from remote areas in Liberia. J Nurs Scholarsh. 2012;44(3):294–301.

61. Munro ML, Lori JR, Boyd CJ, Andreatta P. Knowledge and skill retention of a mobile phone data collection protocol in rural Liberia. J Midwifery Womens Health. 2014;59(2):176–83.

62. Helping Babies Breathe Curriculum. The golden hour. 2013. http://www.helpingbabiesbreathe.org.

63. Nelissen E, Ersdal H, Ostergaard D, Mduma E, Broerse J, Evjen-Olsen B, et al. Helping mothers survive bleeding after birth: an evaluation of simulation-based training in a low-resource setting. Acta Obstet Gynecol Scand. 2014;93(3):287–95.

64. Evans CL, Johnson P, Bazant E, Bhatnagar N, Zgambo J, Khamis AR. Competency-based training "Helping Mothers Survive: Bleeding after Birth" for providers from central and remote facilities in three countries. Int J Gynaecol Obstet. 2014;126(3):286–90.

65. Carlo WA, McClure EM, Chomba E, Chakraborty H, Hartwell T, Harris H, et al. Newborn care training of midwives and neonatal and perinatal mortality rates in a developing country. Pediatrics. 2010;126(5):e1064–71.

66. Carlo WA, Goudar SS, Jehan I, Chomba E, Tshefu A, Garces A, Parida S, Althabe F, McClure EM, Derman RJ, Goldenberg RL, Bose C, Hambidge M, Panigrahi P, Buekens P, Chakraborty H, Hartwell TD, Moore J, Wright LL; First Breath Study Group. High mortality rates for very low birth weight infants in developing countries despite training. Pediatrics. 2010;126(5):e1072–80.

67. Bhutta ZA, Soofi S, Cousens S, Mohammad S, Memon ZA, Ali I, et al. Improvement of perinatal and newborn care in rural Pakistan through community-based strategies: a cluster-randomised effectiveness trial. Lancet. 2011;377(9763):403–12.

68. Wall SN, Lee AC, Niermeyer S, English M, Keenan WJ, Carlo W, et al. Neonatal resuscitation in low-resource settings: what, who, and how to overcome challenges to scale up? Int J Gynaecol Obstet. 2009;107:S47–S64.

69. Singhal N, Lockyer J, Fidler H, Keenan W, Little G, Bucher S, et al. Helping babies breathe: global neonatal resuscitation program development and formative educational evaluation. Resuscitation. 2012;83(1):90–6.

70. Goudar SS, Somannavar MS, Clark R, Lockyer JM, Revankar AP, Fidler HM, et al. Stillbirth and newborn mortality in India after helping babies breathe training. Pediatrics. 2013;131(2):e344–52.

71. Msemo G, Massawe A, Mmbando D, Rusibamayila N, Manji K, Kidanto HL, et al. Newborn mortality and fresh stillbirth rates in Tanzania after helping babies breathe training. Pediatrics. 2013;131(2):e353–60.

72. Hoban R, Bucher S, Neuman I, Chen M, Tesfaye N, Spector JM. 'Helping Babies Breathe' training in Sub-Saharan Africa: educational impact and learner impressions. J Trop Pediatr. 2013;59(3):180–6.

73. Musafili A, Essén B, Baribwira C, Rukundo A, Persson LÅ. Evaluating helping babies breathe: training for healthcare workers at hospitals in Rwanda. Acta Paediatr. 2013;102(1):e34–8.

74. Ashish KC, Målqvist M, Wrammert J, Verma S, Aryal DR, Clark R, et al. Implementing a simplified neonatal resuscitation protocol-helping babies breathe at birth (HBB)—at a tertiary level hospital in Nepal for an increased perinatal survival. BMC Pediatr. 2012;12:159.

75. Wright SW, Mazhani L, Ralston M, Steenhoff AP, Nadkarni VM, Meaney PA, et al. Impact of contextualized pediatric critical care training on pediatric healthcare providers in Botswana. Pediatr Crit Care Med. 2014;15(4):194. doi:10.1097/01.pcc.0000449598.26350.c9.

76. Kilbaugh T, Borasino S, Hales R, Nishisaki A, Nadkarni VM, Meaney PA. A multicultural experience with high fidelity simulation. Proceedings of the 17th Pediatric Critical Care Colloquium, February 20–22; British Columbia, Canada; 2008.

77. Gove S, Tamburlini G, Molyneux E, Whitesell P. Campbell; WHO Integrated Management of Childhood Illness (IMCI) Referral Care Project. Development and technical basis of simplified guidelines for emergency triage assessment and treatment in developing countries. Arch Dis Child. 1999;81:473–7.

78. Tamburlini G, Mario S D, Maggi RS, Vilarim JN, Gove S. Evaluation of guidelines for emergency triage assessment and treatment in developing countries. Arch Dis Child. 1999;81:478–82.

79. Urbano J, Matamoros MM, López-Herce J, Carrillo AP, Ordóñez F, Moral R, et al. A paediatric cardiopulmonary resuscitation training project in Honduras. Resuscitation. 2010;81(4):472–6.

80. Young S, Hutchinson A, Nguyen VT, Le TH, Nguyen DV, Vo TK. Teaching paediatric resuscitation skills in a developing country: introduction of the Advanced Paediatric Life Support course into Vietnam. Emerg Med Australas. 2008;20(3):271–5.

81. Meaney PA, Sutton RM, Tsima B, Steenhoff AP, Shilkofski N, Boulet JR, et al. Training hospital providers in basic CPR skills in Botswana: acquisition, retention and impact of novel training techniques. Resuscitation. 2012;83(12):1484–90.

82. Shirazi M, Sadeghi M, Emami A, Kashani AS, Parikh S, Alaeddini F, et al. Training and validation of standardized patients for unannounced assessment of physicians' management of depression. Acad Psychiatry. 2011;35(6):382–7.

83. Aung T, Montagu D, Schlein K, Khine TM, McFarland W. Validation of a new method for testing provider clinical quality in rural settings in low- and middle-income countries: the observed simulated patient. PLoS One. 2012;7(1):e30196.

84. Sole K, Sawan L. Fostering student clinical skills confidence using obstetric and gynecology hybrid simulation. Presented at: 15th Ottawa Conference: Assessment of Competence in Medicine and Healthcare Professions, March 10; Kuala Lumpur, Malaysia; 2012.

85. Dewhurst D, Borgstein E, Grant ME, Begg M. Online virtual patients—a driver for change in medical and healthcare professional education in developing countries? Med Teach. 2009;31(8):721–4.

86. PRONTO (Programa de Rescate Obstetrico y Neonatal: Tratamiento Optimo y Oportuno) International Curriculum. 2014. http://prontointernational.org.

Simulation for Patient- and Family-Centered Care

26

Maria Carmen G. Diaz, Jennifer L. Arnold and Traci Robinson

Simulation Pearls

1. The four guiding principles of patient- and family-centered care (PFCC) are *respectand dignity, information sharing, participation, and collaboration.* These principles are also the foundation for all simulations for PFCC.
2. Simulation for PFCC may be modified to meet cultural and linguistic needs of the family.
3. The patient and the family are the center of the learning experience in simulation for PFCC and may serve as both learners and educators.
4. Create a home instead of a medical environment for simulations so that patients and home caregivers are able to explore and practice how they would provide care within their own environments and resources.

M. C. G. Diaz (✉)
Division of Emergency Medicine, Nemours Institute for Clinical Excellence, Nemours/Alfred I. duPont Hospital for Children, Wilmington, DE, USA
e-mail: mcdiaz@nemours.org

Department of Pediatrics and Emergency Medicine, Sidney Kimmel Medical College at Thomas Jefferson University, Philadelphia, PA, USA

J. L. Arnold
Simulation Center at Texas Children's Hospital, Houston, TX, USA

Division of Neonatology, Baylor College of Medicine, Houston, TX, USA

T. Robinson
KidSIM Pediatric Simulation Program, Alberta Children's Hospital, Calgary, AB, Canada
e-mail: traci.robinson@ahs.ca

Introduction
What Is Patient- and Family-Centered Care?

PFCC is an approach to healthcare that recognizes the vital role that families play in the health and well-being of infants, children, and family members of all ages. The planning, delivery, and evaluation of this healthcare are grounded in a mutually beneficial partnership among healthcare providers, patients, and families. When implemented, this approach shapes policies, programs, facility design, and daily interactions. Healthcare providers practicing PFCC see healthcare interactions as opportunities to support patients and families in their caregiving and decision-making roles [1–4]. By acknowledging the importance of emotional, social, and developmental support, these healthcare providers are able to engage the family and patient as essential members of the healthcare team. In pediatrics, PFCC practitioners understand that the family is the child's source of strength and support and both the child's and the family's perspectives are important in clinical decision-making. Positive PFCC experiences lead to better outcomes, increased parental confidence in their roles, and greater patient and family satisfaction. It may also encourage children and young adults to take responsibility for their own healthcare [1, 2].

PFCC has four guiding core principles [1]:

1. *Respect and dignity.* PFCC providers listen to and respect each child and family. Care is provided for a person, not a condition. Patient and family values, beliefs, and culture are incorporated into healthcare planning and delivery.
2. *Information sharing.* Complete, honest, unbiased information is shared with patients and families in useful and affirming ways that take into account cultural and linguistic diversity. This ongoing communication encourages patients' and families' effective participation in healthcare and decision-making.

© Springer International Publishing Switzerland 2016
V. J. Grant, A. Cheng (eds.), *Comprehensive Healthcare Simulation: Pediatrics,*
Comprehensive Healthcare Simulation, DOI 10.1007/978-3-319-24187-6_26

3. *Participation.* Patients and families are encouraged and supported to participate in decision-making at the level they choose. Patients and families are empowered to discover their own strengths as they build confidence to participate in healthcare decisions.

4. *Collaboration.* There is collaboration with patients and families at all levels of healthcare including: delivery of care; professional education; policy-making; program development, implementation, and evaluation; and healthcare facility design. PFCC encourages collaboration in safety and quality initiatives, operational issues, and research.

The patient and family are integral members of the healthcare team and should be encouraged to participate in their healthcare plan. Families offer unique insights into the care of their child. Their observations are vital to the development of any care plan. This collaborative process allows for improved clinical decision-making, improved follow-through, more efficient use of resources, and improved patient safety. PFCC also enhances provider, patient, and family satisfaction.

This family participation and collaboration may also extend beyond care of their own child. Patients' and families' perspectives should guide the formation of systems and processes of care as well as patient flow. Additionally, patients and families serve as valuable educators for practitioners. Their viewpoints may offer providers with beneficial lessons for future patient and family interactions. Families' feedback about care rendered and integration of care are helpful tools for practitioners learning about PFCC.

Why Does Simulation Partner Well with Patient- and Family-Centered Care?

It is important to recognize that simulation for PFCC (simPFCC) may be used for purposes other than education. There are at least five other different purposes for healthcare simulation. Given that there are many different ways simulation can be applied, there are also different ways to develop and utilize it for PFCC.

1. Using simulation to improve quality and patient safety

Simulation may serve as a conduit to identify latent safety threats through systems testing and integration (see Chap. 5). Simulation may help perform root cause analysis of a sentinel event by recreating an adverse event, or it may be used to trial new patient care equipment, processes of care, and spaces before implementation to help prevent unpredictable outcomes and potential harms. Here, patients and families may participate in simulation-based system tests as content experts to help uncover threats to patient safety and patient satisfaction by participating in simulations in hospital environments and systems. This provides an opportunity for patients and families to actively *collaborate* in the design of healthcare systems, processes of care, and facility design.

2. Using simulation to assess competency

Validated scenarios and assessment tools may be utilized to evaluate individual or team skills in a realistic and standardized manner (see Chap. 7). In this capacity, patients and/or family members may be the target to assess competency (e.g., assessing a parent's ability to sterilely and properly administer total parenteral nutrition (TPN) through a peripherally inserted central catheter (PICC) line for a child with intestinal issues) or part of the actual assessment process (e.g., a simulation-based assessment of a healthcare provider's ability to discuss bad news using a standardized protocol) [5]. These approaches truly require *participation* from patients and family members in providing care.

3. Using simulation for research

Simulation may be a focus for research, either as a tool for conducting research or as the research study itself (see Chap. 30). Research using patients and family members would not only require the utmost *respect and dignity*, but could also enhance our understanding of how to truly provide PFCC with respect and dignity. Here, participation of a patient or family member would be subject to the same regulations as any human subjects' research study. Examples of simPFCC research are starting to emerge in the literature [6, 7].

Research outside healthcare simulation has shown that positive PFCC experiences lead to better outcomes, increased parental confidence in their roles, and greater patient and family satisfaction. Institutions that promote programs and initiatives aimed at improving PFCC have been shown to have decreased malpractice claims, decreased medical errors, decreased lengths of stay, improved patient satisfaction, and even improved staff satisfaction [8–10]. Although we do not yet fully understand the impact that simulation-based educational efforts may have on improving the patient and family healthcare experience or actual patient care outcomes, this would be a wide open area for research endeavors.

4. Using simulation for advocacy

Healthcare simulation may be purposed for advocacy needs: supporting the larger community with simulation-based activities to educate the general public and promote healthcare simulation through public relations, legislation, and media.

Table 26.1 How simulation aligns with patient- and family-centered care

Patient- and family-centered care principle	Simulation curriculum correlate
Respect and dignity	
Care is provided for a person, not a condition, with patient and family values, beliefs, and culture incorporated into healthcare planning and delivery	Simulation allows for repetitive and deliberate practice at an individual's own pace
	Individualized learning objectives may be met during one-on-one simulations and debriefings
Information sharing	
Complete, honest, unbiased information is shared with patients and families in useful and affirming ways that take into account cultural and linguistic diversity	Immediate, hands-on practice enhances opportunities to discuss and share information related to home care needs
	Trainings may be modified as needed to meet cultural and linguistic needs
	Debriefing provides opportunities to give complete and honest feedback to home caregivers on their ability to provide care
Participation	
Patients and families are empowered to discover their own strengths as they build confidence to participate in healthcare decisions	Simulation is active, hands on requiring the highest level of participation from patients and/or caregivers
	By actively practicing care during simulated events, patients and families are provided an opportunity to be active participants as opposed to bystanders in care
Collaboration	
Collaboration with patients and families at all levels of health care including delivery of care and education	Learner focused debriefings allow for reflection on patient and home caregiver objectives
	Hands-on practice side by side with healthcare providers is congruent with a collaborative approach to education
	Pre-briefing with home caregivers allows for setting individualized patient and family member objectives

Any of these opportunities enhances *information sharing* at the individual, community, and population level. For example, a simulation-based training day focused on decreasing preventable infections may train laypersons on hand-washing techniques and antibiotic dosing. Patients and family members may participate in and/or benefit from these types of activities.

5. Using simulation for education

The most common purpose for healthcare simulation is education. At its core, simulation is a training modality that is utilized by many fields, not just health care, to train individuals and/or teams in new cognitive, technical, and behavioral skills. Simulation is a hands-on educational modality that bridges the gap between classroom learning and real-life clinical experience. It creates a safe, confidential learning environment that offers the participant the opportunity for deliberate practice followed by facilitated feedback and reflection on performance. It creates a safe place for mistakes to be made and learned from. These elements create an educational methodology that is congruent with and closely aligned with PFCC principles (Table 26.1). Healthcare-simulation-based educational activities may be directed to families, patients, and even other home caregivers as the target

learners to help non-healthcare providers learn and practice specific medical issues surrounding the care of themselves or a family member. Examples include families of an infant being discharged on a ventilator with a tracheostomy participating in an airway emergency training program, families with a child being discharged with a seizure disorder learning general seizure management and how to administer a rescue medication, families with an adolescent being discharged with Type 1 diabetes learning how to handle a critical low, among others.

It is important to recognize that home caregivers may also function in the educator role in simulation-based education geared towards healthcare providers. They may serve as the *simulation tool* to help educate healthcare providers on how to better practice PFCC by playing the role of a family member or patient during scenarios (e.g., a simulation-based educational program to train clinicians in disclosure of medical errors). They may also function as simulation educators helping direct learning objectives and debriefing in simulations for PFCC. Healthcare providers or non-healthcare providers alike may serve as the target learner population depending on the need. This chapter, however, will focus on the development and implementation of simulation-based educational activities for home caregivers and patients as the targeted learners.

Logistics of Creating Simulation for Patient- and Family-Centered Care

Who Should Receive Training

Simulation training may be offered to all members of the home caregiver team. This may include family members— parents, siblings, and other relatives; the patients themselves; non-healthcare providers involved in the patients' care such as teachers, nannies, or peers; and out-of-hospital home healthcare providers such as home nursing and prehospital care providers. For example, a teenager with food allergy leading to anaphylaxis would benefit from injectable epinephrine simulation training. Additionally, parents, teachers, and friends may benefit from this same simulation-based education focused on the technical and cognitive skills needed to administer injectable epinephrine if the patient is otherwise incapacitated at the time it is needed.

What Should Be Simulated

The possibilities of what should be simulated are limitless and can focus on cognitive, technical, and/or behavioral skills. Simulation may be extraordinarily useful in teaching technical skills to nonclinical home caregivers (Table 26.2). These may include new tasks that will be performed daily. Simulation-based training will ensure proper performance and increase caregiver confidence with the procedure prior to discharge or after a new diagnosis. Likewise, simulating

Table 26.2 Examples of technical skills that may be taught using Si mPFCC

Daily tasks
Suctioning
Urethral catheterization of a patient with neurogenic bladder
Bolus feeds through gastrostomy-tube
Venting a gastrojejunostomy tube
Wound care
Cast care
Peripherally inserted central catheter (PICC) line care
Administering insulin
Occasionally performed tasks
Change gastrostomy-tube
Change tracheostomy tube
Manage hypoglycemia
Rare tasks
Administer cardiopulmonary resuscitation (CPR)
Administer antiepileptics
Apply an automated external defibrillator

SimPFCC simulation for patient- and family-centered care

tasks that are performed occasionally, or rarely, will also afford some practice of and perhaps some comfort with these events, which could be critical in some high-risk situations.

Simulation may also be used to teach critical decision-making and other cognitive skills. This type of simulation focuses on content knowledge and what the caregiver thinks. These may include recognition of the need for care, knowledge of medical interventions, and cognitive decision-making (Table 26.3).

Simulation-based education for teaching home caregivers critical behavioral skills is quite similar to teaching healthcare providers the same skills. These skills might focus on crisis resource management and interpersonal communication skills (amongst care providers) during high-risk or life-threatening crises (Table 26.4).

Where Should the Simulation Occur

The location of the simulation session is contingent on the goals of the simulation and the type of learner to whom the scenario is being delivered. Depending on the situation, it may be beneficial to provide some preliminary simulation education in the hospital setting. This will afford families ample resources to help hone their technical, cognitive, and behavioral skills prior to discharge. This may occur in a traditional educational space such as a classroom or a simulation lab. Ideally, the space in the hospital setting should be adjusted to mimic the families' home environment. For example, a lounge area in the nursing unit may be altered to mimic the living room in the family's house, or a patient room may be reconstructed to mimic the home nursery (Figs. 26.1 and 26.2).

This added realism may help families better adapt, understand their roles, and recognize their home resources. Finally, simulations may also be conducted outside of the hospital setting, such as in the family's home, at school, or at daycare. This in situ simulation encourages nonclinical caregivers to review and reinforce their skills and to problem solve in their home environment.

When Should the Simulation Occur

When developing simPFCC, timing and frequency issues need to be addressed. There is currently limited data to provide a clear answer to this issue. Existing data from the fields of psychology, education, and simulation suggest that optimal learning occurs when it is dispensed in repetitive and frequent doses as opposed to single or bolus training events [12]. Although curricular decisions on when to implement, frequency of training, and duration of training in healthcare simulation for patients and home caregivers is not

Table 26.3 Some examples of cognitive skills that may be taught using SimPFCC

Clinical example	Recognition of need for care	Knowledge of medical interventions	Decision-making at critical points
Seizures	Identification of signs of a seizure such as tonic-clonic movements, lip smacking, eye rolling	Knowledge of rectal diazepam as treatment for seizures that last longer than 5 min	Understanding when prolonged seizures require further emergent intervention and/or Emergency Medical Services (EMS) call
Anaphylaxis	Identification of symptoms such as lip and tongue swelling, wheezing, and difficulty breathing	Knowledge of how to dose and administer injectable epinephrine immediately	Understanding that if the patient is responsive and able to swallow, diphenhydramine may be given orally while waiting for EMS
Tracheostomy	Identification of signs of respiratory distress such as increased respiratory rate, retractions, and cyanosis	Knowledge of the indications for replacement of a tracheostomy tube	Understanding of management options in emergency situations. If unable to reinsert a tracheostomy tube, a smaller size tube may be used or positive pressure ventilation may be administered via mouth
Gastrostomy tube (G-tube) care	Recognition of signs of malfunctioning G-tube such as burst balloon	Knowledge of indications for when to change G-tube	Understanding when medical care is needed such as abdominal distension or erythema around G-tube

SimPFCC simulation for patient- and family-centered care

Table 26.4 Examples of crisis resource management skills that may be taught using SimPFCC. (Adapted from the behavioral assessment Tool [11])

Crisis resource management skill	Performance goal during care for any clinical situation
Familiarity with the environment	Ability to find emergency equipment and supplies in a timely fashion during a critical situation
Effective communication	Uses closed loop communication with another home caregiver during care
Optimal workload distribution	Assigns appropriate tasks to another caregiver instead of multitasking
Role clarity and leadership	Takes charge of critical situation and takes appropriate steps to manage situation
Effective utilization of resources	Asks for help such as calling EMS in a crisis, uses cognitive aids such as CPR handouts

SimPFCC simulation for patient- and family-centered care, *EMS* Emergency Medical Services, *CPR* cardiopulomonary resuscitation

Fig. 26.1 A backdrop that includes images of the walls and furniture within the home nursery may be used to make the hospital space more closely mimic the home environment. (Photo courtesy of Jen Arnold, MD, Texas Children's Hospital)

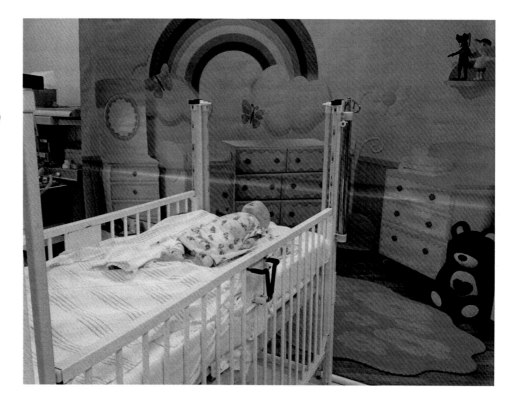

Fig. 26.2 The addition of a few toys, stuffed animals, and baskets from home further transform the hospital room. (Photo courtesy of Jen Arnold, MD, Texas Children's Hospital)

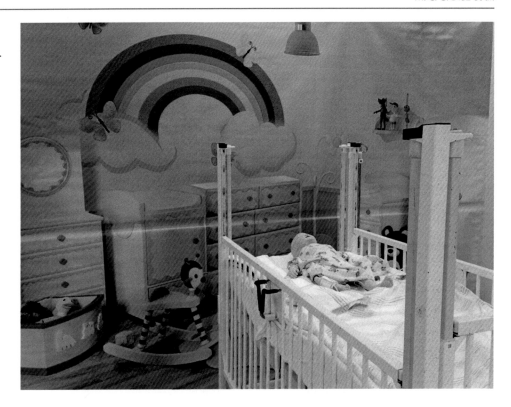

yet known, most educators can make these decisions based on the specific learning objectives of the simulation training, availability of the parents or caregivers, and resources related to instructors, space, and equipment. It is important to stay focused on what an individual family needs when implementing a simulation-based educational program for caregivers and parents. There are many factors to consider for patients and families that could affect when they might be ready and able to learn, whether in a simulated environment or otherwise. A patient or family member may be psychologically or emotionally unprepared for education during a hospital stay depending on the acuity of illness and duration of hospitalization. However, if simulation is felt to be an effective and possibly better educational format than traditional didactic, video, or written methods, certain aspects of education are required prior to discharge for chronic conditions that will require care at home [13, 14]. In one study evaluating a simulation-based training program for parents of children diagnosed with Type I diabetes, parents preferred interspersed education with basic and vital skills taught prior to discharge, complex topics taught 1 month after diagnosis, and review of diabetes management at 3 months post-diagnosis [15]. Interspersed education may provide an opportunity to build knowledge and skills without overburdening an already stressful situation for a patient or caregiver.

Although much research is needed in timing and frequency related to simPFCC, the need for education is paramount. Research has shown that up to 70 % of patients and family members have educational needs that are unmet prior to discharge [16]. In order to help guide these decisions, ask the questions found in Table 26.5 related to the specific medical

complexities that are the focus of the training, and resources available may be helpful.

How Should the Simulation Be Implemented

Begin with Identifying the Objectives for the Teaching Session

There are many critical steps involved in the design and development of simPFCC. Identification of educationally sound learning objectives is critical [17]. These objectives guide the development of the scenario(s). The objectives taught to patients and/or home caregivers during a simulation session can come from multiple sources, both from instructors (medical team and/or educators) and learners (patients and home caregivers). Instructor-driven objectives might include goals from patient treatment plans such as wound care or specific medication administration guidelines. Other instructor-driven objectives might include specific skills required to handle a potential complication or emergency at home such as how to provide CPR or troubleshoot a ventilator in patients going home with tracheostomies and on ventilator support.

In keeping with PFCC principles, all simulation-based educational sessions should also cover learner-focused objectives allowing patients and home caregivers to define their own learning needs. Learner-centered objectives may be identified by interviewing the family prior to the simulation session (Table 26.6) and from the learners' reactions in the debriefing [17]. Allowing patients and home caregivers to have input in creating a climate in which they can most

Table 26.5 Questions to guide decision-making surrounding the timing for simPFCC

1. Is the medical issue a short term or a chronic health issue for the patient and/or home caregivers?
   - Early predischarge simulation training will benefit those dealing with new diagnoses and conditions
   - Frequency of simulation training may be proportional to chronicity of illness and learning needs of caregivers
   - More extensive training is needed when there is a new diagnosis or change in health status
2. Is the patient an inpatient or outpatient at the time of diagnosis?
   - If inpatient, training should occur prior to discharge. If an outpatient, as soon as possible
   - Accessibility to patient and family caregivers in terms of time, travel, and other resources, will help determine frequency and duration of training the inpatient and outpatient settings
     - Access to patients and home caregivers is likely easier when inpatient
     - Patients and home caregivers will have to balance work and other personal priorities to make time for training as outpatients
3. Are the skills to be taught high risk or low risk?
   - Training should occur prior to discharge for inpatients and as soon as possible for outpatients in cases where there is a high risk of poor outcome
   - Training should occur more frequently to help caregivers maintain skills if there is a high risk of poor outcome
   - For more high-risk medical issues, longer durations for training will be needed to achieve and maintain skill mastery
4. What is the emotional state, anxiety level, and level of readiness to learn of the patient and/or home caregivers?
   - Extreme levels of anxiety or stress may inhibit learning and training may need to be postponed until patients/families are ready
   - Standardized assessment tools for anxiety and stress may help determine when patients and/or home givers are ready for training
   - Interspersed, shorter simulations with fewer learning objectives of increasing complexity over time will alleviate issues of readiness when patients and home caregivers are overwhelmed
5. How often will the caregiver perform this skill?
   - The more frequent the skill is required, the sooner training should start, particularly prior to discharge
   - If this skill is anticipated to be used infrequently, more *refresher* opportunities need to be offered
   - Duration of training sessions will likely be less as the patient and home caregiver gain more experience
   - Longer duration training will be needed with high-risk, low-frequency events and skills
6. How complex to learn are the skills that need to be taught?
   - Generally, the more complex the skills being taught, the sooner training should be implemented to allow time for repeat practice
   - Interspersed education with a *ramping* up of complexity may improve learning
7. What is the educational goal of the training, that is, mastery learning versus traditional instruction?
   - If mastery learning is the goal, training should start as early as possible to allow for as much time as needed for achieving learning objectives
   - Mastery learning will require longer training time to allow for true deliberate practice opportunities until caregivers *get it right*
   - More frequent, smaller training sessions with increasing difficulty are needed for achievement of mastery learning

SimPFCC simulation for patient- and family-centered care

fruitfully learn puts the patient and family in the center of the learning experience.

Simulation scenarios for patients and home caregivers should ultimately combine both learner- and instructor-driven objectives to maximize learning outcomes. This blended approach ensures that the discharge teaching plans are tailored to meet the educational needs of both the patient and family, as well as the healthcare professionals overseeing their care.

Table 26.6 Sample questions to help identify learner-centered objectives

What has this experience been like for you so far?
What is your biggest concern taking your son home?
What was it like for your when your daughter had a seizure?
What would you like to learn from this session?
What challenges or struggles have you had when managing your child's condition at home?

Build a Realistic Situation for the Patient and Family

Once specific objectives are identified, the next step is to create a realistic scenario that skillfully engages the learners, in this case the patients and/or home caregivers (see Chap. 2). In health care, we are still trying to understand the relationship between learner engagement and the degree to which the scenario matches the real environment. Some researchers hold that simulation realism must be related and tailored to the specific goals and target population for the simulation [18]. Environmental elements that replicate the home environment enhance the fidelity of the simulation and bring PFCC principles and objectives to life. It is very important to create a home instead of a medical environment for simPFCC so that patients and home caregivers are able to explore and practice how they would provide care within

Table 26.7 Tips for creating a realistic situation

Choose a mannequin or task trainer that is roughly the same size and age of the patient
Teach using the identical equipment and supplies that the family will use at home
Limit props, equipment, and supplies available during simulation to those that the patient and/or home caregivers would use
Recreate a similar environment where the patient and/or home caregivers would most likely use the skills being trained

their own environments and with their own available resources (Table 26.7).

Choose a Simulator (… or Not)

Many types of simulators are available. Learning outcomes can be successfully met through the use of task trainers, partial task trainers and/or whole-body computer-generated, interactive human patient simulators (HPSs) [19, 20]. Unfortunately, as is the case often in pediatrics, there are no simulators available that meet all the specific requirements of the teaching session. As such, modifications and adaptations are required. For example, there are currently no whole-body computer-generated HPS mannequins with a tracheostomy. As a result, simPFCC for tracheostomy teaching may require that modifications be made to the mannequin such as creation of a stoma within the mannequin or placement of a stoma on top of the mannequin's existing trachea. This type of modification may result in voiding of the mannequins' warranty, and as such, educators are advised to check with the manufacturer prior to proceeding. This may also be a way to effectively recycle retired mannequins. This type of education may also require the simultaneous use of more than one type of simulator.

For many purposes, specifically those involving teaching procedural skills, a partial task trainer may be most appropriate. A partial task trainer replicates only that specific portion of the body needed to learn the key elements of a specific skill or procedure. A modified foam pad, for example, may be used to mimic the thigh muscle and be used for teaching intramuscular injections in the setting of anaphylaxis.

There are whole-body computer-generated mannequins that not only have similar capabilities to some of the task trainers, but also have more advanced features such as the ability to breathe, turn blue, generate pulses, vocalize, and even mimic seizure activity. These advanced features allow the learner(s) to become more interactive with the mannequin and respond to changing medical conditions. This can help refine patients' and home caregivers' ability to make decisions and problem solve under time pressure in a more realistic fashion.

The use of confederates/actors to portray various individuals who would participate in a real-life event may be considered in simPFCC. For example, a confederate may play the role of an EMS dispatcher to help families practice communicating their needs to EMS during an emergency at home, or a confederate may portray a home health nurse who assists family members in providing care (see Chap. 8).

Lastly, the environment itself may be the simulation tool. Rooms or spaces within the home may be used or even recreated as home caregivers walk through their anticipated care plans. This allows home caregivers to identify latent safety threats within their home. Literature has shown the benefits of using the environment as a simulation tool [6]. By recreating living spaces or simulated homes, researchers in injury prevention successfully used simulation to help parents identify potential risks and hazards [6].

Pilot the Scenario

Once a simulation scenario is developed, it is important to trial the scenario. It is important to ensure that the intended learning objectives are achievable with the scenario design, props, and equipment chosen. Trialing and practicing scenarios on other experienced home caregivers, who have cared for children with similar medical complexities in the past, allows scenario architects to receive valuable feedback on realism, believability, and applicability.

Prebrief the Learners

Although real-life examples of simulation activities are readily available in our day-to-day lives: batting cages, golf driving ranges, interactive video games, and driving simulators, simulation in health care will most likely be very new to families. As such, they will require an orientation to this type of learning. Best practice in simulation-based education recommends that any learner who participates in simulation be oriented to a safe and confidential learning environment [17]. This is an important consideration because any learner takes some psychological risks when participating in simulation. This is likely to be even more important for a patient or home caregiver, whose stress level and anxiety may be higher as they are learning to handle challenging situations for themselves, let alone for their own child or family member. This would include setting a safe and confidential learning environment by verbalizing that mistakes are expected and accepted. One should also be specific when describing the type of feedback that will be used during debriefing, including the use of video if it is being used for review.

Allowing patients and/or home caregivers to watch a video of a simulated event may also help prepare them for their participation. Learners will need to know what to expect from the session. They need to be instructed to behave

as if this were a real event and verbalize each step of their thinking. It is helpful to encourage them to use the child's name when referring to the mannequin. Allowing families to know that they will have many opportunities to practice until they feel confident will help alleviate anxiety they may have. Patients and/or home caregivers will require an orientation to the specific simulator and to the simulated environment. They will need to know what the capabilities of the simulators are and how the limitations of the mannequin will be overcome. For example, current whole-body mannequins are not able to demonstrate eye rolling or tonic positioning of extremities in a seizure. Describing to families that these findings will be shown in a video or be described by the instructor will help with their engagement, as well as help avoid any confusion during the scenario.

Implementation of the Scenario

The delivery of a simPFCC can take on many different forms. Factors such as the time allotted for the session and selected learning objectives will influence how the scenarios and debriefing are implemented. Some sessions may last longer, 20–90 min, followed by a debriefing focused on allowing learners additional time for reflection and discussion. Other sessions may be much shorter, some less than 10–20 min, with the debriefing focused primarily on providing corrective feedback with little time for reflection. The decision on which path to choose should reflect the objectives of the scenario and the tasks and procedures being asked of the caregiver(s). The duration of the session also depends on the learner, the number of scenarios or tasks practiced, and the time needed for mastery. The use of simPFCC can be just as diverse as that for healthcare providers. A successful combination of mastery learning and deliberate practice was used to study the use of simulation to teach home caregivers seizure management and rescue medication administration as part of their discharge treatment plan [7]. Participants were given multiple opportunities to manage their child's seizures during simulations followed by guided reflection using advocacy/inquiry combined with instructor-driven directive feedback on performance.

Who Should Instruct

The specific instructors for simPFCC depend on the goals of the simulation. There are three components of expertise to consider in simPFCC: clinical content expertise, simulation and debriefing expertise, and PFCC expertise. When patients and home caregivers are the target learners, it is crucial that the debriefers are able to give appropriate feedback on the clinical aspects of the scenario and also answer clinical questions during debriefing. Healthcare learners traditionally come to simulation with background knowledge and skills surrounding a clinical area. A patient or home caregiver, however, may have little to no clinical knowledge or skills prior to taking part in a simulation. As with any simulation educational activity, the instructors should have knowledge and expertise in simulation theory, scenario delivery, and debriefing. Additionally, simulation educators should be ideally trained in the core principles of PFCC. When conducting debriefing for patients and home caregivers, it is important to understand that the training needs to be collaborative and specific to the patient. This is a unique situation where an attempt is made to focus the education to a specific patient, not a condition, and requires a partnership in expertise between the simulation educator and the patient and/or family member. The healthcare provider may be the expert related to clinical content, but the patient and/or home caregiver is the expert related to the patient and their environment. To further illustrate this, simply teaching how to manage an airway emergency in an infant being discharged home with a tracheostomy will not be effective without taking into account the specific medical history and plan of care for that patient, an understanding of the specific symptoms that patient exhibits when in distress, and defining how that care can be provided in the patient's specific home environment. The parent or family member will provide content expertise on how to identify a problem and manage it based on the patient's context and home environment. In this example, signs and symptoms of respiratory distress in their infant, what their resources are at home (i.e., how many people may be in the home to assist and what equipment and supplies are available) will be patient specific. In order for simPFCC to be successful, the training needs to be truly collaborative on every level. Given this unique challenge in simulation for patients and home caregivers, this may be an ideal setting to consider the opportunity to have co-debriefers and include non-healthcare professionals such as family advisors or patients and home caregivers who have been there.

Debriefing: How to Do it in Simulation for Patient- and Family-Centered Care

The debriefing process is vital to effective educational experiences in healthcare simulation. It is felt to be the most important aspect of simulation-based education and has the biggest influence on learning [21–24]. When training non-healthcare providers, just as in training healthcare providers, it is vital to identify and address performance gaps that occur during simulation scenarios [25]. How this is done can be extremely variable as feedback can be given by multiple sources (instructors, peers, the actual simulator, etc.) and at different times during the simulation experience

Table 26.8 Example of a simulation for patient- and family-centered care course template: SimPFCC to train parents of an infant with a seizure disorder on seizure management and medication administration

What: Simulation to train parents of an infant admitted with seizures on how to manage a prolonged seizure at home	
Objective development	
Instructor-centered objectives	Technical:
• Determine technical, cognitive, and behavioral goals of simulation	• Proper administration of intranasal midazolam
	• Proper positioning of patient during a seizure to protect airway
	Cognitive:
	• List the steps of seizure management
	• Describe specific medication side effects that may occur
	Behavioral:
	• Effective communication with EMS
	• Effective workload distribution with another home caregiver
Learner-centered objectives	Example questions to ask learners:
• Identify learner-centered objectives during family interview or during debriefing	• What has this experience been like for you so far?
	• What is your biggest concern about taking your child home?
	• What was it like for you when your child had a seizure?
	• What would you like to gain from this session today?
Who: *should receive training*	
Identify all members of the home caregiver team	Potential learners
	• Mother and father
	• Grandparents
	• Professional caregivers (i.e., nannies)
Consider including the patient in the training depending on the situation and the patient's age	• Siblings
	• Daycare provider
	• Home nurse
Where: *should the simulation be held*	
Need to determine ideal location (in hospital vs. in situ in the home environment)	Recreate an environment similar to where the patient and/or home caregivers would most likely use the skills being trained
	• Recreate the family's living room by transforming the hospital's family lounge. Place pillows on chairs and move furniture in the room to match the family's home setting
When: *should the training take place*	
Determine when to start training based on	In this seizure scenario, this is a new diagnosis for an inpatient expected to have chronic health issues
• Urgency for training	
• Short-term or chronic health issue	Early predischarge simulation training will be beneficial
• New diagnosis or existing diagnosis	
• Inpatient or outpatient	
Duration:	Simulation sessions may need to occur after parent's work hours
• Consider factors such as family accessibility, availability, attention span, stress level	Simulation sessions may need to be short if learners have short attention spans
• Consider goals of training	Home caregivers who are anxious or stressed by the seizure may need shorter simulations with fewer objectives
	Some family members may want to learn with other family members rather than alone
	Mastery learning will take longer
Frequency of training needed: Assess risk of intervention in relation to anticipated frequency of event	One session may suffice if the infant has a short admission. Given the high risk and low frequency of this seizure management skill, recommend a *refresher* session 3–6 months post-discharge

Table 26.8 (continued)

How: should the team develop the simulation	
Build a realistic scenario	
• Choose a mannequin roughly the size and age of the patient	Infant computer-generated mannequin
• Teach using identical equipment and supplies the family will use at home	A *medication pack* that matches what the family would use at home, including needle, syringe, nasal atomizer, alcohol swab, and expired medication vial
• Limit props, equipment, and supplies to those available in the home	Have the mom use her cell phone to time the seizure and call EMS
	Make pillows accessible to the family as they would use this for positioning at home
Pre-brief the family	Explain that simulation is a safe place to make mistakes and everyone maintains confidentiality
Introduction and orientation to the session	Inform the parents that they may stop the scenario at any time to ask for help
	Remind parents to act like they normally would and to think out loud
	Encourage the parents to use the child's name when referring to the mannequin
	Explain that the parents need to draw up the medication and actually administer the medication to the mannequin
	Set clear expectations of the scenario (e.g., the simulation will last for 6 min, and a discussion will follow)
	Demonstrate the mannequin's seizure features to the parents
	Clarify that eye rolling and secretions that are normally present during a seizure will be described by the facilitator instead of visualized on the mannequin
Debrief	
Debriefing: Reactions phase—Open-ended questions to elicit parent's emotional response and thoughts	"How did it feel?"
	"What are your thoughts about today's session?"
Debriefing: Analysis phase	"As I watched, I noticed you drew up the medication perfectly. I am wondering what happened when the medication wasn't given."
Use open-ended advocacy/inquiry questions to address all instructor and learner centered objectives	
Debriefing: Close performance gaps	"So, the next time your child has a seizure, how will you administer the medication differently?"
Follow-up plans	
Schedule further training	Timing will depend of safety issues identified during simulation session and performance gaps that need to be improved
Close the loop with the team—healthcare providers and home caregivers	Document simulation training in medical record
	Discuss training with healthcare and home caregiver team
	Discuss training with healthcare and home caregiver team
	Request feedback about ongoing home care and potential need for further education

EMS Emergency Medical Services

(immediately during simulation or after) [26]. There are still many questions to be answered in healthcare simulation as to the best practice and methodology for simulation education, particularly related to debriefing techniques. The best debriefing methodology to be implemented in simulation for non-healthcare providers is yet to be determined [24]. Specific debriefing techniques are further discussed in Chap. 3. When debriefing simulations for parents and caregivers, we recommend using techniques that are specific and congruent with known healthcare simulation best practice. This would include setting a safe and confidential learning environment, being specific with feedback during debriefings [27], engaging adult learning strategies, using video-review if possible,

and being focused on learning objectives in addition to objectives of the learner(s). Although video-assisted debriefing has been found to be superior in other fields such as sports performance and military, studies from simulation in health care demonstrate mixed results [24]. In our experience, if resources allow for video review during debriefing, learning is enhanced for patients and families. However, we make this recommendation only for facilitators that are comfortable and experienced with use of video during debriefing [28]. Table 26.8 provides a comprehensive example of a template for planning a simPFCC event. Readers are encouraged to use this step-by-step template in the planning and implementation of simulation-based teaching for patients and families.

Conclusions

The future of simPFCC is broad as this is a new and growing field within healthcare simulation. Evaluating the outcomes of programs and facilities that utilize simPFCC as a method for patient education is vital. Understanding how it may improve patient safety and outcomes, improve patient compliance with care plans, and improve hospital efficiency and costs related to patient education, will be essential. Additionally, more research is needed to understand which patient care processes and educational needs should be simulated, what are best practices in implementing simPFCC, and how these trainings affect patient and families psychologically, including their quality of life. The psychosocial consequences of putting parents and caregivers through simulation-based educational experiences are unknown. Research needs to first identify whether training makes caregivers feel reassured by receiving training because it provides them with concrete skills to use in an emergency or whether it actually increases the stress they already feel by reminding them that their child or loved one could experience an emergency at home that they may have to manage [29]. We will then need to identify whether added or decreased stress and anxiety affects their ability to care for their loved one and ultimately patient outcomes.

References

1. Committee on Hospital Care and Institute for Patient- and Family-Centered Care. Patient- and family-centered care and the pediatrician's role. Pediatrics. 2012;129:394–404.
2. O'Malley P, Brown K, Krug S. Patient- and family-centered care of children in the emergency department. Pediatrics. 2008;122: e511–21.
3. Brown K, Mace SE, Dietrich AM, Knazik S, Schamban NA. Patient and family-centred care for pediatric patients in the emergency department. CJEM. 2008;10:38–43.
4. Murphy NA, Carbone PS, Council on Children with Disabilities. Parent-provider-community partnerships: optimizing outcomes for children with disabilities. Pediatrics. 2011;128:795–802.
5. Tobler K, Grant E, Marczinski C. Evaluation of the impact of a simulation-enhanced breaking bad news workshop in pediatrics. Simul Healthc. 2014;9:213–9.
6. Bultas M, Curtis M. Using simulation to teach child injury prevention to mothers recovering from substance abuse. J Community Health Nurs. 2013;30(3):155–63.
7. Sigalet E, Cheng A, Donnon T, Koot D, Chatfield J, Robinson T, Catena H, Grant V. A simulation-based intervention teaching seizure management to caregivers: a randomized controlled pilot study. Paediatr Child Health. 2014; 19(7):373–8.
8. Sodomka P. Patient- and family-centered care. In: The patient- and family-centered care: good values, good business conference. American College of Healthcare Executives Conference, May 17-1-2001; Virginia Beach, VA.
9. Sodomka P, Scott HH, Lambert AM, Meeks BD. Patient and family centered care in an academic medical center: informatics,
partnership and future vision. In: Weaver CA, Delaney CW, Weber P, Carr R, editors. Nursing and informatics for the 21st century: an international look at practice, trends and the future. Chicago: Healthcare Information and Management Systems Society; 2006: 501–6.
10. Patient and Family Centered Care Benchmarking Project. Executive Summary. University Health System Consortium, Oakbrook Terrace, IL 2007.
11. Anderson JM, Murphy AA, Boyle KB, Yaeger KA, Halamek LP. Simulating extracorporeal membrane oxygenation emergencies to improve human performance. Part II: assessment of technical and behavioral skills. Simul Healthc. 2006;1(4):228–32.
12. Mayer RE. Applying the science of learning to medical education. Med Educ. 2010;44(6):543–9.
13. Glascoe FP, Oberklaid F, Dworkin PH, Trimm F. Brief approaches to educating patients and parents in primary care. Pediatrics. 1998;101:e10.
14. Schlittenhart JM, Smart D, Miller K, Severtson B. Preparing parents for NICU discharge: an evidence based teaching tool. Nurs Womens Health. 2011;15:485–94.
15. Sullivan-Bolyai S, Bova C, Lee M, Johnson K. Development and pilot testing of a parent education intervention for type 1 diabetes: parent education through simulation-diabetes. Diabetes Educ. 2012;38:50–7.
16. Moser DK, Dracup KA, Marsden C. Needs of recovering cardiac patients and their spouses: compared views. Int J Nurs Stud. 1993;30(2):105–14.
17. Rudolph JW, Simon R, Raemer DB, Eppich W. Debriefing as formative assessment: closing performance gaps in medical education. Acad Emerg Med. 2008;15:1110–6.
18. Dieckmann P, Gaba D, Rall M. Deepening the theoretical foundations of patient as a social practice. Simul Healthc. 2007;2(3): 183–93.
19. Scholtz AK, Monachino AM, Nadkarni VM, Lengetti E. Central venous catheter dress rehearsals: translating simulation training to patient care outcomes. Simul Healthc. 2013;8(5):31–9.
20. Andreatta P, Saxton E, Thompson M, Annich G. Simulation based mock codes significantly correlate with improved pediatric patient cardiopulmonary arrest survival. Pediatr Crit Care Med. 2011;12(1):33–8.
21. Issenberg SB, McGaghie WC, Petrusa ER, Gordon DL, Scalese RJ. Features and uses of high-fidelity medical simulations that lead to effective learning: a BEME systematic review. Med Teach. 2005;27:10–28.
22. Kolb DA. Experiential learning: experience as the source of learning and development. Englewood Cliffs: Prentice-Hall; 1984.
23. Lederman LC. Debriefing: toward a systematic assessment of theory and practice. Simul Gaming. 1992;23:145–59.
24. Cheng A, Eppich W, Grant V, Sherbino J, Zendejas-Mummert B, Cook D. Debriefing for technology-enhanced simulation: a systematic review and meta-analysis. Med Educ. 2014;48:657–66.
25. Van De Ridder JM, Stokking KM, Mcgaghie WC, Ten Cate OT. What is feedback in clinical education? Med Educ. 2008;42: 189–97.
26. Motola I, Devine LA, Chung HS, Sullivan JE, Issenberg SB. Med Teach. 2013;1–20.
27. Hewson MG, Little ML. Giving feedback in medical education: verification of recommended techniques. J Gen Intern Med. 1998;13:111–6.
28. Fanning RM, Gaba DM. The role of debriefing in simulation-based learning. Simul Healthc. 2007;2(2):115–25.
29. Dracup K, Moser DK, Doering, LV, Guzy PM, Juarbe T. A controlled trial of cardiopulmonary resuscitation training for ethnically diverse parents of infants at high risk for cardiopulmonary arrest. Crit Care Med. 2000;28:3289–95.

Part V

Pediatric Simulation Program Development

Simulation Operations and Administration

Michael Moyer, Joseph O. Lopreiato and Nicola Peiris

Simulation Pearls

1. Pediatric simulation programs have become an accepted and necessary part of pediatric health-provider education.
2. Advisory boards are often established to form a bond between the simulation program stakeholders, community partners, and the simulation program.
3. Program administrators must be flexible and adapt to the changing priorities of a simulation program and its stakeholders.
4. A balance between costs and revenue must be clearly established in order to sustain and successfully build a simulation program.

Introduction

A formal administrative and operations model can take on many different forms within a pediatric simulation program. Some programs are linked to existing educational or clinical institutions, while others are freestanding, remaining responsible for their own activities. This decision is often based on funding models, faculty affiliation, or space considerations [1]. In making any of these choices, it becomes critical to organize operations based on on long-range plans that include

M. Moyer (✉)
Center for Simulation & Education, TriHealth, Cincinnati, OH, USA
e-mail: Michael_moyer@trihealth.com

J. O. Lopreiato
Val G. Hemming Simulation Center, Department of Pediatrics, Uniformed Services University of the Health Sciences, Bethesda, USA MD,
e-mail: joe.lopreiato@simcen.usuhs.edu

N. Peiris
KidSIM Simulation Program, University of Calgary, Alberta Children's Hospital, Calgary, AB, Canada
e-mail: nicola.peiris@ahs.ca

potential strategies for future growth. This can be difficult to forecast but helpful when considering the mission, vision, and goals of the program. This chapter will review the necessary components to address when building a pediatric simulation program, from choosing faculty, advisory board members and staff, to information technology strategies, equipment types, loan agreements, and business models. It is important to note that in this chapter, we refer to simulation organizations as *programs,* meaning that while some institutions may in fact have simulation *centers,* others may rely on in situ simulations as their training model and not have a specific site or property for training.

Organization and Resources

Vision and Mission Statements

Established vision and mission statements supportive of long-term goals are critical to successfully focus on program-related decision-making, planning, and growth. Vision and mission statements need to be crafted early in a program's development in order to steer the direction of its goals and to measure its progress, which in turn pays dividends on subsequent planning for its future. Many community organizations not only look at financial progress over a period of time but also look at successes and failures relative to the established vision and mission statements, specifically as they relate to milestones of evaluation, growth, community presence, benefits, and impact. It is important not to make mission or vision statements too lengthy; rather, they should be realistic and achievable based on a program's size and resources. As such, the vision and missions statements should also parallel a simulation center's business model.

Mission statements, in general, contain information relating to a program's reason for existence and its abilities to advocate simulation. It is a way for programs to invest in

Table 27.1 Example of mission, vision, and values statement for a simulation program. (Courtesy: Uniformed Services University of the Health Sciences in Bethesda, MD)

Mission	To use simulation and technology to enhance medical education, training, and promote safe patient outcomes
Vision	Develop a center of excellence for medical modeling and simulation utilizing clinical simulation technologies to provide a safe learning environment for all members of the interdisciplinary healthcare team to train and sustain the required medical skills ensuring readiness and safe patient care in both fixed and deployed settings
Values	We consistently strive to provide the highest quality of care for our patients and are committed to providing a supportive learning environment for all staff members. Utilizing an interprofessional team training approach, we are an innovative and unique center of excellence. Our employees are critical to the success of our organization, and we value their proficiency, expertise, knowledge, and vision. Driven by the imagination and enthusiasm of our employees, our potential is unlimited

their parts of simulation within a community as well as serve as a measurable for sustainment in the future. Vision statements follow the mission statements closely; however, they describe more of what the program intends on becoming; more or less, the programs' future potentials and realizations of what is to come (Table 27.1).

Stakeholders

Simulation program structures can be very diverse: some defined by faculty members who are part- or full-time and who donate or are remunerated for their time, as compared to larger simulation programs with dedicated staff who are additionally guided by advisory boards (or committees).

Advisory boards can comprise internal stakeholders of one's institution and/or external members who serve as objective advisors and provide expert leadership for decision-making in the sustainability, leadership, and growth of the simulation program. Advisory boards are sometimes created in order to have broad representation from various clinical areas and departments that will be the primary users of the simulation program, as well as external representation from local businesses or community leaders independent of the governing body of the program itself. This forms a connection between the relevant stakeholders, community partners, and the simulation program to help critical decisions about the direction of the program. Pediatric institutions serve valuable roles within the broader community, along with champions that help create partnerships with larger entities, including schools, hospitals, and industry. A strong link in the community is seen as beneficial to both the pediatric institution (represented in this case by the simulation program) and within the surrounding community where the benefits of this training are readily identified. Both internal and external stakeholders are important in connecting the pediatric simulation program and the community, and bring a wealth of expertise to the program, thus helping to foster excellence and innovation within a simulation program.

Space

Most simulation centers are physically linked to and are part of an existing educational system, whether that is college-based, hospital-based, or one that is similar in function. It is important to define both the utility and support of the simulation program, that is, who the simulation center will support with its own resources and who in turn will support the simulation program with monetary resources. Conducting a site assessment outlines the necessity and capacity for skills space, teaching area, audiovisual (AV) implementation, administration, and storage (Table 27.2, Figs. 27.1 and 27.2).

Planning for the various rooms well ahead of time allows for the greatest flexibility going forward, meaning that planning for maximum utilization, such as running concurrent sessions, can be thought of early in the planning phase of all facets of the simulation center. Table 27.2 also gives ideas and reasoning of simulation space in the event that a program does include physical space. While each program will differ, it is important to define space approximations with types and volumes of simulations expected. Space allotment is not a well-defined process, rather it is usually an entity that increases in relation to one's program; the greater volume and variety of simulations correlating to a greater amount and diversity of space needed.

Programs that have dedicated space within a hospital or college can vary in their use and function. Many times, these factors are related directly to their accessibility. As hospital providers inherently benefit and use a dedicated site more widely, it has become common to have programs on-site within a hospital's space. On-site simulation centers allow for healthcare provider training during a regular workday, thus reduce staffing costs associated with freeing up healthcare providers for training [2]. For off-site programs, providing a means of transportation may become a consideration when planning program budgets for simulation training.

Space for storage is one of the most fundamental, yet critically underestimated, pieces of the program equation. Storage is unique in that a growing program will continue to need more space in order to sustain its increase in equipment, which is inevitable as simulations become more warranted or requested.

Table 27.2 Space considerations when planning a simulation center

Simulation labs	Labs need to be designed with the flexibility to mimic a variety of clinical areas
	Spaces may be equipped with gas, air, simulators, monitors, clinical equipment, medication, and telephones
	Designing adaptable spaces to recreate multiple environments for training (e.g., use of curtains mimicking different environments) may provide enhanced flexibility
Control rooms	Sometimes equipped with one-way mirrored glass offering an unobstructed view into the simulation lab
	Control rooms require telephones to receive calls from the simulation lab, overhead and confederate microphones, and computers with the ability to run simulators from the control room, as well as within the active simulation space
Debriefing rooms	Formal debriefing rooms offer a separate, safe environment for learners and instructors to reflect on their experiences and to revisit their learning objectives [3]
	Ideally outfitted with audiovisual recording and playback capabilities
Audiovisual	Integration of an audiovisual recording and playback system into labs and debriefing rooms offering multiple angles for video recordings which can later be used for reflection, teaching, research, and quality assurance purposes
Classrooms	Other designated learning spaces must be made available for teaching, courses, conferences, and skills training
	Flexibility in designing rooms that can be converted into smaller rooms is advantageous in order to host additional simultaneous courses and classes [4]
Administration and offices	Dedicated workspace for primary simulation personnel involved in the daily operations of the center
Reception	This area is the first impression to visitors and should be designed to reflect the vision of the center
	The reception area can be used as a waiting room and to direct learners and staff through the use of daily schedules displayed on media screens
Dropdown space	Workstations equipped with data ports and computers for simulation personnel and learners
Secure storage and utility rooms	Adequate space to store extra simulators, supply carts, clinical equipment, and technical servers
Simulation library	Physically or virtually housed library of scenarios, labs, diagnostic images, supporting documents, and other resources for running simulation scenarios
Outreach storage and parking	Parking for mobile education vehicle and storage for outreach equipment

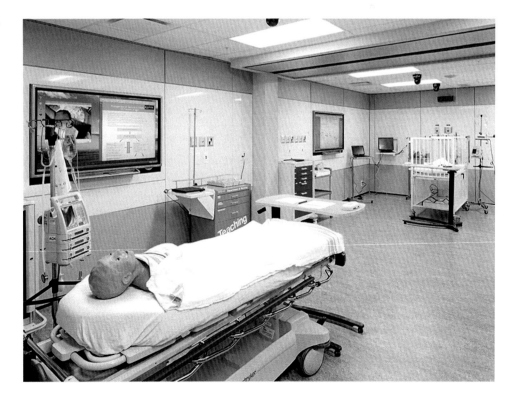

Fig. 27.1 Simulation lab set up with optional retractable wall. (Photo permission courtesy of KidSIM Pediatric Simulation Program, Alberta Children's Hospital)

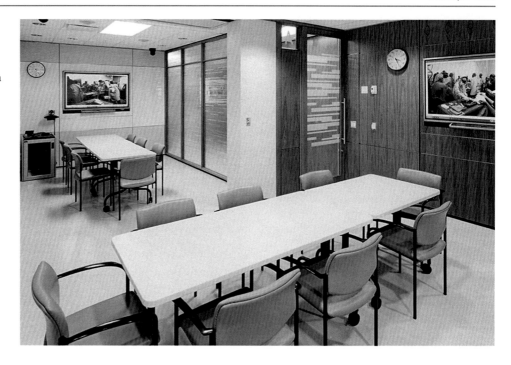

Fig. 27.2 Debriefing and classroom layout with optional retractable wall. (Photo permission courtesy of KidSIM Pediatric Simulation Program, Alberta Children's Hospital)

Programs that do not have dedicated space have unique challenges of their own. While it is certainly possible to utilize clinical spaces through in situ simulation, one must also consider equipment needs, patient safety, and confidentiality issues (see Chap. 12 for details). Other considerations for in situ simulation include the additional time required for transportation and setup of equipment and simulator(s) to the clinical space, as well as ensuring the clinical space is available for the simulation activity.

Teaching Faculty and Staff

Competent and trained faculty are necessary in order to deliver effective simulation-based education. Not only is it imperative to choose the *right* faculty but establishing clear roles for faculty is also important to meet the needs of the various curricula that are run by a simulation program. Based on these established roles, formal faculty development should be identified and provided to ensure that faculty obtain the necessary knowledge and skills to effectively perform those defined roles (see Chap. 14). Without identifying required roles carefully, it is easy to overlook several aspects of successful programs: breadth of courses offered, the target audience(s), course preparation, evaluation and research, quality improvement, growth, and faculty/staff development. Simulation center administrative leaders are encouraged to define the roles required within their program and then create an organizational chart that describes how these roles function within the program (see Table 27.3 and Fig. 27.3).

The development of an organizational chart and governance structure will define how each of the roles listed above fit within the simulation program. Ideally, the organizational chart should be accessible by all simulation program staff to ensure there is a shared and common understanding of the reporting structure and how different individuals are contributing to the overarching goals of the program.

Standard Operating Procedures and Policies

A simulation center should have standard operating procedures (SOPs) in order to clearly define roles, responsibilities, accountability, and the rules of engagement within a program. SOPs set procedure for setup, tear down, and maintenance of simulation equipment and cover a diversity of topics such as (but not limited to): administrative and regulatory procedures, training for new personnel, pay rates, quality assurance, evaluation, confidentiality statements, and orientation of learners. The Society for Simulation in Healthcare offers a Policy and Procedures manual that effectively outlines many standard program concerns, addressing issues in many areas of simulation programs [5].

One of the main responsibilities of a simulation program is to track users for educational and training purposes, as well as certification needs. Ideally, having either hard copies on file or electronic means to gather, store, or access these areas of information are necessary. Many learning management systems are available to aid in this task, as well as draw on the system data to produce statistics that can be helpful in describing the program as a whole.

Table 27.3 Roles and responsibilities within a simulation program

Title/Position	Responsibilities
Director of simulation operations	Oversees the entire program
	Aligns program goals with stakeholders, needs and responds to requests for simulations from all entities (within a center or from outside the center)
	Serves as the key contact for the program
	Determines organizational structure and delegates responsibilities to other members of the program
Program manager (or) operations manager	Responsible for day-to-day operations within the program
	Ensures that all operations within the program are functioning, such as simulators and other equipment, personnel, and scheduling
Business manager	Oversees the fiscal operations of the program
	Responsible for any and all financial obligations and requests and works with the advisory board (if present) or other governing body of the program to ensure financial stewardship
Simulation education coordinator (or) simulation educator	Responsible for the day-to-day activities of simulation with assigned groups
	Develops educational curriculum
	Serves as educator, operator of simulator(s), and/or facilitators in the simulations
Simulation operator	Responsible for operation and troubleshooting of any simulator within the program
	Day-to-day operator of simulators
Simulation technician	Responsible for setup and takedown of simulation events
	This person can also assume the role of an operator within some simulation programs
Simulation research director and/or coordinator	Oversees research activities of the simulation program
	Is also responsible for interaction with the institutional review board (IRB), developing and overseeing research protocols
Administrative assistant(s)	Assumes responsibility of pre-course planning of necessary paperwork, consents (i.e., video releases or confidentiality releases), post-course evaluations and/or summaries
	Responsible for many of the intricate parts of the simulation that deal with overseeing proper collection of documents, processing continuing education, and other critical information entered into program databases, such as learner names and demographics
Audiovisual/biomedical support	This may be two roles or a combined role based on the background of the person performing the role
	Troubleshoots and repairs any problems with the audiovisual or simulation equipment

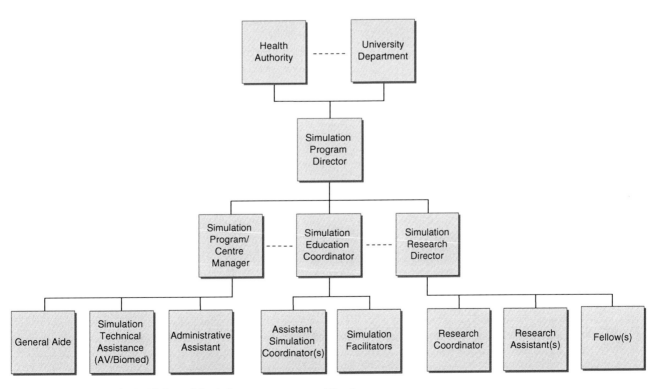

Fig. 27.3 Sample organizational chart of simulation program personnel/faculty

Information Technology

One area that cannot be overlooked in operations is privacy and accountability. As in all areas of healthcare, as well as many areas of business, protecting individual privacy has become the foundation of electronic data keeping. Pediatric simulation programs are not excluded. Early discussions with institutional information technology (IT) experts are quite beneficial in dedicating not only servers for privatizing information but also securing networks for key data transmission to and from those servers. Many simulation centers are also going to engage external vendors for AV products for research, debriefing, and data collection as well as established learning management system databases, both of which are reliant on secure and protected connections. This includes having the external vendors provide secure connections into the simulation centers' IT infrastructure for upgrades, repairs, etc. Much of this discussion needs to be done in advance of installation and should be done between the simulation program representative and IT representatives from the institution and/or vendor.

Data from learners must be secured within the servers and cannot be shared without the consent of the learners. Data should also be considered confidential without the specific consent of the simulation center director and/or the person deemed in charge of the simulation center itself. This is usually confirmed through a binding written agreement (consent) between the learner and the simulation program. Many pediatric institutions will also consider having all learners sign and consent to a confidentiality agreement, which is a soft agreement between the learner and institution that also asks the learner not to share the scenario information that they will experience during their simulation encounter with other students. This is an attempt to preserve the simulation scenarios and to allow other students the ability to be challenged by the scenario without knowing its content ahead of time. This is essential in a testing or high-stakes assessment environment. A soft agreement means that there is no consequence to the learner if this agreement is broken; however, there is an agreement between them and the institution to not discuss this outside the center. Specific written consent must also be obtained for special circumstances, such as video recording the learners, and whether these recordings can be used for education and research purposes (Fig. 27.4). Most institutions have a research ethics review body that requires individual consent forms for each individual study. These consent forms must be stored securely for a defined period of time.

Safety/Security

All SOPs must have specific written plans on safety and security within the simulation environment. The preceding section reviewed security as it pertains to IT. However, it is also critical to keep plans in place when thinking of:

a. Simulators and training mannequins—including where they are to be stored when not in use

b. Storage of other equipment—where additional equipment can be housed, not only in the present but also future considerations as groups become more involved in your program. This can be a unique problem when considering a simulation program with property allocations; however, if the program is entirely built on in situ training, there will still be necessities for storage which must be considered. Considerations must be made for using the same type and model of clinical equipment (e.g., defibrillators, intravenous pumps, etc.) used within a facility.

c. Computers and AV equipment—including security and storage when not in use. In addition, many of these need to be left on and connected to networks for institution updating and security.

d. Safety plans—including accidents or injuries related to any learners, faculty, or visitors to the lab.

e. Medications used during the simulations—whether these are actual medications or are empty vials that are now being refilled with water or saline. Some of these medications can be obtained from a hospital pharmacy where certain medications are housed when expired; or there are commercial distributors of replica medications that are nearly identical to actual medications but usually are quite substantial in cost.

f. Crash carts—whether these are replicas of actual code/crash carts within a medical facility such as a hospital. If they are available in a setting within a lab, are they easily accessible by visitors who might not know the difference in an emergency? Considerations must be made for using the same type, model, and content of true carts used within a facility.

g. After-hours access—includes access to simulators and additional equipment after normal operating hours either within a simulation center or with in situ training.

SOPs on safety and security will need to include clear and consistent labeling of products and equipment used in simulation to avoid any use on a real patient. This needs to be considered in all aspects of your program, whether with medications, defibrillators, or other equipment that should not be used on actual patients. A natural division must take place between *actual* patient equipment and non-patient medical use. This is especially important with in situ simulation.

Specific Policies and Procedures

There are numerous other policies and procedures that can be discussed at length when considering the administration

Video Record Use and Confidentiality Agreement

Our Simulation Center is committed to quality education and training. Toward this end, learners are routinely observed and evaluated directly or through video recordings. Because video recording creates a potentially enduring record of images, the following document describes the policies regarding use of such records, confidentiality, security, and record retention.

These policies must be understood and adhered to by all learners, faculty and staff.

1) All video recordings generated within the Simulation Center are maintained on a private network server within the SC server room.

2) Videoviewing is controlled on a need-to-view basis. Only those Simcenter faculty or staff, with a legitimate educational need will have access to video recordings.

3) Video recordings obtained in the course of education can be used to:

   - Provide feedback to learners to improve their performance;

   - Formally assess learnerachievement and/or competency;

   - Help evaluate and improve the curriculum;

   - Evaluate and improve our teaching and assessment processesusing human and non-human simulations;

   - Aid in the teaching of future learners;

   - Research and scholarly purposes

4) Video Recordings will be maintained in accordance with Simcenter Record Retention and Destruction Policy.

   - Video recordings will be retained until electronically destroyed, normally one year following the end of the course or event.

Fig. 27.4 Sample consent form. (Courtesy Joseph Lopreiato, Uniformed Services University of the Health Sciences)

5)   Any copying, duplication, or other form of distribution of audio or video footage released by the Simcenter

      is prohibited. Violation of this policy may result in learner dismissal or faculty/staff termination.

Consent for Video Recording (for student, faculty, SP)

I, _____ hereby authorize the Simulation Center to video record me for the purpose

of teaching, learning, review, research and evaluation. I hereby assign all rights to the release and retention of video

recordings to the Simulation Center as outlined in this agreement. I understand that video recordings will be used

for educational and research purposes only. Any other use will require specific written permission. _____ Initials

                                        Signature of User   *Date*

                                        Signature of Witness   *Date*

Courtesy: Uniformed Services University of the Health Sciences in Bethesda,MD

Fig. 27.4 (continued)

and operation of a pediatric simulation program. Table 27.4 contains a comprehensive list of various policy examples shared from existing simulation centers in order to stimulate discussion and provide direction and assistance to programs in development. These are general guidelines and are meant to be starting points and content for policy in specific areas for simulation centers only.

Finances and Revenue

Careful planning of finances and potential revenue sources helps to ensure the long-term viability of simulation programs. While specific simulation programs may have unique differences in terms of financial support, there are similarities in the potential sources of overall funding: either from internal (hospital, university) and external (user fees, re-

search funding, and philanthropy) sources. Philanthropic sources are usually good for larger, more expensive items, such as equipment (i.e., simulators and other clinical pieces of equipment) or facilities (construction of a simulation lab or center). Funding from these sources is generally not aimed at operational funding, including salaries and benefits. A long-term solution that involves a combination of internal institutional support and creative use of external support enables some simulation programs to become self-sustaining while also planning for on-going equipment needs and growth over the long term.

Successful philanthropic requests can be one-time gifts or multiyear commitments. Great care and creativity must be taken when approaching external funding sources either directly or through an established foundation. The competition for philanthropic support is significant, so creativity is necessary in making a compelling case and highlighting a clear

Table 27.4 Simulation program policy and procedure examples

Scheduling	Facility use: What can/cannot be booked in the facility
	Process: Intake and confirmation of any request for simulation space and equipment, who is responsible for this, and process, who is responsible for final approval and notification
	Fee schedule (if applicable)
	Priority: A hierarchy of which providers have preferential access to simulations should there be duplicate requests made for space, mannequins, equipment, or trainers
	Cancellation: Process of cancellation for use of space, mannequins, or equipment (user); considerations for closing a center or cancelling a session based on weather or other imminent considerations (including communications plan)
Video recording	General: policies and regulations for when and if sessions can be recorded
	Notification: Informing participants in advance of the intention to video record session, including background information for the purpose and value of video recording and consent for completion
	Distribution/storage: Specific instructions about how video recordings will be used and who will be authorized to review them, who has authority to grant such requests, other legal considerations within individual institutions
	Destruction: When and how video recordings will be destroyed
	Publication: Usually also disclosed within a written agreement; whether video of learners/facilitators will be permissible within a published format, whether as part of a quality improvement session, media (such as PowerPoint), or within a research ethics-approved publication (still photos or photos obtained from video)
Equipment/lab use (daily checklists)	Equipment: Standard equipment use and tests (e.g., gases, monitors, batteries, doors unlocked)
	Gases: May want a separate and more profiled gas checklist
	Simulators: Power on and off procedures
	Paperwork/computers: Data collection is functional and ready
	Malfunctions: Reporting procedures
	Shutdown: Procedures for cleaning up after simulation session is over
	Re-stocking: Lab and equipment
Scenarios	Template use
	Structure and mandatory minimum components
	Authorship rules
	Storage rules
	When can a scenario be used—policy on validation
	Implementation: Recommended procedure; peer review/validation process
Vendor relations	Beta testing: If a vendor expresses interest in using any program equipment or simulators for testing products; legalities of each institution as well as intellectual property considerations
	Gifts: What donations or gifts are acceptable and who must approve any form of reimbursement or services
	Events: Approval process for vendor participation within a program's operations, courses, or use of equipment
	Showcases: Process for approving any displays used within a program
	Grants: Usually a detailed process that must be acted on in an organizational manner; process in place to work towards applying for and/or receiving grants for a program
	Access to facility: Protocols for access to facility during working hours and after hours
Miscellaneous	Observation for course participants: Discussing how courses, classes, and simulations will be conducted; the dynamics of who will be allowed within a simulation session at any given time during a particular session
	Observation for nonparticipants: Will those in attendance of sessions who are not a part of a class or group/department be permitted to observe other participants; are consents needed; disclosure to participants?
	Required disclaimers and pre-event statements/consents

Table 27.5 Potential sources of funding and revenue

Institution	Funding at the organization level
	Requires engagement and buy-in from management early in the development process [6]
Department	Departments with an invested interest in simulation learning objectives pool resources to further fund training and staff
	Generate department interest by highlighting unit-specific goals and engaging content experts
Foundation	Gifts and donations managed and distributed by internal and external foundations
	Research foundation guidelines, application requirements, and deadlines early in the program development process
Grant	Grant funding is becoming increasingly competitive. Find a *niche* to submit a more competitive application [7]
Federal	Federal governments provide funding for the research and development of innovative ideas [7]
	Examples of federal granting agencies are the Canadian Institutes of Health Research (CIHR), the National Institutes of Health (NIH) Office of Extramural Research, the National Science Foundation (NSF), and the Department of Defense (DOD)
Industry	Industry leaders in the world of simulation or healthcare support programs through donation of equipment, equipment discounts, funding, scholarships, and staff training
Self-generated	Revenue generated from the implementation of an internal fee structure, such as charging for space usage, equipment rental, and hosting of paid courses and conferences
Database	Massive databases collectively house searchable research funding opportunities
	Examples include, but are not limited to; Grant.gov, the Sponsored Programs Information Network (SPIN) http://infoedglobal.com/solutions/spin-global-suite/ and pivot http://pivot.cos.com/

need, as well as sharing positive outcomes and inviting them to become active partners in the solution. Inviting members of the public to the simulation setting (and potentially watching or being involved in simulation themselves) can be very helpful in having them understand the need more clearly. A similar approach can be taken with internal funding sources, although more emphasis should be placed on outcomes and organizational benefits. Organizational support helps facilitate success by sharing the value of training initiatives and in turn contributing more simulation resources and funding [6, 7].

Independent of the funding stream being pursued, a clear understanding of the overall vision of the program and, in particular, the simulation center needs (both equipment and personnel) is extremely important early on in the planning of the simulation program/center. A list of available funding sources can be found in Table 27.5.

Facility Fees

One avenue of ongoing funding for simulation centers is charging the end users a facility fee (Table 27.6). This can be an effective way to ensure long-term sustainability of a simulation program by trying to recoup some of the costs of wear and tear on simulation equipment and the need to eventually purchase new simulators, as well as the need to replace clinical supplies and other consumables. However, it is unlikely that facility fees will allow for funding of human resources or new infrastructure. There is no standard simulation facility fee structure that will fit every program as individual costs vary among regions and is dependent on each institution's simulation needs. A fee calculation will also change depending on the amount of operational funding a program already receives from other sources. A rental policy and fee structure should be developed and reviewed with key stakeholders. The fee structure should include use

Table 27.6 Example of program fee structure

	External • Non-charitable • Organizations • Industry	External • Registered charities • Internal • Participant fee • Research	Internal • No participant fee
Simulation center Per room per hour of event time (inclusive of setup and clean-up time)	Priced per simulation room per hour[a]	Priced per simulation room per hour[a]	No fee
Simulation center Staff members	Priced per staff member per hour	Priced per staff member per hour	No fee
External use High-fidelity equipment	Priced per hour of event time	Priced per hour of event time	No fee
External use Low-fidelity equipment	Priced per hour of event time	Priced per hour of event time	No fee

[a] Multiple simultaneous room bookings may qualify for overall discount

of the simulation rooms and clinical equipment, disposable items, access to debriefing rooms, and the need for technical and educational assistance. Even catering for events and courses needs to be considered. The review with stakeholders is important as the implementation of a user fee may impact use of the center by some groups. Some programs create a differential in the fee schedule whether the user group is considered *internal* or *external* and whether the use is during normal business hours or is an after-hours request. Some user group categories to consider when incorporating facility fees into an operations model: internal faculty during business hours, internal faculty outside of business hours, external faculty on-site, external use of equipment and staff, registered charities, noncharitable organizations, industry, and research groups. Researchers should incorporate this fee structure into their grant proposals.

Revenue is crucial in generating a sustainable program, but consider the balance between charging a user fee for external use and the availability of the center to internal groups.

Simulation Program Expenditures

The other side of the equation is simulation center costs, which include mannequins and clinical equipment, disposable clinical items, and human resources. The actual cost of simulation-based training is largely dependent on the target population, purpose of the simulations, and the technology used. The business case will vary widely between regions and countries, and will have differing driving forces and economic strengths [1]. Other variables include the level of fidelity, requirements for space, and the amount of institutional support, which will be key factors in determining a site-specific budget. In addition to the significant costs of mannequins, AV equipment, space design, and large pieces of clinical equipment, it is also advisable to take into consideration additional costs accrued from maintenance, warranties, standardized patients, medical supplies, furniture, computers, and purchase of scenarios among others [8]. Creative options to minimize cost involve using medical supplies and equipment from surplus and using expired medication and other clinical supplies from clinical units [6, 8].

Competent and adequately trained personnel are the most valuable and expensive resource in an organization [6]. Adequate training can be time-consuming and costly, so minimizing staff turnover is significant. Identifying simulation champions early in the development process is essential to generate momentum and buy-in, and eventually program sustainability [6]. It is also very important to identify the program's human resource needs early on as this will affect their inclusion in operational funding. Planning for future growth is equally important, although looking ahead when trying to secure initial operational funding is sometimes difficult, especially when the simulation program use is based solely on estimates. It is also important to include all possible human resource needs: teaching faculty; simulation technicians; managers; administrative assistants; aides; AV, IT, and biomedical support; among others. While simulation and clinical equipment are essential in bringing this education modality to life, simulation center staff is crucial to keeping a program live and sustainable.

Conclusions

The operation and maintenance of a simulation program is a complex and dynamic process involving people, time, space, and money. Balancing these variables while delivering high-quality, credible, and sustainable simulation education is a challenge. With attention to stakeholders' needs, proper planning, and organization of resources, SOPs, and a strong sense of mission and purpose, these challenges can be overcome in order to allow a simulation program to serve the communities' needs. This chapter has provided a foundation for new and existing simulation programs aimed at capitalizing on educational needs within their own institutions and communities.

References

1. Gaba DM. The future vision of simulation in healthcare. Qual Saf Health Care. 2004;13(Suppl 1):i2–10.
2. Brindley PG, Arabi YM. An introduction to medical simulation. Saudi Med J. 2009;30(8):991–4.
3. Fanning RM, Gaba DM. The role of debriefing in simulation-based learning. Simul Healthc. 2007;2(2):115–25.
4. Ross K. Practice makes perfect. Planning considerations for medical simulation centers. Health Facil Manage. 2012;25(11):23–8.
5. Dongilli T, Gavilanes J, Battista D, Shekhter I, Halasz J, Fraga-Sastrias JM, et al. Simulation center policy and procedure manual; 2012. https://ssih.org/resources.
6. Lazzara EH, Benishek LE, Dietz AS, Salas E, Adriansen DJ. Eight critical factors in creating and implementing a successful simulation program. Jt Comm J Qual Patient Saf. 2014;40:21–9.
7. Hanberg A, Brown S, Hoadley T, Smith S, Courtney B. Finding funding: the nurses' guide to simulation success. Clin Simul Nurs Educ. 2007; 3:e5–9.
8. Rothgeb MK. Creating a nursing simulation laboratory: a literature review. J Nurs Educ. 2008;47(11):489–94.

Simulation Education Program Development

28

Marino Festa, Elaine Sigalet, Walter J. Eppich, Adam Cheng and Vincent J. Grant

Simulation Pearls

1. At the outset, the desire to positively impact real patient outcomes and experiences may seem overambitious. Without it the necessary program planning, data collection, and analysis of simulation-based outcomes, such as observations of changed practice in the simulated learning environment may not translate to the real-world setting.

2. It is important to appreciate the interaction between the learner during SBE and the actual process of care experienced by the patient; rather than acting simply as a mode of instruction, the input of the learner in performing and analyzing the task during SBE may be utilized to constantly amend and improve existing care processes to achieve more efficient and safer work practices for the real-world setting.

3. Curricular design is used to plan experiences to impart, improve, or sustain knowledge, skills, and/or behaviors to address an identified problem and/or health need. These may be related to a single or a multitude of internal and external forces affecting the process of care: patient presentations and outcomes, healthcare provider (HCP) competence, population needs, institution needs, systems and processes, or educational curricula and programs.

4. The most significant barrier to sustainability for most simulation programs is the ongoing buy-in and support from the administration of the institution responsible for the simulation program. This buy-in has many forms, from simply allowing SBE to occur on the premises and advocating for staff and physicians to attend to establishing a formal budget for the simulation program and staff, and everything in between.

5. Formal faculty development events within a local program can promote a sense of community and a shared understanding.

6. Beyond the design and implementation of simulation scenarios, a great need exists in simulation programs for educators who are versed in debriefing methodologies appropriate for learning objectives (i.e., clinical decision-making, team behaviors, communication skills, and procedural skills).

M. Festa (✉)
Kids Simulation Australia & Paediatric Intensive Care, Sydney Children's Hospitals Network, Sydney, NSW, Australia
e-mail: marino.festa@health.nsw.gov.au

E. Sigalet
Department of Education, Sidra Research and Medical Center, Doha, Qatar
e-mail: esigalet@sidra.org

W. J. Eppich
Departments of Pediatrics and Medical Education, Department of Pediatric Emergency Medicine, Northwestern University Feinberg School of Medicine, Ann & Robert H. Lurie Children's Hospital of Chicago, Chicago, IL, USA
e-mail: w-eppich@northwestern.edu

A. Cheng · V. J. Grant
Department of Pediatrics, Cumming School of Medicine, University of Calgary, Calgary, AB, Canada

KidSIM Pediatric Simulation Program, Alberta Children's Hospital, Calgary, AB, Canada
e-mail: chenger@me.com

V. J. Grant
e-mail: vjgrant@ucalgary.ca; vincent.grant@ahs.ca

Introduction

This chapter describes important concepts in planning, delivery, and measurement of outcomes from a simulation-based education (SBE) program. At the very outset when planning a SBE program, careful consideration should be given to the overall aim and how the program may fit with existing curriculum and other learning opportunities. Also, from a pediatric program standpoint, the vital importance of including the perspective of the child or parent when deciding on the program's aims cannot be understated. The most successful healthcare SBE programs aim to impact a

© Springer International Publishing Switzerland 2016
V. J. Grant, A. Cheng (eds.), *Comprehensive Healthcare Simulation: Pediatrics,*
Comprehensive Healthcare Simulation, DOI 10.1007/978-3-319-24187-6_28

clear patient-based outcome that any parent would value. These may be termed T3 outcomes in translational medicine, that is, improved patient or public health outcomes directly related to the educational intervention [1]. At the outset, the desire to positively impact real patient outcomes and experiences may seem overambitious. However, without it, the necessary program planning, data collection, and analysis of earlier outcomes, such as observations of changed practice in the simulated learning environment and observations of changed healthcare practices in the real-world setting, may be omitted [2, 3]. Any SBE programs able to document outcomes that include improved patient care would be highly valued by the child or caregiver, the learner, and the organization, and would easily justify future funding.

In order to build an effective and sustainable SBE program, the role of education and training in the *effectiveness hierarchy* of interventions in the healthcare system needs to be scrutinized and well understood. Other elements must be in place and operate in concert with the training initiative for any chance of real and lasting success. These elements include forcing functions, automation and computerization, simplification and standardization, decision-support tools such as reminders and checklists, and rules and policies [4]. While arguably less effective as a stand-alone intervention, the SBE program is a critically important element. In addition to the intrinsic value of the opportunity for deliberate practice and reflection for the individual learner, the SBE program has the power to inform, shape, and bind all other elements into a cohesive, safe, and efficient system of healthcare. It is important to appreciate the interaction between the learner during SBE and the actual process of care experienced by the patient; rather than acting simply as a mode of instruction. The input of the learner in performing and analyzing the task during SBE may be utilized to constantly amend and improve existing care processes to achieve more efficient and safer work practices for the real-world setting (Fig. 28.1).

Fig. 28.1 The simulation learning cycle

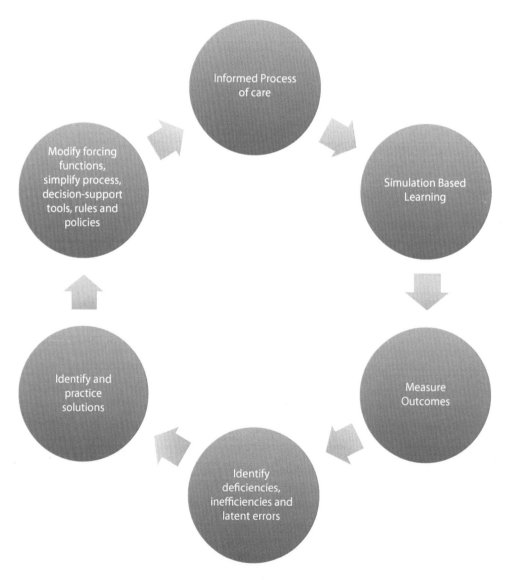

Learning Theories Supporting Simulation-Based Education

To fully appreciate the value of SBE, it is important to review the learning theories and related concepts that underscore the value of using experience to support the learning process: experiential learning theory and reflective practice, deliberate practice, mastery learning, and automaticity.

Experiential learning theory houses the concepts of reflective practice, deliberate practice, mastery learning, and automaticity. The basic premise behind experiential learning theory is that learners learn through doing, and in the process of doing, they experience certain outcomes which inform their thought processes [5, 6]. Experiential learning theory was derived from the intellectual work of John Dewey, Kurt Lewin, and Jean Piaget [5]. It consists of four phases: the *concrete experience, observations and reflection, abstract conceptualization,* and *direct experimentation* to test new concepts. Dewey, the most influential educational theorist of the twentieth century, believed experience was necessary to enhance learning *(concrete experience)*. His intellectual work focused on understanding the dialectical tension between experience, concepts, and purposeful action. Experience informs ideas which inform impulses and resultant behaviors. The experience itself is the impetus for reflection even without facilitated discussion or debriefing [6]. Lewin contributed to the theory by adding to our understanding of organizational behavior. He believed that human behavior is a function of an individual's characteristics and the immediate social situation influenced by the power of group dynamics. For him, stability and change was achieved through reflection on group processes, discussion, and feedback (reflection) to unfreeze poor assumptions or practices in order to change and refreeze new and better practices *(abstract conceptualization)*. He also believed that refreezing only occurred when learners experienced positive outcomes in response to their actions *(direct experimentation)* [7]. Lastly, Piaget defined the process of *abstract conceptualization*. Unanticipated and undesirable outcomes to actions create individual and team tension, underscoring the need to accommodate new understandings or assimilating current understandings and thought processes to achieve desired outcomes [8, 9].

All four phases in the experiential learning cycle are essential and iterative, and learners move through the cycle with all experiences in life. Simulation optimizes a process that occurs naturally with real-life experiences, while allowing some control over the experience to tailor it to meet learner needs [10]. Simulation also allows immediate replay of the experience to allow the learner the opportunity to experience a positive outcome from their behaviors and actions.

The concept of deliberate practice emphasizes attention, reflection, and repetition with feedback to increase one's level of performance. The value of deliberate practice was first espoused by Sir Francis Galton. Galton recognized the need for practice to achieve a desired level of performance even when individuals were perceived to have innate genetically inherited characteristics that predetermine them for greatness [11]. Appreciation for the concept of deliberate practice is also supported by knowledge of the learning curve and the theory of skill acquisition. Research on the learning curve makes explicit the relationship between units of practice and increasing levels of performance which will eventually slow down over time as individuals or teams become more skilled [12]. Skill acquisition theory describes the characteristics of learners as they progress through increasing levels of performance, novice to expert. According to Dreyfus, as individuals become more skilled, they become less reliant on abstract principles and more reliant on concrete experience. Additionally, the complexity of the task or behavior, and the frequency of use by a HCP or team influence the capacity for automaticity, with frequently experienced tasks and behaviors being more susceptible to becoming automated [13]. Bloom highlighted the value of learning in sequence allowing learners to master elementary levels before being tasked with more complex levels of performance [14]. Lastly, the concept of mastery learning, a term also coined by Bloom, is reliant on the learner having the prerequisite knowledge to be successful with the learning objective, learner motivation, and a well-designed rigorous curriculum allowing learners the time needed to achieve the outcome/objectives [14]. SBE curriculum is grounded by experiential learning theory, allowing learners the opportunity to engage in deliberate practice to master learning [15]. When curricula design is underpinned by principles of adult and experiential learning theory, it is more likely to result in learning that is directly transferable to the workplace.

Steps in Curriculum Design and Development

Curricula design for SBE describes the framework for selecting, structuring, sequencing, and managing selected experiences to support learning [16]. Carefully planned experiences provide an opportunity for individual or teams to engage in deliberate practice, applying their knowledge, skills, and behaviors (KSB) to manage a patient care episode to optimize outcomes. It is in this process that learning occurs; the experience in turn further informs an individual or team's KSB

Table 28.1 A modified six-step approach to curriculum design

Steps	Based on Kern et al. [18]	
Step 1	Problem identification and general needs assessment	Obtain a 360 degree view of the problem
Step 2	Targeted needs assessment	Understand the specific needs, prior experience, and learning styles of all learner groups
Step 3	Learning outcomes and learning objectives	Set explicit expectations for learners (explicit, sequential, achievable, and measurable) and develop assessment criteria and tools
Step 4	Educational strategies	Articulate the content and modality needed to deliver the curriculum: Appropriate content and adequate realism for the ability or expertise of the learners
Step 5	Implementation	Identify the required resources for curriculum delivery: profession and institution support, identified committed faculty, SBE faculty development, funding, space, equipment, time, and administrative support
Step 6	Assessment, evaluation, and feedback	Assess and evaluate the program against the desired level of performance and inform lesson and curriculum design with feedback from the SBE event

SBE simulation-based education

[6]. In Latin, the term curricula means "a running or a race course," the pathway for achieving a desired outcome [17]. In current usage, the term curriculum is used to describe the plan of (a) an educational program, (b) a course, (c) a workshop, or (d) any educational activity intended to impart KSB to support learning [18]. Effective curricula design is underscored by the following principles: (a) the experience should be underpinned by the principles of adult learning theory, (b) learning objectives should reflect learner abilities and need, (c) assessment should be based on learning objectives, and (d) evaluation is important because it provides information about the efficacy of curriculum for supporting learning, as well as an opportunity to further improve curriculum design, and ultimately to inform the real-world process of care [1, 19, 20]. In SBE programs, curricula design is used to plan experiences to impart, improve, or sustain KSB to address an identified problem and/or health need. These may be related to a single or a multitude of internal and external forces affecting the process of care: patient presentations and outcomes, HCP competence, population needs, institution needs, systems and processes, or educational curricula and programs.

For the purpose of describing curriculum design in this chapter, we will use a simplified version of Kern's six-step approach [16, 18, 21]. *Learning outcomes* is used here to replace goals in step 3, and *assessment* is added to step 6, in order to make explicit the need for both assessment and evaluation in order to understand the efficacy of the curriculum. Table 28.1 presents this modification of Kern's six-step approach.

The six-step model can be conceptualized as either a linear or circular process with movement in any direction from any step and the outcome of step 6 acting as the precursor for further curriculum. Examples and practical guidance, drawn from experience gained in developing and teaching pediatric interprofessional (IP) curriculum to undergraduate students, are provided below [22–24].

Step 1: Problem Identification and General Needs Assessment

Curricula are generally developed to address a problem or health need. To develop an effective curriculum, program developers should endeavor to obtain a 360-degree view of the problem; first, who is impacted and second, the extent of the impact on patients, the HCP and team, the institution, the system and processes, and the current educational program. This approach should expose the internal and external forces that contribute to the problem [16]. In this approach, these forces are labeled predisposing, enabling, and reinforcing factors [18]. Predisposing factors are elements such as competence levels and attitude that impact a person's desire to change. Enabling factors are forces from the system and the environment that can support or impede change. Lastly, reinforcing factors reflect perceptions of the experience after change. When the experience is valued and positive, it is more likely to be sustained in contrast to when it is not valued. Once the problem and internal and external forces are identified, program developers need to look at current efforts to address the problem from all sources of influence. A review of the current approach and practice and its degree of separation from the desired practice is important to identify existing gaps; this then forms a natural outline for the curriculum. Observations and experiences taken from real practice settings, reviews of adverse events, informal or formal discussions with the various stakeholders, competence assessments, questionnaires, and surveys are all methods that can be used to gather this information.

Example

An IP curriculum was developed in a tertiary-care children's hospital in order to teach critical assessment and treatment skills around routine pediatric emergencies [22–24].

Problem/need: Despite general endorsement of interprofessional education (IPE), very few initiatives exist in undergraduate health professional education [25]. In this children's hospital, groups of nursing, respiratory therapy, and medical students were engaging independently in weekly SBE sessions to learn how to manage common emergencies and presentations, and how to work as a team. However, the sessions were being delivered unprofessionally.

Scope of the problem and predisposing factors: Discussion with relevant leadership from each profession's training program exposed the following forces that underscored the need to engage in an IP curricula. The predisposing factors were: no other exposure to IPE and related concepts, conflicting schedules, and no allocated funding for IPE initiatives. The enabling factors were: All students were at the children's hospital every Wednesday for their clinical experience and all students were required to learn about common pediatric emergencies. Reinforcing factors: Faculty had positive personal experiences with IPE, some resources were in place (simulation program offered to sponsor the curriculum) and IP training added important realism.

Step 2: Targeted Needs Assessment

Development of effective curricula is dependent on understanding the targeted learners' previous experience, levels of competence, learning styles, program resources, and the predisposing, enabling, and reinforcing factors identified in step 1. This information underpins the learning objectives and the scenario design to create the necessary relevance and realism to provide real-world cues and engage the learner in deliberate practice. As outlined in step 1, this information can be gathered through formal or informal methods.

Example

The targeted learners were undergraduate nursing, respiratory therapy, and medical students. The nursing students, in year 3 of a 4-year program, had less experience than the medical and respiratory therapy students, who were in the final year of their respec-

tive programs and had been exposed to more KSB. In particular, the nursing students had very little experience with intravenous medications. This information was used in developing learning objectives around common emergency presentations with a focus on identification of the illness and initiation of treatment that were appropriate and relevant for all learners. It was anticipated that the learners would benefit from an opportunity to learn with students from other professions and gain insight and respect for each other's team roles with an expectation of improved team collaboration [22–24, 26–28]. Wednesday was identified as the ideal time to deliver the IP curriculum as all learners were scheduled to be present in the hospital. The assumption that there would be variation in learning styles makes SBE a suitable modality as it provides visual, auditory, and kinesthetic cues during the experiences. Two faculty leaders from each discipline committed to the IP curriculum and created a pool of instructors. Each session was led by faculty leaders from two of the three professions to provide an expert model for IPE. Competence with SBE was addressed by supporting faculty participation in local simulation faculty-development workshops.

Step 3: Outcomes and Objectives

Competency-based, learner-centered education focuses on outcomes to secure readiness for practice [29]. Learning outcomes are broad statements about learner achievement, in contrast to learning objectives which are more specific and used to delineate the path for achieving the outcome [30]. Outcomes and objectives serve many functions: set explicit expectations for learners and programs, create a template for organized thought, outline content development and resource needs, and, importantly, enable development of assessment criteria and tools [30, 31]. Objectives are drafted to identify the *conditions* under which the *performance* should occur and *the criteria* or standard required to meet the expectation or expected outcome [31]. In the six-step approach, the following five elements are used to simplify the process: who *(stakeholder/learner)* will do *(performance)* how much and how well *(criteria or expected standard)* of what *(conditions)* by when *(conditions)* [18]. The verbs used to describe the level of performance should reflect the appropriate level of complexity of KSB for the targeted learner [19]. Different taxonomies may be used to identify these levels. Bloom uses cognitive, psychomotor, and affective domains to illustrate six levels of progression in complexity of knowledge, skill/behavior, and attitudinal objectives [14]. Miller uses *knows* to *knows how* to *shows* to *does* to differentiate between recalling information, the ability to describe procedures and solve problems, and the demonstration of behaviors in a controlled setting to behaviors in a real practice setting [32, 33]. When learning objectives or outcomes are developed for an IP group of learners, faculty must consider the different elements that define competence of the different professional learners in order to secure relevance and learner engagement [34]. In all cases, the emphasis should be on writing learning objectives or outcomes that make the expectations for learners or programs explicit, sequential, achievable, and measurable.

Example

By the end of the simulation-based learning session (the condition), nursing, respiratory, and medical students will demonstrate effective team management (performance) of a child with a pediatric acute-care presentation (e.g., acute exacerbation of asthma; criteria). Of the students, 90 % will participate in one 3-h IP session during their clinical rotation at the children's hospital and will recommend the experience to their colleagues. Learners will: (a) identify (performance) the clinical signs and symptoms of an acute exacerbation of asthma (criteria), (b) administer (performance) a timely dose of bronchodilator (criteria) as per physician order to improve work of breathing and ventilation, (c) use closed-loop communication (performance) when completing task work (criteria) so that each team member is aware of completed task work, and (d) establish (performance) role clarity ensuring someone is assigned to lead the management, control the airway, document, complete procedures, and administer medications (criteria).

Step 4: Educational Strategies

Educational strategies articulate the content and modality used to deliver the curriculum. Content is developed to support each learning objective. Key instructional design features that may be utilized are discussed here. The provision of enough content detail to support achievement but not overwhelm learners is an important principle, and should be based on the ability or competence level of learners [35]. Scenarios are used to support the learning objectives for individuals and teams. By incorporating key cues characteristic of the event, they create an appropriately realistic context. In this way, scenarios provide realistic (but not real) experiences, with the aim of providing reusable cues to implement strategies, behaviors, and actions for successful outcomes in the real world. Learners of differing KSB or expertise will expect and respond to different elements of the environment

and key cues should be incorporated for all learning objectives [36].

To ensure the best chance of appropriate realism, the specifics of a scenario are often taken from real practice examples. The initial content of most clinical scenarios covers elements common to many clinical encounters, such as, establishing team introductions, roles and positions, locating and checking equipment, and correct donning of personal protective equipment. Attention and feedback on these initial elements of most scenarios has been described as *two-minute training* and has the potential for the development of automaticity for behaviors in learners with repeated exposures to SBE [37]. By detailing specifics of the patient presentation, environment, and available resources, an effective scenario orientates the learners and provides context to enable transfer of learning to the real world. In SBE, an effective scenario details suitable simulation technology to achieve the learning objectives and desired management. Many programs use a template to standardize the approach and create a shared mental model for faculty (see Chap. 2 on Scenario Building).

Final choice of instructional design is dependent on many factors including the learning objectives, participant knowledge, skills, expertise and IP diversity, time available, and program scalability. In some programs (including smaller and less resourced), this may result in greater use of role play [38, 39], whereas in well-funded and resourced education programs, faculty may have access to part task trainers, haptic trainers, low- and high-technology mannequins, and standardized patients (SPs) [40, 41]. Part task trainers and haptic trainers are predominantly used for skill training and hybrid simulations, often in combination with a SP, but require greater faculty involvement in the scenario as feedback from the models is usually limited [42]. SPs are a useful resource, although a costly one, and as such are not used as frequently as other types of simulation technology [43]. Lastly, low- and high-technology mannequins are frequently used for individual and team-focused objectives as they allow faculty to control acuity to align with the learner's level of ability and behaviors [44]. In all cases, and regardless of the level of technology, other elements of the real-world environment, including the need to ensure a family-centered approach, availability of clinical decision-making and clinical care tools, and relevant equipment always need to be incorporated and used in the SBE session to create appropriate realism and context for the learner.

One final consideration is the potential benefit of immediate repetition of the same simulated experience, as it may enable participants to realize and experience successful strategies for a positive outcome, and to rehearse and integrate new information in working memory into existing frames or schema in long-term memory [45]. An understanding of the simulation training dose required for the majority of learners to achieve the desired minimum standard is helpful but rarely known for any specific skill or learning objective and is likely to vary substantially between individuals. A study of chess players showed that some players became masters with relatively few hours of deliberate practice, while others needed up to eight times as long [46]. In SBE, it is likely that several factors will influence the training dose required, including the previous experience and prior skills of the learner, and the complexity of the task or learning objective. As an example, a study of medical students acquiring the skills required for thoracocentesis revealed that between three and four training episodes were required to achieve the mastery standard [47].

Example

A scenario template was used to script four scenarios for the undergraduate IP curriculum: asthma, bronchiolitis, seizure, and septic shock. Pediatric mannequins were used to deliver the scenarios in a simulation center. The environment was set up to reflect an acute-care facility treatment room in an urban center. Student teams were expected to assemble, communicate and assign roles, and to wear appropriate personal protective equipment. In each of the scenarios, teams were expected to complete an airway, breathing, and circulation (ABC) assessment, put the child on a cardiac monitor with measurement of noninvasive blood pressure and oxygen saturation, and perform ongoing monitoring of the child's status. They were also expected to provide hemodynamic support with intravenous access and fluids, and provide medical management with medications as required. Task requirements were congruent with each discipline's scope of practice as expected by individual educational programs. Following group debrief, the same scenario was immediately re-run to allow learners to utilize newly learnt behaviors and management strategies.

Step 5: Implementation

Implementation of a curriculum requires resources: profession and institution support, identified committed faculty, funding, space, equipment, time, and administrative support. Prior training of faculty to ensure appropriate teaching skills for SBE is important. Utilization of available learning spaces, either in a simulation center or in situ within a clinical area of a healthcare facility, will impact scheduling and complexity of coordination of the curriculum. Implementation is the ultimate validation of the feasibility of the curriculum, hence a pilot to better understand the challenges in implementation is generally recommended.

Example

In the IP undergraduate curriculum, piloting provided important information about the amount of operational support needed to effectively implement the curriculum. The pilot exposed the need for additional faculty resources to support the operation of the mannequin, allowing for a greater focus on observation and debriefing.

Step 6: Assessment, Evaluation, and Feedback

The last phase of curricula design is assessment, evaluation, and feedback. While the terms assessment and evaluation are often used interchangeably, there is an important distinction [48]. Assessment is the process of getting information about learner/program achievement, while evaluation is the judgment about the quality of achievement—did the learners/program meet the expectations or criteria articulated in the learning outcomes? The need for assessment (informal vs. formal) and evaluation is often determined by who needs the information and how the information will be used. However, the basic principle of aligning assessment questions and criteria to the outcomes/objectives is essential [30]. Formal assessment of reliability and validity of nominated outcomes in any educational program requires sufficient resources, funding and knowledge of research design, methods and statistical analysis [49, 50].

Another initial challenge is to carefully establish the desired level of performance. This may require a reference group with demonstrated ability or expertise to undertake the task with objective assessment in order to define a band of acceptable performance scores. Checklists, performance scales (sometimes incorporating time taken to achieve role-specific tasks), and questionnaires are all examples of tools used to gather and examine this level of evidence [51].

Kirkpatrick's Four-Level Training Evaluation Model is acknowledged for its contribution to understanding the impact of learning on individuals, teams, and systems [52]. Level one describes how learners responded to a curriculum and is often referred to as learner satisfaction. Level two focuses on the type of learning that occurs with respect to knowledge, skills and/or attitudes. Level three evaluates individual or team behavior change and the capacity to complete task work or interact effectively to provide timely medical management. Level four evaluates cost and benefit for the system and how learning benefited the practice setting, the population, and the health service delivery system.

An alternative approach is to apply a SBE research paradigm and utilize the principles of translational science to demonstrate that results achieved in the educational laboratory (T1) transfer to improved downstream patient care practices (T2) and improved patient and public health (T3) [1] (see Chap. 30 on Research).

Lastly, feedback from the learning event is used to inform curricula design and also in some cases the actual process of care [2].

Example

In the undergraduate IP curriculum, a novel, specific, validated IP attitude questionnaire and team performance scale were used to evaluate the efficacy of the curriculum [22]. Feedback was disseminated internally to all professions and stakeholders and externally through peer-reviewed publications. The results support a relationship between IP SBE and learner behaviors and attitudes (level two of Kirkpatrick's evaluation model). The ultimate goal will be to show a difference in patient outcomes (Kirkpatrick's level four, or alternatively, T3 outcome). The benefits in terms of learner and patient must be weighed against the cost of delivering SBE. As a result, the IP curriculum was found to be efficacious and feasible and has therefore been sustainable.

Curricula design for SBE creates a venue for guiding the educational experience to enhance stakeholder learning. Regardless of which curricula model is used, stakeholders should maintain the basic principles of curricula design presented in the six steps. In all cases, the following factors should be taken into account to ensure the most appropriate instructional design for a successful program:

a. Prior identification of an essential knowledge base for participants to acquire beforehand then refer back to and reflect on during the simulated learning event.

b. Appropriate realism with utilization of tools, communication pathways, and strategies found in the real-world setting, in order to provide reusable cues for required behaviors and actions.

c. Adequate time for feedback and reflection of behaviors and actions; as a rule of thumb, at least 50% of the time available should be allocated to this activity.

d. Opportunity for repetition of the same simulated experience in order to enable participants to realize successful strategies for a positive outcome.

e. Data collection and analysis to capture participant knowledge skills and behaviors integral to successful attainment of learning objectives to be used to inform future curriculum and actual care processes. Careful assessment against predefined outcomes will inform program development and patient care and should strive towards providing evidence in a translational science framework.

Building a Simulation Education Culture

The integration of a new teaching methodology like SBE into established healthcare education culture may be very difficult. Other important educational revolutions like the focus on patient safety and the emergence of IP education, both heavily tied to SBE, share a similar need to invade and influence a pre-established culture. The development and growth of simulation programs can face many challenges in this regard. This section will highlight specific practical ideas on how this invasion, integration, and change can be promoted through specific influences on learners, faculty, administrators, and potential philanthropic funding sources. All of these strategies are means of establishing and growing effective SBE programs.

Culture change in any organization, including healthcare and healthcare education, is difficult. It is well established that it takes time to alter the way people think and behave, and even after sufficient time, the changes seen may be small. It is important that those driving the change recognize the barriers to change and use established strategies to move things forward.

> In building greatness, there is no single defining action, no grand program, no one killer innovation, no solitary lucky break, no miracle moment. Rather the process resembles relentlessly pushing a giant, heavy flywheel in one direction, turn upon turn, building momentum until a point of breakthrough and beyond [53].

Barriers to Change

There are four main common barriers to change in organizations, most of which are applicable to healthcare education and SBE. The first barrier is cognitive, in that *people must understand clearly the reason for change*. The second barrier is the *motivation of all of the stakeholders to change*. Change may be viewed as difficult and/or feared within established organizations. In such cases, behavior is sometimes not affected significantly, even in the face of overwhelming evidence that it should. The third barrier is resources, in that *change will require an inevitable shift of resources from some areas to others*. These resources could be material or human, but will likely have a profound impact on the program(s) affected. The fourth barrier is the *institutional politics,* representing the history of the organization, which can be the most difficult to affect. In particular, strategies that are at odds with the existing culture/history are most likely to fail as culture will likely trump any innovation given the opportunity [54, 55].

Strategies to overcome these barriers include: recognizing that not everyone will be converted immediately; searching for champions who are early adopters or who have a disproportionate amount of influence on their peers and coworkers; celebrating the accomplishments of these champions within a program; redistributing resources to make these areas succeed, especially those requiring few resources but will result in significant change; ensuring that strategies try to honor the strengths of the existing culture; and measuring and monitoring the evolution of the cultural change. Measuring and monitoring any change is particularly important as most people will only shift their beliefs and attitude (i.e., change culture) after that change has led to results that matter. These individual (and organizational) shifts in beliefs and attitudes often take the longest to occur [54, 55]

Engaging Learners from Different Groups

Of all the learning groups participating in SBE, the earliest adopters (i.e., acceptors) of this teaching modality are learners in the formative part of their training: undergraduate students from the various health professions and postgraduate residents and fellows from the medical disciplines. Although these learners may in fact have little choice in terms of their participation, as it is typically part of the formal curricula for their various training programs, they are also a generation of learners who are accustomed to learning in new and novel ways. There is an inherent understanding of the need to practice and rehearse before applying their craft on real patients. They have also been more exposed to the nonclinical expert roles of communication and IP collaboration than previous generations of health profession learners. With the growth of some level of SBE in most undergraduate institutions, the current generation of health professionals have already had some exposure to SBE in their formative training [56]. Based on their acceptance of this methodology, it is most likely they will seek out programs and institutions that have ongoing professional development using SBE. You might say we are currently in an intergenerational shift where the next generation of health professionals will be well versed and trained in, and accepting of, SBE, patient safety, and IP team training. Most simulation programs have had their most substantial growth through the development of learners in the formative part of their training. In order to meet the ongoing needs of these learners, there are several very important areas that must be adequately addressed to ensure that their acceptance of this teaching methodology remains strong and unwavering (Table 28.2).

One group of learners that have been more difficult to engage are those who are already practicing their profession in terms of continuing professional development, especially those considered to be in the senior years of their clinical practice. Combinations of factors are likely to be important barriers to participation in this group. These include the significant difference in how this cohort was trained, the diffi-

Table 28.2 Tools for achieving the buy-in of learners

Objectives	Actions
Start small and grow smartly	Incorporate SBE into scheduled teaching Appropriate areas of established curricula Orientation Morning rounds/report Academic half days Slow clinical days Involve other professionals
Be educationally sound	Curriculum planning Needs assessment Clear objectives Match reasonable expectations to level of learners Evaluations
Build reasonable scenarios	Keep learning as real as possible Do not overlook common presentations and building/gauging fundamentals Use reasonable atypical presentations of common scenarios Use level-appropriate uncommon presentations Include realistic multimedia (pictures, videos, labs, X-rays, ECGs, etc.) Include appropriate and realistic confederates

SBE simulation-based education, *ECGs* electrocardiograms

culty in creating all the necessary cues for adequate realism for expert performers in the simulated learning environment, and their performance anxiety in front of a team of peers or junior colleagues [57]. Some of these barriers to participation are slowly eroding, thanks in large part to the integration of SBE into established courses, such as Pediatric Advanced Life Support, Neonatal Resuscitation Program, and Advanced Trauma Life Support, among others, and to improving SBE design and implementation. Useful strategies to minimize participation anxiety include careful orientation of learners to the simulation environment, allowing the learner group to know the scenario or topic area in advance of the simulation and allowing more senior clinicians to observe a scenario prior to their participation. Reluctance to participate is becoming less and less of an issue as SBE technology and techniques improve and this form of education is utilized in more areas of continuing medical education and continuous professional development. In this way, the complete intergenerational acceptance of SBE as an accepted, appreciated, and desired educational modality is likely to be further buoyed.

Building Capacity Through Faculty Engagement

As programs grow in terms of the various learning groups where SBE is being delivered, there is also the need for growth in the simulation preceptors and facilitators (the faculty) that will help deliver and debrief these education sessions. Although formal faculty development will be addressed later in the chapter, there are some important considerations to consider when planning the establishment or expansion of a program. First, many teachers that come forward to become involved in SBE training are relatively junior in their career and have themselves been taught using SBE. The advantage of this group is that they are young, enthusiastic, and believe in SBE. The main disadvantage is their clinical inexperience and their ability to appropriately debrief and give feedback to more senior learners. It is particularly important that these facilitators receive formal debriefing training and are mentored by more established and experienced simulation educators or partnered with clinically experienced staff to ensure a high level of content expertise. Second, an important barrier to faculty involvement is their availability and the potential for direct remuneration of teachers by the simulation program. Some programs are able to pay their faculty directly through either an operations budget or through money derived from philanthropy or other cost recovery methods. If financial remuneration is a barrier, consider finding champions in clinical areas who already hold a remunerated position within an organization, or at least make their involvement count towards some kind of currency (e.g., annual performance review, certificates of involvement, ongoing faculty development, etc.), including developing *quid pro quo* arrangements such as improved or free access to associated participants based on attendance of the faculty educator.

Finally, there are several logistical issues that act as barriers to faculty participation. These can be addressed by the development of organized guides to demystify the simulation equipment, opening access to existing faculty expertise and know-how by establishing "simulation solutions" drop-in sessions, establishing program guidelines for the involvement of at least two faculty members in each scenario and debriefing, and by incorporating an active mentorship and feedback program.

Getting Buy-in from Hospital Leadership

The final barrier to longevity and sustainability for most simulation programs is the ongoing buy-in and support from the administration of the institution responsible for the simulation program. This buy-in has many forms, from simply allowing SBE to occur on the premises and advocating for staff and physicians to attend to establishing a formal budget for the simulation program and staff, and everything in between. For those struggling to get administration buy-in for their SBE programs, there are several strategies that can be helpful. The first is that SBE is likely to be a significant recruitment and retention tool for staff, especially with the intergenerational shift in acceptance of SBE and its associated elements, including patient safety and IP collaboration. The second is to highlight the obvious advantages in terms

of patient safety, provider confidence, increased efficiency, systems improvement, better team skills, and improved morale. The third, especially for those who do not have an appreciation for what SBE really is, is to showcase the breadth and possibilities of SBE either through observing live simulation in action or through planned demonstrations. These may include the invitation of a known simulation expert to provide objective expertise to leaders of the organization and highlight the merits of SBE over traditional forms of education. This is especially helpful when linking SBE to improved patient outcomes, increased system efficiencies, and improved IP morale. Finally, the last and most important tool to influence administrators is to show research and evaluation of the aforementioned areas. This may include evaluation of patient-based or T3 outcomes that show a difference on a local scale (e.g., repeated medication errors, times to intervention, adequacy and outfitting of clinical spaces, handover/communication problems, intravenous line confusion, etc.) or involvement in larger collaborative research initiatives including multicenter studies, which will provide evidence for the efficiency, effectiveness, and integration of SBE on a more global scale.

Program Funding

Without an identified source of ongoing and sustainable funding, the development of some simulation programs is dependent on their ability to solicit funds via philanthropy. The ability to raise funds for the development of space, the purchase of equipment and even the funding of some elements of the program can be very effective in the area of SBE. Examples of philanthropic targets include hospital charities, companies or corporations with a local connection, and local community charities. Many of these organizations will place immediate value on the appeal of SBE and its effect on the health and welfare of the communities they are involved in. Some may already incorporate simulation-based training or experiential learning practice in their own day-to-day activities. Keys to engaging philanthropic donors are to: (1) give frequent demonstrations using real providers that can speak to the advantages of simulation in their own clinical practice, (2) accumulate evidence of improved patient outcomes, testimonies, and success stories where simulation has made a tangible difference in the community, (3) describe the obvious advantages of simulation on provider confidence, better teamwork and communication, and more efficient and ultimately safer care, (4) demonstrate the effect of the program on recruitment and retention, and (5) highlight simulation as one of the potential solutions to the current crisis in health professional education, namely where all of our formative trainees are going to get adequate and reproducible clinical experience.

Simulation Faculty Development

Faculty development refers to "all activities health professionals pursue to improve their knowledge, skills, and behaviors as teacher and educators, leaders and managers, and researchers and scholars, in both individual and group settings" [58]. Faculty development programs improve educational practice, augment individual strengths, and facilitate positive cultural change within organizations [59–62]. Systematic reviews about faculty development in medical education outline a spectrum of activities, including event-based sessions such as workshops, seminar series, courses or longitudinal programs such as fellowships as well as individualized peer feedback in the context of work-based faculty mentorship [60, 61]. Key features of faculty development activities include effective relationships that promote provision of peer feedback, diverse educational methods, and increasing participation in authentic teaching experiences with support of more expert colleagues [63]. These features are readily applicable to faculty development for SBE.

Defining Competencies for Simulation Educators

Recent trends have highlighted the professionalization of healthcare educators, with simulation being no exception. A useful set of professional standards for medical educators including core values and key general competency domains has been articulated by the Academy of Medical Educators in the UK, which is immediately applicable to simulation faculty development [64]. The competency framework includes: (a) designing and planning learning, (b) teaching and facilitating learning, (c) assessment of learning, (d) educational research and scholarship, and (e) educational management and leadership. The US-based Society for Simulation in Healthcare (SSH) has formulated certification standards for simulation educators [65] that have some overlap with the UK Academy of Medical Educators, including key elements related to:

- Professional values and capabilities (e.g., integrity, motivation, and leadership)
- Knowledge of educational principles, practice, and methodology in simulation (e.g., designing simulation education interventions, realism, simulation modalities, and feedback)
- Implementing, assessing, and managing simulation-based educational interventions, including feedback and debriefing practices.

To become a certified healthcare simulation educator (CHSE), applicants in the USA must complete a knowledge-based exam with over 80% of items related to either (a) educating and assessing learners using simulation (52%) or

(b) demonstrating knowledge of simulation principles, practice, and methodology (34%) [66]. In addition to the written exam, educators validate their proficiency in key domains through reference letters, a personal statement, and submission of their curriculum vitae. Through an additional portfolio-based process, qualified CHSE may apply for advanced status as a sign of their ability to serve as mentors to others in the healthcare simulation field.

Creating Safe Learning Environments for Faculty Development

Formal faculty development events within a local program can promote a sense of community and a shared understanding. A particularly important domain for simulation educators is how to establish a supportive yet challenging learning environment, which is essential to promote psychological safety to enable interpersonal risk taking [67, 68]. Threats to psychological safety can undermine the learning process, which makes the ability to set the scene for the simulation learning activity and to facilitate a pre-briefing before the scenario foundational skills for all simulation educators [68]. A related core principle surrounds issues dealing with realism; how simulation educators anticipate and deal with these issues is essential [69, 70]. See Table 28.3 for specific faculty development strategies for helping educators create safe learning environments. Suggestions for how simulation programs can implement structured local faculty development activities to augment debriefing skills are outlined in Table 28.4 (general debriefing approaches and structure), Table 28.5 (promoting discussion), and Table 28.6 (identifying and exploring performance gaps, preparing debriefing points).

Courses for Training Simulation Educators

While a full discussion of developing educational researchers and leaders is beyond the scope of this chapter, various courses designed by leading simulation programs around the world provide faculty development opportunities for simulation educators in the form of 1–5-day course offerings. A common feature of these courses is that they cover many of the core concepts required to be an effective simulation educator, namely: (a) adult learning theory, (b) curriculum design and development, (c) instructional design for simulation activities, (d) scenario design and development, (e) teamwork and leadership principles, (f) evaluation and assessment, and (g) debriefing. While many of these courses are offered by simulation programs geared at care of the adult patient, several highly regarded courses are also offered by pediatric simulation programs that offer a pediatric focus to

Table 28.3 High yield targets for faculty development in debriefing: pre-briefing and establishing a safe learning environment

Solicit feedback from learners via session evaluation forms
Include items about perceived psychological safety, that is, "I felt comfortable making mistakes and discussing them"—provides valuable programmatic feedback
Standardize the orientation process
Handout/orientation video for participants
Orientation checklist for educators
Checklist before the scenario starts (for educator team)
Participant and faculty introductions
Educator oriented to learning objectives and scenario
Equipment functioning and ready, including video recording as needed
Faculty development sessions
Journal club—read article and discuss
Establishing supportive yet challenging learning environments: read and discuss article
Rudolph, J. W., Raemer, D. B., & Simon, R. Establishing a Safe Container for Learning in Simulation: The Role of the Presimulation Briefing. *Simul Healthc.* 2014;9:339–49
Use of simulated participants—get everyone one on the same page and using the same terminology
Pascucci, R. C., Weinstock, P. H., O'Connor, B. E., Fancy, K. M., & Meyer, E. C. (2014). Integrating actors into a simulation program: a primer. *Simul Healthc, 9*(2), 120–126.
The role of realism
Rudolph, J, Simon R, Raemer D. Which reality matters? Questions on the path to high engagement in healthcare simulation. Simul Healthcare. Fall 2007

Table 28.4 High yield targets for faculty development in debriefing: general debriefing approach

Debriefing
General approach to debriefing
Make this a priority, especially for novice debriefers—give your faculty feedback on structure
Ensure that faculty are doing a reactions phase and giving trainees a chance to speak
Ensure that faculty are giving trainees a chance to state take home messages
Develop/modify a cognitive aid or debriefing script
As a guide for developing a debriefing script, see Eppich WJ, Cheng A. Promoting Excellence And Reflective Learning in Simulation (PEARLS): Development and Rationale for a Blended Approach to Debriefing. *Simul Healthcar.* 2015 (in press)
Faculty development session
Journal club—read article and discuss
DASH
Simon, R., Raemer, D. B, & Rudolph, J. W. (2009). Debriefing assessment for simulation in healthcare: Rater Version. Available at: https://harvardmedsim.org/debriefing-assesment-simulation-healthcare.php
OSAD
Arora, S., Ahmed, M., Paige, J., Nestel, D., Runnacles, J., Hull, L.,… Sevdalis, N. Objective structured assessment of debriefing: bringing science to the art of debriefing in surgery. *Ann Surg,* 2012;256:982–988
3D model of debriefing
Zigmont, JJ, Kappus, LJ, Sudikoff, SN. The 3D model of debriefing: defusing, discovering, deepening. Semin Perinatol, 2011; 35:52–58
PEARLS
Eppich, WJ, Cheng A. Promoting Excellence And Reflective Learning in Simulation (PEARLS): Development and Rational for a Blended Approach to Debriefing. *Simul Healthc.* 2015 (in press)
Mini-workshop on debriefing: simulated debriefings
Have participants view a short video of simulation scenario. Assign roles from the video for participants to play during the simulated debriefing. May debrief alone or co-debrief in pairs. Explicitly practice the debriefing structure
Observers may provide feedback to debriefers before workshop faculty

DASH debriefing assessment for simulation in healthcare, *OSAD* objective structured assessment of debriefing, *PEARLS* promoting excellence and reflective learning in simulation

Table 28.5 High yield targets for faculty development in debriefing: facilitating discussion

Promoting discussion
Promote self-awareness
Record a video of the debriefing and have educators review their own debriefing
Helps educators see the effectiveness of their approach (e.g., use of questions, use of silence, nonverbal communication
Have faculty complete the debriefing assessment tool (DASH or OSAD)
Have more experienced simulation faculty observe more junior faculty during a debriefing of a routine session; tell the faculty member in advance what you are going to give feedback on
Avoid giving too much feedback—be focused on a few key points
Focus on strategies that emphasize an honest yet nonthreatening approach to debriefing
Faculty development session
Journal club (read article and discuss)
McDonnell L, Jobe K, Dismukes R, Ames Research Center. Facilitating LOS debriefings: A training manual. 1997
Classic article on facilitation techniques tailored to levels of participant engagement
Rudolph JW, Simon R, Dufresne RL, Raemer DB. There's no such thing as "nonjudgmental" debriefing: a theory and method for debriefing with good judgment *Simul Healthc.* 2006;1:49–55
Seminal article on a debriefing approach well suited for debriefing teams
Kolbe M, Weiss M, Grote G, Knauth A, Dambach M, Spahn DR, et al. TeamGAINS: a tool for structured debriefings for simulation-based team trainings. BMJ Qual Saf. 2013;22:541–53
Overview of advanced topics related to debriefing, such as guided team self-correction, systemic constructivist methods such as the use of circular questions
Simulated debriefings (as above, focus on promoting discussion through verbal and nonverbal techniques)

DASH debriefing assessment for simulation in healthcare, *OSAD* objective structured assessment of debriefing

Table 28.6 High yield targets for faculty development in debriefing: identifying and exploring performance gaps

Identifying and exploring performance gaps; promoting good performance
Make sure that faculty review the case objectives before the simulation starts (team huddle can be helpful here)
Journal club (read article and discuss)
Rudolph JW, Simon R, Raemer DB, Eppich WJ. Debriefing as formative assessment: closing performance gaps in medical education. *Acad Emerg Med.* 2008 Nov;15(11):1010–6
Overview of debriefing as formative assessment and the concept of performance gaps to help guide the analysis phase of the debriefing
Workshop on identifying performance gaps and prepare debriefing points
Show a video of simulated performance
Facilitate a discussion about the performance gaps (may use plus/delta, important to identify positive aspects of performance as well as those aspects that are in need of improvement)
Facilitate a discussion that helps faculty group performance gaps by potential category (e.g., communication, leadership, etc.)
Generate debriefing points
Practice crafting opening questions for a particular topic
Observe a debriefing during normal teaching and tell the faculty member in advance *what you are going to give feedback on*
Avoid giving too much feedback—be focused on a few key points
Focus on strategies that emphasize addressing gaps in performance as they relate to preestablished learning objectives
Faculty development session
Simulated debriefings (see above, focus on addressing specific performance issues)

their simulation educator training. See Table 28.7 for a sampling of simulation educator training courses.

Beyond the design and implementation of simulation scenarios, a great need exists in simulation programs for educators who are versed in debriefing methodologies appropriate for learning objectives (i.e., clinical decision-making, team behaviors, communication skills, and procedural skills). Various approaches exist and the simulation community is beginning to delineate which approach works best in which context. For example, feedback and debriefing integrated into deliberate practice and mastery learning models are well suited for resuscitation skills [71] and procedural skills training such as central venous catheter insertion [72]. Alternatively, other approaches such as debriefing with good judgment seem well suited for debriefing scenarios focused on clinical decision-making and team behaviors [73]. Providing

Table 28.7 Simulation educator training courses

Name of course	Program/institution	Website
Pediatric simulation educator training courses		

ASSET course
  Foundations course
  Advanced (difficult) debriefing course
  Co-debriefing course
	KidSIM Pediatric Simulation Program, Alberta Children's Hospital	http://www.kidsim.ca

Simulation Instructor Workshop	Boston Children's Hospital Simulator Program	http://simpeds.org/course/pediatric-simula-tion-multi-day-instructor-workshop/
Pediatric SET	PAEDSIM e.V. (courses in German)	http://www.paedsim.org/
Simulation Instructor Program	CAPE, Lucile Packard Children's Hospital	http://cape.stanford.edu/programs/for-health-care-instructors.html
Nuts and Bolts Faculty Training Days	Kids Simulation Australia, Sydney Children's Hospitals Network	http://www.schn.health.nsw.gov.au/health-professionals/work-and-learn/learn-with-us/kids-simulation-australia
Other courses		
SET course (English and French)	Royal College of Physicians and Surgeons of Canada	http://www.royalcollege.ca/por-tal/page/portal/rc/resources/ppi/simulation_education_training_course
Comprehensive Instructor Workshop (English and Spanish)	Center for Medical Simulation, Boston/USA	https://harvardmedsim.org/center-for-medical-simulation-ims.php
Basic and advanced simulation educator courses (English, Dutch, French, and German)	EuSim	http://www.eusim.org/home
iSIM	Collaboration between WISER Center at the University of Pittsburgh and the University of Miami Gordon Center for Medical Education	http://www.isimcourse.com/

ASSET advanced skills for simulation educators and teachers, *SET* simulation educator training, *CAPE* Center for Advanced Pediatric and Perinatal Education, *iSIM* improving simulation instructional methods

feedback and facilitating effective debriefings are core competencies for simulation educators, discussed further in detail in Chap. 3. Developing and augmenting faculty debriefing expertise is a consistent faculty development need that can initially be met through participation in faculty development courses for simulation educators [74]. It can be particularly beneficial if multiple educators from a given program participate in such courses, as this helps educator teams develop shared expectations and common skills.

Work-Based Mentored Faculty Development and Peer Feedback

After such courses, it can be helpful for simulation programs to pair more- and less-experienced simulation educators for routine teaching that promotes work-based faculty development. In work-based mentored faculty development, less experienced educators engage in authentic teaching activities with the support and guidance of more experienced educators, who can provide scaffolding while junior educators gain experience [63]. Role modeling can also play an important role [75], especially during co-debriefing [76]. A key component of work-based faculty development is peer feedback, which can come from various sources, including peer simulation educators with demonstrated expertise [60, 77]. Peer observation of teaching with associated feed-

back in clinical settings has shown benefits [78–80]; similar strategies have the potential benefit of building a culture of feedback in simulation programs, where espoused values of giving and receiving feedback should be practiced by educators and learners alike. Of course, clear communication of expectations related to peer feedback in the context of work-based faculty development is a critical success factor [78]. Using debriefing assessment tools such as the debriefing assessment for simulation in healthcare (DASH) [81, 82] and objective structured assessment of debriefing (OSAD) [83] may provide the basis for a common language to facilitate peer feedback and coaching.

Fellowship Training in Pediatric Simulation

The incredible growth and integration of simulation into pediatric healthcare has spurred the need to train the next generation of pediatric simulation educators. To meet this growing demand, some pediatric simulation programs offer dedicated simulation fellowship training geared at providing a complete, immersive, and longitudinal training for highly motivated individuals seeking a career in pediatric SBE. These fellowship training programs typically range from 6–12 months in duration, although some may be longer and paired with advanced degrees (e.g., Masters or Ph.D.) in specific areas of interest. While some simulation programs offer dedicated fellowship training with purely simulation-based educational and research opportunities, other programs offer the simulation training in conjunction with clinical work in a related field. Table 28.3 lists core content and key activities for a fellowship training program in simulation education and research. See Chap. 29 for a list of pediatric simulation fellowship programs.

Societies, Webinars, and Online Resources

Simulation societies and associations provide another venue for faculty development, both through their annual conferences and online resources such as webinars. The International Pediatric Simulation Society offers frequent webinars featuring leading pediatric simulation educators, researchers, and innovators from around the world, while the SSH has an online learning library of webinars that can be purchased for individual or institutional use. The Royal College of Physicians and Surgeons of Canada offers a series of free podcasts that serve as a primer for seeking to understand the key principles required to become a simulation educator. See Table 28.3 for examples of simulation and healthcare professions educations organizations that support development of simulation educators.

Conclusions

Effective programs of SBE lead to learning through invaluable insights into participants' cognitive processes underpinning observed behaviors and actions in the simulated learning environment. Successful SBE programs are designed to provide opportunities for tacit learning and attainment of new strategies and solutions to inform future curriculum and real-world processes of care. The know-how and resource base required to enable effective simulation design and program delivery is fast becoming established in countries around the world, yet it may be argued that the true power of SBE to influence how we train tomorrow's HCPs to deliver the care of the future is yet to be realized. SBE programs have the potential to help grow a smarter, more cohesive generation of HCPs to provide safer healthcare. Each new technology or medical innovation offering treatments for long established or previously unknown diseases offers the potential for innovative practice to be discovered and realized through SBE. Yet the cost, time, and additional effort required to effectively plan, deliver, debrief, and reconstruct real-world care are not insubstantial and need always to be justified by systematic documentation of educational and meaningful patient-based outcomes. In the future, carefully designed SBE has the capacity to cement its place as an essential element of any safe, efficient, and responsive healthcare system.

References

1. McGaghie WC, Draycott TJ, Dunn WF, Lopez CM, Stefanidis D. Evaluating the impact of simulation on translational patient outcomes. Simul Healthc. 2011;6(Suppl):S42.
2. Draycott TJ, Crofts JF, Ash JP, Wilson LV, Yard E, Sibanda T, Whitelaw A. Improving neonatal outcome through practical shoulder dystocia training. Obstetr Gynecol 2008;112(1):14–20.
3. Barsuk JH, McGaghie WC, Cohen ER, O'Leary KJ, Wayne DB. Simulation-based mastery learning reduces complications during central venous catheter insertion in a medical intensive care unit. Crit Care Med 2009;37(10):2697–701.
4. Cafazzo JA, St-Cyr O. From discovery to design: the evolution of human factors in healthcare. Healthc Q 2012;15:24–9.
5. Kolb DA. Experiential learning: experience as the source of learning and development. Upper Saddle River: Prentice Hall; 1984.
6. Dewey J. Experience and education. Toronto: Collier-MacMillan; 1938.
7. Gold M. The complete social scientist. Washington, DC: American Psychological Association; 1999.
8. Ginsburg S, Opper S. Piaget's theory of intellectual development. California: Englewood; 1969.
9. Piaget J. La Psychologie de l'intelligence. London: Routledge & Kegan Paul; 1950.
10. McGaghie W, Issenberg B, Cohen E, Barsuk J, Wayne D. Does simulation-based medical education with deliberate practice yield better results than traditional clinical education? A meta-analytic comparative review of the evidence. Acad Med. 2011;86:706–11 (Epub).
11. Ericsson K. Deliberate practice and the acquisition and maintenance of expert performance in medicine and related domains. Acad Med. 2004;79(10):S70–81.
12. Pusic M, Kessler D, Szyld D, Kalet AL, Pecaric M, Boutis K. Experience curves as an organizing framework for deliberate practice in emergency medicine learning. Acad Emerg Med. 2012;19(12):1476–80.
13. Dreyfus S, Dreyfus R. A five stage model of the mental activities involved in directed skill acquisition. In: Center OR, editor. Berkley: University of California Berkley; 1980.
14. Bloom BS. Learning for mastery. Instruction and curriculum. Regional education laboratory for the carolinas and virginia, topical papers and reprints, Number 1. Evaluation comment, 1968;1(2), n2.
15. Howard SK, Gaba DM, Fish KJ, Yang G, Sarnquist FH. Anesthesia crisis resource management training: Teaching anesthesiologists to handle critical incidents. Aviat Sp Environ Med. 1992;63(9):763–9.
16. Taba H. Curriculum development: theory and practice. New York: Harcourt, Brace, and World; 1962.
17. Goodson I. The making of curriculum: collected essays. 2nd ed. London: Falmer Press; 1995.
18. Kern DE, Thomas PA, Howard DM, Bass EB. Curriculum development for medical education. Baltimore: John Hopkins University Press; 1998.
19. Bloom B, Englehart M, Furst E, Hill W, Krathwohl D. Taxonomy of educational objectives: handbook 1: the cognitive domain. London: Longmans, Green and Co. Ltd.; 1956.
20. Okuda Y, Bryson E, DeMaria S Jr, Jacobson L, Quinones J, Shen B, et al. The utility of simulation in medical education: what is the evidence? Mt Sinai J Med. 2009;76(4):330–43.
21. Tyler R. Basic principles of curriculum and instruction: syllabus for education. Chicago: University of Chicago Press; 1950.
22. Sigalet E, Donnon T, Cheng A, Cooke S, Robinson T, Bissett W, et al. Development of a team performance scale to assess undergraduate health professionals. Acad Med. 2013;88(7):989–96.
23. Sigalet E, Donnon T, Grant V. Undergraduate students' perceptions of and attitudes toward a simulation-based interprofessional curriculum: the KidSIM ATTITUDES questionnaire. Simul Healthc. 2012;7(6):353–8.

24. Sigalet EL, Donnon TL, Grant V. Insight into team competence in medical, nursing and respiratory therapy students. J Interprof Care. 2015;29(1):62–7.

25. Grace S. Interprofessional competencies in the curriculum: interpretations of educators from five health professions. J Interprof Care. 2014;EPUB(Dec 23 1–2).

26. Leape L. Errors in medicine. Clin Chim Acta. 2009;404(1):2–5.

27. Institute of Medicine. To err is human: building a safer health system. New Engl J Med. 1999;342:1123–5.

28. Hodges B, Albert M, Arweiler D, Akseeer S, Bandiera GW, Byrne N, et al. The future of medical education: a Canadian environmental scan. Med Educat. 2011;45(1):95–106.

29. Frank J, Snell L, ten Cate O, Holmboe C, Swing S, Harris P, et al. Competency-based medical education: theory to practice. Medical Teacher. 2010;32(8):638–45.

30. Harden RM. Learning outcomes and instructional objectives: is there a difference? Med Teach. 2002;24(2):151–5.

31. Mager R. Preparing instructional objectives. Atlanta: The Center for Effective Performance; 1962.

32. Miller G. The assessment of clinical skills/competence/performance. Acad Med. 1990;65(9):S63–7.

33. Issenberg BS, Mcgaghie WC, Petrusa ER, Lee Gordon D, Scalese RJ. Features and uses of high-fidelity medical simulations that lead to effective learning: a BEME systematic review. Med Teach. 2005;27(1):10–28.

34. Freeth D, Hammick M, Reeves S, Koppel I, Barr H. Effective interprofessional education: development, delivery & evaluation. Oxford: Blackwell; 2005.

35. Harden RM. Learning outcomes and instructional objectives: is there a difference? Med Teach. 2002;24(2):151–5.

36. McCormack C, Wiggins MW, Loveday T, Festa M. Expert and competent non-expert visual cues during simulated diagnosis in intensive care. Front Psychol.2014;5:949.

37. Festa M, Leaver J. Chapter 2: communication and teamwork. DETECT Junior manual. NSW Health, July 2011.

38. http://www.cec.health.nsw.gov.au/programs/between-the-flags/education.

39. Round J, Conradi E, Poulton T. Training staff to create simple interactive virtual patients: the impact on a medical and healthcare institution. Med Teach. 2009;31(8):764–9.

40. Barrows HS. An overview of the uses of standardized patients for teaching and evaluating clinical skills. AAMC. Acad Med. 1993;68(6):443–51.

41. Scalese RJ, Obeso VT, Issenberg SB. Simulation technology for skills training and competency assessment in medical education. J Gen Intern Med. 2008;23(1):46–9.

42. Kneebone R, Baillie S. Contextualized simulation and procedural skills: a view from medical education. J Vet Med Educ. 2003;35(4):595–8.

43. Qayumi K, Pachev G, Zheng B, Ziv A, Koval V, Badiei S, et al. Status of simulation in healthcare education: an international survey. Adv Med Educ Pract. 2014;5:457–67.

44. McGaghie W, Issenberg S, Petrusa E, Scalese RJ. A critical review of simulation-based medical education research 2003–2009. Med Educ. 2010;44(1):50–63.

45. Clark RC, Mayer RE. Does practice make perfect? In: Clark RC, Mayer RE, editors. E-Learning & the science of instruction. San Francisco: Jossey-Bass; 2002. p. 148–71.

46. Gobet F, Campitelli G. The role of domain-specific practice, handedness and starting age in chess. Dev Psychol. 2007;43:159–72.

47. Jiang G, Chen H, Wang S, Zhou Q, Li X, Chen K, Sui X. Learning curves and long-term outcome of simulation-based thoracentesis training for medical students. BMC Med Educ. 2011;11(1):39.

48. Astin A. Assessment for excellence: the philosophy and practice of assessment and evaluation in higher education. Westport: The Oryx Press, An Imprint of Greenwood Publishing Group, Inc.; 1991.

49. McGaghie W, Siddal V, Mazmanian P, Myers J. Lessons for continuing medical education from simulation research in undergraduate and graduate medical education: effectiveness of continuing medical education: American college of chest physicians evidence-based educational guidelines. Chest. 2009;135(3):62S–8S.

50. McGaghie WC, Issenberg SB, Cohen ER, Barsuk JH, Wayne DB. Translational educational research: a necessity for effective healthcare improvement. Chest. 2012;142(5):1097–103.

51. Scholtz AK, Monachino AM, Nishisaki A, Nadkarni VM, Lengetti E. Central venous catheter dress rehearsals: translating simulation training to patient care and outcomes. Simul Healthc. 2013;8(5):341–9

52. Kirkpatrick D, Kirkpatrick J. Evaluating training programs: the four levels. San Francisco: Berrett-Koehler; 2006.

53. Collins JC. Good to great: why some companies make the leap— and others don't. New York: Harper Business; 2001.

54. Kim WC, Mauborgne R. Blue ocean strategy. Boston: Harvard Business Review Press; 2005.

55. Katzenbach JR, Steffen I, Kronley C. Cultural change that sticks. Harvard Business Review 2012;90(7/8):110–17.

56. Bandali KS, Craig R, Ziv A. Innovations in applied health: evaluating a simulation-enhanced, interprofessional curriculum. Med Teach. 34(3):e176–84, 2012.

57. McCormack C, Wiggins MW, Loveday T, Festa M. Expert and competent non-expert visual cues during simulated diagnosis in intensive care. Front Psychol. 2014. doi:10.3389/fpsyg.2014.00949.

58. Steinert Y. Faculty development: core concepts and principles. In: Steinert Y, editor. Faculty development in the health professions: a focus on research and practice. Dordrecht: Springer; 2014. p. 3–27.

59. Bligh J. Faculty development. Med Educ. 2005;39(2):120–1.

60. Steinert Y, Mann K, Centeno A, Dolmans D, Spencer J, Gelula M, et al. A systematic review of faculty development initiatives designed to improve teaching effectiveness in medical education: BEME Guide No. 8. Med Teach. 2006;28(6):497–526.

61. Leslie K, Baker L, Egan-Lee E, Esdaile M, Reeves S. Advancing faculty development in medical education: a systematic review. Acad Med. 2013;88(7):1038–45.

62. Jolly B. Faculty development for organizational change. In: Steinert Y, editor. Faculty development in the health professions: a focus on research and practice. Dordrecht: Springer; 2014. p. 119–39.

63. Steinert Y. Learning from experience: from workplace learning to communities of practice. In: Steinert Y, editor. Faculty development in the health professions: a focus on research and practice. Dordrecht: Springer; 2014. p. 141–58.

64. Academy of Medical Educators. Professional standards. 3rd ed. Cardiff: Academy of Medical Educators; 2014. March 1, 2015. http://www.medicaleducators.org/aome/assets/File/AOME%20 Professional%20Standards%202014%281%29.pdf.

65. Certification Standards and Elements2012 January 4, 2015. http://www.ssih.org/Portals/48/Certification/CHSE%20Standards.pdf.

66. SSH Certified Healthcare Simulation Educator Handbook2014 January 4, 2015. http://www.ssih.org/Portals/48/Certification/CHSE_Docs/CHSE%20Handbook.pdf.

67. Edmondson AC. Psychological safety and learning behavior in work teams. Adm Sci Q. 1999;44:350–83.

68. Edmondson AC. Teaming: how organizations learn, innovate, and compete in the knowledge economy. San Francisco: Jossey-Bass; 2012.

69. Rudolph JW, Simon R, Raemer DB. Which reality matters? Questions on the path to high engagement in healthcare simulation. Simul Healthc. 2007;2(3):161–3.

70. Dieckmann P, Gaba D, Rall M. Deepening the theoretical foundations of patient simulation as social practice. Simul Healthc. 2007;2(3):183–93.

71. Wayne DB, Butter J, Siddall VJ, Fudala MJ, Wade LD, Feinglass J, et al. Mastery learning of advanced cardiac life support skills by internal medicine residents using simulation technology and deliberate practice. J Gen Intern Med. 2006;21(3):251–6.

72. Barsuk JH, McGaghie WC, Cohen ER, Balachandran JS, Wayne DB. Use of simulation-based mastery learning to improve the quality of central venous catheter placement in a medical intensive care unit. J Hosp Med. 2009;4(7):397–403.

73. Rudolph JW, Simon R, Dufresne RL, Raemer DB. There's no such thing as "nonjudgmental" debriefing: a theory and method for debriefing with good judgment. Simul Healthc. 2006;1(1):49–55.

74. Cheng A, Grant V, Dieckmann P, Arora S, Robinson T, Eppich W. Faculty development for simulation programs: five issues for the future of debriefing training. Simul Healthc. 2015;10:217–22.

75. Mann K. Faculty development to promote role-modeling and reflective practice. In: Steinert Y, editor. Faculty development in the health professions: a focus on research and practice. Dordrecht: Springer; 2014. p. 245–64.

76. Cheng A, Palaganas JC, Eppich WJ, Rudolph J, Robinson T, Grant V. Co-debriefing for simulation-based education: a primer for facilitators. Simul Healthc. 2015;10:69–75.

77. Boillat M, Elizov M. Peer coaching and mentorship. Faculty development in the health professions: a focus on research and practice. Dordrecht: Springer; 2014. p. 159–80.

78. Sullivan PB, Buckle A, Nicky G, Atkinson SH. Peer observation of teaching as a faculty development tool. BMC Med Educ. 2012;12:26.

79. Finn K, Chiappa V, Puig A, Hunt DP. How to become a better clinical teacher: a collaborative peer observation process. Med Teach. 2011;33(2):151–5.

80. Adshead L, White PT, Stephenson A. Introducing peer observation of teaching to GP teachers: a questionnaire study. Med Teach. 2006;28(2):e68–73.

81. Simon R, Raemer DB, Rudolph JW. Debriefing assessment for simulation in healthcare: rater Version2009 September 27, 2012.

82. Brett-Fleegler M, Rudolph J, Eppich W, Monuteaux M, Fleegler E, Cheng A, et al. Debriefing assessment for simulation in healthcare: development and psychometric properties. Simul Healthc. 2012;7(5):288–94.

83. Arora S, Ahmed M, Paige J, Nestel D, Runnacles J, Hull L, et al. Objective structured assessment of debriefing: bringing science to the art of debriefing in surgery. Ann Surg. 2012;256(6):982–8.

Simulation Research Program Development

29

Yuko Shiima, Jordan M. Duval-Arnould, Adam Dubrowski, Elizabeth A. Hunt and Akira Nishisaki

Simulation Pearls

1. Simulation-based research program development requires: a good understanding of research methodology and issues specific to simulation-based research; establishing mission, vision, and short- and long-term goals; specific organizational structure which enables research administration and mentorship for the next generation of researchers; and ongoing assessment of the process and outcomes of each component of the research program.

2. An individual development plan (IDP) should be established and followed regularly to ensure success for research trainees and aligns with the mission and vision of the research program.

3. An assessment of the research program should take place regularly as a meeting which includes periodic reports of ongoing research projects, ensuring alignment with the program's mission, vision, short- and long-term goals,

abstract and manuscript submission and acceptance, and internal and extramural funding proposal submission and reception of awards.

Introduction

What Is Simulation Research?

The field of pediatric simulation has grown rapidly in the past decade. In general, simulation research is categorized into two types: studies that assess the efficacy of simulation as a *training* methodology and studies where simulation is used as an *investigative* methodology [1]. Research about simulation as a training methodology examines whether the specific features of simulation experiences add to overall educational effectiveness [1], and this has made simulation-based education (SBE) standard in both healthcare provider curricula and for on-the-job training in many hospitals [2, 3]. Increasingly, decision-makers and stakeholders are requesting evidence that supports the use of simulation-based methods for improving learning and patient outcomes. Often the question is not "Does SBE improve performance?" but "Is SBE more effective and more efficient than conventional educational methods?" Simulation-based research is, no doubt, necessary to answer this and other similarly important questions. Therefore, simulation-based research is one of the key factors in advancing the field of SBE in healthcare [4]. The current best practice in educational curriculum development emphasizes six steps (Table 29.1) to identify the problem and perform a comprehensive needs assessment to ensure appropriate allocation of educational and human resources, evaluate the impact of educational intervention, and therefore maximize return on investment from an administrative perspective [5, 6]. It is important to emphasize that each step of the curriculum development process requires assessment, evaluation, and specific feedback; therefore, they are natural targets for educational and simulation research.

A. Nishisaki (✉)
Department of Anesthesiology and Critical Care Medicine, The Children's Hospital of Philadelphia, Philadelphia, PA, USA
e-mail: nishisaki@email.chop.edu

Y. Shiima
Center for Simulation, Advanced Education and Innovation, The Children's Hospital of Philadelphia, Philadelphia, PA, USA
e-mail: shiimay@email.chop.edu

J. M. Duval-Arnould
Department of Anesthesiology & Critical Care Medicine, Division of Health Sciences Informatics, Johns Hopkins University School of Medicine, Baltimore, MD, USA
e-mail: jordan@jhu.edu

E. A. Hunt
Department of Anesthesiology & Critical Care Medicine, Pediatrics & Health Informatics, Pediatric Intensive Care Unit, Johns Hopkins University School of Medicine, Johns Hopkins Hospital, Baltimore, MD, USA
e-mail: ehunt@jhmi.edu

A. Dubrowski
Emergency Medicine and Pediatrics, Memorial University, Newfoundland and Labrador, Canada
e-mail: adam.dubrowski@med.mun.ca

© Springer International Publishing Switzerland 2016
V. J. Grant, A. Cheng (eds.), *Comprehensive Healthcare Simulation: Pediatrics*,
Comprehensive Healthcare Simulation, DOI 10.1007/978-3-319-24187-6_29

Table 29.1 Six-step curriculum development model [5]

Step 1	Problem identification and general needs assessment
Step 2	Needs assessment of targeted learners
Step 3	Goals and specific measureable objectives
Step 4	Educational strategies
Step 5	Implementation
Step 6	Evaluation and feedback

Table 29.2 Sim-PICO model as applied to simulation research [10]

WHO (subjects)	WHAT (methods/ content)	WHEN (timing)	WHERE (environment)	WHY (theory)
Sim: description of simulation experiment				
P: population				
I: intervention				
C: comparator				
O: outcome				

Research using simulation as an investigative methodology leverages the standardization provided by simulation to answer diverse research questions on the performance-shaping factors that otherwise could not be answered feasibly, safely, ethically, or in a timely fashion in clinical settings [1]. Performance-shaping factors enhance or degrade performance and subsequently impact patient safety and quality of care. The standardization by simulation allows for a quantitative and qualitative measurement of those factors to improve safety and reduce errors in clinical medicine. Those performance-shaping factors include individuals, teams, work environment, technology, systems factors, and patient factors [1, 7].

The Current State of Simulation Research

A recent meta-analysis showed that the number of publications describing simulation-based interventions increased substantially after 2006 [8]. Regarding simulation research as an educational intervention, a meta-analysis for technology-enhanced simulation (TES) in 2011 demonstrated moderate to large effect size in knowledge, skills in the simulation environment, clinical behaviors, and clinical outcomes when compared to no intervention [8]. A meta-analysis for TES and pediatric education in 2014 reported that TES for pediatrics is associated with large favorable effects in comparison with no intervention [9]. However, the current literature does little to help identify the optimal method of delivering SBE for pediatrics because of a paucity of comparative studies.

SBE interventional studies should focus on the comparative effectiveness frame: when, for what type of learners, in what context is the simulation-based intervention preferable to *other methods of intervention, as opposed to no intervention* [9]. To delineate this process more clearly, the Sim-PICO model proposed for debriefing research [10] can be extrapolated and applied to simulation-based educational intervention studies in general (Table 29.2).

By contrast, simulation research as an investigative methodology assesses the impact of individual/team factors, clinical environment, and implementation of technology on clinical performance under simulated standardized conditions. Here, simulation serves as an environment for research to evaluate factors affecting human and systems performance in healthcare. Examples include a study where simulation was used to identify latent safety threats (e.g., resources, equipment) in a new pediatric emergency department [11], a study which compared a video-laryngoscope versus traditional laryngoscopy in pediatric intubation success [12], and a study assessing whether or not a use of voice-activated decision support system was associated with increased compliance with American Heart Association (AHA) guidelines [13].

Interpreting and conducting simulation research is an acquired skill. From an organizational perspective, a well-established simulation research program plays a critical role to provide a research-focused environment and to support appropriate activities and training necessary to develop simulation researchers, staff, and trainees. In this chapter, we describe essential components and organizational structure to develop a sound simulation research program and discuss the importance of continuous assessment for maintaining a high-quality simulation research program.

Essential Components of a Simulation Research Program

A simulation research program is an essential component for simulation centers in academic institutions. In this section, we describe several of the essential components that are required to ensure success of a simulation research program.

Mission, Vision, and Goals

Each simulation center should have mission and vision statements. The mission statement is the purpose of the existence of a simulation center. It serves as a guide for all of the center's decision-making. It should help staff and stakeholders within the organization know what decisions and tasks best align with the mission of the simulation center. A vision statement might provide a direction for a simulation center while also noting a commitment to quality of care and training for excellence, for example. In the context of the institution within which a simulation center exists, a simulation research program should be aligned to the institution's overarching mission, vision, and goals. Mission and vision statements specifically address the intent and functions of the simulation program including (1) impacting integrated system improvement, (2) enhancement of the performance of individual teams and organizations, and (3) creating a safer patient environment and improving outcome [14]. A simulation research program can be a vital component of a simulation center, helping to achieve its mission and specific goals based on the mission. Here are examples from two institutions.

The simulation center at The Children's Hospital of Philadelphia developed their mission and vision statements as follows (from their intranet web site; personal communication with hospital administration, June 2015):

Mission Statement

"Advance the quality and safety of healthcare processes and systems for children through discovery, translation and implementation of innovative high quality professional education and pioneering research impacting individual, team and organizational outcomes."

Vision Statement

"We will be the premier pediatric simulation training, education and research center, influencing and promoting simulation to improve healthcare quality and safety locally, nationally and internationally."

Johns Hopkins Medicine Simulation Center tied their mission and vision statement to the entire organizational mission statement (http://www.hopkinsmedicine.org/about/mission.html).

Johns Hopkins Medicine's mission statement (from their website) is: "To improve the health of the community and the world by setting the standard of excellence in medical education, research and clinical care. Diverse and inclusive, Johns Hopkins Medicine educates medical students, scientists, healthcare professionals and the public; conducts biomedical research; and provides patient-centered medicine to prevent, diagnose and treat human illness."

The Johns Hopkins Medicine Simulation Center has a vision statement for the broader program that aligns with that of the entire healthcare system and another that is specific to the Johns Hopkins Simulation Research Program, which again, flows directly from the larger organization's mission (personal communication with Elizabeth A. Hunt, M.D., Ph.D., Director of Johns Hopkins Medicine Simulation Center on June 19, 2015):

"To integrate individuals, environments, technology, experience, and expertise, using simulation theory and applica-

tion, in order to effectively support Johns Hopkins Medicine in achieving a tripartite mission of patient care, education, and research."

The Johns Hopkins Medicine Simulation Center's vision is:

"To be the leading-edge of interdisciplinary healthcare simulation research, while translating novel training methods and new scientific knowledge to the bedside, and sharing our discoveries to advance healthcare education and patient safety around the world."

Focused Areas and Setting Objectives

Mission and vision statements provide overall direction and guidance for a simulation program or center as well as departments/programs housed within it (e.g., a research program). Regardless of the degree to which mission and vision statements exist, research programs should strive to establish focused areas of research, for example, resuscitation, team training, technical skills in acute care, nontechnical skills. As these focused areas are formalized, development of short- and long-term objectives for each will help to guide progress more specifically (and purposefully) than at the mission/vision level of organizational goal setting.

Example: Johns Hopkins Medicine Simulation Center: Resuscitation

The Johns Hopkins community is proud to be the birthplace of cardiopulmonary resuscitation (CPR). Kouwenhoven, Knickerbocker, and Jude published their first paper in the *Journal of the American Medical Association* (JAMA) on July 9, 1960 introducing chest compressions as a method to rescue victims of cardiac arrest [15]. They partnered with Peter Safar who was conducting research resulting in rescue breathing at Baltimore City Hospital, now known as Johns Hopkins Bayview Hospital, to synthesize rescue breathing and chest compressions into modern CPR. Safar then partnered with Asmund Laerdal to develop the first simulator to teach CPR, that is, Resusci-Anne. They were honored to have Drs. Knickerbocker and Jude attend the official opening of the Johns Hopkins Simulation Center and have defined the Simulation Center as a Center for Excellence in Resuscitation Education and Research. They have utilized a variety of simulation-based strategies to better understand the teamwork choreography associated with exquisite in-hospital CPR and ideal training intervals [16], to identify design flaws in current defibrillators [17], to study the impact of cognitive aids on team performance [18], and to develop novel training methods associated with improving resuscitation performance [19, 20]. They have also partnered with other pediatric simulation research programs to contribute to multicenter resuscitation-focused research studies [21,22]. A number of postdoctoral fellows and simulation research fellows have trained in the program to develop a rich understanding of research methodology with a specific focus on advancing the science of resuscitation using simulation-based educational and translational research approaches.

The development of focused areas, along with short- and long-term goals (for each area), will help to ensure that research programs build a body of work that is summative, as opposed to individual projects and studies that are unrelated. Research objectives will ideally be synergistic (or at least consistent and coherent) within a focused area; across focused areas, research methods may inform one another.

Mentorship in Simulation Research

Mentorship is a critical part of postdoctoral training [23]. Although trainees have primary responsibility for their careers, appropriate mentorship is an important component of their training. Each simulation research program should develop a research mentorship structure to enhance and support the research environment and strengthen the trainees. The research mentorship should address the following points:

- Supporting intellectual growth and development
- Supporting the development of simulation research skills for the trainee
- Leveraging the medical/scientific skills of the individual to develop unique or novel skill sets
- Increasing overall job satisfaction among trainees and mentors through natural synergies that foster (1) a productive academic career in simulation research, (2) cultivation of the trainees to become the next generation of research leaders, and (3) professional development and establishment of a productive, independent researcher

The overall goal of a research mentorship is to first develop healthy, successful individuals, guiding them on career paths which follow their personal goals, meet their departments' missions, and utilize their strongest assets. Consequently, a simulation research program will strive to establish, develop, and facilitate positive, enduring, and mutually beneficial mentor–trainee relationships. Appropriate mentorship structure is essential with clear mentor–trainee relationship and should ideally include documented educational goals and an individual development plan (IDP) [24], regular progress reports and meetings, and specific trainee roles such as organizing or presenting at a simulation research conference and simulation journal club.

Responsibilities of the Mentor

The mentor should serve as a source of facilitation, supportive guidance, supervision, constructive criticism, and evaluation. In particular, they will:

1. Ensure that the trainees know what constitutes excellence in research in their field.
2. Formalize goals, objectives, and metrics of success with the trainee, and meet periodically to review progress and attainment of goals.
3. Provide feedback and encouragement on accomplishments. Mentors should actively engage in helping the trainee succeed.
4. Be open and encouraging of evaluation by the trainee with particular attention to objective assessment of whether the mentor meets or exceeds expectations.
5. Identify opportunities for academic and career advancement, collaboration, and personal growth.

Expectation of the Trainee

1. Be expected to participate in research design, implementation, analysis, and publication (manuscript writing, conference poster/podium/workshop) of results.
2. Be expected to set objectives for training and identify opportunities to acquire the necessary knowledge and skills to meet the objectives.
3. Under the direction and guidance of a mentor (principle investigator), be a coinvestigator, assume responsibility for a specific, ongoing research project and the research group.
4. Seek out opportunities for personal growth, academic and career advancement, and collaboration.

Periodic Reviews and Meetings

Simulation research mentees and mentors should strongly consider the usage of a mentoring worksheet based on the IDP of each trainee. This mentoring worksheet can be started by trainees and completed during or after the monthly mentorship meeting with trainees, mentors, educators, and administrators (Fig. 29.1). The following are five areas of focus that may comprise monthly simulation research mentorship meetings:

- Research/creative activity—leadership in innovative research
  Simulation research development and progress, presentations and publications, funding and grant support and application, copyrights and patents, editing, and peer review
- Self-development
  Faculty development activities, leadership programs, language or presentation skill improvement, participation in professional academic associations or societies
- Networking
  Developing and expanding professional contacts and collaborators and utilizing additional mentors in specific areas of focus

Fig. 29.1 Example: Mentoring update worksheet used at The Children's Hospital of Philadelphia. (Used with permission)

The Children's Hospital *of* Philadelphia®

CENTER FOR SIMULATION, ADVANCED EDUCATION & INNOVATION

Progress Update Worksheet

Please complete prior to Monthly Mentoring Meeting and Periodic Reviews with your mentor.

Visiting Scholar/Fellow/Mentee _____ Date of Meeting: _____

Mentor: _____

1) Teaching	☐ Exceeds Expectations	☐ Meets Expectations	☐ Below Expectations
Goals / Expectations for this Month			
Accomplishments			
Obstacles / Barriers			
New Goals for next Month			
2) Research	☐ Exceeds Expectations	☐ Meets Expectations	☐ Below Expectations
Goals / Expectations for this Month			
Accomplishments			
Obstacles / Barriers			
New Goals for next Month			
3) Self Development	☐ Exceeds Expectations	☐ Meets Expectations	☐ Below Expectations
Goals / Expectations for this Month			
Accomplishments			
Obstacles / Barriers			
New Goals for next Month			
4) Networking	☐ Exceeds Expectations	☐ Meets Expectations	☐ Below Expectations
Goals / Expectations for this Month			
Accomplishments			
Obstacles / Barriers			
New Goals for next Month			
5) Work / Life Balance	☐ Exceeds Expectations	☐ Meets Expectations	☐ Below Expectations
Goals / Expectations for this Month			
Accomplishments			
Obstacles / Barriers			
New Goals for next Month			

Notes:

- Work/life balance

  Work as defined by the mentor and trainee and balance defined by the trainee but informed by the mentor's experience and insight on strategies to achieve and pitfalls to avoid

- Teaching—excellence in education

  Student and/or resident teaching, student advising, continuous medical education (CME)/curriculum, teaching/involvement, new course development, etc.

Mentorship Evaluation

The mentorship evaluation assesses the trainees' experience during their mentorship. Specific questions are asked regarding the fulfillment of initial mentorship agreement between a mentor and a trainee and evaluation regarding the effectiveness of the mentorship. The results will be used to gauge the effectiveness of the research training program and the mentorship atmosphere at the simulation center. Through this process, the mentorship program should be revised and remodeled continuously. At the Children's Hospital of

Fig. 29.2 Example: Mentorship evaluation form used at the Children's Hospital of Philadelphia. (Used with permission)

CH The Children's Hospital *of* Philadelphia®

CENTER FOR SIMULATION, ADVANCED EDUCATION & INNOVATION

Mentorship Evaluation Form

To be completed by mentee for primary mentor; additional forms for secondary mentor(s) can be provided if desired.

Mentee: _____ Date: _____

Primary Mentor: _____ Date range of Mentorship: _____

Secondary Mentor(s): _____

This evaluation is for: ☐ Primary Mentor   ☐ Secondary Mentor

Circle One: 1 = Disagree strongly   2 = Disagree   3 = Agree   4 = Agree strongly

Topics	Rating	Comments (additional comments may be written on back of this form)
Intellectual Growth and Development		
Encourages my inventiveness including identification of new research topics and discovery of new methodologies	1 2 3 4	
Helps me develop my capacity for theoretical reasoning and data interpretation	1 2 3 4	
Helps me to be critical and objective concerning my own results and ideas	1 2 3 4	
Helps me become increasingly independent in identifying research questions and conducting and publishing my research	1 2 3 4	
Provides constructive feedback on my experimental designs	1 2 3 4	
Provides thoughtful advice on my research progress and results	1 2 3 4	
Professional Career Development		
Provides counsel for important professional decisions	1 2 3 4	
Provides opportunities for me to meet with visiting scientists, faculty and peers	1 2 3 4	
Maintains balance between supporting his/her own research and developing my own career	1 2 3 4	
Helps me to envision a career plan	1 2 3 4	
Provides guidance in development and presentation of research projects for outside review groups	1 2 3 4	
Ensures that I am firmly grounded in rules regarding ethical behavior and scientific responsibility	1 2 3 4	
Skill Development		
Helps me to work effectively with other individuals	1 2 3 4	

Page 1

Philadelphia, this mentorship evaluation by trainees is required at least twice during the training period. The evaluation form includes topics about intellectual growth and development, professional career development, skill development, personal communication, severing as role model, mentorship program quality, partnership, personal growth, and relationship (Fig. 29.2).

Research Committee and Meetings

At many simulation programs, research conducted within the simulation center is overseen and reviewed by the research committee, chaired by the research director. It is recommended that open research committee meetings are held at a minimum quarterly and are open to any investigator, faculty, or staff member interested in either presenting their research or in participation in the meeting. Regular simulation research committee meetings are an essential activity for a vital simulation-based research program. At the meeting, each active research study is presented, reviewed, and the progress and productivity is monitored. Simulation research meetings should encourage novel, innovative and pioneering research through the use of simulation. These meetings can help to focus efforts toward translation and implementation of a research to improve simulation training, bedside training, and ultimately patient outcomes. Interprofessional, interdisciplinary, interdepartmental, and multi-institutional research activities are highly valued because they may provide insight into the generalizability of the study findings. Lastly, the research director, administrative director, and research program manager meet at least every other month to monitor productivity of the ongoing research.

Simulation Journal Club

Simulation journal club can be an effective venue to expose simulation educators, administrators, mentors, and trainees to emerging evidence in simulation-based research. The role of organizing a simulation journal club is a highly educational experience for simulation research trainees. Preparing the presentation for a journal club requires critical appraisal skills. Project and program management skills are developed as part of the organization of a journal club. These include scheduling, coordinating meeting space (both face-to-face and virtual), identifying and inviting guest presenters, facilitating discussion, disseminating the summary of lessons learned, documenting action items, and ensuring follow-up.

Critical Appraisal and Consideration for Inherent Biases

Critical appraisal is an established method to translate the results of medical research into clinical practice [25]. It is designed to help provide our patients with care that is based on the best evidence currently available (i.e., evidence-based medicine) [25]. This can be easily applied to simulation-based research. Three essential questions are used to help facilitate discussion and critical appraisal of simulation studies (Table 29.3).

Research Administrative Structure Within a Simulation Center

A research program with solid infrastructure and proper resourcing is essential for a simulation center committed to conduct high-quality research. Typical positions that would ideally exist and contribute as standing members of

Table 29.3 Three essential questions in critical appraisal of medical literature [26]

Are the results of the study valid?
This question helps us evaluate the impact of systematic biases. All outcome measures are subject to systematic biases, and we need to evaluate the impact and direction of biases when interpreting each study. Dropout or lost follow-up is a challenge in simulation-based studies. Caution should be exercised especially when the dropout may be potentially related to learning at each learner's level. Failure to capture interpretable data for outcome measures due to technological challenges is also a significant concern in simulation-based studies
What are the results?
This question helps us evaluate the impact (i.e., effect size) of the results and precision of outcome measures
Will the results help me in maximizing the learner's educational experience?
Will this simulation-based intervention produce a similar educational impact in our environment? This question helps us consider study population, context, feasibility, and limitation in generalizability

a research program include research director, administrative assistant or director, research program manager, and research coordinator(s) (Table 29.4).

It is important to note that the administrative assistant/director is responsible for daily administrative/operation-based aspects of the research program. There may be a separate medical director responsible for leadership related to the overall direction and operations of the simulation center, often functioning as a subject matter expert for curriculum development and a liaison to the overarching institution (i.e., school of medicine, hospital, health authority, etc.). These two roles are distinctive and usually independent of the role of the research director. Each of these roles may be part of the research program, and each have different responsibilities within the context of a research program; however, for a research program's overall success all three will have to work together synergistically (Fig. 29.3). This is because many simulation research projects are not stand-alone research projects, and funding sources often come from elsewhere;

Table 29.4 Function, role, and responsibility of the research committee

	Function/role/responsibility
Research director	Multifaceted position with responsibilities for development and oversight of medical simulation and simulation research program in collaboration with the center leadership. The director will also help develop and implement the overall mission, vision, and strategy goals of the center and the institution
Administrative assistant/director	Responsible for day-to-day operations that may include clinical training, research, budgetary, and fundraising
Research program manager	Expected to have sufficient authority, appropriate background, knowledge, training, and accountability to carry out all aspects of the project including assumption of fiscal responsibility and qualified under the eligibility guidelines
Research coordinator(s)	Qualified and trained to perform the procedures as required in the protocol and will be oriented and trained on new protocols

Fig. 29.3 Example of research program administrative structure within a simulation center

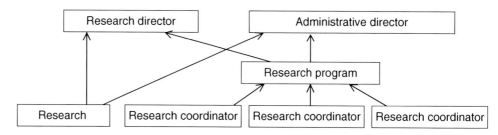

the administrative director needs to provide oversight for resource utilization and perspective on return on investment. Responsibilities of the research program typically include:

1. Review the merit of proposed simulation-based research projects and make suggestions regarding protocol amendments to the initiating investigator
2. Ensure that research conducted is scientifically and ethically sound
3. Act as a resource for developing solutions for delayed progress
4. Monitor productivity of ongoing research
5. Promote, review, and assist the submission and presentation of research conducted at local, regional, national or international forums, and for peer-review publication
6. Act as a resource for promoting current status of projects, presentations, publications, and grants
7. Promote simulation training to improve process of care and outcomes of patients with the findings of simulation-based research
8. Monitor of cross-contamination of participants to ongoing multiple studies

Cross-contaminating subjects within an institution may become an issue when multiple simulation studies are ongoing at single institutions. While some studies have different use of simulation, and co-enrollment is acceptable, others may utilize similar simulation-based educational interventions, which will affect the impact of interventions either positively or negatively. In this situation, co-enrollment is not acceptable. Establishing short- and long-term goals helps to prioritize each project such that the possibility of recruiting the same subjects is reduced. This concept is analogous to co-enrollment of the patient subjects in multiple researches.

Source of Funding (Internal, External)

Financial sustainability is one of the critical components for simulation research programs. A multidimensional strategy has been recommended to achieve a sustainable business model. This strategy includes (1) integration of required simulation-based training and accompanying research into the curricula, (2) the use of simulation for the ideal practice development and training, (3) the use of simulation for diagnosis of system issues, (4) the development of simu-

Table 29.5 External funding resources [28]

NLN Research Grants
http://www.nln.org/research/grants.htm The NLN research grants may be used to investigate any nursing education topic including simulation
US Department of Health and Human Services, HRSA
http://www.hrsa.gov/grants HRSA funds research on a range of healthcare topics. Visit its site to find out about grant opportunities and how to apply
Robert Wood Johnson Foundation
http://www.rwjf.org/ The mission of the Robert Wood Johnson Foundation is to improve the health and healthcare of all Americans
Grants.Gov
http://www.grants.gov/
National Institutes of Health
http://grants.nih.gov/grants/oer.htm
NLN *National League for Nursing*, HRSA *Health Resources and Services Administration*

lation-based research to address national and international priorities, and (5) the development of simulators or related technologies [27].

Internal funding mainly consists of discipline- or clinicalentity-specific support. For example, in the Children's Hospital of Philadelphia, pediatric intensive care unit nurses are oriented with extensive simulation-integrated curriculum. All hospital employees receive a mandatory interprofessional safety training utilizing SBE. Also interprofessional simulation-based training program in trauma resuscitation and neonatal resuscitation have been integrated into the training curriculum in both nursing and residency training. Multiple research projects related to those educational curriculums are being conducted. These tight integrations of SBE in the curricula made the simulation center a strong candidate for internal funding.

External funding includes designated research awards, special purpose funds, and donations from philanthropic sources. These rely on more traditional extramural funding mechanisms. Table 29.5 provides some examples of grant funding sources for SBE [28]. Institutional division or departments may also have administrative research support resources that can be leveraged to help identify requests for proposals that are well suited for simulation-based research.

Collaboration with Other Departments/Divisions

The research program should create and explore extensive but manageable collaborative simulation research projects with other departments and divisions within the university and/or hospital. Each department/division has the need to educate their providers and to evaluate their process of care in a standardized fashion. Through collaboration with simulation research program, each department/division should be able to develop specific needs assessments, SBE, or simulation as an investigative methodology to assess factors affecting clinical care quality. For example, neonatal resuscitation program (NRP) is one of the standard methods for teaching neonatal resuscitation. The simulation research program can assist department of pediatrics, nursing, and respiratory department to collaboratively develop interprofessional SBE with technical and nontechnical skills assessment embedded as a pre- and post-evaluation to document training effectiveness. Another example is a patient handoff simulation. Here environmental, provider, and clinical factors affecting the quality of patient handoffs are evaluated in a standardized simulated environment. A simulation research program can collaboratively develop a handoff tool or specific metrics to evaluate quality of handoff.

Multicenter Collaboration

Simulation research programs should encourage active participation in, and foster collaborative relationships with, research communities and networks external to the program. Multicenter simulation research can be labor intensive, time consuming, and challenging, both logistically and administratively. However, the collaboration of many simulation research programs may be the only way to answer many difficult clinical or educational questions with simulation-based research. Simulation research networks such as the International Network for Simulation-Based Pediatric Innovation, Research, and Education (INSPIRE) have been formed from a variety of disciplines and specialties looking to improve SBE research collaboration, mentorship, and productivity [29]. Another pediatric SBE research network, the Examining Pediatric Resuscitation Education Using Simulation and Scripting (EXPRESS) network, reported that the use of a collaborative research portal has enabled the collaborators to simplify and streamline the management of multicenter SBE research studies. In a single institution, there are significant obstacles to conducting high-quality simulation research, such as limited pool of potential subjects, generalizability, and funding [30,31]. Table 29.6 shows the benefits of research collaboration. Many of these benefits help to overcome the barriers to simulation-based research.

Table 29.6 The benefits of research collaboration [30]

Category	Potential benefit
Recruitment	Recruitment from multiple centers allows larger sample sizes
Generalizability	Multicenter collaboration provides inclusion of various subject populations which expands the generalizability of studies
Funding	Funding opportunities are more accessible when conducting multicenter studies involving experts with existing track records in research
Accessibility	Access to the rich and diverse experience of other network members help protocol design and implementation
Communication	Regular and planned communication within networks allows for groups to develop consensus-derived, well-informed, timely, and relevant research agendas to guide network projects

Table 29.7 Institution list of several pediatric simulation fellowship programs

Alberta Children's Hospital/University of Calgary (Canada)
Boston Children's Hospital (USA)
The Children's Hospital of Philadelphia (USA)
The Hospital for Sick Children (Canada)
The University of North Carolina (USA)

Simulation Fellowships

Several formal simulation research training programs (simulation fellowships) have been developed (Table 29.7). From the simulation program's perspective, fellowship programs are effective ways of attracting talented emerging educators and/or researchers to a program, an excellent way to ensure that new research projects and funding are continuously being brought into the program, and an excellent way of establishing national and international recognition. From a learner perspective, a formal fellowship is an excellent way of gaining extra experience and expertise that would make them more marketable post training, either as a simulation educator or researcher. This includes the ability to write more sophisticated proposals for both internal and extramural grant programs. The training mentoring process should follow each component described in mentorship section. It is important to note that simulation fellowship is not currently recognized by Accreditation Council for Graduate Medical Education (ACGME).

Assessment of Simulation Research Programs

The quality assessment of the simulation research program is necessary for each program to be reflective, to identify strengths and weaknesses, and to identify areas for

Table 29.8 Eight essential elements for evaluating research effectiveness and quality

1. Environment/climate	Safe, healthy, and nurturing environment for all research and participants
2. Administration/organization	Well-developed infrastructure and sound fiscal management to support and enhance worthwhile research activities for all researchers
3. Relationships	Develops, nurtures, and maintains positive relationships and interaction among staff, researchers, and collaborators to support the program's goal
4. Staffing/professionals	Recruits, hires, and trains diverse staff and investigators who value each participant, understand their developmental needs, and work closely with administration, staff, researchers, and collaborative partners to achieve the program goal
5. Administration/researcher/collaborative partnerships	Establish a strong partnership with research communities in order to achieve program goals
6. Program sustainability/growth	A coherent vision/mission and a plan for increasing capacity that supplies continuing growth
7. Measuring outcomes/evaluation	A system for measuring outcomes and using that information for ongoing program planning, improvement, and evaluation
8. Dissemination of information	Ability to interpret study results and present them in a scientifically sound, unbiased and timely manner to the greater research community through local, regional, and international conferences and peer-reviewed publications

improvement. Research investigators or any personnel who participated in any stage of a research and had support from the simulation center should complete the assessment. Research program quality assessments are to be distributed, reviewed, and discussed by members of the research committee on at least an annual basis. At the Children's Hospital of Philadelphia, eight essential elements are evaluated (Table 29.8).

Academic Productivity

Important and useful scholarship in health profession education can be published or presented in many different ways. Table 29.9 lists common scholarly products [32], and Table 29.10 lists several journals that publish simulation-based research. A simulation research program should consider the usage of flexible systems to track and monitor research efforts (past, present, future) and any associated scholarly products. In the simulation research program at The Children's Hospital of Philadelphia, this update is done monthly using Research Electronic Data Capture (REDCap; 33]). This update is shared with educators, research trainees, and directors at simulation operation meetings regularly and can be a useful tool in grant writing, manuscript preparation, and Curriculum Vitae/resume management.

Fellowship Training Outcomes

It should be recognized that the simulation research trainee's progress and training outcomes are one of the important components of the research program assessment. Measurable outcomes should be developed based on each trainee's IDP.

Table 29.9 Common scholarly products in health science education [32]

1. Journal article
2. Book chapter
3. Book or monograph
4. Edited book (collection of chapters)
5. Essay
6. Editorial or statement of opinion
7. Book (or media) review
8. Letter
9. Educational case report
10. Conference report
11. Educational materials
12. Reports of teaching practices
13. Curriculum description
14. Other publication formats (e.g., videos)
15. Simulations (e.g., practice experiences, virtual reality)
16. Simulators (e.g., task trainers, mannequins, computer programs)
17. Web-based tutorials

Examples of the training outcomes include:
- Training evaluation by trainees
  This fellowship program is effective in
  - gaining a clearer sense of the rigors and rewards of a career in simulation research,
  - acquiring a better awareness of expectations for career advancement,
  - developing rapport with other simulation members, and
  - experiencing a shorter transition period from new investigation to mid-career and established research programs.

Table 29.10 Lists of journals that publish simulation-based research

Academic Medicine

Academic Emergency Medicine

American Journal of Surgery

American Journal of Emergency Medicine

Archives of Disease in Childhood: Fetal & Neonatal Edition

BMJ Simulation and Technology-Enhanced Learning

Canadian Journal of Emergency Medicine

Chest

Circulation

Critical Care Medicine

Clinical Simulation in Nursing

Current Opinion in Pediatrics

Family Medicine

Health Informatics Journal

JAMA

JAMA Pediatrics

Journal of Advanced nursing

Journal of Nursing Education

Journal of Pediatric Surgery

Journal of Perinatology

Journal of Perinatal & Neonatal Nursing

Medical Education

Medical Teacher

Pediatrics

Pediatric Anesthesia

Paediatrics & Child Health

Pediatric Emergency Care

Pediatric Critical Care Medicine

Resuscitation

Simulation in Healthcare

Teaching and Learning in Medicine

The Journal of Emergency Medicine

The Journal of Thoracic and Cardiovascular Surgery

Nurse Education Today

JAMA

Journal of the American Medical Association, BMJ *British Medical Journal*

- Academic productivity by trainees: manuscripts, publications, professional presentations nationally or internationally, and grants (written, submitted, or funded).
- Performance of fellowship graduates
  - that needs to be tracked and used as an assessment of the program.

Conclusions

Simulation-based research program development requires collective knowledge and deep understanding of both the strengths and challenges of simulation-based research. This includes the need for further expertise within education and clinical research, including psychometrics and qualitative approaches, clinical epidemiology, health services research and evaluation, and patient outcome research. A specific organizational structure is necessary that enables for appropriate mentorship of trainees as well as quality administrative oversight. Ongoing assessment of the research program is an essential component to both ensure quality assurance and compliance with research rules and guidelines and allow the program to grow responsibly. This includes multicenter collaboration with established networks such as INSPIRE. Focusing the research program to align with the defined mission, vision, and goals; mentoring the next generation of simulation researchers; and measuring research productivity will all lead to a strong research program that ultimately increases the chance of making an important impact on child health.

References

1. Cheng A, Auerbach M, Hunt EA, Chang TP, Pusic M, Nadkarni V. Designing and conducting simulation-based research. Pediatrics. 2014;133:1091–101.
2. Nishisaki A, Hales R, Biagas K, Cheifetz I, Corriveau C, Garber N. A multi-institutional high-fidelity simulation "boot camp" orientation and training program for first year pediatric critical care fellows. Pediatr Crit Care Med. 2009;10(2):157–62.
3. Okuda Y, Bond W, Bonfante G, Mclaughlin S, Spillane L, Wang E. National growth in simulation training within emergency medicine residency programs, 2003–2008. Acad Emerg Med. 2008;15:1113–6.
4. Issenberg SB, Ringsted C, Ostergaard D, Dieckmann P. Setting a research agenda for simulation-based healthcare education. Simul Healthc. 2011;6(3):155–67.
5. Kern DE, Thomas PA, Hughes MT, editors. Curriculum development for medical education. A six-step approach. 2nd ed. Baltimore: The Johns Hopkins University Press; 2009.
6. Jacobs BR, editor. Current concept in pediatric critical care. Society of Critical Care Medicine. 2013.
7. LeBlanc VR, Manser T, Weinger MB, Musson D, Kutzin J, Howard SK. The study of factors affecting human and systems performance in healthcare using simulation. Simul Healthc. 2011;6:S24–9.
8. Cook DA, Hatala R, Brydges R, Zendejas B, Szostek JH, Wang AT. Technology-enhanced simulation for health professions education. A systematic review and meta-analysis. JAMA. 2011;306(9):978–88.
9. Cheng A, Lang TR, Starr SR, Pusic M, Cook DA. Technology-enhanced simulation and pediatric education: a meta-analysis. Pediatrics. 2014;133:e1313–23.
10. Raemer D, Anderson M, Cheng A, Fanning R, Nadkarni V, Savoldelli G. Research regarding debriefing as part of the learning process. Simul Healthc. 2011;6 Suppl:S52–7.

11. Geis GL, Pio B, Pednergrass TL, Moyer MR, Patterson MD. Simulation to assess the safety of new healthcare teams and new facilities. Simul Healthc. 2011;6:125–133.

12. Fonte M, Oulego-Erroz I, Nadkarni L, Sanchez-Santos L, Iglesias-Vasquez A, Rodriguez-Nunez A. A randomized comparison of the glidescope videolaryngoscope to the standard laryngoscopy for intubation by pediatric residents in simulated easy and difficult infant airway scenarios. Pediatr Emerg Care. 2011;27:398–402.

13. Hunt EA, Heine M, Shilkofski NS, Bradshaw JH, Nelson-McMillan, Duval-Arnould J. Exploration of the impact of a voice activated decision support system (VADSS) with video on resuscitation performance by lay rescuers during simulated cardiopulmonary arrest. Emerg Med J. 2013;0:1–6.

14. Society for Simulation in Healthcare [Internet]. To apply for SSH accreditation: 2. Review the SSH accreditation self-study (doc) to determine in which areas you would like to apply for accreditation. http://www.ssih.org/Accreditation/Full-Accreditation. Accessed 13 Nov 2014.

15. Kouwenhoven WB, Jude JR, Knickerbocker GG. Closed-chest cardiac massage. JAMA. 1960;173:1064–7.

16. Sullivan NJ, Duval-Arnould J, Twilley M, Smith SP, Aksamit D, Boone-Guercio P. Simulation exercise to improve retention of cardiopulmonary resuscitation priorities for in-hospital cardiac arrests: a randomized controlled trial. Resuscitation. 2015;86:6–13.

17. Hunt EA, Vera K, Diener-West M, Haggerty JA, Nelson KL, Shaffner DH. Delays and errors in cardiopulmonary resuscitation and defibrillation by pediatric residents during simulated cardiopulmonary arrests. Resuscitation. 2009;80:819–25.

18. Nelson KL, Shilkofski NA, Haggerty JA, Saliski M, Hunt EA. The use of cognitive aids during simulated pediatric cardiopulmonary arrests. Simul Healthc. 2008;3:138–45.

19. Hunt EA, Duval-Arnould JM, Nelson-McMillan KL, Bradshaw JH, Diener-West M, Perretta JS. Resuscitation. 2014;85:945–51.

20. Hunt EA, Cruz-Eng H, Bradshaw JH, Hodge M, Bortner T, Mulvey CL. A novel approach to life support training using "action-linked phrases". Resuscitation. 2015;876:1–5.

21. Cheng A, Brown LL, Duff JP, Davidson J, Overly R, Tofil NM. Improving cardiopulmonary resuscitation with a CPR feedback device and refresher simulations (CPR Cases Study). A randomized clinical trial. JAMA Pediatr. Published Online December 22, 2014.

22. Cheng A, Hunt EA, Donoghue A, Nelson-McMillan K, Nishisaki A, Leflore J. Examining pediatric resuscitation education using simulation and scripted debriefing. A multicenter randomized trial. JAMA Pediatr. 2013;167(6):528–36.

23. Johnson MO, Subak LL, Brown JS, Lee KA, Feldman MD. An innovative program to train health sciences researchers to be effective clinical and translational research mentors. Acad Med. 2010;85(3):484–9.

24. National Institute of General Medical Sciences [Internet]. Individual development plans. http://www.nigms.nih.gov/training/strategicplanimplementationblueprint/pages/IndividualDevelopmentPlans.aspx. Accessed 13 Nov 2014.

25. Evidence-Based Medicine Working Group. Evidence-based medicine. A new approach to teaching the practice of medicine. JAMA. 1992;268(17):2420–5.

26. Andrew DO, Sackett DL, Gordon HG. Use's guides to the medical literature I. How to get started. The Evidence-Based Medicine Working Group. JAMA. 1993;270(17):2093–5.

27. Kahol K. Securing funding for simulation centers and research. In: Levine AI, DeMaria S Jr, Schwartz AD, Sim AJ, editors. The comprehensive textbook of healthcare simulation. New York: Springer; 2014.

28. SIMULATION INNOVATION RESOURCE CENTER [Internet]. Funding; [about 2 screens]. http://sirc.nln.org/mod/page/view.php?id=90. Accessed 13 Nov 2014.

29. INSPIRE [Internet]. http://inspiresim.com/. Accessed 13 Nov 2014.

30. Cheng A, Hunt EA, Donoghue A, Nelson K, Leflore J, Anderson J, et al. EXPRESS-Examining Pediatric Resuscitation Education Using Simulation and Scripting. The birth of an international pediatric simulation research collaborative-from concept to reality. Simul Healthc. 2011;6(1):34–41.

31. Cheng A, Nadkarni V, Hunt EA, Qayumi K, EXPRESS Investigators. A multifunctional online research portal for facilitation of simulation-based research: a report from the EXPRESS pediatric simulation research collaborative. Simul Healthc. 2011;6(4):239–43.

32. McGaghie WC, Webster A. Scholarship, publication, and career advancement in health professions education: AMEE Guide No. 43. Med Teach. 2009;31(7):574–90.

33. Harris PA, Taylor R, Thielke R, Payne J, Gonzalez N, Conde JG. Research electronic data capture (REDCap)-a metadata-driven methodology and workflow process for providing translational research informatics support. J Biomed Inform. 2009;42(2):377–81.

Simulation Research

30

David O. Kessler, Marc Auerbach, Todd P. Chang, Yiqun Lin and Adam Cheng

Simulation Pearls

1. To isolate the variable being studied—standardize as many other aspects of the protocol as possible (e.g., learners, simulators, scenarios, trainers, debriefing, environment, resources, etc.) to avoid confounders.
2. Choose validated outcome measures, like checklists, and when not available, consider doing more basic validation study first before larger trial.
3. Consider multiple sources of funding, such as nonprofit foundations, internal risk management division, multicenter collaborations, or partnerships with public agencies.
4. Make sure your study passes the *who cares* test. Avoid comparing simulation to no intervention or obviously inferior education. Ensure that subjects exposed to different interventions have a similar time on task and have *educational equipoise*.

D. O. Kessler (✉)
Department of Pediatrics, Columbia University College of Physicians and Surgeons, New York Presbyterian Hospital, Columbia University Medical Center, New York, NY, USA
e-mail: dk2592@cumc.columbia.edu

M. Auerbach
Department of Pediatrics, Section of Emergency Medicine, Yale University School of Medicine, New Haven, CT, USA
e-mail: marc.auerbach@yale.edu

T. P. Chang
Department of Pediatrics, Division of Emergency Medicine & Transport, University of Southern California Keck School of Medicine, Children's Hospital Los Angeles, Los Angeles, CA, USA
e-mail: Dr.toddchang@gmail.com

Y. Lin
Department of Community Health Science, Faculty of Medicine, KidSIM Simulation Education and Research Program, University of Calgary, Alberta's Children's Hospital, Calgary, AB, Canada
e-mail: jeffylin@hotmail.com

A. Cheng
Department of Pediatrics, Cumming School of Medicine, University of Calgary, Calgary, AB, Canada

KidSIM Pediatric Simulation Program, Alberta Children's Hospital, Calgary, AB, Canada
e-mail: chenger@me.com

Types of Simulation Research

The use of simulation as an educational methodology for pediatrics has been accompanied by the use of simulation-based research (SBR) to answer clinically important questions related to the care of infants and children. SBR falls into two different categories. First, simulation can be used as an investigative methodology, or the *environment* for research, to study questions that relate to human factors, system factors, and new technology, amongst other things. Secondly, simulation can be the subject of a research study designed to evaluate the *impact* of a simulation-based educational intervention. In this chapter, we discuss the two different types of simulation research, highlight the advantages and disadvantages of SBR, describe standardization strategies and outcomes for SBR, and suggest methods to obtain funding.

Simulation Used as Investigative Methodology

Research using simulation as an investigative methodology allows researchers to study research questions that otherwise could not be answered safely, ethically, or timely in clinical settings [1]. Simulation can be best leveraged as an investigative methodology either to standardize the environment or as a standardized outcome measure.

Simulation as Standardized Environment
The simulated environment can be used as an experimental model to study factors affecting human and system performances in healthcare. A simulated setting in a simulation lab may imitate clinical spaces, such as the resuscitation room, intensive care unit, or operating room. Alternatively, simulated resources (such as medications or equipment) can

© Springer International Publishing Switzerland 2016
V. J. Grant, A. Cheng (eds.), *Comprehensive Healthcare Simulation: Pediatrics*,
Comprehensive Healthcare Simulation, DOI 10.1007/978-3-319-24187-6_30

be used to help standardize assessments in the clinical environment (i.e., in situ simulation). A mannequin connected to a computer that controls its vital signs, physiological parameters, and physical findings can provide healthcare professionals with a realistic clinical experience.

Human Factors

Human interaction is a key element in the clinical process and an essential contributor to accidents and errors in healthcare. Human factors can be assessed or described using simulation in a risk-free environment at both the individual and team level. Most of the studies at the individual level have focused on fatigue, stress, and aging. In one study, simulation was used to compare sleep-deprived anesthesiology residents with rested residents in order to evaluate the effect of sleep deprivation on psychomotor skill performance, mood, and sleepiness [2]. Simulation has also been used to study relationships between team processes and team performance (e.g., leadership, communication, etc.). For example, simulation was utilized to address hierarchy-related errors in medical practice in pediatric intensive care and pediatric emergency departments [3]. Group conformity of behavior among medical students has also been studied with a knee arthrocentesis task trainer [4]. Most of the human factor research using simulation reveals factors that degrade performance. Built on these existing works, future studies could potentially look at a solution to these issues, including how to avoid group conformity or hierarchy-related errors.

Environment

Simulation can be applied to study the impact of the surrounding environment on performance, such as loud noises causing interruption and distraction. The impact of distractions on simulated surgical performance has been demonstrated with a simulated environment [5]. Furthermore, simulation can be brought to the real patient care environment, also known as in situ simulation. Investigators can then identify and correct latent safety threats (e.g., malfunctioning devices, locked resuscitation cart, excessive crowding) to prevent adverse events from occurring on real patients [6]. In situ simulation has also been used to test feasibility and refine processes before the opening of a new pediatric emergency department [7]. Future environment factor studies could consider exploring the optimal setting for work environments (e.g., resuscitation room, layout of equipment).

New Technologies

Simulation provides an ideal platform for comparative efficacy studies to assess behavior and performance with new technologies. For instance, in simulated scenarios depicting normal and difficult airways in infants, video laryngoscopy did not improve intubation performance by pediatric residents compared to standard laryngoscopy [8]. Sylvia et al. reported a similar comparison in pediatric and emergency medicine residents [9]. These studies involved new technology (video laryngoscope) used to complete a life-saving procedure (intubation) done by relatively inexperienced health professionals (pediatric and emergency medicine residents). These critical procedures would be unethical and/or very difficult to conduct without the use of simulation.

System Factors

Discrete event simulation and computer models that include many interrelated complex systems have been used to predict what factors may affect system-level operations. A patient flow model (PFM) has been used in a pediatric emergency department to predict the impact of adding volunteers, triage nurses, and/or extra physician shifts on patients' waiting times before triage and time to be seen by a physician [10]. A similar technique has been used to compare two different triage approaches on patient wait times [11]. Beyond conventional mannequin-based simulation (MBS), researchers are able to develop a computer model and/or use the existing model to answer research questions. With immediate results from simulated changes in the department, hospital administrators can readjust staffing and resources in the system to achieve optimal outcome. However, the accuracy of the results depends on the quality of the model. Further, the process of model fitting could be time-consuming and need additional training and expertise.

Patient Factors

Simulation can be applied to explore performance gaps for uncommon patient conditions. Pediatric cardiac arrest is one such example. One study [12] demonstrated that nearly two thirds of pediatric residents failed to initiate timely chest compressions in a simulated pediatric cardiac arrest scenario, and half of them failed to recognize pulseless ventricular tachycardia after 3 min. These studies were mostly descriptive but very informative, effectively revealing the gaps in clinical knowledge and skills that would be less feasible and more costly to investigate with actual patients.

Simulation Used as a Standardized Outcome

It is not always ethical or feasible to measure the desired clinical outcome in an interventional study. Investigators have utilized simulation as a reasonable proxy outcome measure in numerous situations. A good example of this would be evaluating the quality of chest compressions. Although some studies have reported on quality of chest compressions on real patients, many studies are mannequin-based because the data on quality of cardiopulmonary resuscitation (CPR) can be captured on mannequins, cases can be standardized, and data can be collected in a timely fashion from multiple participants. Mannequins are used to assess the metrics of CPR quality (e.g., depth, rate, residual learning, and chest compression fraction). For instance, the effectiveness of high-frequency, low-dose booster training on CPR skill retention was studied on a CPR torso trainer along with an attached device with data collection capability [13]. Quite a few studies have also looked at the effect of using real-time feedback during training on CPR skill performance and retention [14].

The categories mentioned earlier are not independent of each other, as human, environment, technology, and systems act together in healthcare. These interactions could be studied using simulation. For example, when examining the anesthesiology residents' reaction to equipment failure [15], we could explore environmental factors (equipment failure), human factors (team performance, crisis resource management), and system-level factors (equipment maintenance) simultaneously. Also, simulation could be used as both a standardized environment and for standardized outcomes. A recent multicenter study [16] has examined the effect of real-time feedback (new technology) and just-in-time training (potential system policy or environment factor) on quality of chest compressions on a mannequin (proxy measures and standardized outcome) in a simulated pediatric cardiac arrest scenario (standardized environment).

Simulation as the Subject of a Research Study

Research assessing the efficacy of simulation as a training or assessment modality for pediatric healthcare providers has grown exponentially since the first study supporting the effectiveness of simulation in teaching procedural skills was published in the 1970s [17]. In the past 30 years, it has been well established that simulation-based education (SBE) is effective and complements the training of pediatric healthcare providers. A pediatric SBR meta-analysis mirrored a larger comprehensive review from all specialties, demonstrating that SBE is associated with large effect sizes compared to no intervention [18, 19]. The reviewers noted large impacts on knowledge, skills, and behaviors when simulation was compared to no intervention. Few comparative studies with rigorous designs such as randomized trials have been conducted in pediatric SBR [18].

Many of the current SBR studies are repeating prior work and limited in scope to exploring the efficacy of SBE compared to no intervention, to simple pre- and post- designs and to outcomes related to the participants' satisfaction, knowledge, skills, and attitudes [20]. The current research must serve as a stepping-off point to guide rigorous work in novel areas of inquiry. SBR must transition from *if* SBE is effective in asking questions that address ways to optimize

effectiveness and examine *how, why, what, who, when, and where* to utilize SBE.

How?

Pediatric SBR is now leveraging theoretical frameworks from other areas of inquiry such as instructional design, cognitive psychology, industrial engineering, organizational psychology, and human factors. Tools such as the Medical Education Research Study Quality Instrument describe the key elements of quality medical education research [21]. While this tool can be applied to SBR, there are other important elements that must be considered in reporting on this topic. These elements include a detailed description of the various elements of an intervention, including the type of simulator being used, the specific elements of the scenario program, the debriefing techniques that are used (i.e., plus-delta vs. advocacy inquiry), the infrastructure (i.e., audio and video recording systems), and the human resources required (i.e., facilitators, technicians). Failure to describe or standardize these elements may influence educational outcomes. For example, failure to standardize simulator realism across recruitment sites in a multicenter study may be an issue, as a pediatric meta-analysis revealed that simulators with higher levels of physical realism had moderate effect sizes on outcomes when compared with low physical realism simulators [18]. The consistent reporting of methodological elements will require the development of a framework or guidelines for reporting SBR. Standardized reporting will guide the development of reproducible SBE interventions. While there is a growing body of literature describing best practices in SBE, continued rigorous inquiry is required. Some of the more common designs for SBE and the associated advantages and disadvantages are highlighted in Table 30.1.

Why?

Research on SBE must be grounded in the larger context of health services education. The goal of health services education is to transmit knowledge, impart skills, and embody the values of medicine that will improve health outcomes [22]. SBE is a technique that can be leveraged for healthcare practitioners to develop and maintain knowledge and skills that will transfer to the clinical environment and result in improvements in outcomes for patients. The pediatric SBR research connecting SBE to patient outcomes is limited and has largely been conducted in the areas of cardiopulmonary arrest, intubation, and procedural skills [23, 24, 25–28]. In particular, Andreatta's work demonstrated improved hospital arrest survival by 50% after cardiac arrest. The American Academy of Pediatrics' Helping Babies Breath program demonstrated reduced neonatal mortality by up to 50% [29]. In summary, SBE must be developed within the broad context of health services education and with continuous

Table 30.1 Common study designs

Design	Notation	Advantage	Disadvantage
Single group, posttest only (descriptive)	X–O	Simple, economical, can be used to document process (i.e., program development), can elicit suggestion for improvement (pilot study)	Effect may be result of natural maturation. Result may be due to factors other than intervention
Single group, pretest–posttest (before–after comparison)	O1–X–O2	Simple, economic, can demonstrate changes with intervention	Effect may be result of natural maturation. Bias due to confounding, temporal effect, or Hawthorne effect[a]
Pretest–posttest with control group (quasi-experimental)	E: O1–X–O2 C: O1–N–O2	Control for temporal effect and known factors that might affect the outcome	Relatively complex and resource-intensive, potential selection bias, unable to control unintentional confounders
Posttest only with control group and randomization (true experimental)	E: X–O R O: N–O	Control for potential confounding (intentional or unintentional), less resource-intensive than pretest–posttest design, but preserving the benefits of randomization	Complex and resource-intensive, unable to demonstrate changes in learners, unable to demonstrate equivalence in two groups at baseline
Pretest–posttest with control and randomization (true experimental)	E: O1–X–O2 R C: O1–N–O2	Control for potential confounding, most strict design	Most complex and resource-intensive

X intervention of interest, *O* observation/measurement, *E* experimental/intervention group, *C* control group, *N* no intervention or comparative intervention, *R* randomization

[a] Modification of participant behavior due to awareness of being observed

reflection on the potential downstream impact on improving health outcomes in real patients.

What?

The features of effective SBE described by Cook and Issenberg support the following instructional design components: feedback/debriefing, repetitive and distributive practice, curriculum integration, range of difficulty, clinical variation, active and individualized learning, and design that involves multiple learning strategies [30, 31]. These components require comparative research to explore the impact of specific instructional design features when used for different learning objectives (i.e., psychomotor skills vs. team training), by different instructor groups, by different learner groups, and in different learning environments. Examples of comparative pediatric SBR studies examining instructional design features are described in Table 30.2 [32].

When?

The integration of SBE into preexisting pediatric curricula can be challenging. Finding the time for SBE is difficult due to limitations in duty hours. For example, what will be eliminated from an already full curriculum in order to make time for simulation? Comparative studies examining the efficiency and effectiveness of simulation compared to existing pedagogical techniques will inform these decisions. Didactic sessions such as morning reports that have existed for many years could be transformed into SBE as the cornerstone of future training programs. Innovative techniques such as regional boot camps at the start of training can provide for a common starting point for all trainees as they enter a pro-

Table 30.2 Pediatric simulation-based research (SBR) examining instructional design elements

Instructional design feature	Example of a comparative study
Curricular integration	Comparing simulation-based procedural training occurring within the clinical workplace during an ED rotation to training occurring in a simulation center outside of the ED rotation
Distributed practice	Comparing a single day of simulation for 8 h to eight 1-h sessions distributed over time
Feedback	Comparing scripted to non-scripted debriefing for teamwork and leadership skills
Repetitive practice	Comparing repeating a specific simulation case multiple times in a single session to a single occurrence with a longer debriefing

ED emergency department

gram. Ongoing training should be individualized to learners' needs based on their clinical exposure and experience. For example, if a trainee is doing a clinical rotation in the summer, they may need simulation for bronchiolitis as it is a seasonal illness. SBR must explore questions related to the optimal frequency and duration of training required for the acquisition of sufficient knowledge, skills, and attitudes for healthcare providers to safely and effectively care for patients. This type of work has the potential to improve the efficiency and effectiveness of training that is customized and adaptive to each individual's clinical experience and career development arc.

Where?

The majority of SBR projects have been conducted in the controlled environment of a simulation lab or center. A number of investigators are beginning to explore how to best adapt the setting to better mirror the clinical environment. A growing number of projects are being conducted in situ (at the point of clinical care). While this maximizes the realism of the environment, it has also raised some concerns about the potential impact on real patients and the psychological safety of the participants [33]. SBR must examine the pros and cons to the learners, patients, and the health system of each of these environments. For example, a study could compare simulations in a simulation center to an in situ environment for CPR skills training. A novice medical student would likely benefit from the opportunity for repetitive deliberate practice of CPR skills in a simulation center while an experienced fellow would require greater contextual fidelity of performing this skill in the clinical environment for maximal effect. Future work could also examine the use of virtual environments and computer-based solutions that allow for SBE at home on a tablet or smartphone. The environment should be matched to the specific goals and objectives of the program in order to maximize learning.

Who?

SBE involves the interaction of participants, instructors, and simulators. The majority of SBE focuses on undergraduate and postgraduate trainees; however, little is known about the application of SBE for continuing healthcare education. Furthermore, the current literature falls short in describing how differences in training backgrounds and levels of experience impact learning outcomes from SBE. The researcher can approach topics from the lens of each of these individually or in combination. For example, if we want to compare two different types of simulators, we would do our best to control for the trainee and instructor characteristics. In contrast, in order to research debriefing techniques, we might vary the trainee and instructor interactions while keeping the simulation/simulator constant. Research must examine the demographic characteristics and experiences of the participants and instructors in order to maximize the impact of SBE for the various different types of participants and instructors.

Advantages and Disadvantages of SBR

One may ask: "Why should I conduct SBR?" The answer to this question lies in the understanding of the advantages and disadvantages of SBR, particularly when compared to clinical research. In this section, we highlight the main advantages of SBR and describe some of the disadvantages associated with SBR that may limit its applicability in certain contexts.

Advantages of SBR

To date, most of the SBR conducted in pediatrics has been in the context of assessing MBS as an educational intervention [18]. Using MBS allows the researcher to standardize selected aspects of the clinical research environment, which is often difficult to achieve in multicenter clinical trials. For example, a clinical trial assessing the performance of chest compressions in various pediatric intensive care units across North America may be subject to various confounders, such as mattress type and compressibility, type of defibrillator and/or monitors, availability and location of resuscitation drugs, among many others. A similar study done using simulation could easily control for some or all of these factors, thus helping to eliminate them as potential confounders.

In clinical research, studies are often reliant upon specific patient types (e.g., age, clinical presentation) to meet criteria for enrollment. This makes clinical studies difficult to conduct with rare conditions. SBR allows the researcher to create the specific type of patient (e.g., cardiac arrest), and tailor the age, clinical status, and other characteristics to the needs of the study [32]. Doing so ensures consistent and uniform exposure to all healthcare providers recruited to participate in the study. Furthermore, simulated patients can be provided on an on-demand basis, while clinical studies are often at the mercy of a rare presentation (e.g., cardiac arrest) or seasonal variation (e.g., bronchiolitis in the winter), or other variables that influence clinical presentations.

By standardizing the simulated clinical environment for research, the research team can carefully account for all of the potential confounding variables, such as clinical diagnosis, clinical progression, equipment, confederate actors, etc. [34]. This also provides researchers the chance to build in aspects of care unique to pediatrics, including the presence of family members and/or alternate caregivers, the age and size of the patient, and the variable sizes of equipment [32]. Perhaps the biggest difference between clinical research and SBR is that with most clinical research, the subjects are patients, while with SBR, the subjects are typically healthcare providers. As such, a major advantage of SBR is that recruitment of individuals and/or teams of healthcare professionals is typically more predictable and reliable than real patients. Furthermore, recruitment for clinical research can be inhibited by the challenges of obtaining consent in the context of clinical care, while obtaining consent from healthcare providers is potentially less complicated. Finally, there is no risk for patient harm in SBR, which cannot be said for many

Table 30.3 Characteristics of simulation-based versus clinical research studies

Research characteristic	Simulation-based research	Clinical research
Standardization of research environment	Capability to standardize all aspects of the clinical research environment	Very challenging to standardize all aspects of clinical research environment, particularly for multicenter studies
Patient selection	Patient/clinical case can be offered on demand and when required	Patient/clinical cases are recruited based on presentation and are at the mercy of seasonal variation
Subjects	Typically healthcare providers (and not patients)	Variable, but may be patients, healthcare providers, family members, etc.
Risk for patient harm	No risk for patient harm	Potential risk for patient harm
Recruitment	Simulators as proxy patients easy to schedule Recruiting healthcare providers dependent upon provider schedules and availability	Recruiting patients reliant upon multiple variables that are typically not under control of researcher Recruiting healthcare providers dependent upon provider schedules and availability plus competing clinical demands
Authenticity	Simulated environment not completely authentic, which may influence subject behavior(s)	Clinical environment is always 100% authentic (with exception of Hawthorne[a] effect)
Physiological responsiveness	Physiological responses are either controlled by operator, or property of simulator (chest recoil) or programming (e.g., virtual reality algorithm)	Physiological response are real but may not always be measurable
Resources and expertise	Simulation resources and expertise required	Research expertise required

[a] Modification of participant behavior due to awareness of being observed

clinical studies [32]. Table 30.3 compares and contrasts SBR with clinical research studies.

Disadvantages of SBR

SBR is not without its downsides or limitations. The simulated clinical environment often suffers from a lack of authenticity or realism, which may adversely influence specific behaviors of research subjects [32]. Although simulated patients can be provided on-demand, they lack the physiologic variability and responsiveness of real patients. In SBR, the physiological responses in the simulated patient are controlled by the operator, which may or may not accurately represent how a real patient may respond. This makes it hard or impossible to do certain types of research in the simulated environment (i.e., effect of a drug on patient outcome). Lastly, the conduct of SBR requires an investment in simulation-specific resources and expertise (in addition to research expertise), which may be prohibitive in some institutions (Table 30.3).

Standardization Strategies for SBR

Careful attention to the standardization of the SBR environment allows the researcher to isolate the independent variable and reduce simulation-specific confounding variables that are threats to the internal validity of the study. In a re-

cent review article, these threats are described in detail and strategies are offered to mitigate each of these threats [32]. Controlling these confounding variables is particularly critical for multicenter studies, where site-specific variability can potentially have a negative impact on outcomes. The key variables to consider in SBR are: simulator selection, scenario design, standardized patients (SP)/actors, and debriefing.

Simulator Selection

The type of simulator used for SBR should be carefully selected to ensure that the physical attributes (i.e., physical realism) provide sufficient functionality required for the study. As there is a diverse selection of pediatric simulators, all of which have varying degrees of functionality, the researcher should carefully review and select the simulator with the most appropriate features. One example would be a study where the primary outcome is the ability to properly bag–mask–ventilate a hypoventilating patient; the researcher should select a mannequin that allows for this task to be observed and performed in the most realistic manner. If simulation realism and functionality is not carefully considered, the simulator choice may become a confounding variable that adversely influences the outcome of the study [32].

Scenario Design

Studies utilizing simulated clinical scenarios as the context for research should ensure that the simulated scenarios are designed and delivered in a consistent fashion. Effective strategies to ensure scenario standardization include: (a) limit the duration of the scenario; (b) set transitions in clinical status at predetermined time intervals (i.e., independent of provider management); (c) set transitions in clinical status dependent upon provider management; and (d) detailed scenario scripts with pilot testing to detect potential issues [32].

Standardized Patients (SPs)

SPs are often used to help engage subjects and enhance the emotional realism of the simulated clinical encounter. When used as part of a research study, SP behaviors should be carefully scripted and controlled to prevent them from being confounding variables for the outcome of interest. Several potential ways to standardize SP behaviors include: (a) scripting of SP behaviors at all time points in the simulated clinical scenario; (b) providing SP training prior to initiation of the study; (c) pilot testing scenarios to ensure SP compliance with pre-scripted roles; and (d) cue cards to help SPs adhere to their roles [32].

Debriefing

Debriefing is a critical component of SBE and frequently a part of simulation-based educational interventions that are the subject of research [31, 35]. In a review of the debriefing literature, the key features of debriefing are described as the 5 Ws of debriefing research: Who (debriefer characteristics), What (content and methods of debriefing), When (timing), Where (environment), and Why (theory) [36]. This was expanded in a recent review article that suggested descriptive components for each of these features that should be described in all simulation studies incorporating debriefing [35]. For example, if video is being used as an adjunct to debriefing, it should be used in the same manner (e.g., criteria for video clip selection, duration of video clips, number of video clips, etc.). This is particularly crucial if the study is assessing the impact of one element of debriefing (i.e., a study comparing different methods of debriefing).

Choosing Outcome Measures

Like any protocol, outcome measures in SBR are determined by the research question being asked. First and foremost, outcome measures should be credibly connected to the intervention in a causal relationship. In addition, they must be pertinent to whatever is being studied, or else the findings will not be considered relevant. Finally, attention must be paid to how measurable the outcomes are, both in terms of precision and reliability [32]. In general, the outcome measures differ depending on whether simulation is the subject of research or method of research. And in certain cases, simulation technology may even serve as the outcome measure itself.

Outcome Measures with Simulation as the Subject of Research

When studying the efficacy of simulation as an educational strategy, it is useful to apply Kirkpatrick's learning and training evaluation theory. Originally published in 1959, Kirkpatrick describes four levels of rigor in evaluating the success of a training or educational intervention [37]. Each level is typically more complex than the last in terms of resources needed to conduct the assessment, but the quality of the outcome is also considered more robust evidence of the success of an intervention. The most basic level measures the reactions and attitudes of learners and may include outcome measures such as satisfaction with an intervention or self-confidence. The second level measures learning, and usually involves testing knowledge before and after the intervention. Adding measures of knowledge retention or even learning curves can give a more realistic sense of how the intervention is impacting learners' knowledge [38, 39]. The third level of evaluation measures the learners' behaviors, looking for a sustained application of the knowledge or skill attained in the work environment. The final and most robust level of evidence is to measure actual results or clinical outcomes that occur due to an educational intervention. Kalet et al. point out the challenges in capturing the true impact of education including time lag, multiple confounding clinical variables, patient activation, and the naturally nested nature of subjects within academic hierarchies of supervision. To this point, the authors advocate selecting outcomes in longitudinal educational research that are educational sensitive and can be plausibly linked more directly to the intervention [40]. Transfer of clinical procedural skills from simulation training intervention is a good example of an outcome that is educationally sensitive, in that it has a good chronologic relationship to the intervention, is biologically plausible, and can be easily reproduced [41].

At every level of evaluation, there are different tools and methods one can use to evaluate the success of an intervention (see Table 30.4). Generally, these methods can be categorized in three main themes: (1) simulation technology as an outcome measurement tool, (2) observational checklists, and (3) clinical translational outcomes [32].

Simulation Technology as Outcome Measurement Tool

Technology-enhanced education often comes with an added bonus that simulators, virtual games, and other gadgets often give instructors the option to record and analyze learner performance metrics. The majority of pediatric simulators are able to record actions of participants alongside the physiologic state of the simulator. This gives investigators

Table 30.4 Outcome measurement examples by Kirkpatrick type

Level	Type	Description	Examples of evaluation tools and methods	Resource utilization	A sample of examples in the literature
1	Reaction	Measures how participants feel about the intervention or learning experience	Satisfaction survey (Likert scales) Qualitative interviews or focus groups	Quick, easy, and inexpensive to create, collect, and analyze	Twelve mock codes were conducted at a new facility to test the system and gain familiarity with the space. Sixty-nine percent of the participants reported that the training was beneficial [60]
2	Learning	Measures changes in knowledge, skills, or attitudes	Knowledge test (MCQ) Skills assessment checklists Self-efficacy scores (Likert)	Quick, easy, and inexpensive to create, but depending on the construct is more challenging/expensive/timely to validate	Three NRP simulations followed by a facilitated debriefing was associated with improvements in NRP performance (pretest 82.5% vs. posttest 92.5%, mean difference 10% [95% CI, 1.5–18.5]) [38]
3	Behavior	Measures application of learning in practice	Observed behavior in simulated setting as proxy Clinical behaviors as measured by -Observation -Chart review -Checklists -Self -Patient -Peers	Simulation checklist require validation studies Clinical studies complex, often require large numbers, etc.	In a comparison of instructor-modeled learning to self-directed learning during a clinical simulated experience, individuals demonstrated improvement using the Behavioral Assessment Tool [61]
4	Results	Measures impact of learning in clinical environment and/or actual patients	Clinical outcomes measured by usual processes: -Observation -Chart review -Interviews	Requires coordination/cooperation of clinical administrators. (more expensive and complex)	A simulation-based mastery learning program increased residents' skills in simulated central venous catheter insertion and decreased complications related to central venous catheter insertions in actual patient care [62]

MCQ multiple choice questions, *NRP* Neonatal Resuscitation Program, *CI* confidence interval

the ability to test hypotheses about interventions that might impact any of the outcomes that can be recorded, such as the performance of airway maneuvers or chest compression accuracy. The simulated setting can also serve to study the impact of an intervention on timeliness of skill performance [42–44].

The reliability of measurements and calculations made by computers or simulators may seem good, but if not disclosed by a manufacturer's research and development section, investigators may wish to conduct small pilot trials to validate measurements being used as a primary outcome. For example, the accuracy of compression depth as a metric varies greatly depending on the technology and manufacturer of the product being used to record this outcome. Furthermore, little is known about the predictive validity of measurements in the simulated environment and whether such proxy measures truly reflect the real world constructs they aim to replace.

Observational Checklists

Observational checklists are often used to represent concepts or constructs that are otherwise difficult to capture with a biologic or other more concrete measurement. Such check-

lists are especially common in human factors research to assess behavioral performance [34]. Another common place for using checklists is to assess clinical or procedural skills. If validated instruments do not already exist for the behavior, skill, or construct that is the subject of study, researchers should take a systematic approach to developing checklists in order to ensure their internal and external validity and reliability [45, 46].

Some observational checklists are designed to be used in the live setting, while others are specifically meant for use with video review. There is no perfect checklist, and selecting or designing a checklist is heavily reliant upon the specific objectives of a study. Chapter 7 provides a detailed list of pediatric assessment tools for use in the simulated and/or real clinical environment.

Clinical Translational Outcomes

Clinical outcomes are not always feasible or even possible in educational research. However, the most meaningful outcome to measure is the impact of an intervention on actual patients. Oftentimes, such studies are possible but unrealistic due to the size, cost, or time of conducting them. Less than 2% of all published simulation studies involve a clinical outcome [47]. Aside from funding, one of the challenges to showing a statistical difference in clinical outcomes often relates to having enough of a sample size. Multicenter research networks have evolved, in part to work together to achieve adequate sample size to conduct patient-oriented outcome studies, in addition to improving external validity [48].

Outcome Measures with Simulation as the Method of Research

When simulation is being used as the method of research, the outcome measures will depend upon what is being studied. For example, a simulated environment was used as the laboratory for a comparative efficacy study of glidescope in the procedure of direct laryngoscopy [49]. In this case, time to intubation was used as the outcome measure on three different-sized pediatric simulators revealing faster times with direct laryngoscopy on child and neonatal airways, but no difference for infant size. Researchers interested in exploring elements of human factors or environmental design may similarly use the simulated environment to test theories using validated instruments as outcome measures [4]. Primary outcomes when simulation is used as a method of research are similar to those in any other research setting and limited only by the creativity of the researcher.

Funding Opportunities Within Simulation

SBR often has a large, up-front equipment or development cost, without which research cannot be performed. Having prior access to simulators helps, but existing equipment or software may not be appropriate or sufficient depending on research goals. Funding is required for larger-scale or more resource-intensive studies, particularly those that extend to a multicenter network. Funding agencies generally use two principles when deciding to provide monetary support for research.

Responsible Research and Innovation (RRI)

RRI is a concept applied to innovative technologies, first described for future technologies such as robotics, artificial intelligence, and virtual reality [50, 51]. Embracing RRI means that discoveries on new technologies should be responsive to societal needs and improve society as a whole [50]. Funding agencies that use this principle fund SBR based on its potential for an innovative product, particularly with potential for the product to directly improve the well-being of society.

Broad Impact

Broad impact is the concept that research should attempt to improve disadvantaged groups and create sustainability for science within the community [50]. Foundations that identify disadvantaged communities and children use this principle for funding. *Helping Babies Breathe* is an example of a SBR principled on broad impact [52]. This is a program using low-cost mannequins simulating neonates as a training tool for basic neonatal resuscitation following delivery in resource-limited settings. A low-cost model with reasonable anatomic representation of a baby's nasal and oral airway was essential to ensure broad applicability and generalizability in resource-limited countries.

Funding for Simulation as Method

When simulation is used to discover provider-, patient-, or system-level problems and innovations, there is more interest in further discovering and diagnosing safety concerns that could threaten health or healthcare and, more importantly, how to solve or prevent them. Typical simulation-based studies that use this methodology focus on patient safety, such as latent safety threats analysis [53]. Although patient outcomes are still the end goal of this type of SBR, funding agencies generally concentrate on patient safety, quality of care, and system issues. In the USA, the Agency for Healthcare Research and Quality (AHRQ) and agencies interested in the business, policy, or hospital system functioning are typical funding sources.

Funding for Simulation as the Subject of Research

These studies test or validate simulation-based training programs that improve provider-related knowledge, skills, or attitudes leading to improved patient or population outcomes. It is perceived as an educational intervention. Medical education intervention studies—including non-simulation-based interventions—are poorly funded at this time by traditional national entities such as the National Institutes of Health in the USA [54, 55]. However, funding for simulation as an educational intervention tends to be attractive to foundations whose philosophies and goals are based on RRI. The American Heart Association, whose core educational products use CPR simulators, has funded research using CPR simulation as an educational intervention. Foundations that represent simulators (e.g., Laerdal, Gaumard, etc.) and medical equipment (e.g., Ethicon, Zoll, Phillips) are also good starting points. Funders focusing on general innovation (e.g., Google, etc.) may also qualify.

The important lesson is that simulation-based intervention research is *translational research*. Like traditional translational research, a discovery found in the biomedical laboratory setting (T1) needs to be tested with actual subjects (T2), and the outcomes to patients, populations, and systems also studied (T3) [56]. Simulation is understood to already be effective at the T1 level and research using simulation as an intervention tends to be funded at the T2 or T3 level. That is, funding agencies are more interested in measurable healthcare provider outcomes and patient outcomes, rather than just a new intervention.

Sources of Funding

Public

Government-based healthcare funding agencies primarily use the principle of broad impact, particularly for children within their jurisdiction. The National Institutes of Health (USA), the Canadian Institute for Health Research (Canada), National Health Services (UK), and the Australian Institute of Health and Welfare (Australia) are examples of very large national public funding agencies. Other agencies with more focused missions or local healthcare agencies are also potential funding sources. These tend to fund clinician scientists and scientists alike. Because the principle of broad impact across the entire jurisdiction is often used, SBR that concentrates on children has a slight innovation advantage over non-pediatric studies.

Other public agencies focus more on technology and software. These can also be potential funding sources if a novel simulator, screen-based simulator, or haptic simulator is being developed. For example, Knight et al. developed a major incident triage training screen-based simulation that was funded by the UK government's Technology Strategy Board [21, 57].

Military-based funding agencies are receptive to SBR, using the RRI principle. Most expect some level of innovative product to be deployed in a military healthcare setting, either for the benefit of civilians or armed personnel. A research protocol need not have soldiers as the target patient population to fit into a military-based funding opportunity.

Private Nonprofit

Nonprofit foundations have very specific missions. Some use broad impact principles and target a disadvantaged population, perhaps identified by socioeconomic status. General nonprofit foundations tend to cluster around poor healthcare services or access, which can be targeted by simulation-based interventions. RBaby Foundation in the USA, for example,

targets funding towards improving pediatric acute care among healthcare providers [58, 59]; these lend themselves to SBR and interventions using the RRI principle. Disease-specific foundations may be sources for research that can tie simulation-based interventions to improving patient outcomes, such as improving colonoscopy skills for providers treating Crohn's disease patients, for example. Cardiac arrest is also a disease, as funded by American Heart Association, as another example.

Industry

Corporate partners who manufacture MBSs or screen-based simulation software are a unique source of funding for healthcare research that other clinician-scientists do not have access to. This is akin to pharmaceutical company-sponsored research. Corporate funding uses RRI principles but not necessarily broad impact. This means corporate funding does not necessarily require measuring patient outcomes, though patient outcome studies are still funded. Funding is more prevalent when particular modifications to mannequins are tested for feasibility and novelty.

Multicenter Collaboration

The sample size advantage of multicenter research also provides incentive for funding agencies based on the principles that we have already discussed. This means multicenter research networks that have the infrastructure and support for scalable SBR improve funding opportunities. Funding for educational studies, for example, is directly affected by the rigor of study design, which includes sampling methods; a multicenter study, when executed well, tends to improve its rigor, which in turn should be better candidates for larger funding. Furthermore, specific funding opportunities, such as the NIH U-series of grants, are only awarded to larger networks as infrastructure funding.

References

1. LeBlanc VR, Manser T, Weinger MB, Musson D, Kutzin J, Howard SK. The study of factors affecting human and systems performance in healthcare using simulation. Simul Healthc. 2011;6:24–9.
2. Howard S, Gaba D, Smith B, et al. Simulation study of rested versus sleep-deprived anesthesiologists. Anesthesiology. 2003;98(6):1345–55.
3. Calhoun AW, Boone MC, Porter MB, Miller KH. Using simulation to address hierarchy-related errors in medical practice. Perm J. 2014;18(2):14–20.
4. Beran TN, McLaughlin K, Ansari A A, Kassam A. Conformity of behaviors among medical students: impact on performance of knee arthrocentesis in simulation. Adv Health Sci Educ. 2013;18(4):589–96.
5. Feuerbacher RL, Funk KH, Spight DH, Diggs BS, Hunter JG. Realistic distractions and interruptions that impair simulated surgical performance by novice surgeons. Arch Surg. 2012;147(11):1026–30.

6. Lighthall G, Poon T, Harrison T. Using in situ simulation to improve in-hospital cardiopulmonary resuscitation. Jt Comm J Qual Patient Saf. 2010;36:209–16.

7. Geis G, Pio B, Pendergrass T, et al. Simulation to assess the safety of new healthcare teams and new facilities. Simul Healthc. 2011;6(3):125–33.

8. Fonte M, Oulego-Erroz I, Nadkarni L, Sánchez-Santos L, Iglesias-Vásquez A, Rodríguez-Núñez A. A randomized comparison of the GlideScope videolaryngoscope to the standard laryngoscopy for intubation by pediatric residents in simulated easy and difficult infant airway scenarios. Pediatr Emerg Care. 2011;27(5):398–402.

9. Sylvia MJ, Maranda L, Harris KL, Thompson J, Walsh BM. Comparison of success rates using video laryngoscopy versus direct laryngoscopy by residents during a simulated pediatric emergency. Simul Healthc. 2013;8(3):155–61.

10. Hung GR, Whitehouse SR, O'Neill C, Gray AP, Kissoon N. Computer modeling of patient flow in a pediatric emergency department using discrete event simulation. Pediatr Emerg Care. 2007;23(1):5–10.

11. Connelly LG, Bair AE. Discrete event simulation of emergency department activity: a platform for system-level operations research. Acad Emerg Med. 2004;11(11):1177–85.

12. Hunt E, Vera K, Diener-West M, Haggerty J, Nelson KL, Shaffner DH, et al. Delays and errors in cardiopulmonary resuscitation and defibrillation by pediatric residents during simulated cardiopulmonary arrests. Resuscitation. 2009;80(7):819–25.

13. Sutton RM, Niles D, Meaney P, Aplenc R, French B, Abella BS, et al. Low-dose, high-frequency CPR training improves skill retention of in-hospital pediatric providers. Pediatrics. 2011;128(1):e145–51.

14. Yeung J, Meeks R, Edelson D, Gao F, Soar J, Perkins GD. The use of CPR feedback/prompt devices during training and CPR performance: a systematic review. Resuscitation. 2009;80(7):743–51.

15. Waldrop W, Murray D, Boulet J, Kras J. Management of anesthesia equipment failure: a simulation-based resident skill assessment. Anesth Analg. 2009;109:426–33.

16. Cheng A, Brown L, Duff J, et al. Improving cardiopulmonary resuscitation with a CPR feedback device and refresher simulations (CPRCARES Study): a multicenter, randomized trial. JAMA Pediatr. 2015;169(2):1–9. doi:10.1001/jamapediatrics.2014.2616.

17. Penta FB, Kofman S. The effectiveness of simulation devices in teaching selected skills of physical diagnosis. J Med Educ. 1973;48(5):442–5.

18. Cheng A, Lang TR, Starr SR, Pusic M, Cook DA. Technology-enhanced simulation and pediatric education: a meta-analysis. Pediatrics. 2014;133(5):e1313–23.

19. Cook DA, Hatala R, Brydges R, Zendejas B, Szostek JH, Wang AT, et al. Technology-enhanced simulation for health professions education: a systematic review and meta-analysis. JAMA. 2011;306(9):978–88.

20. Cook DA. How much evidence does it take? A cumulative meta-analysis of outcomes of simulation-based education. Med Educ. 2014;48(8):750–60.

21. Reed DA, Cook DA, Beckman TJ, Levine RB, Kern DE, Wright SM. Association between funding and quality of published medical education research. JAMA. 2007;298(9):1002–9.

22. Cooke O'Brien I. Carnegie foundation: educating physicians: a call for reform of medical school and residency. 2010.

23. Isaranuwatchai W, Brydges R, Carnahan H, Backstein D, Dubrowski A. Comparing the cost-effectiveness of simulation modalities: a case study of peripheral intravenous catheterization training. Adv Heal Sci Educ Theory Pract. 2014;19(2):219–32.

24. Zendejas B, Brydges R, Wang AT, Cook DA. Patient outcomes in simulation-based medical education: a systematic review. J Gen Intern Med. 2013;28(8):1078–89.

25. Thomson M, Heuschkel R, Donaldson N, Murch S, Hinds R. Acquisition of competence in paediatric ileocolonoscopy with virtual endoscopy training. J Pediatr Gastroenterol Nutr. 2006;43(5):699–701.

26. Nishisaki A, Donoghue AJ, Colborn S, Watson C, Meyer A, Brown CA 3rd, et al. Effect of just-in-time simulation training on tracheal intubation procedure safety in the pediatric intensive care unit. Anesthesiology. 2010;113(1):214–23.

27. Andreatta P, Saxton E, Thompson M, Annich G. Simulation-based mock codes significantly correlate with improved pediatric patient cardiopulmonary arrest survival rates. Pediatr Crit Care Med. 2011;12(1):33–8.

28. Gaies MG, Morris SA, Hafler JP, Graham DA, Capraro AJ, Zhou J, et al. Reforming procedural skills training for pediatric residents: a randomized, interventional trial. Pediatrics. 2009;124(2):610–9.

29. Vossius C, Lotto E, Lyanga S, Mduma E, Msemo G, Perlman J, et al. Cost-effectiveness of the "helping babies breathe" program in a missionary hospital in rural Tanzania. PLoS One. 2014;9(7):e102080.

30. Cook DA, Hamstra SJ, Brydges R, Zendejas B, Szostek JH, Wang AT, et al. Comparative effectiveness of instructional design features in simulation-based education: systematic review and meta-analysis. Med Teach. 2013;35(1):e867–98.

31. Issenberg SB, McGaghie WC, Petrusa ER, Lee Gordon D, Scalese RJ. Features and uses of high-fidelity medical simulations that lead to effective learning: a BEME systematic review. Med Teach. 2005;27(1):10–28.

32. Cheng A, Auerbach M, Hunt E, Chang TP, Pusic M, Nadkarni V, et al. Designing and conducting simulation-based research. Pediatrics. 2014;133(6):1091–101.

33. Raemer DB. Ignaz semmelweis redux? Simul Healthc. 2014;9(3):153–5.

34. Cheng A, Hunt E, Donoghue A, Nelson-McMillan K, Nishisaki A, Leflore J, et al. Examining pediatric resuscitation education using simulation and scripted debriefing: a multicenter randomized trial. JAMA Pediatr. 2013;167(6):528–36.

35. Cheng A, Eppich W, Grant V, Sherbino J, Zendejas-Mummert B, Cook D. Debriefing for technology-enhanced simulation: a systematic review and meta-analysis. Med Educ. 2014;48:657–66.

36. Raemer D, Anderson M, Cheng A, Fanning R, Nadkarni V, Savoldelli G. Research regarding debriefing as part of the learning process. Simul Healthc. 2011;6:S52–S7.

37. Kirkpatrick DI. Evaluating training programs: the four levels. 2nd ed. San Francisco: Berrett-Koehler; 1998.

38. Sawyer T, Sierocka-Castaneda A, Chan D, Berg B, Lustik M, Thompson M. Deliberate practice using simulation improves neonatal resuscitation performance. Simul Healthc. 2011;6(6):327–36.

39. Pusic MV, Kessler D, Szyld D, Kalet A, Pecaric M, Boutis K. Experience curves as an organizing framework for deliberate practice in emergency medicine learning. Acad Emerg Med. 2012 Dec;19(12):1476–80.

40. Kalet AL, Gillespie CC, Schwartz MD, Holmboe ES, Ark TK, Jay M, et al. New measures to establish the evidence base for medical education: identifying educationally sensitive patient outcomes. Acad Med. 2010;85(5):844–51.

41. Dawe SR, Pena GN, Windsor JA, Broeders JAJL, Cregan PC, Hewett PJ, et al. Systematic review of skills transfer after surgical simulation-based training. Br J Surg. 2014;101(9):1063–76.

42. Schunk D, Ritzka M, Graf B, Trabold B. A comparison of three supraglottic airway devices used by healthcare professionals during paediatric resuscitation simulation. Emerg Med J. 2013;30(9):754–7.

43. Rahman T, Chandran S, Kluger D, Kersch J, Holmes L, Nishisaki A, et al. Tracking manikin tracheal intubation using motion analysis. Pediatr Emerg Care. 2011;27(8):701–5.

44. Martin P, Theobald P, Kemp A, Maguire S, Maconochie I, Jones M. Real-time feedback can improve infant manikin cardiopulmonary resuscitation by up to 79 %—a randomised controlled trial. Resuscitation. 2013;84(8):1125–30.

45. Schmutz J, Eppich WJ, Hoffmann F, Heimberg E, Manser T. Five steps to develop checklists for evaluating clinical performance: an integrative approach. Acad Med. 2014;89(7):996–1005.

46. Cook D, Beckman TJ. Current concepts in validity and reliability for psychometric instruments: theory and application. Am J Med. 2006;119(2):166.e7–16.

47. Cook D, Brydges R, Zendejas B, Hamstra SJ, Hatala R. Technology-enhanced simulation to assess health professionals: a systematic review of validity evidence, research methods, and reporting quality. Acad Med. 2013;88(6):872–83.

48. INSPIRE | International Network for Simulation-based Pediatric Innovation, Research, & Education. http://inspiresim.com/.

49. Johnston LC, Auerbach M, Kappus L, Emerson B, Zigmont J, Sudikoff SN. Utilization of exploration-based learning and video-assisted learning to teach GlideScope videolaryngoscopy. Teach Learn Med. 2014;26(3):285–91.

50. Davis M, Laas K. "Broader Impacts" or "Responsible Research and Innovation"? A comparison of two criteria for funding research in science and engineering. Sci Eng Ethics. 2014;20(4):963–83.

51. Schomberg R Von. Towards responsible research and innovation in the information and communication technologies and security technologies fields. Available SSRN 2436399. 2011. http://papers.ssrn.com/sol3/papers.cfm?abstract_id=2436399.

52. Singhal N, Lockyer J, Fidler H, Keenan W, Little G, Bucher S, et al. Helping Babies Breathe: global neonatal resuscitation program development and formative educational evaluation. Resuscitation. 2012;83(1):90–6.

53. Wheeler DS, Geis G, Mack EH, LeMaster T, Patterson MD. High-reliability emergency response teams in the hospital: improving quality and safety using in situ simulation training. BMJ Qual Saf. 2013;22(6):507–14.

54. Reed DA, Cook DA, Beckman TJ, Levine RB, Kern DE, Wright SM. Association between funding and quality of published medical education research. JAMA. 2007;298(9):1002–9.

55. Reed DA, Kern DE, Levine RB, Wright SM. Costs and funding for published medical education research. JAMA. 2005;294(9):1052–7.

56. Dougherty D, Conway PH. The "3T's" road map to transform US healthcare: the "how" of high-quality care. JAMA. 2008;299(19):2319–21.

57. Knight JF, Carley S, Tregunna B, Jarvis S, Smithies R, de Freitas S, et al. Serious gaming technology in major incident triage training: a pragmatic controlled trial. Resuscitation. 2010;81(9):1175–9.

58. Gerard JM, Kessler DO, Braun C, Mehta R, Scalzo AJ, Auerbach M. Validation of global rating scale and checklist instruments for the infant lumbar puncture procedure. Simul Healthc. 2013 Jun;8(3):148–54.

59. Kessler DO, Arteaga G, Ching K, Haubner L, Kamdar G, Krantz A, et al. Interns' success with clinical procedures in infants after simulation training. Pediatrics. 2013;131(3):e811–20.

60. Villamaria FJ, Pliego JF, Wehbe-Janek H, Coker N, Rajab MH, Sibbitt S, et al. Using simulation to orient code blue teams to a new hospital facility. Simul Healthc. 2008;3(4):209–16.

61. LeFlore JL, Anderson M, Michael JL, Engle WD, Anderson J. Comparison of self-directed learning versus instructor-modeled learning during a simulated clinical experience. Simul Healthc. 2007;2(3):170–7.

62. Barsuk JH, McGaghie WC, Cohen ER, O'Leary KJ, Wayne DB. Simulation-based mastery learning reduces complications during central venous catheter insertion in a medical intensive care unit. Crit Care Med. 2009;37:2697–701.

Part VII

The Future of Pediatric Simulation

The Future of Pediatric Simulation

David J. Grant, Vincent J. Grant and Adam Cheng

Simulation Pearls

1. The future of pediatric simulation is bright, but there are many opportunities for improving how simulation is used to optimize healthcare outcomes.
2. The opportunities for improvement relate to optimizing simulation resources, integration, innovation, investigation, and inspiring future leaders.
3. Collaboration between individuals, programs, and institutions will be critical to ensuring the future growth of simulation in pediatrics.

Introduction

Over the past three decades, there have been a wide array of drivers for simulation-based education (SBE). Some of these drivers include medical education reform, professional regulation, professional accountability, and societal expectations. It has been widely recognized that many health-profession trainees are ill prepared for their roles as practicing clinicians. In addition to their well-documented deficiencies in a range of skills [1–4], there have been reports of significant stress resulting from inadequate preparation for their

D. J. Grant (✉)
Bristol Royal Hospital for Children, University Hospitals Bristol NHS Foundation Trust, Bristol, UK
e-mail: david.grant@nhs.net

Bristol Paediatric Simulation Programme, Bristol Medical Simulation Centre, Bristol, UK

V. J. Grant · A. Cheng
Department of Pediatrics, Cumming School of Medicine, University of Calgary, Calgary, AB, Canada

KidSIM Pediatric Simulation Program, Alberta Children's Hospital, Calgary, AB, Canada
e-mail: vjgrant@ucalgary.ca; vincent.grant@ahs.ca

A. Cheng
e-mail: chenger@me.com

roles [5]. These skill deficiencies have occurred alongside a changing pattern of healthcare delivery, which has seen significant changes to the clinical experience of undergraduates and a greater role for interprofessional practice [6, 7]. The need to better prepare students at an undergraduate level for the changing patterns of healthcare delivery has driven the medical education reform agenda. In addition, the need for postgraduate education to adopt a more integrated educational approach that extends into continued professional education following training has been identified [8].

In medical education specifically, the evolution of professional regulation has introduced variables such as working time restrictions and the move toward a more streamlined, shorter duration of postgraduate training [9–11]. Though well intentioned, the introduction of these measures has caused increased concern related to the amount of direct clinical experience necessary to achieve competency during training [12, 13]. The reduction in opportunities for individuals to gain experience and for teams to practice managing clinical cases together has led to the integration of SBE into training curricula to ensure that sufficient opportunities for deliberate practice is provided for both common and rare conditions and procedures [14].

A move to increase professional accountability coupled with increased societal expectations has seen patient safety coming to the forefront of health care. It is no longer acceptable for individuals to practice on real patients, and educational strategies must aim to move the steep part of the learning curve away from the patient to an environment that is safe for both the patient and the healthcare professional. In this manner, SBE provides the ideal solution, a customizable educational strategy tailored to ever-evolving healthcare system needs [15].

SBE allows users at all levels, from novice to expert, to practice and develop skills with the knowledge that mistakes carry no penalties. This provides the learner with early and frequent exposure to the broad spectrum of possible clinical presentations, thus accelerating the journey along the

© Springer International Publishing Switzerland 2016
V. J. Grant, A. Cheng (eds.), *Comprehensive Healthcare Simulation: Pediatrics,*
Comprehensive Healthcare Simulation, DOI 10.1007/978-3-319-24187-6_31

learning curve. Furthermore, titrating the nature, frequency, and difficulty of SBE to the needs of the individual learner helps mitigate the effect of time and chance that is associated with traditional healthcare education. This chapter reviews some of the key aspects of simulation in health care and describes the future role of simulation for improving the care of neonates, infants, and children. Having argued the growing need for integrated interprofessional simulation education, we will explore the future development of pediatric simulation in several thematic areas: *optimizing simulation resources, integration, innovation, investigation,* and *vision*.

Optimizing Simulation Resources

Mannequins

In recent years, the focus on mannequins as simulated patients has moved away from defining high-fidelity as high-technology and toward a setting of high-fidelity appropriate-technology. This has been driven by the belief that high-fidelity is achievable with lower technology mannequins, given the appropriate environment and a well-designed simulated experience. This is a vital mind shift to enable the implementation of high-fidelity simulation across all healthcare systems, in both developed and developing countries across the world.

Currently many elements of commercially available pediatric and neonatal mannequins do not provide cues that are used routinely by practitioners in normal clinical practice. For example, one of the most common pitfalls during the assessment of perfusion is the lack of ability to assess capillary refill time and skin temperature. In addition, the haptic feedback during airway manipulation differs distinctly due to the different characteristics of tissue elasticity. There is a growing body of evidence that suggests that the cues utilized during information acquisition strategies are different between expert and novice learners. It would therefore appear that one of the elements that should be considered with regard to fidelity is the level of expertise within the learner group [16]. Furthermore, current pediatric mannequins are weakly equipped with respect to interventional procedures and clinical tasks. Many educators overcome this issue by using part task trainers to form a hybrid simulation when tasks are performed separately on the task trainers. This is often disruptive to the flow of simulated patient management and detracts from the fidelity of the experience.

In order to facilitate improvement in mannequin design and functionality, novel ideas will need to be tested and implemented by leading mannequin manufacturers. One strategy might include a modular approach to mannequin manufacturing that allows adaptation dependent on the technology required to achieve optimal fidelity for specific learner groups or educational sessions. A potential additional benefit would be the ability to have more affordable mannequins within the same range of products allowing for global implementation of SBE.

Sensory Integration

Learners interact with their simulation environment through engagement of all five of their senses. Future simulation environments will integrate haptic (touch), olfactory (smell), taste, auditory, and visual stimuli to deliver the highest fidelity simulation experience possible. Although many of these technologies already exist, they have yet to be integrated in a fashion that combines them all in a single coordinated fashion.

Augmented or virtual reality technologies are a rapidly developing field. Virtual reality technologies completely obscure the real world, while augmented reality technologies add cues onto the already existing real world through embedding computer graphics (Chap. 9). In practice, the characteristics of many of the technologies fall on a spectrum between virtual and augmented reality. Augmented and virtual reality technology systems are typically implemented in one of the three ways: head-mounted displays, environment-fixed displays (EFDs), and handheld displays (HHDs). Head-mounted displays require accurate tracking of the position and orientation of the user's head and include non-see-through, video-see-through, and optical-see-through devices. Non-see-through displays block out all cues from the real world and provide the most immersion for virtual reality. In contrast, video-see-through and optical-see-through displays enable computer-generated cues to be overlaid onto the visual field and provide the ideal augmented reality experience.

EFDs deliver graphics and/or audio via surfaces and speakers that do not move with the head. EFDs may take many forms. They range from standard monitors to those that completely surround the user. Although the display surfaces are usually flat, more complex shapes can be used. EFDs provide a completely immersive and artificial environment, where the only real-world cue is the user or learner engaged in the simulation. HHDs are tracked devices, held by hand, that do not require precise alignment with the eyes or head. The popularity of handheld augmented reality has increased exponentially with the development of smartphones and tablets. The coordinated integration of such technologies into simulation environments and educational curricula may provide the next frontier of enhanced fidelity.

Improved Educational Quality Control and Quality Assurance

After a prolonged gestation, recent advances have made available affordable technologies that enable the reproduction of clinical events with sufficient fidelity that engage learners in a realistic and meaningful way. Current literature has shown us that despite using resources with similar fidelity, not all training has the same degree of educational impact and transference to clinical practice [17, 18]. Fidelity is only one element of the simulation educational experience that influences the quality of learning. Other elements include, but are not limited to, the integration of simulation into curriculum, development and delivery of simulation educational material, and the quality of the facilitator and debriefer [19].

Apart from the efficacy of the educational experience, the emotional impact of the simulation experience on the learner should not be underestimated. Caine's brain-based learning theory describes the elements required to facilitate learning as an orchestrated immersion in a complex experience (i.e., well-designed and facilitated simulation scenario) followed by an opportunity to actively process the experience in a setting of relaxed alertness (i.e., debriefing). Relaxed alertness is defined as an educational climate that eliminates fear but remains challenging [20]. In her book *Being Wrong,* Kathryn Shultz explores the phenomenon of being wrong. She postulates that the act of being wrong itself has no emotional impact until we actually realize that we were wrong. In simulation environments, candidates are often made aware of being wrong during the debriefing, which may potentially have significant emotional consequences [21]. Keeping this in mind, it therefore stands to reason that successful education in a simulated environment relies on skilled facilitators who can effectively persuade the learners to suspend disbelief, accept the educational contract, and allow themselves to become fully engaged in the simulation experience. Orchestrating a simulation scenario that immerses the learner in a complex high-fidelity experience and facilitating a debriefing that challenges the learners without imparting fear provides a learning environment best suited to enhance learning outcomes [22, 23].

Without quality assurance processes in place to ensure high-quality development and delivery of educational material delivered by educators, it is impossible to assure that each learner's educational experience is sufficiently rich to optimize transfer of newly acquired knowledge, skills, and attitudes to clinical practice. In the early adoption phase of SBE, it was not uncommon for simulation education to be delivered by untrained faculty with no quality control and/or quality assurance processes in place. Quality control refers to elements focused on educational outputs such as faculty development and setting standards for course development, delivery, and debriefing. Quality assurance, on the other hand, refers to the administrative and procedural activities implemented to ensure that requirements and goals for the educational activity are fulfilled. It is the systematic measurement, comparison with a standard, monitoring of processes, and an associated feedback loop that allows continuing improvement of educational delivery.

The educational quality assurance journey starts with a robust educational needs assessment, followed by the design of robust curricula and programs with specified outcomes and standards. After the delivery of the curricula, feedback is gathered from learners and stakeholders, which, in turn, is used to modify programs, teaching, learning, and assessment approaches. In the future, pediatric simulation programs should aim to implement quality control and quality assurance measures to help inform the modification of elements with the program to optimize the impact on patient outcomes.

Open Platform Sharing of Simulation Educational Resources

The phenomena of Massive Open Online Courses (MOOC) aimed at large-scale interactive participation via the web or other network technologies are a recent development in distance education. MOOC are part of the movement toward the globalization of healthcare education. The future will see both improved links between centers to allow real-time and asynchronous participation in simulation events and the ability to develop and share simulation resources on open platforms. This will enable us to accelerate the learning curve of newly established simulation programs and stop the phenomenon of reinventing the wheel.

It therefore stands to reason that in order to optimize our current resources, four elements need to be addressed:

- Simulation educators should aim to collaborate with the simulation industry to optimize the fidelity of the simulation mannequins.
- Simulation programs must invest in high-quality faculty development strategies that continue to develop adaptable simulation educators.
- Quality control and quality assurance processes need to be put in place to ensure that requirements and goals for the educational activity are fulfilled and regularly reviewed and updated.
- The development of an international pediatric simulation educator community through organizations like the International Pediatric Simulation Society will provide the capacity to link programs and share existing resources.

Integration

In the past, simulation has often been perceived solely as an educational tool for undergraduate and postgraduate education in developed countries. The future, facilitated by technological advances and disruptive simulation technologies, will bring a globalization of simulation as educational and research methodologies are further developed to improve health care and patient safety.

Integration into Clinical Governance and Clinical Practice Development

Clinical governance is a system through which healthcare organizations are accountable for continuously improving the quality of their services and safeguarding high standards of care by creating an environment in which excellence in clinical care will flourish [24]. This definition defines three key aspirations: high standards of care, transparent responsibility and accountability for those standards, and a constant strive for improvement. The most commonly described pillars of a clinical governance infrastructure include risk management and patient safety, clinical audit, clinical effectiveness (evidence-based care), patient liaison services, and education training and continuing professional development. In order to optimize the efficacy of such an infrastructure, it is vital to establish a bidirectional relationship between these pillars. In many instances, this relationship does not exist at a departmental or organizational level.

Simulation delivered in a clinical setting with native teams is a powerful tool to evaluate systems proactively and to identify latent threats that can be communicated to clinical leaders within specific pillars of the clinical governance structure. Latent threats should be reported through the organizations' risk reporting system to inform risk management and patient safety as well as communicated to the clinical effectiveness pillar to allow for review of elements threatening patient safety and adherence to institutional guidelines and/or protocols. Integration of simulation in this manner helps to capitalize on its use as a tool for proactive identification of latent patient safety threats.

Simulation provides an opportunity to review clinical practice and treatment protocols in an environment that is safe for the patients and the practitioners. In this manner, simulation acts as a focus for facilitated reflection and active review of organizational protocols and practice in relation to current best evidence. Learners may conclude that current protocols and practice are consistent with best practice and set a revised review date. Alternatively, they may conclude that current protocols and practice are not in line with the best practice leading to an update in organizational protocols. Additional processes might include the use of simula-

tion in a clinical setting to evaluate the feasibility of implementing new clinical practice protocols into clinical practice. By integrating interprofessional simulation into an organization's change management plan, leaders can help to facilitate widespread adoption of new protocols and standards for clinical practice.

Integration of Simulation into Family-Centered Care

In pediatrics, patient and parental education as well as family-centered care are important means for empowering families to share in the responsibility of managing the patient's overall healthcare needs. This is particularly important for children suffering from chronic illnesses, where there may be a need to prepare family members and providers for discharge. Discharge teaching may include day-to-day routine skills such as tracheostomy care or suctioning, and also may include emergencies such as the management of seizures [25], a hypoglycemic episode, a blocked tracheostomy, or home ventilator malfunction. The future will see simulation education integrated as a key component family-centered care in the form of patient, parental, and caregiver education.

Integration of Simulation as an Assessment Tool

The use of simulation as an assessment tool is an area of growing interest among all spheres of healthcare education and regulating bodies. Though the use of simulation in formative assessment is well established, there are still many educators who have reservations about the introduction of simulation as a summative assessment tool. This concern is driven by an appreciation that the outcome of such summative evaluations informs high-stakes decisions of real consequence to the candidate. It may involve the candidate passing a course, gaining certification/recertification or licensure. As such, highly reliable data that permit valid inferences about the competence of the candidates are a necessity. Satisfying this prerequisite requires a specialized approach to the design and delivery of the standardized simulation assessment scenario. The use of simulation as a summative assessment tool should only be undertaken by individuals and organizations that have expertise in both the fields of assessment and simulation education.

In healthcare education, summative assessment using part task trainers, low-fidelity simulators, and simulated patients as part of objective structured clinical examinations (OSCEs) has been well established since the 1970s [26]. However, the majority of the elements evaluated relate to basic psychomotor and communication skills. The reliable evaluation of higher levels of expertise in such a setting may prove far more difficult [27]. Not surprisingly, as the skills become more complex, so too does the challenge of assessment in the simulated environment. Despite this, there is mounting evidence of the successful implementation of such assessment strategies [28, 29, 30]. The use of simulation in high-stakes healthcare assessment will increase exponentially as the technology advances and as the expertise of simulation educators increases to allow measurement methods to become more precise and valid [31].

Innovation

The meteoric development of the global information and technology (I&T) industry combined with society's embracement of technology has created opportunities to enhance educational delivery. Similarly, consumer expectations have increased the demand for the creation and delivery of learning materials incorporating the latest I&T developments. This has created an entirely new knowledge economy, with a novel world of learning emerging through computer-based learning, online learning, e-learning, and distance learning. It is essential that healthcare educational systems and simulation programs learn to harness the full potential of I&T to allow them a wider reach and their learners access to a broader knowledge base. The application of I&T to education is only limited by the imagination of the educators and their knowledge of new technologies. In order to optimize the efficacy of pediatric simulation programs and improvement of patient-care outcomes, the pediatric simulation community needs to find innovative ways to incorporate I&T solutions into their educational plans. In this section, we share a few examples of how I&T solutions can enhance the impact of SBE.

Fusion of Synchronous and Asynchronous Education

In healthcare education, there is an increasing focus on lifelong learning. This requires the capacity to deliver education to large numbers of busy clinicians, and thus also requires the delivery of SBE in the setting of limited learner availability. These challenges will not be met through traditional classroom-based educational interventions and will require an increased focus on the fusion of innovative synchronous and asynchronous healthcare education modalities. Synchronous education is defined as education delivered in real time with the physical presence of an instructor who facilitates education. With synchronous education, the pace and duration of learning are determined by the instructor and all learners being present at the same time and able to communicate directly with the instructor and each other. In contrast,

asynchronous education is education delivered without the physical presence of an educator (or other learners) with virtual access to educators (and other learners) through online bulletin boards, discussion groups, and/or e-mail. Course content can be delivered through online videos via Internet-based technology, and learners determine the pace of learning and the duration of educational experience. Enhanced student learning does not flow from the technology itself but relies on educators to shape the learning environment to best exploit the features of the technology [32].

Information and information processing are central in most conceptions of learning. Three major phases can be distinguished: information presentation, information processing, and information integration [33, 34]. During information presentation, the learner selects and stores the information in their short-term memory. Information processing that involves the organization of information in the working/short-term memory follows this and, in turn, is followed by information integration involving the construction of cognitive structures, also called schemas or mental models. Combining the asynchronous delivery of information (presentation) via I&T with the delivery of simulation education allows the creation of a synchronous, on-demand clinical experience that allows the learner to implement information processing and integration during debriefing. In this form, the combination of asynchronous and synchronous learning can help enhance educational efficacy.

Establishing Simulation Education Management Systems

In order to implement the marriage between asynchronous education and synchronous simulation delivery, an effective learning management system (LMS) is required. There are many examples of commercially available LMS, defined as a software application used for administration, documentation, tracking, reporting and delivery of electronic educational technology, courses or training programs. In addition, there are project management software solutions that facilitate the development of educational materials. The desired functionality of such a system is depicted in Table 31.1.

An example of a purposefully designed system that combines features of a traditional LMS and project management functionality is the Instructor Resource Innovation and Sharing (iRIS) platform developed by Health Education England Southwest in the UK. It fulfills the criteria outlined in Table 31.1 and is central to ensuring equity of access to simulation education programs for all healthcare practitioners across the Southwest of England. It allows educators to collaborate in an asynchronous fashion to develop and share educational resources and establishes the ability for experienced simulation educators to share their resources with those who are in an earlier phase of the development of their program. Collaboration in this fashion allows for newer programs to develop and implement their curriculum at a much faster rate. If we are to maximize the impact of simulation education on patient outcomes, such initiatives must be implemented on a regional, national, and international level across the globe.

Distance Learning

Healthcare education in the twenty-first century is facing a number of challenges that impact the 100-year old apprenticeship model of education. A reduction in work hours, coupled with a drive to deliver safe and efficient care, has reduced work-based experiential learning opportunities. A reduction in workplace learning opportunities, coupled with the growth in Internet-based innovative technology and a focus on knowledge exchange across the global healthcare community, has brought distance learning to the forefront of healthcare education discussion [35].

Though the majority of distance learning is still paper-based, the development of inexpensive disruptive technologies is likely to influence rapid change in the future. An example of such an initiative is the open-access, peer-reviewed, not-for-profit Internet-based learning application, OPEN-Pediatrics. Developed as a collaborative effort between the World Federation of Pediatric Intensive and Critical Care Societies and Harvard Medical School, it was designed to promote postgraduate educational knowledge exchange for physicians, nurses, and others caring for critically ill children worldwide [35].

Though there are anecdotal reports of distance learning applied to simulation education, it has not yet been widely adopted. In order to keep pace with the drive for knowledge exchange across the global healthcare community, simulation programs will have to find novel ways to apply distance learning to simulation education. The use of video links might allow learners from one institution to watch a clinical scenario taking place at another host center. The educational principle of Legitimate Peripheral Participation (LPP) implies that learners who watch the simulated clinical event from a distance become members of the team and become acquainted with the tasks, vocabulary, and organizing principles of the community [36]. However, special care should be taken to ensure the psychological safety of learners. In order to further individualize their learning experience, learners from both sites should be involved in the debriefing of the scenarios.

With regard to procedural technical skills, several institutions that have used inexpensive voice-over-Internet audiovisual solutions to deliver deliberate practice education that allowed the learner to observe the expert performing a particular task prior to performing it. In turn, the expert is then able to view the learner performing the task, allowing them to correct performance deficits via directive feedback. Though the application of technology using video review of the learners' performance to support deliberate practice and mastery learning of a skill is commonplace in the sports coaching world, it has not yet been adopted widely in healthcare education. In order to meet the challenges of the twenty-first century, healthcare educators should seek ways of implementing such techniques to improve the quality and breadth of SBE.

Table 31.1 Desired functionality for simulation learning management systems

Simulation learning management system	
Educator focused	Learner focused
1. Educational materials and resources	1. Pre-learning/information presentation
a Facility for asynchronous collaborative development of educational material and resources	a Electronic lecture notes
	2. Communication systems
	a Collaborative learning—connecting course participants
b Facility to share completed educational material and resources	b Enabling real-time chat or threaded discussions
c Facility to review and update educational material and resources	c Connecting learners and educators to allow post-action reflection beyond action
2. Course management	3. Learner feedback
a Database management system to organize course materials	4. Self-assessment
3. Educational quality assurance	
a Guidance to ensure development of consistently high-quality educational material	
b Frequent review to ensure materials up to date	
c Audit trail of updates and the rationale for them	
4. Student management	
a Database management system that organizes student information	
b Track individual user so that customized services can be provided	

Developing Safer Clinical Environments of the Future

Simulation has been used in combination with human factors to evaluate specific elements of the healthcare system, including newly constructed healthcare environments prior to clinical use. These events simulate a functional clinical environment prior to opening for patient care and aim to identify latent threats in the environment allowing them to be addressed prior to exposing patients to these risks [37–39]. Though human factors and teamwork training form an integral part of most established simulation programs, very few apply human factors theory to help inform the integration of new technology and medical equipment. We believe that in future simulation will form an integral part of the design process of new healthcare environments and equipment.

Investigation

The pediatric simulation community has been a leader in using simulation as a tool to improve patient care and outcomes. The establishment of the International Network for Simulation-based Pediatric Innovation, Research and Education (INSPIRE) has allowed for researchers with similar interests to come together and conduct robust, multicenter studies addressing some of the most pertinent issues in clinical care that may be difficult to answer with clinical studies. The benefits of simulation as a research tool are multifold and include (1) ability to recreate and study any clinical presentation, (2) ability to customize the clinical presentation to the needs of the study, (3) ease of recruitment of clinical subjects, (4) ease of collaboration within existing research networks provided that equipment is available, and (5) no concerns related to patient confidentiality. As such, there has been a recent explosion of pediatric simulation studies, with more and more research published each year addressing pertinent clinical issues [40].

Research in pediatric simulation can be grouped into two broad categories: studies where simulation is used as an educational intervention targeted to improve a specific area of patient care and studies where simulation is used as the environment for research [41]. A recent systematic review described a series of studies conducted demonstrating the positive impact of simulation as an educational tool for teaching pediatric healthcare providers [40]. These studies included those using simulation to teach pediatric resuscitation and life support, neonatal life support, trauma management, team training, and procedural skills. Simulation was found to be effective in improving the acquisition of knowledge, skills, and behaviors when compared to no intervention [40]. Future work in this area should aim to identify the best means

of designing simulation-based educational interventions, including how to tailor the degree of realism to the learning needs and learning context.

Other studies have used simulation as the environment for research. In these studies, the simulated environment is used to assess new protocols, equipment, patient-care processes, or clinical spaces [41]. Alternatively, the simulated environment can be a venue to describe or document specific aspects of provider performance and how providers interact with their environment. Given the growth in healthcare innovations, simulation will play a critical role in the future to determine how these innovations influence healthcare providers and processes, and whether these new innovations truly have a positive impact on patient-care outcomes.

Pediatrics is a field that is ripe for innovative simulation-based research. Future opportunities for pediatric research include the use of simulation to train for informed consent, disclosure of medical error, or conversations around death and dying. As pediatric patients come in a variety of sizes, future research should also aim to define how procedural skills can be best taught to ensure that providers are competent in these skills across age ranges. Finally, work in our field can help to address how simulation-based education can be designed to help accelerate the learning curve for pediatric-specific competencies.

Vision: SBE to Achieve a Positive Impact on a Global Scale

In recent years, there has been a growing focus on developing healthcare simulation solutions to address global healthcare issues. Pediatric SBE has led the field through projects such as the Helping Babies Breathe project. It is an example of an educational initiative delivered as a consistent program in collaboration with local healthcare providers who deliver ongoing training and mentoring to improve clinical management and patient outcomes. Implementation of this program has resulted in a 47% reduction in neonatal mortality and a 24% reduction in fresh stillbirths in some areas [42]. Further evidence of the growing collaboration between individuals and societies to help global partners develop resources for simulation education is the partnership between the International Pediatric Simulation Society (IPSS), the World Federation of Pediatrics and Critical Care Societies (WFPICS), and the Malawi Department of Health. These groups are in the process of implementing a simulation-based program to address the infant and under-five mortality in Malawi that adheres to the principles outlined in the Helping Babies Breathe program [43]. As a pediatric simulation community, we should learn from such programs and remember that simulation is an educational modality underpinned by the educational concept of experiential learning and that its application to improve Global Child health is only limited by our imagination [44].

In order for pediatric simulation to successfully impact child health on a global scale, the following issues will need to be addressed:

1. Resource Limitations

Given the financial constraints associated with training in certain regions of the world, it is imperative that the pediatric simulation community focuses the use of simulation technology to arenas where its educational impact will be optimized in a cost-effective way. This will require healthcare professionals, educators, and researchers from across the continuum of the healthcare system to engage health-systems partners in defining priorities for SBE moving forward. Defining priorities in SBE will reduce redundancies in curriculum development and design for specific professional or specialty training programs, and bring with it an economy of scale to help with more widespread dissemination. In addition, a larger focus on the delivery of in situ SBE may allow for integration of educational processes and facilitation of multi-professional and interprofessional education.

2. Collaboration

The creation and growth of a community of pediatric simulation educators through the IPSS and the INSPIRE network have been central to ensuring that the full potential of pediatric SBE and research is achieved. IPSS and the INSPIRE network have given simulation educators a means to gather, collaborate, and innovate during annual conferences and in an asynchronous fashion to develop and share educational resources. Furthermore, IPSS and INSPIRE have established the ability for experienced simulation educators to share their resources with other programs that are earlier on in their developmental phase.

3. Technological Limitations

Existing simulators often fail to meet pediatric-specific needs with respect to the degree of realism, variety (e.g., size and skin color), and cost. They fail to span age, anatomic and physiologic ranges found in real pediatric patients. In addition, higher technology simulators can be prohibitively expensive and are often not durable or appropriate for austere environments. Another important consideration is that numerous incompatibilities between existing simulators and medical equipment exist, often presenting a barrier for those programs trying to implement simulation-based testing of new technology into clinical environments.

Societies or consumer groups should work collectively to address prohibitive costs through shared purchasing models.

Research and development should be encouraged by leveraging policy makers to incentivize industry cooperation with academic centers. The development of interdisciplinary and/or interinstitutional collaboration may optimize cost–benefit ratios. Research identifying the appropriate level of realism for particular applications of SBE also has the potential to help control costs. Identifying and correcting compatibility between medical devices and medical simulation equipment can help drive better systems integration, scalability, and realism. It is essential that technology—the simulators themselves, the technology of the healthcare environment and that of the educational experience—be thoughtfully developed to maximize the impact on clinical outcomes.

4. Research Collaboration

Much like education, it will be imperative for the pediatric simulation community to define priorities for future research in the area. Doing so will map out a collective plan for the community moving forward, allowing the most important research questions to be addressed in systematic and collaborative manner. Through the INSPIRE network and other networks of researchers, multicenter trials can be organized and conducted to ensure there is sufficient sample size to contribute to meaningful results that can be generalized across sites and countries.

5. Lack of Translational Research Evidence

While the evidence supporting simulation-based education is growing, there still exists a paucity of research linking simulation to improved clinical performance, safe processes of care, patient outcomes, or cost effectiveness. Researchers must develop the methods and infrastructure to assess the translation between simulation and clinical care. Future studies should control for potentially confounding factors in this complex healthcare system that impact patient outcomes so that we can understand the impact of simulation on patient care. Over time, researchers must develop and rigorously evaluate the most effective components of simulation-based interventions from a patient-centered perspective. Analysis must be conducted to identify the most cost-effective approaches to the deployment of simulation resources and explore issues related to decay rates and retraining intervals. Funding of such research is essential to define best practices in simulation that improve clinical outcomes and to justify subsequent funding.

6. Integration, Implementation, and Sustainability

The lack of systematic integration and consideration of long-term sustainability of simulation across the healthcare spectrum has limited the potential growth of SBE. This may be related to the fact that the impact, cost, and return on investment of SBE have not yet been sufficiently defined. In order to translate the benefits of SBE to front-line providers and their patients in a sustainable way, SBE must become an integral part of optimal healthcare delivery, and no longer regarded as supplemental.

A review and synthesis of 19 empirical health-related studies reports five important factors influencing the extent of sustainability: (a) program modification, (b) presence of a champion, (c) fit with organizational mission and strategic plan, (d) perceived benefits to staff members and/or clients, and (e) stakeholders' support. In order to gain institutional support from key stakeholders, demonstration of the superior effectiveness of SBE over traditional training methods and active engagement of leadership as champions are necessary. Cost-effectiveness data are needed to provide organizations with relevant information to make financial decisions and allocate appropriate educational resources to SBE. In addition, working directly with institutional leaders to align simulation curricula or research with organizational goals can improve the perceived fit between the two. Finally, consideration of adult learning theory principles in terms of ensuring that simulation curriculum is timely, easily accessible, and directly relevant to the front-line providers is essential.

Conclusions

The future of pediatric simulation is dependent on the ability of our community to come together and tackle the most pertinent issues in our field. This will include working with each other to (1) optimize our resources, (2) identify new ways to integrate simulation into our healthcare systems, (3) innovate and develop new technologies and methods to enhance healthcare outcomes with simulation, (4) investigate the most burning healthcare questions using simulation-based methodologies that are most likely to have a positive impact on patient outcomes, and (5) to inspire and lead the healthcare community by advancing our field to positively impact global health.

References

1. Carter R, Aitchison M, Mufti G, Scott R. Catheterisation: your urethra in their hands. BMJ. 1990;301:905.
2. Cartwright MS, Reynolds PS, Rodriguez ZM, Breyer WA, Cruz JM. Lumbar puncture experience among medical school graduates: the need for formal procedural skills training. Med Educ. 2005;39(4):437.
3. Feher M, Harris-St John K, Lant A. Blood pressure measurement by junior hospital doctors—a gap in medical education? Health Trends. 1992;24(2):59–61.
4. Maguire GP, Rutter DR. History taking for medical students. 1. Deficiencies in performance. Lancet. 1976;2:556–8.
5. Williams S, Dale J, Glucksman E, Wellesley A. Senior house officers' work-related stressors, psychological distress, and confidence in performing clinical tasks in accident and emergency: a questionnaire study. BMJ. 1997;314:713–8.
6. McManus I, Richards P, Winder B, Sproston K, Vincent C. The changing clinical experience of British medical students. Lancet. 1993;341:941–4.
7. McManus I, Richards P, Winder B. Clinical experience of UK medical students. Lancet. 1998;351:802–3.
8. Braley P. The history of simulation in medical education and possible future directions. Med Educ. 2006;40:254–62.
9. MacDonald R. How protective is the working time directive? BMJ. 2004;329:301–2.
10. Fletcher KE, Saint S, Mangrulkar RS. Balancing continuity of care with residents' limited work hours: defining the implications. Acad Med. 2005;80(1):39–43.
11. Romanchuk K. The effect of limiting residents' work hours on their surgical training: a Canadian perspective. Acad Med. 2004;79(5):384–5.
12. Chikwe J, de Souza AC, Pepper JR. No time to train the surgeons. BMJ. 2004;328:418–9.
13. Talbot M. Good wine may need to mature: a critique of accelerated higher specialist training. Evidence from cognitive neuroscience. Med Educ. 2004;38(4):399–408.
14. Gordon JA. High-fidelity patient simulation: a revolution in medical education. In: Dunn WF, Editor. Simulators in critical care and beyond. Des Plaines: Society of Critical Care Medicine; 2004. pp. 3–6.
15. Cheng A, Grant V, Auerbach M. Using simulation to improve patient safety: dawn of a new era. JAMA Pediatrics. March 9, 2015. Published online. doi:10.1001/jamapediatrics.2014.3817.
16. McCormack C, Wiggins MW, Loveday T, Festa M. Expert and competent non-expert visual cues during simulated diagnosis in intensive care. Front Psychol. 2014;5:949.
17. Grobman WA, Miller D, Burke C, Hornbogen A, Tam K, Costello R. Outcomes associated with introduction of a shoulder dystocia protocol. Am J Obstet Gynecol. 2011;205:513–7.
18. Draycott TJ, et al. Improving neonatal outcome through practical shoulder dystocia training. Obstet Gynecol. 2008;112(1):14–20.
19. Issenberg SB, et al. Features and uses of high-fidelity medical simulations that lead to effective learning: a BEME systematic review. Med Teach. 2005;27(1):10–28.
20. Caine RN, Caine G. Making connections. Menlo Park: Addison-Wesley; 1994.
21. Schulz K. Being wrong: adventures in the margin of error. NY: HarperCollins Publishers; 2010.
22. Dieckman P, Manser T, Wehner T, et al. Reality and fiction cues in medical patient simulation: an interview study with anesthesiologists. J Cogn Eng Decis Mak. 2007;1:148–68.
23. Rudolph J, Simon R, Raemer DB. Which reality matters? Questions on the path to high engagement in healthcare simulation. Simul Healthc. 2007;2:161–3.
24. Scally G, Donaldson LJ. Clinical governance and the drive for quality improvement in the new NHS in England. Br Med J. 1998;317(7150):61–5.
25. Sigalet E, Cheng A, Donnon T, Catena H, Robinson T, Chatfield J, Grant VA. Simulation-based intervention teaching seizure management to caregivers: a randomized controlled study. Pediatr Child. 2014;19(7):373–8.
26. Harden RM, Gleeson FA. Assessment of clinical competence using an objective structured clinical examination (OSCE). Med Educ. 1979;13:41–54.
27. Hodges B, McNaughton N, Regehr G, Tiberius R, Hanson M. The challenge of creating new OSCE measures to capture the characteristics of expertise. Med Educ. 2002;36:742–8.

28. Gallagher AG, Cates CV. Approval of virtual reality training for carotid stenting: what this means for procedural-based medicine. JAMA. 2004;292:3024–6.

29. Berkenstadt H, Ziv A, Gafni N, Sidi A. Incorporating a simulation-based objective structured clinical examination into the Israeli national board examination in anaesthesiology. Anesth Analg. 2006;102:853–8.

30. Berkenstadt H, Ziv A, Gafni N, Sidi A. The validation process of incorporating simulation-based accreditation into the anaesthesiology Israeli national board exams. Isr Med Assoc J. 2006;8:728–33.

31. Pugh CM. Simulation and high-stakes testing. In: Kyle RR, Murray WB, editors. Clinical simulation: operations, engineering, and management. Burlington: Academic; 2008. pp. 655–66.

32. Mark A. Freeman MA, Capper J. Exploiting the web for education: an anonymous asynchronous role simulation. Aust J Educ Technol. 1999;15(1):95–116.

33. Mayer RE. Multimedia learning. New York: Cambridge University Press; 2001.

34. Paivio A. Mental representations: a dual coding approach. Oxford: Oxford University Press; 1986.

35. Wolbrink TA, Kissoon N, Burns JP. The development of an internet-based knowledge exchange platform for pediatric critical care clinicians worldwide. Pediatr Crit Care Med. 2014;15:197–205.

36. Lave J, Wenger E. Situated learning: legitimate peripheral participation. Cambridge: Cambridge University Press; 1991. ISBN: 0-521-42374-0.

37. Kaji AH, Bair A, Okuda Y, et al. Defining systems expertise: effective simulation at the organizational level—implications for patient safety, disaster surge capacity, and facilitating the systems interface. Acad Emerg Med. 2008;15:1098–103.

38. Villamaria FJ, Pliego JF, Wehbe-Janek H, et al. Using simulation to orient code blue teams to a new hospital facility. Simul Healthc. 2008;3:209–16.

39. Kobayashi L, Shapiro MJ, Sucov A, et al. Portable advanced medical simulation for new emergency department testing and orientation. Acad Emerg Med. 2006;13:691–5.

40. Cheng A, Lang T, Starr S, Pusic M, Cook D. Technology-enhanced simulation and pediatric education: a meta-analysis. Pediatrics. 2014;133:e1313–23.

41. Cheng A, Auerbach M, Chang T, Hunt EA, Pusic M, Nadkarni V, Kessler D. Designing and conducting simulation-based research. Pediatrics. May 12, 2014. Published online. doi:10.1542/peds.2013-3267.

42. Msemo G, Kidanto HL, Massawe A, et al. Newborn mortality and fresh still-birth rates in Tanzania after helping babies breathe training. Pediatrics. 2013;131:e353–60.

43. http://www.helpingbabiesbreathe.org. Accessed 6th Nov 2015

44. McKee M, Karanikolos M, Belcher P, Stuckler D. Austerity: a failed experiment on the people of Europe. Clin Med. 2012;12(4):346–50.

Index

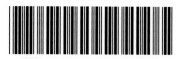